Rare Diseases of the Immune System

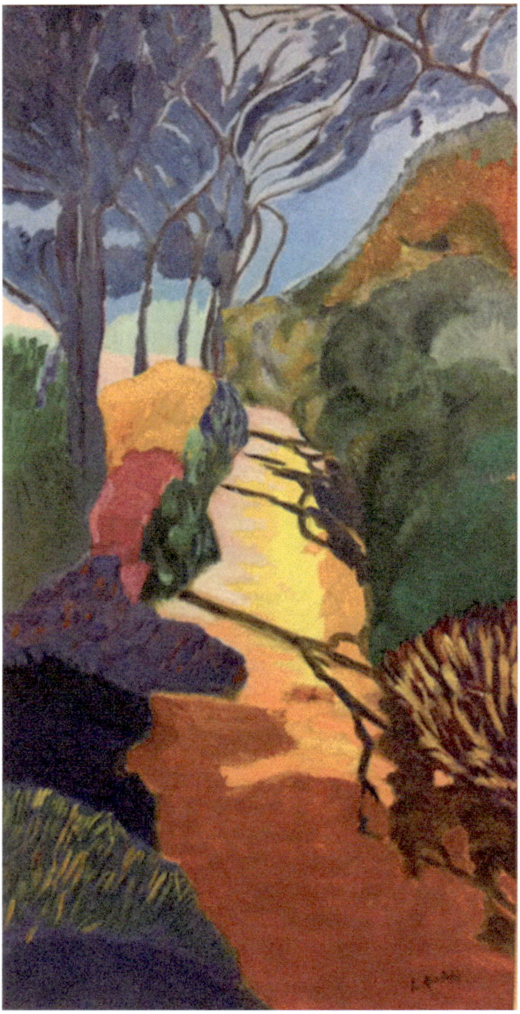

Sentiero al mattino Laura Maddii Emmi (Private collection)

Mario Milco D'Elios • Marta Rizzi
Editors

Humoral Primary Immunodeficiencies

Springer

Editors
Mario Milco D'Elios
Careggi Hospital
Department of Clinical and Experimental Medicine, University of Florence
Firenze
Italy

Marta Rizzi
University Medical Centre Freiburg
Department of Rheumatology and Clinical Immunology and Center for Chronic Immunodeficiency
Freiburg
Germany

ISSN 2282-6505 ISSN 2283-6403 (electronic)
Rare Diseases of the Immune System
ISBN 978-3-319-91784-9 ISBN 978-3-319-91785-6 (eBook)
https://doi.org/10.1007/978-3-319-91785-6

Library of Congress Control Number: 2018962559

This Springer imprint is published by the registered company Springer Nature Switzerland AG
The registered company address is: Gewerbestrasse 11, 6330 Cham, Switzerland

Dedicated with love to our children
Emilia, Carlo, and Flavia
and
Sofia, Emanuele, Alessandro, and Bernardo;
to all of our patients with primary
immunodeficiencies and their families;
to our nurses;
and to all of our students.

Preface

Primary immunodeficiencies are rare diseases. Nevertheless, the study of patients with primary immunodeficiencies has provided the chance to understand how the immune system really works. This journey into the pathogenetic mechanisms behind primary immunodeficiencies started many years ago, inspired by several giants in the field of immunology. One of them, Charles Janeway, Jr., spent his life discussing how the immune system functions and the importance of the pioneering discoveries made by his father, Charles Janeway, Sr., the first person to use gammaglobulin to treat patients with humoral immunodeficiencies.

When we think about antibodies, our minds drift immediately to vaccination responses (with the question as to whether or not they are protective), to the power of our antibody repertoire to defend ourselves from reinfection with specific viruses (e.g., rubella or measles), or to the pathogenic potential of self-reactive antibodies and their contributions to disease manifestation in autoimmune diseases. We live in a time of controversy in which public opinion against vaccination is very strong, thanks to fake, only half-true, or distorted information, spread via the media and via social media. Thanks to this discussion, there is public awareness of the rare group of patients who benefit greatly from herd immunity against common infections that are harmless for most people but possibly deadly for weak individuals. Those weak individuals carry some sort of fault in their immune system. In the great majority of cases this may be acquired (secondary) because of severe illnesses (e.g., cancer), treatment (e.g., immune suppression in cases of autoimmunity), or transplantation; or it may simply be due to age (in newborn or elderly patients). In more rare situations, subjects with a weak immune system carry a primary immune defect. The prevalence of such patients in western countries is around 40–50 patients per 100,000 inhabitants, with more than half of them having B cell immunodeficiencies. Hence, the awareness of primary immunodeficiency has increased in the community, and this has occurred in parallel with the creation of national and supranational registries (e.g., the European Society for Immunodeficiencies (ESID) registry), patient advocacy, research, and discovery.

Indeed, we have witnessed a blossoming of research into primary immunodeficiency in the past 25 years; many genetic defects related to immunodeficiency have been discovered, and since the advent of high-throughput sequencing a new genetic defect is discovered almost monthly. This is especially true for the group of patients who carry humoral immunodeficiency or common variable immunodeficiency disorders. In this group of patients the main clinical features are a reduced level of immunoglobulin in the serum and inability to mount vaccination responses. Infection is not the only feature in these patients, who may present with a complicated course of disease, with lymphoproliferation, autoimmunity, cancer, lung involvement, or gastrointestinal involvement.

The perception of humoral immune diseases as a complex entity and the identification of specific defects leading to that phenotype represent major contributions to the understanding of the human immune system in past years. The discovery of genetic defects has also aided the identification of new therapeutic targets and the forecasting of adverse events that may occur with targeted therapies.

Nevertheless, many molecular, cellular, and clinical aspects of primary immunodeficiencies (e.g., the roles of epigenetics, the microbiome, and gene therapy) are yet to be disclosed, making primary immunodeficiency one of the most exciting fields to work in. Indeed, we hope that this book will boost the curiosity of young students approaching immunology for the first time, as well as being of interest to specialists and researchers in clinical immunology.

Firenze, Italy Mario Milco D'Elios
Freiburg, Germany Marta Rizzi

Contents

The B-Side of the Immune Response 1

Laura Patrussi, Nagaja Capitani, Mario Milco D'Elios, and Cosima T. Baldari

1.1 Introduction

B cells are the central cellular players in humoral immunity. The main effector B cells, namely, the plasma cells, produce indeed antibodies which permeate extracellular spaces to protect against infection. We now know that B cells are also critical to cellular immunity by participating in T-cell activation via antigen presentation, co-stimulation, and cytokine production. Both humoral and cellular immunities depend on the formation of intercellular structures, known as immune synapses, between B cells and other cell types, the main ones being the specialized phagocytic cells localized in secondary lymphoid organs, which exploit immune synapse formation to transfer antigen to B cells, and the helper T cells, which exploit the immune synapse to promote B-cell differentiation and maturation to plasma cells.

We describe in this chapter the recognition of antigen by B cells, either in a soluble form or presented by professional cells through the immune synapse (B-synapse), and its processing and presentation to T cells, with a final section regarding the formation of immune synapses with T cells (T-synapse).

L. Patrussi (✉) · C. T. Baldari
Department of Life Sciences, University of Siena, Siena, Italy
e-mail: patrussi2@unisi.it

N. Capitani (✉)
Department of Life Sciences, University of Siena, Siena, Italy

Department of Experimental and Clinical Medicine, University of Florence, Florence, Italy
e-mail: capitani2@unisi.it

M. M. D'Elios
Department of Experimental and Clinical Medicine, University of Florence, Florence, Italy

M. M. D'Elios, M. Rizzi (eds.), *Humoral Primary Immunodeficiencies*,
Rare Diseases of the Immune System, https://doi.org/10.1007/978-3-319-91785-6_1

1.2 B-Cell Traffic: How B Lymphocytes Reach Their Specific Environmental Niches

During their lifetime, mature B cells circulate through the secondary lymphoid organs approximately every 24 h, with a half-life of few days in the absence of antigen. Their transit from the vascular system to lymph nodes is carried out via specialized endothelia of high endothelial venules [1] which they cross to reach the discrete follicular compartment localized within the cortical region of the lymph node (Fig. 1.1). This transit was thought to be primarily regulated by gradients of chemokines and their associated G protein-coupled receptors (GPCRs) that work in a concerted manner to govern immune cell positioning in time and space. CCL19 and CCL21, the ligands of CCR7, are produced by the stromal fibroblastic reticular cells (FRC) and attract B cells to home into secondary lymphoid organs, while CXCL12, the only known ligand of CXCR4, mainly attracts B cells to the stroma of the bone

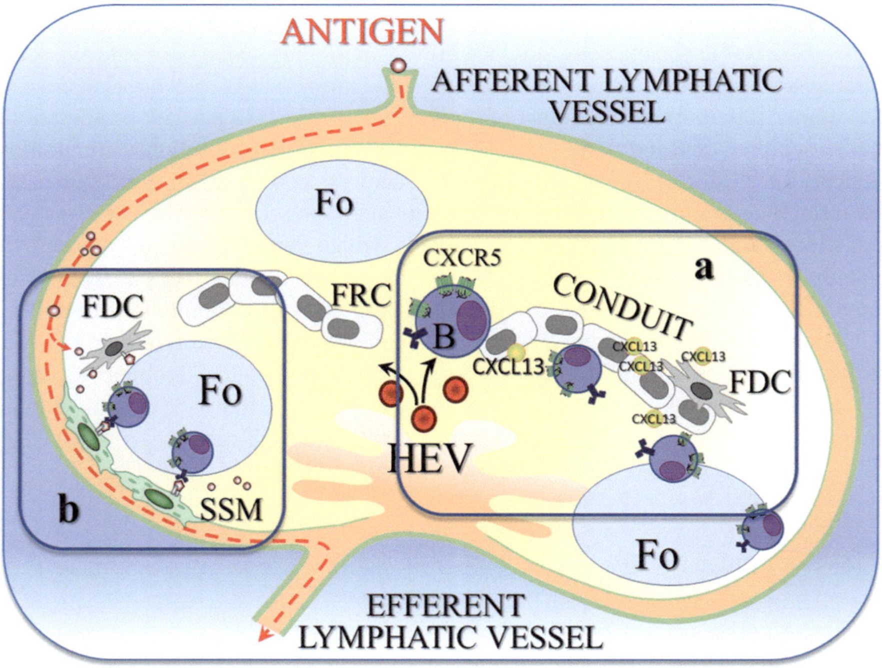

Fig. 1.1 B cells enter the secondary lymphoid organs via high endothelial venules (HEV) and are attracted toward the follicles (Fo), thanks to a gradient of the chemokine CXCL13, which is produced by fibroblastic reticular cells (FRC) and follicular dendritic cells (FDC) and percolates through special channels enveloped by FRCs, known as conduits, which provide a directional highway for B cells to reach the follicles (**a**). In the peripheral zone of the follicles, B cells come in contact with antigens (**b**), which enter the secondary lymphoid organs through afferent lymphatic vessels, either directly via small gaps in the floor of the lymph node sinus (low-molecular-mass antigens) or indirectly with the help of macrophages lining the subcapsular sinus (SSM) and FDCs residing in lymph nodes which act as antigen-presenting cells

marrow [2]. B cells are moreover attracted to the follicles by the CXCR5 ligand CXCL13 released by FRCs and by other specialized stromal cells of the follicles known as follicular dendritic cells (FDC) [3], a process which has been long believed to occur essentially through random migration across the stroma of secondary lymphoid organs. Thanks to recent technical advances, which allowed a more complete understanding of the complex regulation of lymphocyte trafficking, we now know that B cells non-randomly traffic to reach the follicles along a system of *conduits* [4–7], channels composed of a core of collagen fibers surrounded by extracellular matrix and enveloped by FRCs, which produce the extracellular matrix [8], often associated to FDC which can extend short sensor protrusions into the conduits [5]. CXCL13 secreted within the B-cell area by FRCs percolates through the conduit system providing an attractant factor to B cells [9]. Thus, conduits may provide a highway for B cells to navigate through the follicles [4].

1.3 Antigen Dynamics Dictate How and Where B Cells Come in Contact with Antigens

B cells spend most of their life in the stroma of secondary lymphoid organs, where specific B-cell areas are organized (Fig. 1.1). Each B cell carries BCRs of unique antigenic specificity that, once activated, trigger multiple intracellular signaling cascades that ultimately lead to B-cell differentiation into antibody-secreting plasma cells or memory B cells.

How B cells encounter and recognize antigens depends therefore on the molecular characteristics of the different types of antigens and by the routes they employ to access these areas. Multiphoton microscopy techniques have been valuable tools to address how antigens enter into the B-cell follicles within peripheral lymph nodes [10]. Recent studies using this technology have shown that the *size and nature of antigens* influence their pathway of entry.

1.3.1 Direct Antigen Binding to the BCR

Particulate antigens that access the blood circulation can simply diffuse into the lymphoid tissue and reach the B-cell population residing in the MZ of the spleen [11] which quickly differentiates into IgM-secreting cells offering immediate protection against the pathogen in a manner which is independent of antigen presentation to T cells but is promoted by a local population of neutrophils [12].

Small soluble antigens originated by infection of peripheral tissues employ instead afferent lymphatic vessels to rapidly access draining lymph nodes. Once arrived in the subcapsular sinus, they reach B cells through two alternative pathways. Pape and colleagues reported that low-molecular-mass antigens directly enter the follicles via small gaps in the floor of the lymph node sinus where they immediately come in contact with B cells [13] (Fig. 1.1). Several electron microscopy studies have indeed identified pores of ~0.1–1 μm diameter in regions of the subcapsular sinus that are adjacent to the lymph node parenchyma [14–16]. These pores might allow small soluble antigens that enter the lymph nodes, such as low-molecular-mass toxins, to directly diffuse into the follicle and gain access to B cells [13], without requiring cell-mediated presentation. However, the existence of these pores remains controversial, as they simply may be sites generated by cells that have recently migrated through the sinus wall. More recently conduits have been suggested to represent the alternative mechanism exploited by small soluble antigens to reach the follicles. Anderson and colleagues, who first described conduits in rat lymph nodes in the 1970s [17], proposed that this extensive network of fibers is important for antigen distribution into the parenchyma of lymph nodes. The conduits drain indeed antigens deep into B-cell follicles, where they directly bind to B cells [4, 18]. However, notwithstanding the fact that the overall diameter of conduits is relatively large (0.5–1.0 μm), they are full of tightly packaged collagen fibers, which strongly limits the size of molecules that can access the tubes (approximately 5–8 nm). This has opened a dispute on whether conduits permit B-cell traffic or act as molecular sieves which only accept structures less than 5–8 nm in diameter, providing a rich source of antigens for B cells [4].

1.3.2 Need of an Intermediary: The Antigen-Presenting Cell (APC)

Although B cells are fully able to recognize soluble antigens in the absence of presenting cells, these encounters usually happen with the help of innate immune system components. Macrophages, dendritic cells (DC), and FDCs lie at the heart of adaptive response by efficiently providing antigens to B cells, especially in case of large soluble antigens originated by infection of peripheral tissues, such as viruses or antigens that are coated with antibodies and complement which, due to their relatively large size, cannot directly reach B-cell follicles. They are therefore first captured from the lymph by specific APCs (Fig. 1.1). Macrophages lining the subcapsular (SSM) or medullary (MM) sinus [4, 19–21] and FDCs residing in lymph nodes [22, 23] display a variety of receptors, such as Fc receptors, complement receptors, and C-type lectins, to capture the antigens [23].

Each APC presents antigens for a limited timeframe. SSM are indeed unable to maintain antigens on their surface for long periods [10] and overcome this limitation by transferring the captured antigens on the complement receptor CR2 of *non-cognate* naïve B cells. They in turn act as carriers to transport the transferred antigens to the core of B-cell follicles where they are deposited onto Fc receptors and on the complement receptors CR1 and CR2 of FDCs [20, 24]. These professional APCs retain antigens for long periods (several weeks) by promoting a switch in the subcellular localization from the plasma membrane to the endosomal compartment through a nonstop recycling process [25] which contributes to keep them available for recognition by *cognate* B cells for long time [26, 27].

1.4 B-Cell Response to Antigen: The Immune Synapse

B-cell fate relies primarily on the BCR, a multimeric complex composed of the antigen-specific surface immunoglobulin (Ig) and the Igα/Igβ heterodimers (CD79a and CD79b) [28]. In the resting state, B cells survive, thanks to tonic signals delivered from the BCR [29]. These signals depend on BCR distribution on the cell surface, which is in equilibrium between clusters and monomers, and on its ability to laterally diffuse along the plasma membrane. According to the so-called "picket-fence" model, diffusion of the BCR in resting cells is constrained in zones of the plasma membrane of approximately 30–700 nm in diameter enriched in selected transmembrane proteins which act as pickets defining confinement zones and are reversibly linked to the underlying actin/ezrin-radixin-moesin (ERM) cytoskeleton [30]. Alteration of the actin cytoskeleton by exposure of B cells to depolymerizing agents such as latrunculin A or cytochalasin D leads to BCR signaling in the absence of antigen and increases the diffusion rate of the BCR [31, 32]. However, whether the unstimulated BCR is in a monomeric state [32, 33] or is mainly organized in closed autoinhibited oligomers in the membrane [34] remains still debated.

Antigen recognition happens when the BCR meets specific antigen appropriately presented by APCs. This is a fundamental step in the entire life not only of the naïve B cell, which profoundly changes its metabolism, proliferation, and gene expression profile, but also of the activated B cell, which repeatedly binds antigen during the antibody affinity maturation process, ensuring the development of plasma cells that secrete high-affinity antibodies [35]. During antigen recognition, a close communication takes place through a signaling area that forms at the contact between the B cell and the APC, which is referred to as the *immune synapse* [18, 19, 36]. This highly specialized membrane region, built through the tightly regulated sequential recruitment of receptors and signaling molecules, controls not only B-cell activation but also the subsequent gathering and acquisition of membrane-bound antigens for processing and presentation to $CD4^+$ T cells [36, 37]. Two concentric regions referred to as the central supramolecular activation cluster (cSMAC), enriched in BCRs, and the peripheral SMAC (pSMAC) that contains adhesion molecules, such as LFA-1, bound to their ligands [36], are easily recognizable in the immune synapse. Of note, the most peculiar feature of the immune synapse is that, although its structure is stable both temporally and spatially, its molecular components are highly dynamic due to the action of continuous driving forces controlled by complex cytoskeletal rearrangements [37].

It is generally accepted that antigen binding leads to BCR clustering; however, the steps required for BCR clustering and whether clustering is required for B-cell activation remain to be understood [33, 38]. Studies on insect cells reconstituted with the BCR complex indicate that BCRs, which in resting cells are organized in autoinhibited oligomeric complexes, upon ligand binding undergo a conformational change to a monomeric "active" state [31]. Furthermore, the nature of antigen is critical in determining B-cell activation. Multivalent antigens, which can cross-link the BCR, are versed in triggering B-cell activation, although monovalent antigens can also elicit B-cell activation provided that early signals exceed a threshold required to elicit optimal BCR downstream signaling and expression of activation markers, leading to BCR clustering [39, 40]. Moreover membrane-bound antigens are considered the most efficient at triggering BCR signals and at antigen presentation to T cells, possibly due to a high local concentration of antigen in the two-dimensional structure of the immune synapse compared to soluble antigens [36, 38, 41].

1.5 Two-Phase Assembly of the Immune Synapse

1.5.1 Phase 1: Early Events that Control B Cell Spreading over the APC

Potent imaging techniques, among which the total internal reflection microscopy (TIRFM) on synthetic lipid bilayers stands out [38], revealed that the earliest events associated with successful antigen stimulation include the formation of microclusters of 50–500 BCR complexes at the plasma membrane [42, 43] which become focal signaling sites [38]. A series of molecular events starts indeed close to the engaged BCRs within seconds. These include:

- The phosphorylation and activation of the BCR-proximal kinase Lyn and the subsequent phosphorylation of immunoreceptor tyrosine-based activation motifs (ITAMs) in the non-covalently associated Igα and Igβ heterodimers
- The recruitment and phosphorylation of the kinases spleen tyrosine kinase (Syk) and Bruton's tyrosine kinase (Btk)
- The activation of downstream components such as PLCγ2, Vav, and PI3K and the adaptors B-cell linker protein (BLNK) and CD19 [43]
- The generation of second messengers—calcium ion release from endoplasmic reticulum, production of diacylglycerol, and inositol-1,4,5-trisphosphate

All of these molecules (and many others) contribute to build what was first known as a multicomponent assembly known as "signalosome" [44–46] which now, thanks to modern imaging techniques, has been shown to consist of many "micro-signalosomes" focused at the engaged BCRs [47].

One of the most important tasks of the microsignalosomes is the association between engaged BCRs and local cortical actin cytoskeleton which reorganizes to drive consecutive changes in B-cell shape [42]. B cells spread indeed over the surface of the APC, with the specific goal to increase the number of triggered BCRs by enlarging the synaptic area between the two interacting cells—the larger the area of the synapse, the more antigen the B cell can reach, internalize, and present to T cells [42]. To this end, actin first depolymerizes, a process which involves the small GTPase Rap1 and the actin-depolymerizing protein Cofilin-1 downstream of PLCγ2 [48], and detaches from the plasma membrane, which results from the dephosphorylation of the ERM complex [30, 49]. Subsequently actin polymerizes in branched actin filaments which extend the cell membrane to form lamellipodia (Fig. 1.2). Actin polymerization capitalizes on the guanine nucleotide exchange factor Vav,

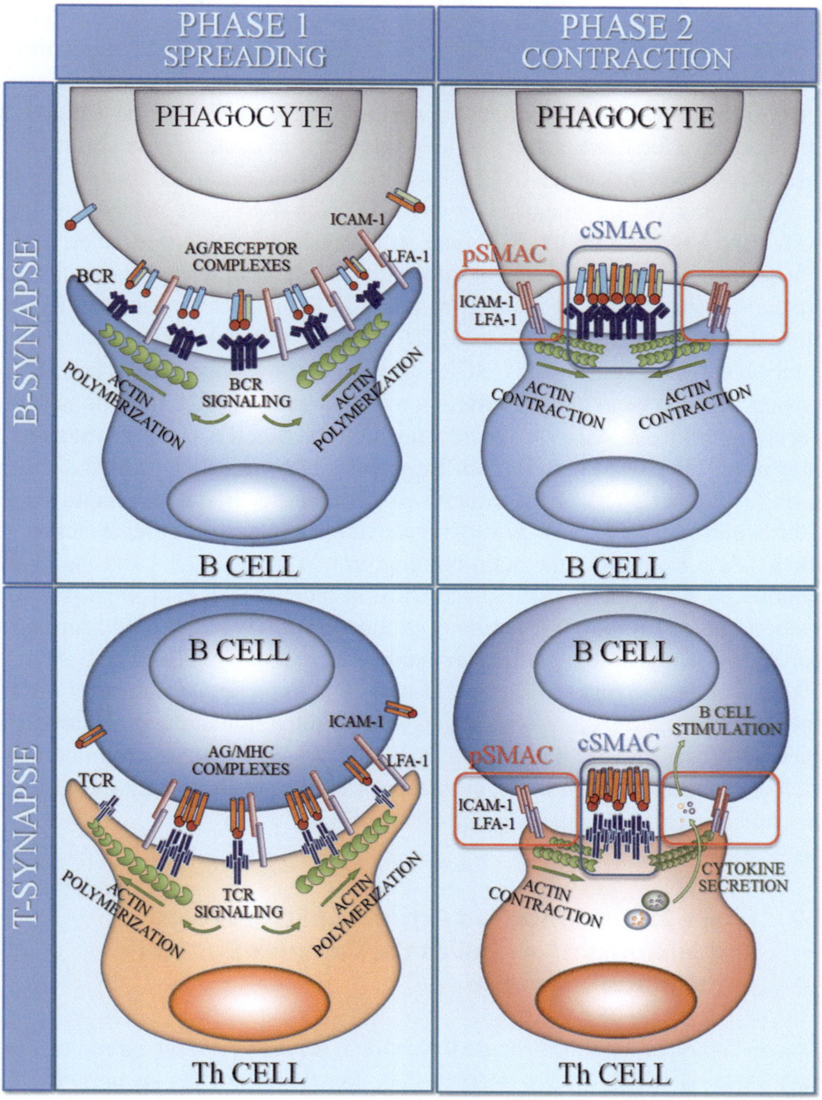

Fig. 1.2 Two-phase assembly of the immune synapse. *Phase 1*. Adhesion molecules, such as LFA-1/ICAM-1 complexes, mediate the first contact between phagocytes and the B cell (B-synapse) or between B cells and the helper T cell (Th) (T-synapse). Antigens (Ag) presented on the surface of antigen-presenting cells then bind either the B-cell receptor (BCR) or the T-cell receptor (TCR) which reorganize into microclusters. These activate a signaling cascade which induces the reorganization of the actin cytoskeleton that promotes B- and T-cell spreading over the antigen-presenting surface. *Phase 2*. After spreading, BCR and TCR microclusters converge toward the center of the contact area with the antigen-presenting cell through the contraction of actin filaments, forming the central supramolecular activation cluster (cSMAC), while adhesion molecules such as LFA-1/ICAM-1 complexes accumulate in the peripheral SMAC (pSMAC). The secretion of cytokines into the intermembrane space of the T-synapse stimulates B cells to undertake their differentiation process to either plasma cells or memory B cells

which is activated at the microsignalosomes and in turn activates the Rho GTPases Rac and Cdc42, two well-known regulators of cytoskeleton polymerization through the actin nucleation complex Arp2/3 [50–52]. Extension of lamellipodia along the surface of the APC now creates new opportunities for BCRs to bind antigens and leads to positive feedback loops that help the B cell to center the synapse over the highest density of the antigen [42]. B-cell lamellipodia also adhere to the APC through binding of the integrins LFA-1 and VLA-4 to their respective ligands ICAM-1 and VCAM-1 on the APC, an extra adhesion which is particularly important when antigen concentration is low [53, 54]. It is noteworthy that integrins expressed on the surface of naïve B cells are in their inactive state and require a conformational change triggered by BCR signaling to reach their active state and become able to bind their ligands. BCR signaling thus not only induces lamellipodia extension but also lamellipodia adhesion to the target cell [53]. Integrin activation has been in turn proposed to lower the threshold for B-cell activation when antigen avidity is low [53]. Once activated the integrins create indeed the pSMAC, an adhesion ring in the periphery of the synapse which enhances immune synapse stability and the achievement of *phase 2*. Integrin activation depends on several factors such as the GTPase Rap1 [55], the actin-binding protein vinculin [56] and the guanine nucleotide exchange factor Dock8, whose loss of function in B cells impairs pSMAC formation and results in poor antibody production in vivo [57], underscoring the importance of B-synapse organization in humoral immunity (Fig. 1.2).

Phase 1 of the B-synapse, which helps therefore to increase the number of BCR-antigen encounters, lasts for 2–5 min and ends by retraction of the lamellipodia and antigen gathering into BCR signaling microclusters which are transported toward the center of the synapse, in which co-receptors and cytosolic signaling components are recruited to form the microsignalosomes [47].

1.5.2 Phase 2: The Concerted Action of Microtubules and Microfilaments Builds the Complex Structure of the Mature Synapse

The second phase of immune synapse formation is driven by prolonged contraction of the cytoskeleton which allows microclusters containing antigen-engaged BCRs to move along actin fibers and to converge toward the center of the contact area, where they accumulate into the dense central disk of the cSMAC [36] (Fig. 1.2). This contraction is caused by the concerted actions of (i) polymerization of the cortical actin cytoskeleton to create a peripheral ring of F-actin enclosing a central actin low zone [30] and (ii) reorganization of the microtubular network, which brings the microtubule-organizing center (MTOC) toward the immune synapse platform [47, 58].

Although some aspects of the mechanisms that initiate the coordinated reorganization of the actin and microtubule networks at the B- as well as the

T-synapse remain poorly understood, the synaptic polarization of the MTOC is accompanied by clearance of F-actin from the cSMAC [59] and its accumulation at the pSMAC (Stinchcombe et al. 2006) and involves the small GTPase Cdc42, its downstream effector atypical protein kinase C zeta (aPKCζ), and the Par polarity complex [58, 60–64]. Wang and colleagues recently added a tile to the puzzle of the B-synapse reporting that Rap1, an evolutionarily conserved regulator of cell polarity, and Cofilin-1, the actin-severing downstream target of Rap1 [48], together coordinate actin remodeling and MTOC polarization at the B-synapse [65].

The most likely scenario is that B cells relocalize the MTOC to the cSMAC to allow microtubules to extend along the inner face of the plasma membrane at the contact site [66]. Dynein motor complexes, which are recruited to antigen-bound BCRs through the adaptors Grb2 and Dok-3, then propel BCR microclusters along these juxta-membrane microtubules toward the MTOC to reach the central zone of the synapse [64, 66–70].

It is noteworthy that the two phases of assembly of the immune synapse are strictly interconnected. The BCR/antigen transport to the cSMAC begins indeed already during lamellipodia extension, when antigen clusters are carried by centripetal flow of lamellipodial actin. B cells deficient in regulators of actin polymerization, such as WASP, N-WASP, and Abp1, show disruption of the actin patterns at immune synapses and delayed centralization of the antigen [71, 72].

Antigen gathering during synapse formation is thus an active process, driven by BCR signaling and executed by the mechanical activity of the cytoskeleton. In addition to the BCR and integrins, antigen gathering is also modulated by chemokine/chemokine receptor axes, and an interesting interplay exists between signals provided by the CXCL13/CXCR5 and antigen/BCR axes. CXCL13, which is produced by FDCs and stromal cells in B-cell follicles [22], has been indeed implicated in ruffling of B-cell lamellipodia and in LFA-1-supported adhesion, processes which require both functional actin cytoskeleton and myosin II motor protein. These mechanisms have been suggested to enhance the possibility of antigen encounter while also promoting antigen gathering in the central region of the immune synapse [73].

1.6 B Cells as APCs

Once they have recognized specific antigen and built a mature synapse, B cells have the unique opportunity to change their lifestyle, from cells which take advantage of APCs to APCs per se. This drastic change, which has a fundamental role in initiating T-cell responses, is performed through an articulated process, subdivided into three different steps: (i) extraction of antigen from the cSMAC, (ii) antigen processing and loading on major histocompatibility complex (MHC) molecules, and (iii) antigen presentation to $CD4^+$ or $CD8^+$ T cells at the plasma membrane.

1.6.1 Antigen Extraction

B cells, bound to APCs through antigen/BCR forces, now grab antigens from the APC, a process named "extraction." Two mechanisms have been proposed to mediate extraction of antigens from the synaptic surface of antigen-bearing cells. The first mechanism involves the fusion of degradative vesicles with the membrane of the pSMAC, a process driven by MTOC polarization, which allows the release of lysosomal proteases and lipases into the intermembrane area of the synaptic region and determines its acidification, facilitating antigen removal from the presenting cell [64]. The second mechanism is based on mechanical forces through which B cells physically pull out synaptic antigen through the BCR and deform flexible membranes to promote antigen internalization [74, 75]. It is noteworthy that these two mechanisms are non-exclusive and can coexist at the B-synapse to promote antigen extraction, assisted by co-stimulatory signals provided by engaged adhesion molecules, such as ICAM-1 and LFA1, which activate signaling cascades that regulate cytoskeleton organization contributing to immune synapse organization and function [55, 76].

1.6.2 Antigen Processing and Loading on MHC Molecules

Antigen extraction is followed by its internalization through clathrin-dependent BCR-mediated endocytosis [74, 77]. Clathrin-coated pits nucleate indeed close to BCR/antigen clusters and are mediated by the molecular adaptor AP-2, which is phosphorylated following BCR stimulation and co-localizes with BCR/antigen clusters [78]. Once internalized BCR/antigen complexes move to the endosomal compartment that contains the required processing machinery (proteases, MHC and H2-DM molecules) to cleave antigens in peptides loadable onto MHC molecules [47]. Microtubule-dependent reorientation of the vesicular apparatus toward the mature immune synapse has been proposed to facilitate delivery of extracted antigens to these compartments [64, 76].

Endocytosed antigens follow a degradative process which transforms them in peptides. In this form they are ready to be loaded onto MHC class II (MHC-II) or MHC class I (MHC-I) molecules to be presented to $CD4^+$ or $CD8^+$ T cells, respectively. Of note, antigens must follow different degradative pathways to be loaded on different MHC molecules: peptides derived from proteins degraded by the lysosomal pathway are indeed primarily presented by MHC-II molecules, while peptides generated by the ubiquitin-proteasome pathway are presented by MHC-I molecules [79] (Fig. 1.3). An exception is represented by the "cross-presentation," which specifically concerns professional APCs, whereby peptides derived from proteins that have entered the lysosomal pathway gain access to MHC-I molecules [80].

A complex series of molecular events regulates antigen loading on *MHC-II molecules*, αβ heterodimers generated in the endoplasmic reticulum and associated to the invariant chain Ii, a specialized chaperone which prevents the loading of MHC-II molecules with endogenous peptides and directs their trafficking to endo-lysosomes.

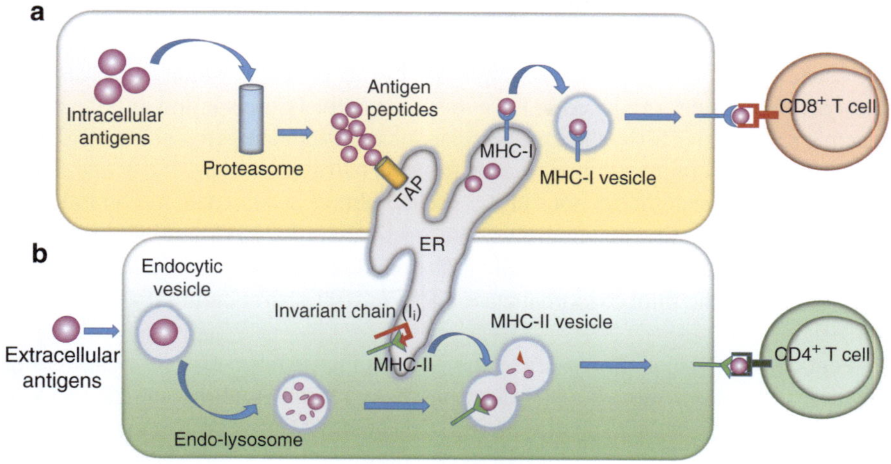

Fig. 1.3 The main steps of antigen processing and presentation on class I and class II major histocompatibility complex (MHC). Peptides generated by the ubiquitin-proteasome pathway are presented by MHC-I molecules (**a**), while peptides derived from proteins degraded by the lysosomal pathway are primarily presented by MHC-II molecules (**b**)

It contains indeed a peptide, named class II-associated invariant chain peptide (CLIP), which allows its non-covalent binding to the MHC-II groove [81]. A dileucine motif on its cytosolic tail enables moreover αβ/Ii sorting to clathrin-coated vesicles and their localization to "MHC-II compartments" (MIICs), which are specialized endosomal structures enriched in proteolytic enzymes and disulfide reductases [77, 82, 83]. To allow loading of antigen peptides onto MHC-II molecules, Ii must be processed by specific proteases [84], and the remaining 25-aa CLIP fragment must be exchanged with the digested peptide antigen [85, 86].

This complex reaction is tightly controlled by both positive and negative regulators. In addition to the classical MHC molecules, B cells and the other professional APCs express the nonclassical class II molecule HLA-DM (DM) which, despite the close structural similarity with the MHC-II molecule, appears unable to directly bind peptides [87] and rather transiently associates with MHC-II, stabilizing it in a peptide-receptive form [88, 89]. Interestingly, HLA-DM promotes the loading of high-affinity peptides on MHC-II facilitating removal of the weak ones, such as CLIP [90], through a pH-dependent process that encounters the optimal conditions in the MIICs [91–94]. Among negative regulators, the nonclassical class II molecule HLA-DO (DO) mimics MHC-II by binding to the same site on HLA-DM and blocking its catalytic activity on MHC-II/peptide complexes [87, 95–97].

MHC-I molecules, expressed on the plasma membrane of most cell types, load and present peptides to cytotoxic $CD8^+$ T cells. Of note, as opposed to MHC-II, MHC-I molecules load peptides generated by proteolysis of cytosolic antigens through, with few exceptions [98], the ubiquitin-proteasome pathway. The covalent attachment of multiple copies of the 76-residue protein ubiquitin to free amino groups by a multimolecular complex, which includes the substrate-specific ubiquitin-protein ligase E3, the ubiquitin-activating enzymes E1 and E2, and the additional conjugation factor E4 [99], targets antigens to the proteasome where they are broken down into peptides ranging from 2 to 25 residues, which are released in the cytosol. Peptides produced in the cytosol are actively transported into the endoplasmic reticulum (ER) by the transporter associated with antigen processing (TAP), a heterodimeric complex composed of the two half-transporters TAP1 and TAP2 that form a transmembrane pore in the ER membrane whose opening and closing depend on ATP binding and hydrolysis, respectively [100, 101].

Four ER chaperone proteins finally assist peptide loading on MHC-I molecules: calnexin [102], the thiol oxidoreductase ERp57 [103], calreticulin [104], and tapasin [105].

Peptide/MHC-I complexes leave the ER within vesicles that cross the Golgi apparatus, migrate to the cell membrane, and fuse with it. This allows the ER-resident chaperones to be released and the peptide bound to the MHC-I groove to be exposed extracellularly. Here the peptide/MHC-I complex can be recognized by and interact with the cognate TCR on $CD8^+$ T cells [106].

1.6.3 Antigen Presentation to $CD4^+$ or $CD8^+$ T Cells: The T-Synapse

The principal objective of antigen presentation by MHC molecules on the surface of B cells is the stimulation of B cells themselves which, with the help of T cells, differentiate in either "long-lived memory B cells" or "antibody-secreting plasma cells" [107], although a marginal role is ascribed to B cells in the stimulation of naïve T cells.

B-/T-cell interactions take place within secondary lymphoid tissues and are guided by the expression of chemokine receptors and corresponding ligands [108]. Naïve B cells, which express CXCR5, are retained within defined areas of lymph nodes, known as "primary lymphoid follicles" or "B-cell zones," by the CXCR5 ligand CXCL13 produced by FDCs [108]. Following antigen recognition, antigen-bearing B cells migrate toward the edge of the follicles in specific areas defined as "the B-cell-T-cell boundaries," a process which depends on CCR7 [109]. There they have the opportunity to encounter and engage T cells with matched antigen specificity [110, 111]. It is noteworthy that the outcome of this interaction depends on the binding affinity between TCRs and peptide/MHC complexes. When the binding affinity is low, neither the T nor the B cell receives a signal, and both cells move on [112], while when the binding affinity is high the contact transforms into a functional platform known as the T-synapse (Fig. 1.2).

Similar to the B-synapse, several coordinated events occur during T-synapse formation—polarization of TCRs, adhesion molecules and kinases, and rearrangement of the cytoskeleton and organelles—which organize the intercellular platform at the cSMAC and pSMAC [113]. Although B cells that present antigen to T cells have long been known to become activated, thanks to the polarized secretion of cytokines such as interferon-γ and interleukin-2, interleukin-4, and interleukin-5 by the activated helper T cell [114, 115] (Fig. 1.2), the molecular events that occur on the

B-cell side of the synapse are as yet poorly defined. A new mechanism has been recently proposed by Gardell and Parker [116], whereby the T cell transfers the costimulatory molecule CD40L, bound to the receptor CD40 on the surface of the B cell, to the interacting B cell in the context of a productive T-synapse, allowing the B cell to receive help by the T cell and making of the synapse a focal point not only of exocytosis but also of endocytosis [117].

Initial T-cell contact drives B-cell activation and differentiation through either extrafollicular or follicular pathways. B cells can indeed develop into extrafollicular plasmablasts and early memory B cells without entering the follicles (extrafollicular pathway). Alternatively, they can return to the follicles through B-cell lymphoma 6 (Bcl6) upregulation (follicular pathway), where they are retained by the expression of sphingosine-1-phosphate receptor 2 and where they differentiate into centroblasts and form germinal centers (GCs). In the B-cell-rich dark zones of the GC, the centroblasts, sustained by IL-21 and costimulatory signals derived from T cells, undergo somatic hypermutation, generating clonal variants with modified antigen affinity and specificity [107]. Centroblasts further differentiate into centrocytes and enter the GC light zone, where they encounter FDCs. Centrocytes with higher affinity for antigen are selectively preserved, whereas those with reduced BCR affinity are deleted. Additionally, a subset of centrocytes undergoes class-switch recombination for expression of IgG, IgA, or IgE [107, 118]. While MHC-II/peptide complexes on the surface of centroblasts become ubiquitinated and targeted for degradation to prevent the accumulation of older MHC-II/peptide complexes in GC centroblasts, MHC-II/peptide complexes on the surface of centrocytes become stabilized to facilitate productive interactions with $CD4^+$ T cells [119]. Centroblasts and centrocytes circulate between the light and dark zone until they achieve the optimal level of BCR affinity and further undergo differentiation steps to reach the alternative stages of "long-lived memory B cells" or "antibody-secreting plasma cells" [107]. Plasma cells migrate in a CXCR4-dependent manner to the BM, where they reside in survival niches supported by stromal cells secreting CXCL12 and cytokines and produce antibodies maintaining serologic memory independent of further antigen exposure [120].

Memory B cells, which will survive for long time, recirculate and form extrafollicular aggregates in lymphoid tissues. In case of a second antigen encounter, they will become again selectively activated by B-/T-cell cognate interactions to rapidly generate plasmablasts or reenter GCs upon antigen rechallenge resulting in further diversified secondary antibody responses [121, 122]. Hence both memory B cells and plasma cells generate high-affinity immunoglobulin class-switched diversified antibodies, which are the basis of long-lived humoral immunity.

$CD8^+$ T cells have the peculiar ability to specifically recognize MHC-I molecules loaded with peptides derived from intracellular nonself-proteins [106]. Through this system of intracellular surveillance, which enables the immune system to eradicate viruses and other intracellular pathogens, $CD8^+$ T cells build a functional T-synapse with a B cell and promote a cytotoxic response by releasing the pore-forming protein perforin and several granzyme proteases into the synaptic cleft, a mechanisms which has been suggested to limit the diffusion of toxic molecules and to maintain the specificity of the killing response [35, 60, 123].

1.7 Conclusions and Perspectives

Years of study unveiled the fundamental features of B cells and of their relationship with the other members of the immune system. Of note, the new era of studies on B cells is focused on their relationship with cells that B cells encounter during their entire life and which include non-hematopoietic cells whose activity profoundly affects B-cell responses. The capacity to establish effective immune responses requires indeed the presence of organized peripheral lymphoid organs, where hematopoietic cells are arranged into discrete anatomical territories created by sessile non-hematopoietic cells that form the three-dimensional tissue architecture [124, 125]. Of mesenchymal origin, they include FDCs, FRCs, marginal reticular cells, and endothelial cells. This class of cells is commonly identified by the word "stromal," a generic noun that does not account for their great variety of functions, which can be classified as *direct interaction-based* or *secretion-based.*

Stromal cells act indeed by secreting in the environment soluble factors, such as cytokines and chemokines, which mediate not only survival but also immune cell trafficking and localization, which are essential for bringing cognate leukocytes together to start building the GC. They moreover directly interact with B cells to promote their activation and differentiation by supplying antigen and in some instances by presenting cytokines and chemokines at their surface to promote B-cell proliferation, somatic hypermutation, and affinity maturation [125].

More recently, a new class of cells known as innate lymphoid cells has been described which also includes NK cells, generated by the diversification of committed lymphoid precursor cells independently of clonally rearranged antigen receptor genes. Their important contribution to inflammation and protection against pathogens in a tissue-specific manner and how they also influence the onset of immune responses in tissue-specific fashion are still under debate and raise the possibility of tissue-specific interplay between stromal and innate lymphoid cells [125].

The implication of stromal cells in the onset and development of pathologies pertaining B cells, among which the oncologic ones, is currently an area of active investigation. The lymphoma microenvironment is characterized by a heterogeneous population of stromal cells, which interact with neoplastic cells to promote tumor growth, survival, and drug resistance through multiple mechanisms among which angiogenesis is recognized as an important factor associated with disease progression [126].

Another example is the interesting dialogue existing between the stromal cells of secondary lymphoid organs and tumoral cells in chronic lymphocytic leukemia (CLL), a widespread hematological malignancy where tumoral cells depend on survival signals that they receive in lymphoid tissues from neighboring nonneoplastic cells within the cancer microenvironment [127]. CLL cells follow chemokine gradients in lymph nodes, forming atypical "proliferation centers" where they take extreme advantage of nonmalignant stromal cells to prolong their survival [128].

Although many questions remain to be answered about lymphoid tissue stromal cells, due to the difficulty in isolating these cells types, a better understanding of stromal cell functions within lymphoid tissues may lead to useful therapeutic applications. Targeting stromal cells might on one hand promote vaccine responses as well as limit autoimmune reactions and on the other hand help developing new drugs helpful for the treatment of B-cell malignancies, some of which remain, to date, incurable.

Acknowledgments The CTB lab is supported by grants from AIRC (IG 2014-15220), Telethon-Italy (Grant GGP1102) and ITT-Regione Toscana. The MMDE lab is supported by grants from the University of Florence and the Italian Ministry of Health.

References

1. von Andrian UH, Mempel TR. Homing and cellular traffic in lymph nodes. Nat Rev Immunol. 2003;3(11):867–78.
2. Schröttner P, Leick M, Burger M. The role of chemokines in B cell chronic lymphocytic leukaemia: pathophysiological aspects and clinical impact. Ann Hematol. 2010;89(5):437–46.
3. Cyster JG, Ansel KM, Reif K, Ekland EH, Hyman PL, Tang HL, et al. Follicular stromal cells and lymphocyte homing to follicles. Immunol Rev. 2000;176:181–93.
4. Roozendaal R, Mempel TR, Pitcher LA, Gonzalez SF, Verschoor A, Mebius RE, et al. Conduits mediate transport of low-molecular-weight antigen to lymph node follicles. Immunity. 2009;30(2):264–76.
5. Gretz JE, Anderson AO, Shaw S. Cords, channels, corridors and conduits: critical architectural elements facilitating cell interactions in the lymph node cortex. Immunol Rev. 1997;156:11–24.
6. Sixt M, Kanazawa N, Selg M, Samson T, Roos G, Reinhardt DP, et al. The conduit system transports soluble antigens from the afferent lymph to resident dendritic cells in the T cell area of the lymph node. Immunity. 2005;22(1):19–29.
7. González SF, Degn SE, Pitcher LA, Woodruff M, Heesters BA, Carroll MC. Trafficking of B cell antigen in lymph nodes. Annu Rev Immunol. 2011;29:215–33.
8. Schmidt EE, MacDonald IC, Groom AC. Comparative aspects of splenic microcirculatory pathways in mammals: the region bordering the white pulp. Scanning Microsc. 1993;7(2):613–28.
9. Cyster JG. B cell follicles and antigen encounters of the third kind. Nat Immunol. 2010;11(11):989–96.
10. Gonzalez SF, Pitcher LA, Mempel T, Schuerpf F, Carroll MC. B cell acquisition of antigen in vivo. Curr Opin Immunol. 2009;21(3):251–7.
11. Martin F, Oliver AM, Kearney JF. Marginal zone and B1 B cells unite in the early response against T-independent blood-borne particulate antigens. Immunity. 2001;14(5):617–29.
12. Puga I, Cols M, Barra CM, He B, Cassis L, Gentile M, et al. B cell–helper neutrophils stimulate the diversification and production of immunoglobulin in the marginal zone of the spleen. Nat Immunol. 2011;13(2):170–80.
13. Pape KA, Catron DM, Itano AA, Jenkins MK. The humoral immune response is initiated in lymph nodes by B cells that acquire soluble antigen directly in the follicles. Immunity. 2007;26(4):491–502.
14. Clark SL. The reticulum of lymph nodes in mice studied with the electron microscope. Am J Anat. 1962;110(3):217–57.
15. Farr AG, Cho Y, De Bruyn PP. The structure of the sinus wall of the lymph node relative to its endocytic properties and transmural cell passage. Am J Anat. 1980;157(3):265–84.
16. van Ewijk W, Brekelmans PJ, Jacobs R, Wisse E. Lymphoid microenvironments in the thymus and lymph node. Scanning Microsc. 1988;2(4):2129–40.
17. Anderson AO, Anderson ND. Studies on the structure and permeability of the microvasculature in normal rat lymph nodes. Am J Pathol. 1975;80(3):387–418.
18. Batista FD, Harwood NE. The who, how and where of antigen presentation to B cells. Nat Rev Immunol. 2009;9(1):15–27.

19. Carrasco YR, Batista FD. B cells acquire particulate antigen in a macrophage-rich area at the boundary between the follicle and the subcapsular sinus of the lymph node. Immunity. 2007;27(1):160–71.
20. Phan TG, Grigorova I, Okada T, Cyster JG. Subcapsular encounter and complement-dependent transport of immune complexes by lymph node B cells. Nat Immunol. 2007;8(9):992–1000.
21. Junt T, Moseman EA, Iannacone M, Massberg S, Lang PA, Boes M, et al. Subcapsular sinus macrophages in lymph nodes clear lymph-borne viruses and present them to antiviral B cells. Nature. 2007;450(7166):110–4.
22. Suzuki K, Grigorova I, Phan TG, Kelly LM, Cyster JG. Visualizing B cell capture of cognate antigen from follicular dendritic cells. J Exp Med. 2009;206(7):1485–93.
23. Gonzalez SF, Lukacs-Kornek V, Kuligowski MP, Pitcher LA, Degn SE, Kim Y-A, et al. Capture of influenza by medullary dendritic cells via SIGN-R1 is essential for humoral immunity in draining lymph nodes. Nat Immunol. 2010;11(5):427–34.
24. Ferguson JS, Weis JJ, Martin JL, Schlesinger LS. Complement protein C3 binding to Mycobacterium tuberculosis is initiated by the classical pathway in human bronchoalveolar lavage fluid. Infect Immun. 2004;72(5):2564–73.
25. Heesters BA, van der Poel CE, Das A, Carroll MC. Antigen presentation to B cells. Trends Immunol. 2016;37(12):844–54.
26. Cinamon G, Zachariah MA, Lam OM, Foss FW, Cyster JC, Cyster JG. Follicular shuttling of marginal zone B cells facilitates antigen transport. Nat Immunol. 2008;9(1):54–62.
27. Hoogeboom R, Tolar P. Molecular mechanisms of B cell antigen gathering and endocytosis. Cham: Springer; 2015. p. 45–63.
28. Hobeika E, Maity PC, Jumaa H. Control of B cell responsiveness by isotype and structural elements of the antigen receptor. Trends Immunol. 2016;37(5):310–20.
29. Kraus M, Alimzhanov MB, Rajewsky N, Rajewsky K. Survival of resting mature B lymphocytes depends on BCR signaling via the Igα/β heterodimer. Cell. 2004;117(6):787–800.
30. Treanor B, Depoil D, Bruckbauer A, Batista FD. Dynamic cortical actin remodeling by ERM proteins controls BCR microcluster organization and integrity. J Exp Med. 2011;208(5):1055–68.
31. Yang J, Reth M. Oligomeric organization of the B-cell antigen receptor on resting cells. Nature. 2010;467(7314):465–9.
32. Treanor B, Depoil D, Gonzalez-Granja A, Barral P, Weber M, Dushek O, et al. The membrane skeleton controls diffusion dynamics and signaling through the B cell receptor. Immunity. 2010;32(2):187–99.
33. Tolar P, Sohn HW, Pierce SK. The initiation of antigen-induced B cell antigen receptor signaling viewed in living cells by fluorescence resonance energy transfer. Nat Immunol. 2005;6(11):1168–76.
34. Schamel WW, Reth M. Monomeric and oligomeric complexes of the B cell antigen receptor. Immunity. 2000;13(1):5–14.
35. Basu R, Huse M. Mechanical communication at the immunological synapse. Trends Cell Biol. 2017;27(4):241–54.
36. Batista FD, Iber D, Neuberger MS. B cells acquire antigen from target cells after synapse formation. Nature. 2001;411(6836):489–94.
37. Yuseff MI, Lankar D, Lennon-Duménil AM. Dynamics of membrane trafficking downstream of B and T cell receptor engagement: impact on immune synapses. Traffic. 2009;10(6):629–36.
38. Tolar P, Sohn HW, Liu W, Pierce SK. The molecular assembly and organization of signaling active B-cell receptor oligomers. Immunol Rev. 2009;232:34–41.
39. Avalos AM, Bilate AM, Witte MD, Tai AK, He J, Frushicheva MP, et al. Monovalent engagement of the BCR activates ovalbumin-specific transnuclear B cells. J Exp Med. 2014;211(2):365–79.
40. Avalos AM, Ploegh HL. Early BCR events and antigen capture, processing, and loading on MHC class II on B cells. Front Immunol. 2014;5:1–5.
41. Lanzavecchia A. Receptor-mediated antigen uptake and its effect on antigen presentation to class II-restricted T lymphocytes. Annu Rev Immunol. 1990;8(c):773–93.

42. Fleire SJ, Goldman JP, Carrasco YR, Weber M, Bray D, Batista FD. B cell ligand discrimination through a spreading and contraction response. Science. 2006;312(5774):738–41.
43. Depoil D, Fleire S, Treanor BL, Weber M, Harwood NE, Marchbank KL, et al. CD19 is essential for B cell activation by promoting B cell receptor–antigen microcluster formation in response to membrane-bound ligand. Nat Immunol. 2008;9(1):63–72.
44. Wang J, Sohn H, Sun G, Milner JD, Pierce SK. The autoinhibitory C-terminal SH2 domain of phospholipase C-2 stabilizes B cell receptor signalosome assembly. Sci Signal. 2014;7(343):ra89.
45. Xu S, Huo J, Chew W-K, Hikida M, Kurosaki T, Lam K-P. Phospholipase Cgamma2 dosage is critical for B cell development in the absence of adaptor protein BLNK. J Immunol. 2006;176(8):4690–8.
46. Scharenberg AM, Humphries LA, Rawlings DJ. Calcium signalling and cell-fate choice in B cells. Nat Rev Immunol. 2007;7(10):778–89.
47. Yuseff M-I, Pierobon P, Reversat A, Lennon-Duménil A-M. How B cells capture, process and present antigens: a crucial role for cell polarity. Nat Rev Immunol. 2013;13(7):475–86.
48. Freeman SA, Lei V, Dang-Lawson M, Mizuno K, Roskelley CD, Gold MR. Cofilin-mediated F-actin severing is regulated by the Rap GTPase and controls the cytoskeletal dynamics that drive lymphocyte spreading and BCR microcluster formation. J Immunol. 2011;187(11):5887–900.
49. Pore D, Parameswaran N, Matsui K, Stone MB, Saotome I, McClatchey AI, et al. Ezrin tunes the magnitude of humoral immunity. J Immunol. 2013;191(8):4048–58.
50. Arana E, Vehlow A, Harwood NE, Vigorito E, Henderson R, Turner M, et al. Activation of the small GTPase Rac2 via the B cell receptor regulates B cell adhesion and immunological-synapse formation. Immunity. 2008;28(1):88–99.
51. Burbage M, Keppler SJ, Gasparrini F, Martínez-Martín N, Gaya M, Feest C, et al. Cdc42 is a key regulator of B cell differentiation and is required for antiviral humoral immunity. J Exp Med. 2015;212(1):53–72.
52. Weber M, Treanor B, Depoil D, Shinohara H, Harwood NE, Hikida M, et al. Phospholipase C-gamma2 and Vav cooperate within signaling microclusters to propagate B cell spreading in response to membrane-bound antigen. J Exp Med. 2008;205(4):853–68.
53. Carrasco YR, Fleire SJ, Cameron T, Dustin ML, Batista FD. LFA-1/ICAM-1 interaction lowers the threshold of B cell activation by facilitating B cell adhesion and synapse formation. Immunity. 2004;20(5):589–99.
54. Carrasco YR, Batista FD. B-cell activation by membrane-bound antigens is facilitated by the interaction of VLA-4 with VCAM-1. EMBO J. 2006;25(4):889–99.
55. Lin KBL, Freeman SA, Zabetian S, Brugger H, Weber M, Lei V, et al. The Rap GTPases regulate B cell morphology, immune-synapse formation, and signaling by particulate B cell receptor ligands. Immunity. 2008;28(1):75–87.
56. Saez de Guinoa J, Barrio L, Carrasco YR. Vinculin arrests motile B cells by stabilizing integrin clustering at the immune synapse. J Immunol. 2013;191(5):2742–51.
57. Randall KL, Lambe T, Johnson AL, Johnson A, Treanor B, Kucharska E, et al. Dock8 mutations cripple B cell immunological synapses, germinal centers and long-lived antibody production. Nat Immunol. 2009;10(12):1283–91.
58. Reversat A, Yuseff M-I, Lankar D, Malbec O, Obino D, Maurin M, et al. Polarity protein Par3 controls B-cell receptor dynamics and antigen extraction at the immune synapse. Mol Biol Cell. 2015;26(7):1273–85.
59. Ritter AT, Asano Y, Lippincott-Schwartz J, Griffiths GM, Stinchcombe JC, Dieckmann NMg, et al. Actin depletion initiates events leading to granule secretion at the immunological synapse. Immunity. 2015;42(5):864–76.
60. Stinchcombe JC, Majorovits E, Bossi G, Fuller S, Griffiths GM. Centrosome polarization delivers secretory granules to the immunological synapse. Nature. 2006;443(7110):462–5.
61. Bertrand F, Esquerre M, Petit A-E, Rodrigues M, Duchez S, Delon J, et al. Activation of the ancestral polarity regulator protein kinase C at the immunological synapse drives polarization of Th cell secretory machinery toward APCs. J Immunol. 2010;185(5):2887–94.

62. Huse M. Microtubule-organizing center polarity and the immunological synapse: protein kinase C and beyond. Front Immunol. 2012;3:235.
63. Stowers L, Yelon D, Berg LJ, Chant J. Regulation of the polarization of T cells toward antigen-presenting cells by Ras-related GTPase CDC42. Cell Biol. 1995;92:5027–31.
64. Yuseff M-I, Reversat A, Lankar D, Diaz J, Fanget I, Pierobon P, et al. Polarized secretion of lysosomes at the B cell synapse couples antigen extraction to processing and presentation. Immunity. 2011;35(3):361–74.
65. Wang JC, Lee JY-J, Christian S, Dang-Lawson M, Pritchard C, Freeman SA, et al. The Rap1-cofilin pathway coordinates actin reorganization and MTOC polarization at the B-cell immune synapse. J Cell Sci. 2017;130(6):1094–109.
66. Schnyder T, Castello A, Feest C, Harwood NE, Oellerich T, Urlaub H, et al. B cell receptor-mediated antigen gathering requires ubiquitin ligase Cbl and adaptors Grb2 and Dok-3 to recruit dynein to the signaling microcluster. Immunity. 2011;34(6):905–18.
67. Combs J, Kim SJ, Tan S, Ligon LA, Holzbaur ELF, Kuhn J, et al. Recruitment of dynein to the Jurkat immunological synapse. Proc Natl Acad Sci U S A. 2006;103(40):14883–8.
68. Martín-Cófreces NB, Robles-Valero J, Cabrero JR, Mittelbrunn M, Gordón-Alonso M, Sung CH, et al. MTOC translocation modulates IS formation and controls sustained T cell signaling. J Cell Biol. 2008;182(5):951–62.
69. Quann EJ, Merino E, Furuta T, Huse M. Localized diacylglycerol drives the polarization of the microtubule-organizing center in T cells. Nat Immunol. 2009;10(6):627–35.
70. Yi J. Centrosome repositioning in T cells is biphasic and driven by microtubule end-on capture-shrinkage. J Cell Biol. 2013;202(5):779–92.
71. Seeley-Fallen MK, Liu LJ, Shapiro MR, Onabajo OO, Palaniyandi S, Zhu X, et al. Actin-binding protein 1 links B-cell antigen receptors to negative signaling pathways. Proc Natl Acad Sci U S A. 2014;111(27):9881–6.
72. Liu C, Bai X, Wu J, Sharma S, Upadhyaya A, Dahlberg CIM, et al. N-WASP is essential for the negative regulation of B cell receptor Signaling. PLoS Biol. 2013;11(11):e1001704.
73. Sáez de Guinoa J, Barrio L, Mellado M, Carrasco YR. CXCL13/CXCR5 signaling enhances BCR-triggered B-cell activation by shaping cell dynamics. Blood. 2011;118(6):1560–9.
74. Natkanski E, Lee W-Y, Mistry B, Casal A, Molloy JE, Tolar P. B cells use mechanical energy to discriminate antigen affinities. Science. 2013;340(6140):1587–90.
75. Nowosad CR, Spillane KM, Tolar P. Germinal center B cells recognize antigen through a specialized immune synapse architecture. Nat Immunol. 2016;17:870–7.
76. Yuseff MI, Lennon-Duménil AM. B cells use conserved polarity cues to regulate their antigen processing and presentation functions. Front Immunol. 2015;6:251.
77. Roche PA, Furuta K. The ins and outs of MHC class II-mediated antigen processing and presentation. Nat Rev Immunol. 2015;15(4):203–16.
78. Cocucci E, Aguet F, Boulant S, Kirchhausen T. The first five seconds in the life of a clathrin-coated pit. Cell. 2012;150(3):495–507.
79. Yewdell JW. Not such a dismal science: the economics of protein synthesis, folding, degradation and antigen processing. Trends Cell Biol. 2001;11(7):294–7.
80. Joffre OP, Segura E, Savina A, Amigorena S. Cross-presentation by dendritic cells. Nat Rev Immunol. 2012;12(8):557–69.
81. Bakke O, Dobberstein B. MHC class II-associated invariant chain contains a sorting signal for endosomal compartments. Cell. 1990;63(4):707–16.
82. McCormick PJ, Martina JA, Bonifacino JS. Involvement of clathrin and AP-2 in the trafficking of MHC class II molecules to antigen-processing compartments. Proc Natl Acad Sci U S A. 2005;102(22):7910–5.
83. Neefjes J. CIIV, MIIC and other compartments for MHC class II loading. Eur J Immunol. 1999;29(5):1421–5.
84. Manoury B, Mazzeo D, Li DN, Billson J, Loak K, Benaroch P, et al. Asparagine endopeptidase can initiate the removal of the MHC class II invariant chain chaperone. Immunity. 2003;18(4):489–98.

85. Lennon-Duménil A-M, Bakker AH, Maehr R, Fiebiger E, Overkleeft HS, Rosemblatt M, et al. Analysis of protease activity in live antigen-presenting cells shows regulation of the phagosomal proteolytic contents during dendritic cell activation. J Exp Med. 2002;196(4):529–40.
86. Denzin LK, Cresswell P. HLA-DM induces CLIP dissociation from MHC class II alpha beta dimers and facilitates peptide loading. Cell. 1995;82(1):155–65.
87. Guce AI, Mortimer SE, Yoon T, Painter CA, Jiang W, Mellins ED, et al. HLA-DO acts as a substrate mimic to inhibit HLA-DM by a competitive mechanism. Nat Struct Mol Biol. 2013;20(1):90–8.
88. Denzin LK, Hammond C, Cresswell P. HLA-DM interactions with intermediates in HLA-DR maturation and a role for HLA-DM in stabilizing empty HLA-DR molecules. J Exp Med. 1996;184(6):2153–65.
89. Pashine A, Busch R, Belmares MP, Munning JN, Doebele RC, Buckingham M, et al. Interaction of HLA-DR with an acidic face of HLA-DM disrupts sequence-dependent interactions with peptides. Immunity. 2003;19(2):183–92.
90. Bryant P, Ploegh H. Class II MHC peptide loading by the professionals. Curr Opin Immunol. 2004;16(1):96–102.
91. Jiang W, Strohman MJ, Somasundaram S, Ayyangar S, Hou T, Wang N, et al. pH-susceptibility of HLA-DO tunes DO/DM ratios to regulate HLA-DM catalytic activity. Sci Rep. 2015;5(1):17333.
92. Kropshofer H, Arndt SO, Moldenhauer G, Hämmerling GJ, Vogt AB. HLA-DM acts as a molecular chaperone and rescues empty HLA-DR molecules at lysosomal pH. Immunity. 1997;6(3):293–302.
93. Sloan VS, Cameron P, Porter G, Gammon M, Amaya M, Mellins E, et al. Mediation by HLA-DM of dissociation of peptides from HLA-DR. Nature. 1995;375(6534):802–6.
94. Yin L, Maben ZJ, Becerra A, Stern LJ. Evaluating the role of HLA-DM in MHC class II–peptide association reactions. J Immunol. 2015;195(2):706–16.
95. Denzin LK, Sant'Angelo DB, Hammond C, Surman MJ, Cresswell P. Negative regulation by HLA-DO of MHC class II-restricted antigen processing. Science. 1997;278(5335):106–9.
96. Chen X, Laur O, Kambayashi T, Li S, Bray RA, Weber DA, et al. Regulated expression of human histocompatibility leukocyte antigen (HLA)-DO during antigen-dependent and antigen-independent phases of B cell development. J Exp Med. 2002;195(8):1053–62.
97. Mellins ED, Stern LJ. HLA-DM and HLA-DO, key regulators of MHC-II processing and presentation. Curr Opin Immunol. 2014;26:115–22.
98. Craiu A, Akopian T, Goldberg A, Rock KL. Two distinct proteolytic processes in the generation of a major histocompatibility complex class I-presented peptide. Proc Natl Acad Sci U S A. 1997;94(20):10850–5.
99. Koegl M, Hoppe T, Schlenker S, Ulrich HD, Mayer TU, Jentsch S. A novel ubiquitination factor, E4, is involved in multiubiquitin chain assembly. Cell. 1999;96(5):635–44.
100. Arora S, Lapinski PE, Raghavan M. Use of chimeric proteins to investigate the role of transporter associated with antigen processing (TAP) structural domains in peptide binding and translocation. Proc Natl Acad Sci U S A. 2001;98(13):7241–6.
101. Higgins CF, Linton KJ. The ATP switch model for ABC transporters. Nat Struct Mol Biol. 2004;11(10):918–26.
102. Diedrich G, Bangia N, Pan M, Cresswell P. A role for calnexin in the assembly of the MHC class I loading complex in the endoplasmic reticulum. J Immunol. 2001;166(3):1703–9.
103. Hughes EA, Cresswell P. The thiol oxidoreductase ERp57 is a component of the MHC class I peptide-loading complex. Curr Biol. 1998;8(12):709–12.
104. Sadasivan B, Lehner PJ, Ortmann B, Spies T, Cresswell P. Roles for calreticulin and a novel glycoprotein, tapasin, in the interaction of MHC class I molecules with TAP. Immunity. 1996;5(2):103–14.
105. Momburg F, Tan P. Tapasin-the keystone of the loading complex optimizing peptide binding by MHC class I molecules in the endoplasmic reticulum. Mol Immunol. 2002;39(3–4):217–33.

106. Leone P, Shin E-C, Perosa F, Vacca A, Dammacco F, Racanelli V. MHC class I antigen processing and presenting machinery: organization, function, and defects in tumor cells. J Natl Cancer Inst. 2013;105(16):1172–87.
107. Victora GD, Nussenzweig MC. Germinal centers. Annu Rev Immunol. 2012;30(1):429–57.
108. Cyster JG. Chemokines, sphingosine-1-phosphate, and cell migration in secondary lymphoid organs. Annu Rev Immunol. 2005;23:127–59.
109. Okada T, Cyster JG. B cell migration and interactions in the early phase of antibody responses. Curr Opin Immunol. 2006;18(3):278–85.
110. Kerfoot SM, Yaari G, Patel JR, Johnson KL, Gonzalez DG, Kleinstein SH, et al. Germinal center B cell and T follicular helper cell development initiates in the interfollicular zone. Immunity. 2011;34(6):947–60.
111. Green JA, Cyster JG. S1PR2 links germinal center confinement and growth regulation. Immunol Rev. 2012;247(1):36–51.
112. Mempel TR, Henrickson SE, von Andrian UH. T-cell priming by dendritic cells in lymph nodes occurs in three distinct phases. Nature. 2004;427(6970):154–9.
113. Dustin ML, Choudhuri K. Signaling and polarized communication across the T cell immunological synapse. Annu Rev Cell Dev Biol. 2016;32(1):303–25.
114. Kupfer H, Monks CR, Kupfer A. Small splenic B cells that bind to antigen-specific T helper (Th) cells and face the site of cytokine production in the Th cells selectively proliferate: immunofluorescence microscopic studies of Th-B antigen-presenting cell interactions. J Exp Med. 1994;179(5):1507–15.
115. Kupfer A, Mosmann TR, Kupfer H. Polarized expression of cytokines in cell conjugates of helper T cells and splenic B cells. Proc Natl Acad Sci U S A. 1991;88(3):775–9.
116. Gardell JL, Parker DC. CD40L is transferred to antigen-presenting B cells during delivery of T-cell help. Eur J Immunol. 2017;47(1):41–50.
117. Griffiths GM, Tsun A, Stinchcombe JC. The immunological synapse: a focal point for endocytosis and exocytosis. J Cell Biol. 2010;189(3):399–406.
118. Klein U, Dalla-Favera R. Germinal centres: role in B-cell physiology and malignancy. Nat Rev Immunol. 2008;8(1):22–33.
119. Bannard O, McGowan SJ, Ersching J, Ishido S, Victora GD, Shin J-S, et al. Ubiquitin-mediated fluctuations in MHC class II facilitate efficient germinal center B cell responses. J Exp Med. 2016;213(6):993–1009.
120. Nutt SL, Hodgkin PD, Tarlinton DM, Corcoran LM. The generation of antibody-secreting plasma cells. Nat Rev Immunol. 2015;15(3):160–71.
121. McHeyzer-Williams LJ, Milpied PJ, Okitsu SL, McHeyzer-Williams MG. Class-switched memory B cells remodel BCRs within secondary germinal centers. Nat Immunol. 2015;16(3):296–305.
122. Kurosaki T, Kometani K, Ise W. Memory B cells. Nat Rev Immunol. 2015;15(3):149–59.
123. Stinchcombe JC, Griffiths GM. Secretory mechanisms in cell-mediated cytotoxicity. Annu Rev Cell Dev Biol. 2007;23(1):495–517.
124. Randall TD, Carragher DM, Rangel-Moreno J, Randall T. Development of secondary lymphoid organs. Annu Rev Immunol. 2008;26:627–50.
125. Kellermayer Z, Vojkovics D, Balogh P. Innate lymphoid cells and their stromal microenvironments. Immunol Lett. 2017;189:3–9.
126. Blonska M, Agarwal NK, Vega F. Shaping of the tumor microenvironment: stromal cells and vessels. Semin Cancer Biol. 2015;34:3–13.
127. Ten Hacken E, Burger JA. Microenvironment interactions and B-cell receptor signaling in chronic lymphocytic leukemia: implications for disease pathogenesis and treatment. Biochim Biophys Acta. 2015;1863(3):401–13.
128. Kipps TJ, Stevenson FK, Wu CJ, Croce CM, Packham G, Wierda WG, et al. Chronic lymphocytic leukaemia. Nat Rev Dis Primers. 2017;3:17008.

Mucosal B Cells

2

Arianna Troilo, Nagaja Capitani, Laura Patrussi,
Cosima T. Baldari, and Mario Milco D'Elios

2.1 Origin and Development of B Lymphocyte Lineage Subsets

The dynamic life of B lymphocytes starts in the bone marrow (or in the fetal liver before birth), where a tightly controlled sequence of maturation steps transforms common lymphoid progenitors in (1) pro-B, (2) pre-B, and (3) immature B cells (Fig. 2.1). The latter are released into the circulation and reach specific organs where they complete their differentiation process to mature B cells, which are conventionally subdivided in three principal populations on the basis of their ontogeny and anatomic localization: *B1 cells*, *marginal zone (MZ) B cells*, *and follicular (FO) B cells.*

A. Troilo
Department of Rheumatology and Clinical Immunology, Medical Center – University of Freiburg, Freiburg, Germany

Department of Clinical and Experimental Medicine, University of Florence Careggi Hospital, Firenze, Italy

N. Capitani
Department of Clinical and Experimental Medicine, University of Florence Careggi Hospital, Firenze, Italy

Department of Life Sciences, University of Siena, Siena, Italy

L. Patrussi · C. T. Baldari
Department of Life Sciences, University of Siena, Siena, Italy

M. M. D'Elios (✉)
Department of Clinical and Experimental Medicine, University of Florence Careggi Hospital, Firenze, Italy
e-mail: delios@unifi.it

M. M. D'Elios, M. Rizzi (eds.), *Humoral Primary Immunodeficiencies*, Rare Diseases of the Immune System, https://doi.org/10.1007/978-3-319-91785-6_2

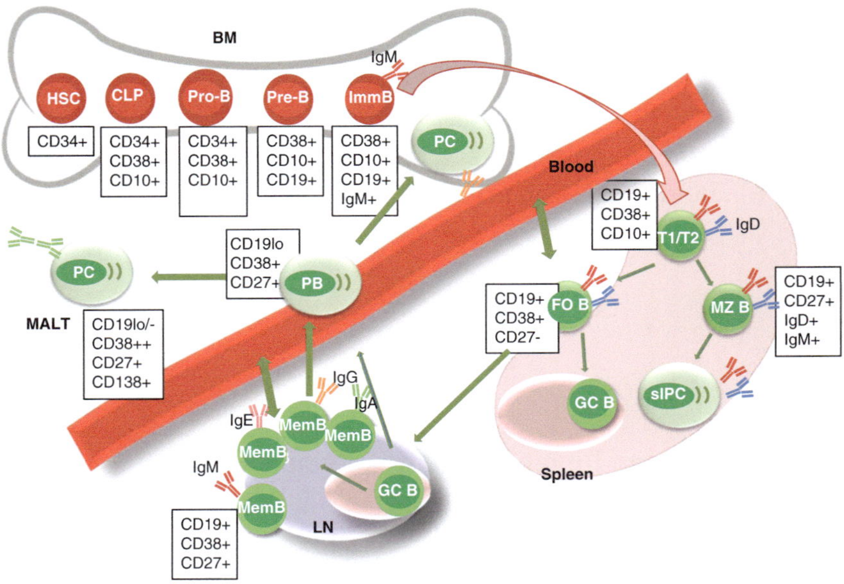

Fig. 2.1 Origin and development of B lymphocyte lineage subsets. B-cell development starts in the bone marrow (BM) from hematopoietic stem cells (HSC) that through a controlled sequence of maturation steps reach the stage of common lymphoid progenitors (CLP), pro-B, pre-B, and immature (Imm) B cells. At this stage, the cells start expressing IgM on their surface and are ready to migrate to the spleen as transitional B cells (T1/T2), where they complete the first stage of development as marginal zone (MZ) B cells or follicular (FO) B cells. MZ B cells develop into short-lived plasma cells (slPC). FO B cells are activated by antigen binding and develop in GCs into memory (Mem) B cells or plasma cells (PC). Plasma cells (PC) then home to specific areas of secondary lymphoid tissue and BM. Principal surface markers from each B cell subset are shown

Little is known about human *B1 lymphocytes*, which originate from B1 progenitors in the fetal liver, with little input from the bone marrow beyond the perinatal period [1, 2]. Our scant knowledge comes from studies on mouse B1 cells; these are also defined as T-independent B cells as they produce antibodies without any help of T lymphocytes and secrete IgM antibodies that selectively recognize altered self-antigens contributing to tissue homeostasis [3]. In addition to IgM, B1 cells also produce polyreactive IgA antibodies that contribute to mucosal immunity [4]. The existence of B1 cells as a distinct lineage in humans remains controversial, and B cells expressing CD5 are mostly considered as B1 cells [5, 6].

Immature B cells that exit the bone marrow and migrate to the spleen differentiate into either transitional B cells, which mature into MZ or FO B cells, respectively. *MZ B cells* develop in the marginal sinus of the spleen through the specific binding of their surface molecule neurogenic locus notch homolog protein 2 (NOTCH2) with the specific ligand Delta-like 1 on endothelial cells, which promotes their subsequent retention within the marginal sinus of the spleen where they reside for most of their life. MZ B cells express a polyreactive B-cell antigen receptors (BCR), thereby producing polyreactive IgM antibodies [7]. Similar to B1 cells, MZ B cells constitutively express Toll-like receptors and can readily respond to pathogen-associated or endogenous Toll-like receptor ligands. MZ B cells also participate in responses to T-dependent protein antigens, generating high-affinity isotype-switched antibodies [2, 7].

FO B cells, the most abundant of all B-cell lineages, originate through BCR-mediated differentiation signals and reside in spleen and lymph nodes where they are considered the conventional B lymphocytes of the adaptive immune system [8]. FO B cells are primarily responsible for the generation of long-lasting, high-affinity IgG antibodies with the help of T lymphocytes, critical for the classical humoral immunity which mediates protection after infection or vaccination. As opposed to spleen-resident MZ B cells, FO B cells continuously recirculate populating various secondary lymphoid tissues (e.g., lymph nodes, tonsils, and mucosal-associated lymphoid tissues).

The transition of B cells from pro-B to pre-B stage and finally to immature B cells proceeds through a complex series of genomic DNA rearrangements undertaken by the immunoglobulin heavy- and light-chain gene segments (variable, V; diversity, D; and joining, J), which culminate in the expression of a surface IgM, the BCR, that can bind antigen [9]. These rearrangements generate B cells expressing a vast repertoire of BCRs capable of recognizing a huge variety of antigens. Since the recombination process occurs through the random assembly of V, D, and J segments, 75% of the resulting BCRs are self-reactive [10] and must be eliminated to avoid autoimmunity. Most self-reactive clones are eliminated before their exit from the bone marrow by clonal deletion and receptor editing, a process termed **central tolerance**, and additional selection mechanisms occur within the spleen to remove the remaining autoreactive clones that recognize peripheral self-antigens. Transitional B cells that strongly recognize self-antigens through their BCRs can indeed either undergo clonal deletion or attain a state of hyporesponsiveness termed "anergy," which dramatically shortens their survival (1–5 days) [11]. Elimination of the few self-reactive B lymphocytes that escape clonal deletion, receptor editing, or anergy relies either on $CD41^{+}$ T cells via Fas receptor-Fas ligand or on CD40-CD40L interactions or even on T and B cells with regulatory properties. Failure of one or more of the self-tolerance checkpoints is central to the development of autoimmune diseases [12].

2.2 Mucosal B Cells: The MALT

The mucosa-associated lymphoid tissue (MALT) is a secondary lymphoid organ that includes more or less organized lymphoid structures. It includes multiple subregions, the most important being the gut-associated lymphoid tissue (GALT), the nasal-associated lymphoid tissue (NALT), and the bronchus-associated lymphoid tissue (BALT). In the human airway of adults, evidence of an organized lymphoid tissue is still lacking, even though such structures have been described in infants and during inflammation.

The MALT is characterized by the presence of inductive sites and effector sites that are specific for different regions, even though anatomically separated districts are in some cases functionally connected. It was in fact shown that IgA secretion at a specific site can be induced by antigen presentation at a different mucosal region.

Systemic and mucosal immune systems have distinct functional structures and can be activated and regulated in an independent fashion [13, 14]. Common characteristics of the MALT are the presence of different cell types, such as B cells, $CD4^+$ and $CD8^+$ T cells, dendritic cells (DC), and in some case macrophages and eosinophils, that permit the organization of an efficient immune response. Other common characteristics of the MALT are the lack of afferent lymphatics as well as the presence of high endothelial regions [15].

The most well-known region is the GALT, which is often used as a paradigm to describe structures and functions of the mucosal immune system (Fig. 2.2).

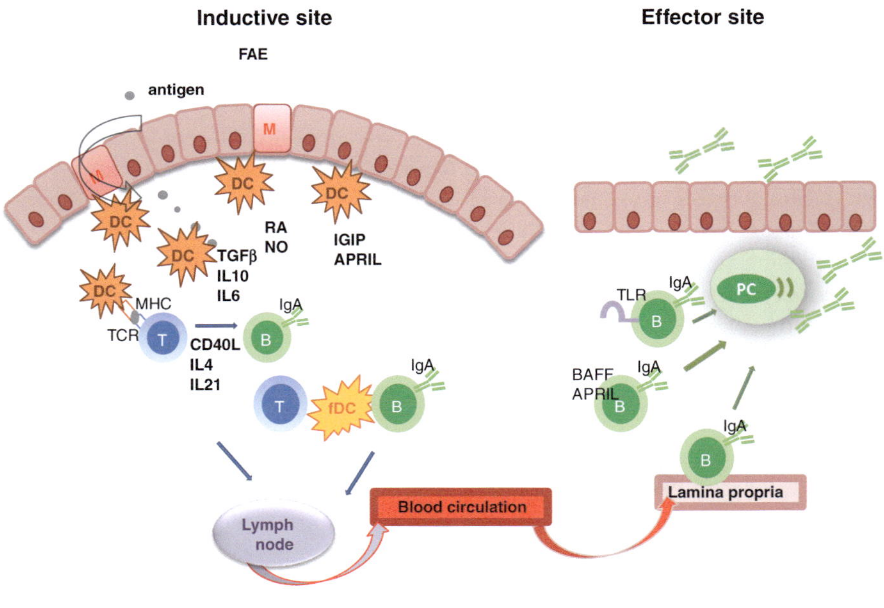

Fig. 2.2 Depiction of mucosal inductive and effector sites. Antigens are sampled from the mucosal lumen through specialized M cells in the follicle-associated epithelium (FAE). Dendritic cells (DCs) capture and process the antigens, transport them to the T-cell zone, and produce cytokines that initiate T-cell-dependent B cell activation and factors like IGIP and APRIL that induce switching to IgA. They also secrete retinoic acid (RA) that induces expression of mucosal-imprinting molecules such as CCR9 and $\alpha 4\beta 7$. Peyer patches (PPs) also contain follicle dendritic cells (fDCs) whose main function seems to be to facilitate the positive selection of high-affinity B cells by antigen. Generated plasmablasts move through blood circulation to the lamina propria where they differentiate to plasma cells (PC). In the lamina propria also T-independent IgA production takes place via TLR-dependent activation or mediated by cytokines such BAFF and APRIL

The GALT is characterized by the presence of several different lymphoid structures, the most important in humans being Peyer's patches (PPs) and isolated lymphoid follicles that are randomly located through the mucosa of the gastrointestinal tract but at higher density in the terminal ileum and in the appendix [16].

Human PPs' development begins during embryonic life and requires signals from IL-7. Their number increases progressively to reach its maximum in teenage years and then progressively decreases with age [16–18].

The epithelium of the gastrointestinal tract is characterized by physical barriers, consisting of tight junctions and a dense layer of mucins [19], and biochemical barriers provided by antimicrobial peptides [19–21]. At variance, the follicle-associated epithelium (FAE) is characterized by the presence of microfold (M) cells [22, 23]. B cells seem to be crucial in the development of M cells. It was in fact shown that M cells are not able to develop in the FAE of PPs in B-cell-deficient mice [24]. M cells are characterized by a peculiar morphology, with an irregular brush border, few microvilli, and decreased glycocalyx [22]. They permit the sampling of pathogens and soluble molecules and their exhibition to the antigen presenting cells (APC) in the subepithelial dome (SED). The subepithelial area is rich in DCs that play a central role in the organization of the mucosal immune response and in the induction of class switch recombination (CSR) via IgA-inducing protein (IGIP) and a proliferation-inducing ligand (APRIL) secretion [25].

Lymphoid structures in the GALT contain, as mentioned, many different cell types, and in the small intestine, germinal centers (GC) structures were identified, in which B cells are surrounded by follicle DCs, follicular T helper (fTh) cells, and macrophages, surrounded by a mantle zone of $CD27^{-}IgM^{+}IgD^{+}$ mature naïve B cells, surrounded by a marginal zone (MZ) of IgDlow B cells that infiltrate the FAE [26].

While naïve and memory B cells appear to be present only in organized lymphoid structures, in the lamina propria, the most represented B cell subsets are antibody-secreting cells (ASC), plasma cells, and plasmablasts mainly producing IgA [27].

Scattered $IgA^{+}CD27^{+}$ cells were also identified in the lamina propria by flow cytometry, and even though a contamination cannot be excluded, the fact that they express low levels of CD40 and are able to proliferate in response to CD40L and to produce IgA in vitro [28] suggests that they could receive T cell help also in vivo and act as local memory cells.

ASC have been identified by various authors as recently recruited plasmablasts on the base of HLAII, CD45RA, CD19, and Ig expression [27–29].

Plasma cells are also present only in the lamina propria, where they are characterized by IgA and IgM expression. This differentiates them from BM plasma cells that mainly express IgG. In the past, PC in the gut had been considered short living [30–33].

Data from intestinal biopsy cultures showed that IgM and IgA plasma cells could survive more than 4 weeks [34], and it was recently shown by Landsverk et al. that PCs, identified as CD38hi CD27hi $CD138^{+}$ $CD20^{-}$ large cells, can be classified in three distinct subsets: a $CD19^{+}$ PC subset and two $CD19^{-}$ subsets, $CD45^{+}$ and $CD45^{-}$, that can persist for decades in the gut. The $CD45^{-}$ subset exhibits no replacement, while the $CD45^+$ subset shows only little replacement and appears to be an intermediate developmental stage between $CD19^+$ and $CD45^-$ [35]. These subsets are similar to BM PC subsets from a phenotype and functional point of view [36, 37].

In human upper airways, a proper NALT was identified only in infants [38], as most of the associated lymphoid structures are located at the level of the Waldeyer's ring [38–40]. Cells histologically similar to the M cells of the gut were described in this region in tonsils and adenoids, even though evidence of a similar function of these cells in the airways is still lacking [41, 42].

Tonsils contain specialized tissue compartments contributing to immune functions, in particular GCs that start to be present shortly after birth, via B-cell activation induced by exogenous antigens, while terminal differentiation of effector B cells to extrafollicular PCs can be detected 2 weeks after birth [43].

In a study from Quiding-Jarbrink et al., the ability of tonsillar and nasal mucosal lymphoid tissues to serve as induction sites of local and/or distant B-cell responses in humans was evaluated. Subjects immunized by the tonsillar route presented a higher number of vaccine-specific ASC in removed tonsils compared to peroral and parenteral immunization with cholera and tetanus [44]. Both intratonsillar and intranasal immunizations were able to evoke specific ASC responses at the mucosal site and in peripheral blood, but specific ASC could not be identified at the duodenum level. Intranasal immunization could not induce efficient Ab secretion in the tonsils but could evoke ASC response in the adenoids [44]. This study and others indicate that in the mucosal immune system, IgA-inductive sites may serve as expression sites of locally induced antibody responses and support the development of immunological memory [44–47].

Laryngeal associate lymphoid tissue (LALT) has also been described in humans and was demonstrated also in healthy adults, even if after the age of 20 years it is present at a lower frequency, probably because of declining primary response to antigens [48].

BALT has not been described in healthy humans [49], but bronchial lymphoid structures were identified in children who died from SIDS [50] and in adults with chronic inflammation [51–53], with autoimmune diseases [54], smokers [55], or affected by lung neoplasia [56]. BALT characterized by lymphoid infiltration of the overlying epithelium, HEV, and partly active germinal centers was found in 44% of children who died because of trauma, malformation, or other non inflammatory causes [50, 57].

2.3 Production of IgA and Their Relevance for Host Protection

During lymphocyte differentiation, antibody diversification results from three main processes: VDJ recombination, class-switch recombination (CSR), and somatic hyper-mutation (SHM). VDJ recombination occurs in the BM and is initiated by the RAG1-RAG2 endonuclease complex [58]. After completing this process, B cells express IgM on their surface and are able to migrate to the peripheral lymphoid structures where they come in contact with the antigens and differentiate into plasma cells and memory cells. CSR takes place in the periphery, allowing the production of different Ig classes, such as IgG, IgE, IgA, and IgD [59, 60], without changing the antigen-binding specificity of the antibodies [61–63].

Antibody affinity maturation is induced by SHM process that introduces point mutations in the variable portions of Ig genes. Both CSR and SHM are antigen-dependent genetic alteration processes catalyzed by the same DNA-editing enzyme, the activation-induced cytidine deaminase (AID), that is able to target different regions [64].

Different mucosal regions are characterized by the presence of different Ab classes. In the urogenital and intestinal mucosa, IgA antibodies are the most represented, while IgD were described prevalently in the respiratory tract. IgE are usually present in case of allergy [59, 65, 66]. Humans present two different classes of IgA: IgA1 is detectable in systemic and mucosal compartments, while IgA2, which seems to be more resistant to bacterial proteases, is more present in mucosal districts colonized by microbiota [67, 68].

In the intestinal mucosa, high- and low-affinity IgA were described, with possible different functions. The role of mucosal IgA is on the one hand to neutralize dangerous and high inflammatory pathogens and microbial toxins and, on the other hand, to regulate the commensal microbiota and confine the symbiotic pathogens to specific areas of the intestinal lumen. A different role for low- and high-affinity IgA in selecting invasive pathogens from symbionts had been proposed, but the distinction is not always clear [17, 18].

Dimeric IgA facilitate the interplay between host and commensal flora not only in the intestinal lumen but also in PPs [18]. Secreted IgA appear to be able to entrap microbial organisms in the mucus layer on the epithelial cells surface [15, 69, 70], a process known as immune exclusion [71]. They are also capable of neutralizing intracellular proinflammatory components, such as LPS [69], and to facilitate antigen sampling by binding to receptors on M cells [72]. IgA dimers released by plasma cells transport bacteria that trespass the epithelial barrier back to the lumen via pIgR [73] or promote their phagocytosis through FcαRI (CD89) [70, 74], a high affinity IgA receptor expressed on DC and neutrophils, but not (or only a little) by intestinal macrophages [73]. The transferrin receptor (CD71) on enterocytes is also able to bind IgA1 and can mediate retrotranscytosis of intact gliadin peptides in celiac disease [75, 76].

In humans, the importance of IgA function is clearly demonstrated in vivo in patients affected by primary antibody deficiencies (PAD). The impairment in IgA production is associated with recurrent respiratory, gastrointestinal, and urogenital infections, but also allergy, autoimmunity, and lymphoid nodular hyperplasia, possibly due to aberrant B-cell activation, are possible complications [77, 78] (specifically described in Chap. 16). Compensatory mechanisms possibly exist, given the high incidence of isolated IgA deficiency (1:400 in Western countries) and given that not every patient affected by PAD is highly or at all symptomatic [79].

Also in the respiratory tract, IgA is the most represented immunoglobulin: IgA1 is predominant, but IgA2 is less represented in the NALT than in the BALT. Unlike in the gut, in the airway mucosa, IgD seems to have an important protective role. IgD are secreted in human nasal mucosa and tonsils by IgD+ IgM- plasmablasts, are polyreactive, and are able to bind to pathogens like *Haemophilus influenzae* and *Moraxella catarrhalis* as well as to interact with cells from the innate immune system [59].

IgA production can be elicited through both T-cell-dependent and T-cell-independent pathways. T-cell-dependent reactions need at least 1 week to lead to IgA production and take place in GCs in PPs, where CSR and SHM also occur. Stimulation of CD40 receptor on B cells by CD40L on fTh cells, associated with BCR and CKS receptor activation, is crucial for the induction of AID expression [80–83].

The T-independent pathway leads to a faster IgA production and takes place in response to highly conserved microbial structure recognition by TLRs. This pathway involves B1 cells in mice, but a clear counterpart of these cells has not been yet identified in humans. Possible pathways that lead to T-independent IgA production are direct B-cell activation via TLR and indirect B-cell stimulation via BAFF and APRIL released by cells of the innate immune system. TLR signaling via NFκB, requiring MyD88, induces both AID expression in B cells and BAFF and APRIL production in different cell types [83].

This pathway is active in isolated lymphoid follicles and in the lamina propria, where in situ CSR was described, even though this is a controversial matter [84, 85]. In the lamina propria B cell can undergo CSR [86] and IgA can be generated via an T independent pathway [87, 88].

2.4 Lymphoma of Mucosa-Associated Lymphoid Tissue

Mucosal B cells are crucial for the host defense; however they can undergo neoplastic transformation and give raise to mucosa-associated lymphoid tissue (MALT) lymphoma, especially in patients with primary immunodeficiencies (see Chap. 23). Extranodal marginal zone B-cell lymphoma of MALT represents the third most common form of non-Hodgkin lymphoma [89–91]. The most frequent site of MALT lymphomas is the stomach, where they were first recognized as a distinct entity [92]. A link of *H. pylori* infection with gastric MALT lymphoma was provided by the identification of *H. pylori* in the majority of the lymphoma specimens [93]. *H. pylori*-related low-grade gastric MALT lymphoma represents a model for studying the interplay between chronic infection, immune response, and lymphomagenesis. This lymphoma represents the first described neoplasia susceptible of regression following antibiotic therapy resulting in *H. pylori* eradication [94]. A prerequisite for lymphomagenesis is the development of secondary inflammatory MALT induced by *H. pylori*. Tumor cells of low-grade gastric MALT lymphoma (MALToma) are memory B cells still responsive to differentiation signals, such as CD40 costimulation and cytokines produced by antigen-stimulated Th cells, and dependent for their growth on the stimulation by *H. pylori*-specific T cells [95–97]. In early phases, this tumor is sensitive to withdrawal of *H. pylori*-induced T-cell help, providing an explanation for both the tumor's tendency to remain localized to its primary site and its regression after *H. pylori* eradication. The analysis of the antigen-induced B-cell help by *H. pylori*-reactive gastric T-cell clones provided detailed information on the molecular and cellular mechanisms associated with the onset of low-grade gastric MALToma. In the stomach of MALToma patients, a high percentage of Th cells were specific for *H. pylori*. Each *H. pylori*-specific Th clone derived from gastric MALToma produced IL-2 and a variety of B-cell-stimulating cytokines, such as IL-4 and IL-13 [98]. In vitro stimulation with the appropriate *H. pylori* antigens induced *H. pylori*-specific Th clones derived from gastric MALToma to provide powerful help for B-cell activation and proliferation [98]. B cells from MALToma patients proliferate in response to *H. pylori*, but the B-cell proliferation induced by *H. pylori* antigens was strictly T dependent because it could not take place with *H. pylori* and without T helper cells [98]. Furthermore other cytokines and B-cell growth factors are able to sustain B-cell growth in gastric MALT lymphomas. Gastric MALT lymphoma expresses high levels of APRIL and B-cell activating factor, which are crucial cytokines for B-cell proliferation [99, 100]. APRIL is produced almost exclusively by gastric lymphoma-infiltrating macrophages located in close proximity to neoplastic B cells. Macrophages produced APRIL on direct stimulation with both *H. pylori* and *H. pylori*-specific T cells [100].

2.5 Conclusions

B-cell life starts in the bone marrow. Following B-cell development through pro-B, and pre-B stage, immature B cells are released in the circulation and reach specific organs, where their differentiation proceeds to mature B cells, which can be subdivided into B1 cells, marginal zone B cells, and follicular B cells, on the basis of their anatomic localization and their ontogeny.

The mucosae represent the largest part of the body in which immune responses against pathogens occur. Mucosal B cells are located in different subregions, the most important being GALT, BALT, and NALT. Mucosal B cells are crucial for the host defense mainly via the production of mucosal IgA. The importance of IgA function is clearly demonstrated in vivo in patients affected by primary antibody deficiencies. The impairment in IgA production is associated with recurrent respiratory, gastrointestinal, and urogenital infections. IgA deficiency might be associated also with allergy, autoimmunity, and lymphoid nodular hyperplasia. Immune compensatory mechanisms exist, given that not every patient affected by PAD is symptomatic. Mucosal B cells may undergo neoplastic transformation and give raise to MALT lymphoma, which is quite frequently observed in patients with humoral PAD. Hence mucosal B cells are the principal guardians protecting us from the majority of harmful pathogens that try to enter the body through ingestion, inhalation, or sexual contact.

References

1. Montecino-Rodriguez E, Dorshkind K. B-1 B cell development in the fetus and adult. Immunity. 2012;36:13–23.
2. Baumgarth N. The double life of a B-1 cell: self-reactivity selects for protective effector functions. Nat Rev Immunol. 2011;11(1):34–46.
3. Grönwall C, Vas J, Silverman GJ. Protective roles of natural IgM antibodies. Front Immunol. 2012;3:66.
4. Suzuki K, Maruya M, Kawamoto S, Fagarasan S. Roles of B-1 and B-2 cells in innate and acquired IgA-mediated immunity. Immunol Rev. 2010;237:180–90.
5. Griffin DO, Holodick NE, Rothstein TL. Human B1 cells in umbilical cord and adult peripheral blood express the novel phenotype CD20+ CD27+ CD43+ CD70. J Exp Med. 2011;208(1):67–80.
6. Tangye SG. To B1 or not to B1: that really is still the question! Blood. 2013;121(26):5109–10.
7. Cerutti A, Cols M, Puga I. Marginal zone B cells: virtues of innate-like antibody-producing lymphocytes. Nat Rev Immunol. 2013;13(2):118–32.
8. Pillai S, Cariappa A. The follicular versus marginal zone B lymphocyte cell fate decision. Nat Rev Immunol. 2009;9(11):767–77.
9. Thomas MD, Srivastava B, Allman D. Regulation of peripheral B cell maturation. Cell Immunol. 2006;239:92–102.
10. Wardemann H, Yurasov S, Schaefer A, Young JW, Meffre E, Nussenzweig MC. Predominant autoantibody production by early human B cell precursors. Science. 2003;301(5638):1374–7.
11. Cambier JC, Gauld SB, Merrell KT, Vilen BJ. B-cell anergy: from transgenic models to naturally occurring anergic B cells? Nat Rev Immunol. 2007;7(8):633–43.
12. Meffre E, Wardemann H. B-cell tolerance checkpoints in health and autoimmunity. Curr Opin Immunol. 2008;20:632–8.
13. Mei HE, Yoshida T, Sime W, Hiepe F, Thiele K, Manz RA, et al. Blood-borne human plasma cells in steady state are derived from mucosal immune responses. Blood. 2009;113(11):2461–9.
14. Weitkamp JH, Kallewaard NL, Bowen AL, Lafleur BJ, Greenberg HB, Crowe JE Jr. VH1-46 is the dominant immunoglobulin heavy chain gene segment in rotavirus-specific memory B cells expressing the intestinal homing receptor alpha4beta7. J Immunol. 2005;174(6):3454–60.
15. Macpherson AJ, McCoy KD, Johansen FE, Brandtzaeg P. The immune geography of IgA induction and function. Mucosal Immunol. 2008;1(1):11–22.
16. Cornes JS. Number, size, and distribution of Peyer's patches in the human small intestine: Part I The development of Peyer's patches. Gut. 1965;6(3):225–9.
17. Peterson DA, McNulty NP, Guruge JL, Gordon JI. IgA response to symbiotic bacteria as a mediator of gut homeostasis. Cell Host Microbe. 2007;2(5):328–39.
18. Obata T, Goto Y, Kunisawa J, Sato S, Sakamoto M, Setoyama H, et al. Indigenous opportunistic bacteria inhabit mammalian gut-associated lymphoid tissues and share a mucosal antibody-mediated symbiosis. Proc Natl Acad Sci U S A. 2010;107(16):7419–24.
19. Baker J, Garrod D. Epithelial cells retain junctions during mitosis. J Cell Sci. 1993;104(Pt 2):415–25.
20. Peters BM, Shirtliff ME, Jabra-Rizk MA. Antimicrobial peptides: primeval molecules or future drugs? PLoS Pathog. 2010;6(10):e1001067.
21. Dann SM, Eckmann L. Innate immune defenses in the intestinal tract. Curr Opin Gastroenterol. 2007;23(2):115–20.
22. Kraehenbuhl JP, Neutra MR. Epithelial M cells: differentiation and function. Annu Rev Cell Dev Biol. 2000;16:301–32.
23. Wolf JL, Rubin DH, Finberg R, Kauffman RS, Sharpe AH, Trier JS, et al. Intestinal M cells: a pathway for entry of reovirus into the host. Science. 1981;212(4493):471–2.
24. Golovkina TV, Shlomchik M, Hannum L, Chervonsky A. Organogenic role of B lymphocytes in mucosal immunity. Science. 1999;286(5446):1965–8.
25. Endsley MA, Njongmeta LM, Shell E, Ryan MW, Indrikovs AJ, Ulualp S, et al. Human IgA-inducing protein from dendritic cells induces IgA production by naive IgD+ B cells. J Immunol. 2009;182(4):1854–9.

26. Spencer J, MacDonald TT, Finn T, Isaacson PG. The development of gut associated lymphoid tissue in the terminal ileum of fetal human intestine. Clin Exp Immunol. 1986;64(3):536–43.
27. Benckert J, Schmolka N, Kreschel C, Zoller MJ, Sturm A, Wiedenmann B, et al. The majority of intestinal IgA+ and IgG+ plasmablasts in the human gut are antigen-specific. J Clin Invest. 2011;121(5):1946–55.
28. Farstad IN, Carlsen H, Morton HC, Brandtzaeg P. Immunoglobulin A cell distribution in the human small intestine: phenotypic and functional characteristics. Immunology. 2000;101(3):354–63.
29. Di Niro R, Mesin L, Raki M, Zheng NY, Lund-Johansen F, Lundin KE, et al. Rapid generation of rotavirus-specific human monoclonal antibodies from small-intestinal mucosa. J Immunol. 2010;185(9):5377–83.
30. Stevens RH, Macy E, Morrow C, Saxon A. Characterization of a circulating subpopulation of spontaneous antitetanus toxoid antibody producing B cells following in vivo booster immunization. J Immunol. 1979;122(6):2498–504.
31. Brieva JA, Roldan E, Rodriguez C, Navas G. Human tonsil, blood and bone marrow in vivo-induced B cells capable of spontaneous and high-rate immunoglobulin secretion in vitro: differences in the requirements for factors and for adherent and bone marrow stromal cells, as well as distinctive adhesion molecule expression. Eur J Immunol. 1994;24(2):362–6.
32. Munoz JL, Insel RA. In vitro human antibody production to the Haemophilus influenzae type b capsular polysaccharide. J Immunol. 1987;139(6):2026–31.
33. Sen ML, Garcia-Alonso A, Brieva JA. Human B lymphocytes capable of spontaneous Ig production in short-term cultures: characterization in the circulation and lymphoid tissues. Cell Immunol. 1986;98(1):200–10.
34. Mesin L, Di Niro R, Thompson KM, Lundin KE, Sollid LM. Long-lived plasma cells from human small intestine biopsies secrete immunoglobulins for many weeks in vitro. J Immunol. 2011;187(6):2867–74.
35. Landsverk OJ, Snir O, Casado RB, Richter L, Mold JE, Reu P, et al. Antibody-secreting plasma cells persist for decades in human intestine. J Exp Med. 2017;214(2):309–17.
36. Mei HE, Wirries I, Frolich D, Brisslert M, Giesecke C, Grun JR, et al. A unique population of IgG-expressing plasma cells lacking CD19 is enriched in human bone marrow. Blood. 2015;125(11):1739–48.
37. Pellat-Deceunynck C, Bataille R. Normal and malignant human plasma cells: proliferation, differentiation, and expansions in relation to CD45 expression. Blood Cells Mol Dis. 2004;32(2):293–301.
38. Debertin AS, Tschernig T, Tonjes H, Kleemann WJ, Troger HD, Pabst R. Nasal-associated lymphoid tissue (NALT): frequency and localization in young children. Clin Exp Immunol. 2003;134(3):503–7.
39. Bienenstock J, McDermott MR. Bronchus- and nasal-associated lymphoid tissues. Immunol Rev. 2005;206:22–31.
40. Dolen WK, Spofford B, Selner JC. The hidden tonsils of Waldeyer's ring. Ann Allergy. 1990;65(4):244–8.
41. Verbrugghe P, Kujala P, Waelput W, Peters PJ, Cuvelier CA. Clusterin in human gut-associated lymphoid tissue, tonsils, and adenoids: localization to M cells and follicular dendritic cells. Histochem Cell Biol. 2008;129(3):311–20.
42. Ogasawara N, Kojima T, Go M, Takano K, Kamekura R, Ohkuni T, et al. Epithelial barrier and antigen uptake in lymphoepithelium of human adenoids. Acta Otolaryngol. 2011;131(2):116–23.
43. Brandtzaeg P. Translocation of immunoglobulins across human epithelia: review of the development of a transport model. Acta Histochem Suppl. 1987;34:9–32.
44. Quiding-Jarbrink M, Granstrom G, Nordstrom I, Holmgren J, Czerkinsky C. Induction of compartmentalized B-cell responses in human tonsils. Infect Immun. 1995;63(3):853–7.
45. Brandtzaeg P, Prydz H. Direct evidence for an integrated function of J chain and secretory component in epithelial transport of immunoglobulins. Nature. 1984;311(5981):71–3.

46. Fukuizumi T, Inoue H, Anzai Y, Tsujisawa T, Uchiyama C. Sheep red blood cell instillation at palatine tonsil effectively induces specific IgA class antibody in saliva in rabbits. Microbiol Immunol. 1995;39(5):351–9.
47. Moldoveanu Z, Russell MW, Wu HY, Huang WQ, Compans RW, Mestecky J. Compartmentalization within the common mucosal immune system. Adv Exp Med Biol. 1995;371A:97–101.
48. Hiller AS, Tschernig T, Kleemann WJ, Pabst R. Bronchus-associated lymphoid tissue (BALT) and larynx-associated lymphoid tissue (LALT) are found at different frequencies in children, adolescents and adults. Scand J Immunol. 1998;47(2):159–62.
49. Pabst R, Gehrke I. Is the bronchus-associated lymphoid tissue (BALT) an integral structure of the lung in normal mammals, including humans? Am J Respir Cell Mol Biol. 1990;3(2):131–5.
50. Tschernig T, Kleemann WJ, Pabst R. Bronchus-associated lymphoid tissue (BALT) in the lungs of children who had died from sudden infant death syndrome and other causes. Thorax. 1995;50(6):658–60.
51. Meuwissen HJ, Hussain M. Bronchus-associated lymphoid tissue in human lung: correlation of hyperplasia with chronic pulmonary disease. Clin Immunol Immunopathol. 1982;23(2):548–61.
52. Sato A, Chida K, Iwata M, Hayakawa H. Study of bronchus-associated lymphoid tissue in patients with diffuse panbronchiolitis. Am Rev Respir Dis. 1992;146(2):473–8.
53. Suda T, Chida K, Hayakawa H, Imokawa S, Iwata M, Nakamura H, et al. Development of bronchus-associated lymphoid tissue in chronic hypersensitivity pneumonitis. Chest. 1999;115(2):357–63.
54. Sato A, Hayakawa H, Uchiyama H, Chida K. Cellular distribution of bronchus-associated lymphoid tissue in rheumatoid arthritis. Am J Respir Crit Care Med. 1996;154(6 Pt 1):1903–7.
55. Richmond I, Pritchard GE, Ashcroft T, Avery A, Corris PA, Walters EH. Bronchus associated lymphoid tissue (BALT) in human lung: its distribution in smokers and non-smokers. Thorax. 1993;48(11):1130–4.
56. Delventhal S, Brandis A, Ostertag H, Pabst R. Low incidence of bronchus-associated lymphoid tissue (BALT) in chronically inflamed human lungs. Virchows Arch B Cell Pathol Incl Mol Pathol. 1992;62(4):271–4.
57. Tschernig T, Pabst R. Bronchus-associated lymphoid tissue (BALT) is not present in the normal adult lung but in different diseases. Pathobiology. 2000;68(1):1–8.
58. Jung D, Giallourakis C, Mostoslavsky R, Alt FW. Mechanism and control of V(D)J recombination at the immunoglobulin heavy chain locus. Annu Rev Immunol. 2006;24:541–70.
59. Chen K, Cerutti A. New insights into the enigma of immunoglobulin D. Immunol Rev. 2010;237(1):160–79.
60. Chen K, Xu W, Wilson M, He B, Miller NW, Bengten E, et al. Immunoglobulin D enhances immune surveillance by activating antimicrobial, proinflammatory and B cell-stimulating programs in basophils. Nat Immunol. 2009;10(8):889–98.
61. Schlissel MS. Regulating antigen-receptor gene assembly. Nat Rev Immunol. 2003;3(11):890–9.
62. Muramatsu M, Kinoshita K, Fagarasan S, Yamada S, Shinkai Y, Honjo T. Class switch recombination and hypermutation require activation-induced cytidine deaminase (AID), a potential RNA editing enzyme. Cell. 2000;102(5):553–63.
63. Randall TD, Carragher DM, Rangel-Moreno J. Development of secondary lymphoid organs. Annu Rev Immunol. 2008;26:627–50.
64. Manis JP, Tian M, Alt FW. Mechanism and control of class-switch recombination. Trends Immunol. 2002;23(1):31–9.
65. Stavnezer J. Antibody class switching. Adv Immunol. 1996;61:79–146.
66. Hodge LM, Marinaro M, Jones HP, McGhee JR, Kiyono H, Simecka JW. Immunoglobulin A (IgA) responses and IgE-associated inflammation along the respiratory tract after mucosal but not systemic immunization. Infect Immun. 2001;69(4):2328–38.
67. Cerutti A. The regulation of IgA class switching. Nat Rev Immunol. 2008;8(6):421–34.
68. Hapfelmeier S, Lawson MA, Slack E, Kirundi JK, Stoel M, Heikenwalder M, et al. Reversible microbial colonization of germ-free mice reveals the dynamics of IgA immune responses. Science. 2010;328(5986):1705–9.

69. Fernandez MI, Pedron T, Tournebize R, Olivo-Marin JC, Sansonetti PJ, Phalipon A. Anti-inflammatory role for intracellular dimeric immunoglobulin a by neutralization of lipopolysaccharide in epithelial cells. Immunity. 2003;18(6):739–49.
70. Phalipon A, Corthesy B. Novel functions of the polymeric Ig receptor: well beyond transport of immunoglobulins. Trends Immunol. 2003;24(2):55–8.
71. Phalipon A, Cardona A, Kraehenbuhl JP, Edelman L, Sansonetti PJ, Corthesy B. Secretory component: a new role in secretory IgA-mediated immune exclusion in vivo. Immunity. 2002;17(1):107–15.
72. Mantis NJ, Cheung MC, Chintalacharuvu KR, Rey J, Corthesy B, Neutra MR. Selective adherence of IgA to murine Peyer's patch M cells: evidence for a novel IgA receptor. J Immunol. 2002;169(4):1844–51.
73. Brandtzaeg P, Baekkevold ES, Morton HC. From B to A the mucosal way. Nat Immunol. 2001;2(12):1093–4.
74. Pasquier B, Launay P, Kanamaru Y, Moura IC, Pfirsch S, Ruffie C, et al. Identification of FcalphaRI as an inhibitory receptor that controls inflammation: dual role of FcRgamma ITAM. Immunity. 2005;22(1):31–42.
75. Matysiak-Budnik T, Moura IC, Arcos-Fajardo M, Lebreton C, Menard S, Candalh C, et al. Secretory IgA mediates retrotranscytosis of intact gliadin peptides via the transferrin receptor in celiac disease. J Exp Med. 2008;205(1):143–54.
76. Moura IC, Centelles MN, Arcos-Fajardo M, Malheiros DM, Collawn JF, Cooper MD, et al. Identification of the transferrin receptor as a novel immunoglobulin (Ig)A1 receptor and its enhanced expression on mesangial cells in IgA nephropathy. J Exp Med. 2001;194(4): 417–25.
77. Molaei M, Kaboli A, Fathi AM, Mashayekhi R, Pejhan S, Zali MR. Nodular lymphoid hyperplasia in common variable immunodeficiency syndrome mimicking familial adenomatous polyposis on endoscopy. Indian J Pathol Microbiol. 2009;52(4):530–3.
78. Schaefer PS, Friedman AC. Nodular lymphoid hyperplasia of the small intestine with Burkitt's lymphoma and dysgammaglobulinemia. Gastrointest Radiol. 1981;6(4):325–8.
79. Macpherson AJ. IgA adaptation to the presence of commensal bacteria in the intestine. Curr Top Microbiol Immunol. 2006;308:117–36.
80. Breitfeld D, Ohl L, Kremmer E, Ellwart J, Sallusto F, Lipp M, et al. Follicular B helper T cells express CXC chemokine receptor 5, localize to B cell follicles, and support immunoglobulin production. J Exp Med. 2000;192(11):1545–52.
81. Boles KS, Vermi W, Facchetti F, Fuchs A, Wilson TJ, Diacovo TG, et al. A novel molecular interaction for the adhesion of follicular CD4 T cells to follicular DC. Eur J Immunol. 2009;39(3):695–703.
82. Reinhardt RL, Liang HE, Locksley RM. Cytokine-secreting follicular T cells shape the antibody repertoire. Nat Immunol. 2009;10(4):385–93.
83. Cerutti A, Rescigno M. The biology of intestinal immunoglobulin A responses. Immunity. 2008;28(6):740–50.
84. Bergqvist P, Gardby E, Stensson A, Bemark M, Lycke NY. Gut IgA class switch recombination in the absence of CD40 does not occur in the lamina propria and is independent of germinal centers. J Immunol. 2006;177(11):7772–83.
85. Fagarasan S, Kinoshita K, Muramatsu M, Ikuta K, Honjo T. In situ class switching and differentiation to IgA-producing cells in the gut lamina propria. Nature. 2001;413(6856):639–43.
86. Shang L, Fukata M, Thirunarayanan N, Martin AP, Arnaboldi P, Maussang D, et al. Toll-like receptor signaling in small intestinal epithelium promotes B-cell recruitment and IgA production in lamina propria. Gastroenterology. 2008;135(2):529–38.
87. Mora JR, von Andrian UH. Role of retinoic acid in the imprinting of gut-homing IgA-secreting cells. Semin Immunol. 2009;21(1):28–35.
88. Vinuesa CG, Sanz I, Cook MC. Dysregulation of germinal centres in autoimmune disease. Nat Rev Immunol. 2009;9(12):845–57.
89. Zucca E, Bertoni F. The spectrum of MALT lymphoma at different sites: biological and therapeutic relevance. Blood. 2016;127(17):2082–92.

90. Swerdlow SH, Campo E, Pileri SA, Harris NL, Stein H, Siebert R, Advani R, Ghielmini M, Salles GA, Zelenetz AD, Jaffe ES. The 2016 revision of the World Health Organization classification of lymphoid neoplasms. Blood. 2016;127:2375–90.
91. Bergman MP, D'Elios MM. Cytotoxic T cells in H. pylori-related gastric autoimmunity and gastric lymphoma. J Biomed Biotechnol. 2010;2010:104918. https://doi.org/10.1155/2010/104918.
92. Isaacson P, Wright DH. Malignant lymphoma of mucosa-associated lymphoid tissue. A distinctive type of B-cell lymphoma. Cancer. 1983;52(8):1410–6.
93. Wotherspoon AC, Ortiz-Hidalgo C, Falzon MR, Isaacson PG. Helicobacter pylori-associated gastritis and primary B-cell gastric lymphoma. Lancet. 1991;338(8776):1175–6.
94. Wotherspoon AC, Doglioni C, Diss TC, Pan L, Moschini A, de Boni M, Isaacson PG. Regression of primary low-grade-B-cell gastric lymphoma of mucosa-associated lymphoid tissue type after eradication of Helicobacter pylori. Lancet. 1993;342(8871):575–7.
95. Hussell T, Isaacson PG, Crabtree JE, Spencer J. The response of cells from low-grade B-cell gastric lymphomas of mucosa-associated lymphoid tissue to Helicobacter pylori. Lancet. 1993;342(8871):571–4.
96. Hussell T, Isaacson PG, Crabtree JE, Spencer J. Helicobacter pylori-specific tumour-infiltrating T cells provide contact dependent help for the growth of malignant B cells in low-grade gastric lymphoma of mucosa-associated lymphoid tissue. J Pathol. 1996;178(2):122–7.
97. Greiner A, Knörr C, Qin Y, Sebald W, Schimpl A, Banchereau J, Müller-Hermelink HK. Low-grade B cell lymphomas of mucosa-associated lymphoid tissue (MALT-type) require CD40-mediated signaling and Th2-type cytokines for in vitro growth and differentiation. Am J Pathol. 1997;150(5):1583–93.
98. D'Elios MM, Amedei A, Del Prete G. Impaired T-cell regulation of B-cell growth in Helicobacter pylori-related gastric low-grade MALT lymphoma. Gastroenterology. 1999;117(5):1105–12.
99. Munari F, Lonardi S, Cassatella MA, Doglioni C, de Bernard M, D'Elios MM, Vermi W. Tumor-associated macrophages as major source of APRIL in gastric MALT lymphoma. Blood. 2011;117:6612–6.
100. Munari F, Fassan M, Capitani N, Troilo A, Baldari CT, D'Elios MM, de Bernard M. Cytokine BAFF released by *Helicobacter pylori*-infected macrophages triggers the Th17 response in human chronic gastritis. J Immunol. 2014;193(11):5584–94.

CVID

3

Ulrich Salzer

3.1 Definition

Primary antibody deficiencies of unknown etiology are usually referred to as common variable immunodeficiency. Apart from the very heterogeneous and still mostly unclear genetic background the clinical term common variable immunodeficiency (CVID) covers patients with antibody deficiency syndromes of various etiology and diverse clinical as well as immunological features. Clinical hallmarks are hypogammaglobulinemia and severe and/or frequent, chronic-recurring bacterial infections especially affecting the respiratory tract. However additional immunological and clinical presentations are by far more diverse and—since CVID per se is not a monogenetically defined disorder—there is a high chance of missed or incorrect diagnosis, since the "clinical picture perfect CVID patient" rarely encounters us in real life. The previous diagnostic guidelines for CVID of the European and Pan-American Society for Immunodeficiencies [1] (ESID/PAGID, www.esid.org) therefore were revised in 2014 to include additional clinical and immunological criteria and are shown in Table 3.1. Especially the early identification and exclusion of patients with concomitant severe T-cell defect is very important, since these patients have a worse disease course and are in need of intensified treatment and follow-up strategies that differ from "plain" CVID [2, 3]. The definitions of the T-cell deficiency, however, probably still need refinement and should include also clinical criteria, e.g., like the occurrence of opportunistic infections [3].

U. Salzer (✉)
Faculty of Medicine, Department of Rheumatology and Clinical Immunology, Medical Center—University of Freiburg, Freiburg im Breisgau, Germany

Faculty of Medicine, Center for Chronic Immunodeficiency (CCI), Medical Center—University of Freiburg, Freiburg im Breisgau, Germany
e-mail: ulrich.salzer@uniklinik-freiburg.de

M. M. D'Elios, M. Rizzi (eds.), *Humoral Primary Immunodeficiencies*, Rare Diseases of the Immune System, https://doi.org/10.1007/978-3-319-91785-6_3

Table 3.1 Diagnostic criteria of CVID according to ESID (www.esid.org)

Clinical criteria for a probable diagnosis of CVID (= clinical diagnosis)	
At least one of the following:	• Increased susceptibility to infection • Autoimmune manifestations • Granulomatous disease • Unexplained polyclonal lymphoproliferation • Affected family member with antibody deficiency
AND	• Marked decrease of IgG and marked decrease of IgA with or without low IgM levels (measured at least twice; <2SD of the normal levels for their age)
AND at least one of the following:	• Poor antibody response to vaccines (and/or absent isohemagglutinins), i.e., absence of protective levels despite vaccination where defined • Low switched memory B cells (<70% of age-related normal value)
AND	• Secondary causes of hypogammaglobulinemia have been excluded (see Table 3.2)
AND	• Is established after the 4th year of life (but symptoms may be present before)
AND	• No evidence of profound T-cell deficiency, defined as 2 out of the following (y = year of life): • CD4 numbers/microliter: 2–6y <300, 6–12y <250, >12y <200 • % naïve CD4: 2–6y <25%, 6–16y <20%, >16y <10% • T-cell proliferation absent

It is nevertheless mandatory to search for differential diagnoses, e.g., hypogammaglobulinemia in context of other defined primary immunodeficiencies and secondary hypogammaglobulinemia caused by immunosuppression (see Table 3.2). Although the latter are usually revealed easily by the patient's clinical history, it may sometimes be more difficult since the final diagnosis of CVID may be preceded by diseases requiring anti-inflammatory or immunosuppressive treatment (e.g., autoimmune thrombocytopenia). In the case of long-term glucocorticoid therapy-induced hypogammaglobulinemia, a careful examination of immunoglobulin subtypes in serum is helpful in the differentiation from CVID [4].

CVID describes the largest group of symptomatic primary immunodeficiencies in adults with an estimated incidence in the western hemisphere between 1: 10,000 and 1: 50,000 [1, 5]. There are considerable regional or ethnic differences in the incidence, which is lower among Asians and African Americans [6–8]. Women and men are almost equally affected. The onset of the disease is usually the early adult age between 20 and 40 years, even though a second peak of onset in childhood can be recognized [6, 9, 10].

3.2 Etiology

The genetic basis of CVID and specific genetic defects associated with CVID-like phenotypes are described in more detail in Chap. 5 and the following chapters of this book. Still, for more than 80% of the CVID cases, no causal or associated

Table 3.2 Differential diagnosis of hypogammaglobulinemia

Secondary hypogammaglobulinemia	
Lymphoma	Chronic lymphatic leukemia (CLL)
	Immunodeficiency and thymoma (Good's syndrome)
	Other malignant non-Hodgkin lymphoma
Serum protein loss	Marked serum protein loss (renal, enteral)
	IgG hypercatabolism (e.g., proximal myotonic myopathy, PROMM)
Drug induced	Antiepileptic drugs (carbamazepine, phenytoin)
	Gold salts
	Glucocorticoids
	δ-Penicillamine
	Antimalarials
	Methotrexate
	Alkylating agents (e.g., cyclophosphamide)
Infections	Congenital with CMV, rubella, and *Toxoplasma gondii*; neonatal HIV infections
	Epstein-Barr virus infections
Primary immunodeficiencies with hypogammaglobulinemia	
	X-chromosomal agammaglobulinemia (BTK)
	Hyper-IgM syndromes (CD40, CD40L, AID, UNC)
	X-chromosomal lymphoproliferative syndrome (SAP, XIAP)
	DNA repair defects Ataxia telangiectasia Nijmegen breakage syndrome ICF (immunodeficiency, chromosomal instability, facial abnormalities) syndrome
	Autosomal recessive severe combined immunodeficiency (SCID), X-chromosomal SCID
	WHIM (warts, hypogammaglobulinemia, infections, myelokathexis) syndrome
	Selective IgA deficiency and IgG subclass deficiency
	DiGeorge syndrome
	Hemophagocytic lymphohistiocytosis

genetic alteration can be determined. The majority of cases diagnosed in Europe are sporadic. A positive family history is present in only about 15% of CVID cases [6, 7], of which more than two thirds show an autosomal dominant inheritance pattern. Variable penetrance and different expressiveness are reflected in families in which, besides affected individuals with CVID, selective IgA deficiency and intermediate forms of antibody deficiency are also present [11, 12]. Autosomal recessive familial cases are rare in Caucasians but appear more frequent in populations with increased consanguineous marriages [7, 13]. If the family pedigree suggests a possible X-chromosomal inheritance, one should consider, depending on the clinical presentation, X-linked agammaglobulinemia, X-linked lymphoproliferative syndrome and X-linked hyper IgM syndrome (see Table 3.2).

Genetic linkage analyses of large CVID/sIgAD families [14–16] revealed three different genetic loci on the chromosome 4q [16], chromosome 6 [14, 15], and chromosome 16q [17]. Candidate gene-oriented studies have previously identified several monogenetic defects or rare genetic polymorphisms associated with the clinical and immunological picture of CVID. These will be elaborated on in separate following chapters. Epigenetic changes including changes in DNA methylation and posttranscriptional gene regulation occur during immune cell differentiation. These and other nonheritable factors contribute much to the individual variability of the immune system [18], and disturbances of these processes are possible additional pathomechanisms contributing to the etiology of CVID. In addition to preexisting genetic susceptibility lesions, environmental factors may promote these epigenetic changes in immune cells that govern the outbreak of disease symptoms and course. The frequent late-onset and sporadic occurrence of CVID may support these basic approaches, but this is currently not well studied. So far only one monozygotic twin study in CVID investigated the epigenetic changes in lymphocyte subsets and found indeed significant changes of methylation patterns of several genes important in B-cell differentiation [19].

3.2.1 Immunopathology in CVID

Numerous phenotypic and functional studies of the immune system in patients with CVID demonstrated distinctive features both in the adaptive and inborn immune system. However, the large number of different manifestations, their different distribution within the CVID cohort, and the lack of controlled parallel studies of these disorders in large patient numbers make it impossible in most cases to generalize the observed immunopathology in distinct CVID subcohorts into an integrated picture of CVID as a whole. Nevertheless, based on the detected disturbances of T cells and B cells, different classification models of CVID have been proposed and applied [20–23]. In cases with severe disturbances of cellular immunity and opportunistic infections, a combined immune defect must be considered [see LOCID, Chap. 4]. In male CVID patients with B lymphocytes below 1%, BTK associated agammaglobulinemia may be suspected.

3.2.2 T-Cell Abnormalities in CVID

Disturbances of peripheral T-cell subset distribution and functions play an important role in the pathogenesis of individual CVID syndromes. Pathological changes affect both CD4+ and CD8+ T cells, as well as regulatory T cell populations. In up to 70% of CVID patients, there is a decrease in total CD4+ T-cell counts or at least the CD4+CD45RA+ naïve subpopulation [24–27]. In addition to reduced expression of activation markers and costimulatory molecules such as CD40L, L-selectin, and attractin [28–30], impaired secretion of cytokines such as IL-2, IL-4, IL-6, IL-7, IL-9, IL-10, IL-13, IL-17, and IFN-gamma is also reported [31–37]. Furthermore dysregulation of cytokine production, such as IFN-gamma secretion by follicular T helper cells skewed to TH1, may contribute to the impaired B-cell function [38, 39]. A potential cause of the functional defects may be defective T-cell receptor (TCR) signaling, which has been described in some CVID patients [40]. There is reduced recruitment of ZAP70 to the TCR, potentially caused by reduced Vav expression and "lipid raft" formation [41–43].

Several studies show that regulatory CD4+/CD25+/FoxP3+ T cells in CVID patients are significantly reduced [43–46]. This is clinically associated with autoimmunity, granulomas, splenomegaly, and specific changes in B-cell subpopulations (increased CD21 low B cells) [46].

CD8+ T cells are often chronically activated in subgroups of CVID patients and, in contrast to the CD4+ T cells, are partially expanded. This explains the inverted CD4/CD8 cell ratio commonly found in CVID patients. One study attributes the expansion of these predominantly CCR7 positive cytotoxic effector memory cells to increased IL-7 levels [47]. This expansion of CD8+/DR+ cells is associated with a loss of memory B cells and a more severe clinical progression [48]. However, chronic and recurrent infections with herpes viruses, in particular cytomegalovirus, may also promote the observed changes in CD8+ T cells [49, 50]. Finally, a subset of CVID patients show polyclonal expansions of "large granular lymphocytes" which is associated with increased CD8+ T-cell counts and splenomegaly [51].

These diverse disorders of the T-cell system are being unified in classification systems to compare these with other immunological parameters and the clinical features of the affected patients. Giovanetti et al. distinguished three subgroups of CVID patients by the extent of reduction of naïve CD4+/CD45RA+ [23]. Group I, with severely reduced naïve T-cell counts, demonstrated massive activation of T cells with a limited oligoclonal repertoire, splenomegaly, and a predominantly more severe clinical course. In addition, these patients had the most significant associated disturbances in the memory B-cell subpopulation. By in vitro studies and gene expression analysis on isolated T cells, each group was assigned a characteristic profile of cytokine production, T-cell turnover and susceptibility to apoptosis, as well as T-cell repertoire and gene expression [23, 52].

Distinct from these mostly phenotypic changes is clinically manifest T-cell deficiency. As shown by the French DEFI cohort study group, a subgroup of CVID patients suffers from a late-onset combined immunodeficiency (LOCID), which is referred to in Chap. 4. [2]. The inclusion criteria required CD4 T-cell counts below 200/μL or evidence of opportunistic infection, which was approximately 3.5% and 5.4% in the studied patient cohort. Importantly, the two subgroups showed only a small overlap (10%), suggesting that T-cell number reduction alone is not a good predictor of impaired T-cell function. The LOCID patients were more often born to consanguineous marriages, more often had granulomas, gastrointestinal disease, splenomegaly, and lymphomas. In summary, LOCID patients had more severe disease, had higher mortality, were hospitalized more frequently, and required more frequent antibiotic treatment [2, 3].

3.2.3 B-Cell Abnormalities in CVID

The total number of B cells in CVID patients is slightly reduced in about 50% of patients [22]. In some CVID patients, total B-cell counts are even increased, especially when patients suffer from increased polyclonal lymphoid infiltrates and autoimmunity [10]. About 10% of CVID patients have severely diminished or even absent B cells in peripheral blood [22]. They show a more progressive course of the disease and a worse prognosis [6, 53]. In these patients, hypomorphic and late-onset variants of agammaglobulinemias must be excluded (XLA and autosomal recessive agammaglobulinemias) [54, 55]. In addition, thymoma should be excluded if complete B-cell aplasia is present (Good syndrome, see Chap. 19). Also some of the patients with ICOS deficiency [56] (Chap. 6) and BAFF-R deficiency [57] (Chap. 11) belong to the group of patients with low B-cell counts. A subset of CVID patients shows an incomplete block of early B-cell development in the bone marrow at the pre-BI to pre-BII stage [58]. A subset of the studied bone marrow biopsies also showed nodular T-cell infiltrates which were more frequently observed in CVID patients with autoimmune cytopenias [58].

The major cellular phenotype correlating with the hypogammaglobulinemia in CVID affects terminal differentiation of B lymphocytes in blood, secondary lymphoid organs, and bone marrow. In consequence a vast majority of CVID patients has a significant reduction in circulating class-switched memory B cells and plasma blasts [22]. Although these changes are not specific to CVID, they have been now introduced as a secondary, optional diagnostic criterion and have been widely used to classify CVID. After exclusion of CVID patients with less than 1% circulating B cells, the original "Freiburg" classification relied on the surface markers CD19, IgM, IgD, and CD27 to first subdivide patients into two main groups (type I and type II) [20]. The group of type I patients, defined by having less than 0.4% of CD27+/IgM/IgD− class-switched memory B cells of total lymphocytes, encompasses about 75% of all CVID patients. By additionally staining of CD21, an atypical B-cell population (called CD21low B cells) can be differentiated, which expresses very low or no CD21. Thereby, type I patients are further subdivided into Ia (CD21low B cells >20%) and Ib (CD21low B cells <20%). About 25% of the CVID patients belong to the prognostically more favorable group II with more than 0.4% of class-switched memory B cells of total lymphocytes. The "Paris" classification also distinguishes three slightly different defined groups of CVID patients by analysis of IgD and CD27 [21]. MB2 refers to patients with normal numbers of CD27+ memory B cells. MB1 refers to patients with decreased class-switched (IgD−/CD27+) but normal non-class-switched memory B cells (IgD+/CD27+). Group MB0 includes patients with very few or no memory B cells at all. Both classification systems allow the heterogeneous CVID cohort to be grouped into more homogeneous groups that share clinical and immunological characteristics, e.g., those patients with splenomegaly or granuloma. In a perspective, the classification systems, if further refined, may allow the identification of predictive markers for disease progression [20, 21]. Indeed several follow-up studies have shown that the classification based on the memory B-cell subpopulations is useful for the identification of clinical subtypes of the disease, adaptation of therapeutic regimens, and the definition of certain disease risks [59–64].

In 2008, both classification systems were merged and validated within a European multicentric study creating the EUROclass classification which is extended by further parameters [22] like CD38 to allow the identification of transitional B cells and plasmablasts. In CVID patients and related antibody deficiency syndromes with very low or absent memory B cells, the functionally immature, transitional B cells accumulate over time [65] and are relatively abundant, e.g., also in BAFF-R deficiency [57].

The results of the EUROclass trial confirmed the clinical association of decreased memory B cells with increased risk of splenomegaly and granulomas [22]. The expansion of CD21low cells was correlated with splenomegaly and the expansion of transitional B cells with lymphadenopathy. There was no clear correlation between CD21low B cells and autoimmunity or autoimmune cytopenias in particular in the EUROclass trial.

The lack of class-switched memory B cells in CVID points toward a disturbance of the germinal center reaction as one major pathophysiological mechanism. Indeed, histological studies identify large and ill-defined germinal centers, correlating with the proportion of CD21low B cells [66]. This is further supported by the finding of significantly less somatic hypermutations (SHM) in CD27+ B cells in a large proportion of CVID patients compared to healthy subjects [67, 68]. Within the CVID cohort, patients with the lowest SHM rates developed chronic lung damage at higher rates [68] or noninfectious complications in general [69, 70]. The consecutive disturbed terminal differentiation of plasma cells in various tissues (intestine, lymph nodes, bone marrow) has been shown in several studies [58, 71, 72]. While the development up to the stage of centroblasts/centrocytes, as well as the sequential expression of BCL-6 and Blimp-1 are detectable in CVID patients' B cells, further development to antibody-secreting plasmablasts and plasma cells was blocked [72]. This differentiation defect could be demonstrated in vitro in most patients [72, 73]. Indeed, based on the replication history, studied by K-deleting recombination excision circles (KRECs) PCR, and on the amount of somatic hypermutation, the patients` defect can be functionally classified as being more likely a bone marrow, pre-germinal center, germinal center, and post-germinal center defect [74].

Beside defined genetic defects, several functional defects underlying the antibody deficiency have been described. Most of the functional defects regard signaling pathways important for B-cell activation. Hyperactivation of BCR signaling, manifested as constitutive phosphorylation of Syk and PLCgamma2, was described in CVID with noninfectious complications [75], and also constitutive activation of pErk was described in naïve and IgM+ memory cells of CVID patients [76]. NF-kB activation, defined by the IKB alpha degradation and p65 phosphorylation, and calcium signaling in response to BCR stimulation are impaired in CVID patients B cells and especially in CD21low B cells [77, 78]. CVID patients B cells have a lower expression of CD73 (ecto-5′-nucleotidase) and are therefore deficient in the hydrolysis of ATP to adenosine that promotes class-switch recombination in B cells [79]. In addition, the response to TLR stimulation is defective in B cells from CVID patients with a more severe course of disease [80, 81].

Cytokine secretion of B cells may also be disturbed in CVID patients as exemplified by the reduced the generation and function of IL-10 producing B cells which may contribute to the increased organ inflammation that is observed in some patient groups [82, 83].

In conclusion, CVID patients carry defects in the maturation, activation, cytokine secretion and signaling of B cells leading finally to a failure in the generation of antibody producing plasma cells.

3.2.4 Disturbances of Antigen-Presenting Cells in CVID

Dendritic cells and other professional antigen-presenting cells interact with naïve T cells in the T-cell areas of the secondary lymphoid organs. This interaction is part of the germinal center reaction, as these T cells cooperate with B cells to facilitate their further differentiation. In addition, plasmacytoid dendritic cells (pDCs) can directly induce Ig class switch and terminal differentiation of B cells outside of germinal centers via T-cell-independent signals via Toll-like receptors (TLR) and the cytokines BAFF/APRIL and their receptors [84, 85]. These two signaling pathways are closely linked, as exemplified at the level of TLR9 and the BAFF/APRIL receptor TACI [86–90].

Dendritic cells (DC) of CVID patients showed a maturation defect when cultured and differentiated in vitro, as evidenced by reduced IL-12 production and impaired upregulation of costimulatory molecules. This may limit the ability of DCs to interact successfully with T cells [91–93]. These in vitro results are supported by the findings of altered tissue distribution and diminished cell numbers of myeloid (mDC) and plasmacytoid dendritic cells (pDC) in CVID [94, 95]. The reduction in pDCs was most pronounced in CVID patients with low memory B-cell counts and granulomatous complications [94]. Low mDC numbers were instead associated with low memory B-cell counts and low overall B-cell counts. There was also a correlation with autoimmunity, splenomegaly, and granulomatous inflammation [95]. Finally, CVID patients also showed impaired in vitro activation of pDCs by CpG DNA. In addition TLR9 expression and response of B cells to CpG stimulation is diminished [96, 97]. The TLR-mediated signals play an important role in the B cells as the third signal of activation [98, 99] and may be involved as polyclonal stimulators supporting the longevity of B memory cells and antibody responses [100]. More recent reports confirmed the lower frequency of naturally occurring pDCs and mDCs but revealed normal responses in vitro to TLR7 or TLR9 agonists [101].

Beyond the dysfunction of TLR9, the TLR7 and TLR8 signaling pathway is also disturbed in CVID patients [102]. Upon stimulation with the TLR7/8 agonist loxoribine, CVID B cells showed significantly lower growth rates and poorly differentiated into class-switched antibody-producing cells in contrast to B cells from healthy individuals. These defects could be rescued by the addition of IFNa, while other TLR responses were normal [102]. Given the known direct connection between TACI and the TLR9 signaling pathway [86], one can assume that defects of the TLR system are of pathophysiological relevance in CVID patients, even if no causal relationship has yet been established (e.g., by detecting genetic mutations) [103].

3.2.5 Innate Immunity

Innate lymphoid cells (ILCs) are immune cells that belong to the lymphoid lineage but do not express antigen-specific receptors. These cells have important functions in innate immune responses to infectious microorganisms and in the regulation of homeostasis and inflammation. They are categorized in three main groups, ILC1, 2, and 3, defined by the expression of key transcription factors and the cytokines that they secrete. The role of ILCs in immune responses is complex as they may contribute both to promote and control inflammation depending on the context [104]. In addition, while in mouse models ILCs show potent immunological functions, the function of ILCs in humans appears to be highly redundant, if T and B cells are present and their function is preserved [105]. However, in case of defective B- or T-cell function, ILCs may become relevant, likewise in patients with CVID. There are conflicting reports as for the frequency and function of ILCs in CVID. Some studies report an increase of ILCs in patients with systemic inflammation [106], while others reported a decreased frequency and defective in vitro expansion of ILC2 and 3 in CVID patients [107]. Also invariant NK T cells (iNKT) seem to be reduced [108]. Further studies will be needed to interpret the clinical relevance of these findings.

3.3 Clinical Manifestations

3.3.1 Infections

CVID patients have an increased susceptibility of the mucous membranes of the respiratory tract and, to a lesser extent, of the gastrointestinal tract to infections by bacterial pathogens, especially encapsulated species [7]. Upper respiratory tract infections—sinusitis and bronchitis—occur in about two third, and more than half of patients had at least one pneumonia at the time of diagnosis. The disease manifestation and infection pattern is different in children and adults. Pediatric-onset CVID patients have more frequent diagnoses of otitis media, developmental delay, and failure to thrive compared with adult-onset CVID patients. Adult CVID patients are more frequently diagnosed with bronchitis, arthritis, depression, and fatigue [109]. As a consequence of the burden of infections, about one third of patients have already developed bronchiectasis. *Streptococcus pneumoniae*, *Haemophilus influenzae*, *Staphylococcus aureus*, and *Moraxella catarrhalis* are often isolated from patient' specimens. Chronic and difficult to treat diarrhea is frequent, but pathogens like *Giardia lamblia*, *Salmonella*, and *Campylobacter jejuni* may only be detectable in about half of these cases. Acute and chronic gastritis caused by *Helicobacter pylori* is also common in CVID patients [6]. Ten percent of CVID patients suffer from recurrent herpes zoster infections. Other viral infections like CMV infection are much rarer although they may be present in some patients [110]. Unusual bacterial and fungal infections are uncommon in CVID and usually are found as secondary complications (e.g., candidiasis after long-term antibiotic therapy or aspergillosis in patients with severe structural lung damage). Of importance, opportunistic infections do usually not belong to the clinical picture of CVID and rather point twoards combined immune deficiency, e.g., LOCID (see Chap. 4) [2, 3, 110].

3.3.2 Noninfectious Manifestations

3.3.2.1 Lung Disease in CVID

Chronic and recurrent infections are sometimes difficult to differentiate from and may even coexist together with inflammatory diseases of the respiratory and gastrointestinal tracts, which are also common in CVID. Up to 20% of CVID patients develop an interstitial, often granulomatous, lung disease. Usually no pathogen can be confirmed in these patients. Although a US study reported the detection of HHV8, this has not been confirmed in larger cohorts [111], and the cause remains unknown and presumably is multifactorial. This type of pulmonary involvement worsens the prognosis of affected CVID patients [112, 113]. The granulomatous lung disease is clinically similar to sarcoidosis in some aspects, and in addition to the lung, granulomas can be found in the lymph nodes but also in the skin, liver, upper and lower gastrointestinal tract, as well as central nervous system [114].

3.3.2.2 Gastrointestinal Disease in CVID

Gastrointestinal complaints are frequent in patients with CVID, but often nonspecific [115]. Diarrhea is a frequent symptom, and a celiac disease-like presentation is common, but also chronic inflammatory bowel involvement may be present. Celiac disease-like villous atrophy is generally not gluten-sensitive in CVID and, in some cases, is more likely to be a distinct autoimmune enteropathy. This is underscored by a distinct immune profile and a lack of association with celiac disease HLA risk haplotypes [115, 116]. The involvement of the colon in CVID, although similar to Crohn's disease and ulcerative colitis clinically, is also a histologically distinct entity [117, 118]. Severe forms of these gastrointestinal disorders are associated with malabsorption. In contrast, nodular lymphatic hyperplasia (NLH), occurring both in the duodenum and the ileum, is often asymptomatic [6, 117]. Chronic liver disease and abnormal liver function tests in the blood are found in 10% of CVID patients [6, 119]. The most common hepatopathy associated with CVID is nodular regenerative hyperplasia (NRH) of the liver tissue [119–121] present at a frequency of about 5% [120]. Although liver function is still preserved, portal hypertension is frequent [121], and a substantial part of affected patients develops an autoimmune hepatitis-like disease with infiltration of T cells [120]. There is also an association with lymphoproliferation, granulomas, lymphocytic enteropathies, and other autoimmune manifestations [119, 121], indicating that the presence of NRH may be another "red flag" that identifies CVID patients at higher risk for disease-associated morbidity and mortality [120].

3.3.2.3 Autoimmunity

Autoimmune manifestations occur in about a third of CVID patients and sometimes precede the manifestation of infection susceptibility but may occur at any time of the disease course [6, 22, 122]. Autoimmune thrombocytopenia (approximately 10–12%) and autoimmune hemolytic anemia (approximately 5–7%) are particularly common. There is a significant association with splenomegaly [22, 123]. Autoimmune neutropenia is less common (1–3%), but often associated with other cytopenias and a more severe form of disease [124]. Autoimmune cytopenias including autoimmune neutropenia are linked to pathological lymphocyte phenotypes, like elevated proportions of CD21low B cells [124, 125], and cluster with other noninfectious complications [22, 124, 125]. Autoimmune thyroid disease, vitiligo, pernicious anemia, psoriasis, rheumatoid arthritis, and SLE are seen at decreasing frequencies in CVID patients [6, 22, 10]. In contrast to CVID patients suffering from infections only, patients with autoimmune or other complications have increased morbidity and decreased life span [53, 122, 125, 126]. Immunologically, autoimmune cytopenias are associated with low numbers of class-switched memory B cells and regulatory T cells, an expansion of CD21low B cells [20, 127], and diffuse and nodular T-cell infiltration of the bone marrow [58]. In addition, those CVID patients with a concomitant T-cell deficiency, characterized by reduced naïve T-cell numbers and T-cell repertoire, are prone to develop autoimmune manifestations [125, 128]. The underlying causes and pathophysiology of autoimmunity in CVID are poorly understood. At the immunological level, both defects in central and peripheral tolerance have been described. Genetically defined immune dysregulatory syndromes may mimic a CVID-like phenotype and therefore must be carefully ruled out as differential diagnosis in these patients [129–132]. Genetic risk factors include mutations in TNFRSF13B/TACI ([133–136] and see Chap. 9). Monogenetic traits with high incidence of autoimmunity include CTLA4 and LRBA deficiency ([137–141] and see Chaps. 5 and 10).

3.3.2.4 Lymphoproliferation

About 50% of patients have splenomegaly, and about 10–20% show local or diffuse lymphadenopathy as signs of benign lymphoproliferation [22, 10]. Follicular lymphatic hyperplasia is equally common. Upon histopathological examination in some patients, follicular hyperplasia is found and granulomatous inflammation in others.

3.3.2.5 Cancer

As with many primary immunodeficiencies, the incidence of cancer is higher in CVID. Several factors contribute to this susceptibility, apart from insufficient targeting and elimination of malignant cells by an insufficient immune system. This includes increased radiosensitivity [12, 142], increased primarily benign lymphoproliferation, and decreased defense against tumor-promoting pathogens like Epstein-Barr virus. Thus there is an increased risk of developing lymphomas [6, 10, 143], most of which are B-NHL type [6]. Gastric carcinomas are a second common malignant manifestation and may be associated with *Helicobacter pylori* infections and pernicious anemia [6, 10, 122, 144, 145].

3.4 Diagnosis

CVID defines—as a clinical diagnosis of exclusion—a very heterogeneous antibody deficiency syndrome. The low incidence and high clinical variability still cause significant delay in the diagnosis between 4 [146] and 9 years [122] from the onset of the first symptoms. The diagnostic delay also varies considerably between different European countries and is larger in patients with early-onset disease [9]. Clinically, most patients have the classic susceptibility to infection by encapsulated bacteria as described above. Opportunistic, fungal and severe viral infections are uncommon. A significant part of CVID patients initially manifests with autoimmune cytopenias. Therefore, CVID should be excluded by checking immunoglobulin serum concentrations in patients with autoimmune cytopenias, especially in the presence of splenomegaly. Although hypogammaglobulinemia and bacterial infections are rare in typical autoimmune lymphoproliferative syndrome (ALPS), one should take it into consideration as differential diagnosis in patients presenting with the triad of autoimmune cytopenias, splenomegaly/lymphadenopathy, and hypogammaglobulinemia. A combined usage of ALPS biomarkers is helpful to make a distinction between these two disorders [132, 147].

The first step toward diagnosis of CVID is the quantitative determination of serum immunoglobulins, which is a widely available and inexpensive test. Occasionally, CVID is diagnosed by chance if the determination of immunoglobulins is made in a different context, but it is a valuable screening tool for the targeted examination of family members of CVID patients.

The novel diagnostic criteria of CVID are summarized in Table 3.1. Mandatory for the diagnosis of CVID is the reduction of at least two isotypes (IgG and IgA or IgM). IgG is usually below 5 g/L (reference range 7–16 g/L), and IgA is significantly reduced or undetectable in most patients. IgM is also below reference in up to 80% of patients. The diagnosis of CVID can only be made after a number of other causes of hypogammaglobulinemia have been ruled out (see Table 3.2). These include drug-induced hypogammaglobulinemia as well as other genetically defined primary immunodeficiencies with hypogammaglobulinemia. The differential diagnosis of other genetically defined immunodeficiencies should be made in a specialized center. To exclude renal or gastrointestinal protein loss, qualitative and quantitative examination of urine and serum proteins is usually helpful. A difficult differential diagnosis is lymphoma with secondary hypogammaglobulinemia, since CVID patients often present with benign lymphoproliferation and may only be differentiated histologically by lymph node biopsy and bone marrow aspiration from genuine lymphoma patients.

In addition to the quantitative determination of serum immunoglobulins, basic laboratory tests at diagnosis should include differential blood counts, liver and kidney function parameters, and CRP. In a second step, this is complemented by the determination of specific antibodies such as isohemagglutinins and vaccine antibodies against protein antigens (tetanus, diphtheria, and in vaccinated patients also HBV, HAV) and antibodies against pneumococcal capsule polysaccharides. The results of these investigations are particularly meaningful if the patient has been vaccinated for diagnostic purposes before starting immunoglobulin substitution, but this should only be performed if the clinical condition of the patient allows a delay of the necessary immunoglobulin therapy by 4 weeks.

The next level of diagnostic testing is the flow cytometric analysis of lymphocyte subpopulations. These should include absolute numbers of total CD3+ T cells, CD4+ and CD8+ T-cell subsets, as well as B and NK cells. This helps to delineate late-onset agammaglobulinemias and combined immunodeficiencies with CD4+ T-cell counts below 200/μL. The assessment of B-cell subpopulations now serves as optional diagnostic criteria and may be used for classification of the disease. Bone marrow aspiration is indicated if lymphoma is suspected or to rule-out non autoimmune cytopenias. In younger patients with very low B-cell counts [58], the detection of abnormalities in early B-cell precursor development may guide a diagnosis towards agammaglobulinemia and related disorders.

Genetic testing is currently reserved for the exclusion of other primary immunodeficiencies, familial cases, and patients with a strong clinical and immunological suspicion for an underlying known genetic defect. However there is no general recommendation to test for the known gene defects or even search for unknown genetic causes in every CVID patient in the routine setting. A full genetic work-up may however be useful, if the disease progresses in spite of therapy and stem cell transplantation is envisaged.

For therapy planning, monitoring, and prognosis, the recording and follow-up of clinical manifestations are very important. The complete infectious history should include the type, duration, and frequency of individual infections. Not only the frequency of infections but also the severity, the development of complications (e.g., empyema, bronchiectasis), and the inadequate response to therapy may indicate the need for a change or reinforcement of the therapeutic regimen. Direct detection of pathogens by PCR or culture is necessary to detect specific pathogens, install targeted antibiotic treatment, and avoid the development of antibiotic resistance.

In general, pathogen detection should always be done directly (e.g., by microbial culture, PCR, antigen ELISA), since serological results are not safe to use in CVID patients. In the case of cytopenia, lymphoproliferation, or hepatitis, infections with EBV or CMV should be excluded by PCR.

Further diagnostic measures cover the examination of organ systems that are significantly affected in CVID. The initial and annual lung function tests are used to record and control for secondary, especially interstitial lung changes. If there is a suspicion of such changes, a high-resolution CT scan of the lungs has to be performed. Clinical or pulmonary function tests are unreliable indicators of progression of granulomatous involvement and bronchiectasis; follow-up CTs of the lungs should be done every 2–3 years in affected patients.

X-ray, CT, and ultrasound imaging are used to monitor lymphoproliferation. Initially, and depending on findings and individual complaints, a gastroscopy should be performed to exclude *Helicobacter pylori* infection, nodular lymphoid hyperplasia (NLH), celiac-like disease, *Giardia lamblia* colonization of the duodenum, and mucosa-associated lymphoid tissue (MALT) lymphoma. In case of lower gastrointestinal tract complaints and inconspicuous findings in gastroscopy, colonoscopy should be performed.

3.5 Management

Therapeutic management consists of the following: (1) continuous replacement therapy with immunoglobulins, (2) targeted antibiotic treatment of (breakthrough) infections, (3) adequate therapy of complications, and (4) allogenic peripheral stem cell transplantation is considered today in patients with severe hematological changes (chronic transfusion-dependent anemia, leukopenia, thrombocytopenia), malignancies, and overall prognostically poor outcome despite adequate immunoglobulin substitution [148, 149].

Immunoglobulin replacement therapy is the pillar of therapy in 90% of CVID patients [150, 151]. It can be administered either monthly intravenously or weekly subcutaneously. The intramuscular administration of immunoglobulins for substitution purposes is obsolete, as effective levels are not achieved due to the limited administrable dose. The subcutaneous form of therapy has been introduced in the Scandinavian countries and is widely available in Europe since the end of the 1990s [152, 153] and is now used by roughly 50% of patients [150]. Typical current dosage ranges are 400–600 mg/kg administered intravenously every 3–4 weeks. When subcutaneous administration is chosen, this corresponds to 100–150 mg/kg/week. The goal of therapy is of the control of infections. This is usually achieved with individually different IgG trough levels. In general the IgG trough level should be above 7 g/L before the next infusion. Patients with existing chronic lung disease (e.g., bronchiectasis) or increased protein loss/increased Ig catabolism usually require higher Ig doses to reach this target levels. Individual trough levels of up to 10–12 g/L may be necessary in some patients to achieve adequate protection from infection. In case of chronic sinusitis, however, this can often only be achieved in combination with thorough local therapy (saline rinsing, expectorant, and mucosal decongestant therapy).

Treatment of secondary complications should be planned in collaboration with specialized immunodeficiency centers. Autoimmune cytopenia is primarily treated with steroids; second line are other immunosuppressants (e.g., cyclosprin A) and biologicals including rituximab. The decision for splenectomy must be carefully considered because of the additional infection risk this imposes on the patient. Granulomatous manifestations affecting the lungs, liver, and intestine respond only insufficiently to immunoglobulin substitution therapy and often require additional immunosuppressive therapy.

The results of allogeneic hematopoetic stem cell transplantation (HSCT) have been first reported in four patients. In two cases, the indication was secondary hematological complications. Of the three long-term survivors, two continued to be dependent on regular immunoglobulin substitution [148]. In a second multicenter study describing the outcome of HSCT in 25 CVID patients between 8 and 50 years of age at the time of transplantation, the overall survival rate was 48%, and the survival rate for patients undergoing transplantation for lymphoma was 83%. The major causes of death were treatment-refractory graft-versus-host disease accompanied by poor immune reconstitution and infectious complications. Immunoglobulin substitution was stopped in 50% of surviving patients. In 92% of surviving patients, the decisive condition for HSCT was resolved [149]. This multicenter study demonstrated that HSCT in patients with CVID was beneficial in most surviving patients; however, there was a high mortality associated with the procedure. Therefore further studies will be needed to assess patient selection, time point of transplantation, and conditioning regimen, thereby improving outcome.

Life expectancy [10, 122] has greatly improved compared to older studies and is now well over 50 years [6]. However, especially patients with additional complications still show increased morbidity and mortality [10]. Reduced survival is associated with age at diagnosis, lower baseline IgG, higher IgM, and low peripheral B cells. The risk of death is 11 times higher for patients with noninfectious complications (hazard ratio = 10.95; $P < 0.0001$). Mortality is associated with lymphoma, any form of hepatitis, functional or structural lung impairment, and gastrointestinal disease with or without malabsorption, but not with bronchiectasis, autoimmunity, other cancers, granulomatous disease, or previous splenectomy [53].

References

1. Conley ME, Notarangelo LD, Etzioni A. Diagnostic criteria for primary immunodeficiencies. Representing PAGID (Pan-American Group for Immunodeficiency) and ESID (European Society for Immunodeficiencies). Clin Immunol. 1999;93(3):190–7.
2. Malphettes M, et al. Late-onset combined immune deficiency: a subset of common variable immunodeficiency with severe T cell defect. Clin Infect Dis. 2009;49(9):1329–38.
3. Bertinchamp R, et al. Exclusion of patients with a severe T-cell defect improves the definition of common variable immunodeficiency. J Allergy Clin Immunol Pract. 2016;4(6):1147–57.
4. Wirsum C, et al. Secondary antibody deficiency in glucocorticoid therapy clearly differs from primary antibody deficiency. J Clin Immunol. 2016;36(4):406–12.
5. Bonilla FA, et al. Practice parameter for the diagnosis and management of primary immunodeficiency. Ann Allergy Asthma Immunol. 2005;94(5 Suppl 1):S1–63.
6. Cunningham-Rundles C, Bodian C. Common variable immunodeficiency: clinical and immunological features of 248 patients. Clin Immunol. 1999;92(1):34–48.
7. Oksenhendler E, et al. Infections in 252 patients with common variable immunodeficiency. Clin Infect Dis. 2008;46(10):1547–54.
8. Tseng CW, et al. The incidence and prevalence of common variable immunodeficiency disease in Taiwan, a population-based study. PLoS One. 2015;10(10):e0140473.
9. Gathmann B, et al. Clinical picture and treatment of 2212 patients with common variable immunodeficiency. J Allergy Clin Immunol. 2014;134(1):116–26.
10. Chapel H, et al. Common variable immunodeficiency disorders: division into distinct clinical phenotypes. Blood. 2008;112(2):277–86.
11. Vorechovsky I, et al. Family and linkage study of selective IgA deficiency and common variable immunodeficiency. Clin Immunol Immunopathol. 1995;77(2):185–92.
12. Aghamohammadi A, et al. Progression of selective IgA deficiency to common variable immunodeficiency. Int Arch Allergy Immunol. 2008;147(2):87–92.
13. Aghamohammadi A, et al. Clinical and immunological features of 65 Iranian patients with common variable immunodeficiency. Clin Diagn Lab Immunol. 2005;12(7):825–32.
14. Schroeder HW Jr, et al. Susceptibility locus for IgA deficiency and common variable immunodeficiency in the HLA-DR3, -B8, -A1 haplotypes. Mol Med. 1998;4(2):72–86.
15. Kralovicova J, et al. Fine-scale mapping at IGAD1 and genome-wide genetic linkage analysis implicate HLA-DQ/DR as a major susceptibility locus in selective IgA deficiency and common variable immunodeficiency. J Immunol. 2003;170(5):2765–75.

16. Finck A, et al. Linkage of autosomal-dominant common variable immunodeficiency to chromosome 4q. Eur J Hum Genet. 2006;14(7):867–75.
17. Schaffer AA, et al. Analysis of families with common variable immunodeficiency (CVID) and IgA deficiency suggests linkage of CVID to chromosome 16q. Hum Genet. 2006;118(6):725–9.
18. Brodin P, et al. Variation in the human immune system is largely driven by non-heritable influences. Cell. 2015;160(1–2):37–47.
19. Rodriguez-Cortez VC, et al. Monozygotic twins discordant for common variable immunodeficiency reveal impaired DNA demethylation during naive-to-memory B-cell transition. Nat Commun. 2015;6:7335.
20. Warnatz K, et al. Severe deficiency of switched memory B cells (CD27(+)IgM(−)IgD(−)) in subgroups of patients with common variable immunodeficiency: a new approach to classify a heterogeneous disease. Blood. 2002;99(5):1544–51.
21. Piqueras B, et al. Common variable immunodeficiency patient classification based on impaired B cell memory differentiation correlates with clinical aspects. J Clin Immunol. 2003;23(5):385–400.
22. Wehr C, et al. The EUROclass trial: defining subgroups in common variable immunodeficiency. Blood. 2008;111(1):77–85.
23. Giovannetti A, et al. Unravelling the complexity of T cell abnormalities in common variable immunodeficiency. J Immunol. 2007;178(6):3932–43.
24. De Vera MJ, Al-Harthi L, Gewurz AT. Assessing thymopoiesis in patients with common variable immunodeficiency as measured by T-cell receptor excision circles. Ann Allergy Asthma Immunol. 2004;93(5):478–84.
25. Isgro A, et al. Bone marrow clonogenic capability, cytokine production, and thymic output in patients with common variable immunodeficiency. J Immunol. 2005;174(8):5074–81.
26. Goldacker S, Warnatz K. Tackling the heterogeneity of CVID. Curr Opin Allergy Clin Immunol. 2005;5(6):504–9.
27. Stuchly J, et al. Common variable immunodeficiency patients with a phenotypic profile of immunosenescence present with thrombocytopenia. Sci Rep. 2017;7:39710.
28. Farrington M, et al. CD40 ligand expression is defective in a subset of patients with common variable immunodeficiency. Proc Natl Acad Sci U S A. 1994;91(3):1099–103.
29. Nordoy I, et al. Adhesion molecules in common variable immunodeficiency (CVID)--a decrease in L-selectin-positive T lymphocytes. Clin Exp Immunol. 1998;114(2):258–63.
30. Pozzi N, et al. Defective surface expression of attractin on T cells in patients with common variable immunodeficiency (CVID). Clin Exp Immunol. 2001;123(1):99–104.
31. Ferrer JM, et al. Alterations in interleukin secretion (IL-2 and IL-4) by CD4 and CD4 CD45RO cells from common variable immunodeficiency (CVI) patients. Clin Exp Immunol. 1995;102(2):286–9.
32. Fischer MB, et al. Defective interleukin-2 and interferon-gamma gene expression in response to antigen in a subgroup of patients with common variable immunodeficiency. J Allergy Clin Immunol. 1993;92(2):340–52.
33. Holm AM, et al. Impaired secretion of IL-10 by T cells from patients with common variable immunodeficiency—involvement of protein kinase A type I. J Immunol. 2003;170(11):5772–7.
34. Holm AM, et al. Abnormal interleukin-7 function in common variable immunodeficiency. Blood. 2005;105(7):2887–90.
35. North ME, Webster AD, Farrant J. Role of interleukin-2 and interleukin-6 in the mitogen responsiveness of T cells from patients with 'common-variable' hypogammaglobulinaemia. Clin Exp Immunol. 1990;81(3):412–6.
36. Taraldsrud E, et al. Defective IL-4 signaling in T cells defines severe common variable immunodeficiency. J Autoimmun. 2017;81:110–9.
37. Berron-Ruiz L, et al. Impaired selective cytokine production by CD4(+) T cells in common variable immunodeficiency associated with the absence of memory B cells. Clin Immunol. 2016;166–167:19–26.

38. Unger S, et al. The T_H1 phenotype of follicular helper T cells indicates an IFN-gamma-associated immune dysregulation in patients with CD21low common variable immunodeficiency. J Allergy Clin Immunol. 2018;141(2):730–40.
39. Cunill V, et al. Follicular T cells from smB(−) common variable immunodeficiency patients are skewed toward a Th1 phenotype. Front Immunol. 2017;8:174.
40. Fischer MB, et al. A defect in the early phase of T-cell receptor-mediated T-cell activation in patients with common variable immunodeficiency. Blood. 1994;84(12):4234–41.
41. Boncristiano M, et al. Defective recruitment and activation of ZAP-70 in common variable immunodeficiency patients with T cell defects. Eur J Immunol. 2000;30(9):2632–8.
42. Paccani SR, et al. Defective Vav expression and impaired F-actin reorganization in a subset of patients with common variable immunodeficiency characterized by T-cell defects. Blood. 2005;106(2):626–34.
43. Arumugakani G, Wood PM, Carter CR. Frequency of Treg cells is reduced in CVID patients with autoimmunity and splenomegaly and is associated with expanded CD21lo B lymphocytes. J Clin Immunol. 2010;30(2):292–300.
44. Horn J, et al. Decrease in phenotypic regulatory T cells in subsets of patients with common variable immunodeficiency. Clin Exp Immunol. 2009;156(3):446–54.
45. Melo KM, et al. A decreased frequency of regulatory T cells in patients with common variable immunodeficiency. PLoS One. 2009;4(7):e6269.
46. Yu GP, et al. Regulatory T cell dysfunction in subjects with common variable immunodeficiency complicated by autoimmune disease. Clin Immunol. 2009;131(2):240–53.
47. Holm AM, et al. Gene expression analysis of peripheral T cells in a subgroup of common variable immunodeficiency shows predominance of CCR7(−) effector-memory T cells. Clin Exp Immunol. 2004;138(2):278–89.
48. Viallard JF, et al. CD8+HLA-DR+ T lymphocytes are increased in common variable immunodeficiency patients with impaired memory B-cell differentiation. Clin Immunol. 2006;119(1):51–8.
49. Raeiszadeh M, et al. The T cell response to persistent herpes virus infections in common variable immunodeficiency. Clin Exp Immunol. 2006;146(2):234–42.
50. Kuntz M, et al. Analysis of bulk and virus-specific CD8+ T cells reveals advanced differentiation of CD8+ T cells in patients with common variable immunodeficiency. Clin Immunol. 2011;141(2):177–86.
51. Holm AM, et al. Polyclonal expansion of large granular lymphocytes in common variable immunodeficiency—association with neutropenia. Clin Exp Immunol. 2006;144(3):418–24.
52. Wong GK, et al. Accelerated loss of TCR repertoire diversity in common variable immunodeficiency. J Immunol. 2016;197(5):1642–9.
53. Resnick ES, et al. Morbidity and mortality in common variable immune deficiency over 4 decades. Blood. 2012;119(7):1650–7.
54. Weston SA, et al. Assessment of male CVID patients for mutations in the Btk gene: how many have been misdiagnosed? Clin Exp Immunol. 2001;124(3):465–9.
55. Gaspar HB, Conley ME. Early B cell defects. Clin Exp Immunol. 2000;119(3):383–9.
56. Warnatz K, et al. Human ICOS deficiency abrogates the germinal center reaction and provides a monogenic model for common variable immunodeficiency. Blood. 2006;107(8):3045–52.
57. Warnatz K, et al. B-cell activating factor receptor deficiency is associated with an adult-onset antibody deficiency syndrome in humans. Proc Natl Acad Sci U S A. 2009;106(33):13945–50.
58. Ochtrop ML, et al. T and B lymphocyte abnormalities in bone marrow biopsies of common variable immunodeficiency. Blood. 2011;118(2):309–18.
59. Alachkar H, et al. Memory switched B cell percentage and not serum immunoglobulin concentration is associated with clinical complications in children and adults with specific antibody deficiency and common variable immunodeficiency. Clin Immunol. 2006;120(3):310–8.
60. Detkova D, et al. Common variable immunodeficiency: association between memory B cells and lung diseases. Chest. 2007;131(6):1883–9.
61. Ko J, Radigan L, Cunningham-Rundles C. Immune competence and switched memory B cells in common variable immunodeficiency. Clin Immunol. 2005;116(1):37–41.

62. Vodjgani M, et al. Analysis of class-switched memory B cells in patients with common variable immunodeficiency and its clinical implications. J Investig Allergol Clin Immunol. 2007;17(5):321–8.
63. Berglund LJ, Wong SW, Fulcher DA. B-cell maturation defects in common variable immunodeficiency and association with clinical features. Pathology. 2008;40(3):288–94.
64. Sanchez-Ramon S, et al. Memory B cells in common variable immunodeficiency: clinical associations and sex differences. Clin Immunol. 2008;128(3):314–21.
65. Cuss AK, et al. Expansion of functionally immature transitional B cells is associated with human-immunodeficient states characterized by impaired humoral immunity. J Immunol. 2006;176(3):1506–16.
66. Unger S, et al. Ill-defined germinal centers and severely reduced plasma cells are histological hallmarks of lymphadenopathy in patients with common variable immunodeficiency. J Clin Immunol. 2014;34(6):615–26.
67. Bonhomme D, et al. Impaired antibody affinity maturation process characterizes a subset of patients with common variable immunodeficiency. J Immunol. 2000;165(8):4725–30.
68. Andersen P, et al. Deficiency of somatic hypermutation of the antibody light chain is associated with increased frequency of severe respiratory tract infection in common variable immunodeficiency. Blood. 2005;105(2):511–7.
69. Almejun MB, et al. Noninfectious complications in patients with pediatric-onset common variable immunodeficiency correlated with defects in somatic hypermutation but not in class-switch recombination. J Allergy Clin Immunol. 2017;139(3):913–22.
70. Almejun MB, Borge M. Somatic hypermutation defects in common variable immune deficiency. Curr Allergy Asthma Rep. 2017;17(11):76.
71. Herbst EW, et al. Intestinal B cell defects in common variable immunodeficiency. Clin Exp Immunol. 1994;95(2):215–21.
72. Taubenheim N, et al. Defined blocks in terminal plasma cell differentiation of common variable immunodeficiency patients. J Immunol. 2005;175(8):5498–503.
73. Bryant A, et al. Classification of patients with common variable immunodeficiency by B cell secretion of IgM and IgG in response to anti-IgM and interleukin-2. Clin Immunol Immunopathol. 1990;56(2):239–48.
74. Driessen GJ, et al. B-cell replication history and somatic hypermutation status identify distinct pathophysiologic backgrounds in common variable immunodeficiency. Blood. 2011;118(26):6814–23.
75. Taraldsrud E, et al. Patterns of constitutively phosphorylated kinases in B cells are associated with disease severity in common variable immunodeficiency. Clin Immunol. 2017;175:69–74.
76. Visentini M, et al. Dysregulated extracellular signal-regulated kinase signaling associated with impaired B-cell receptor endocytosis in patients with common variable immunodeficiency. J Allergy Clin Immunol. 2014;134(2):401–10.
77. Keller B, et al. Disturbed canonical nuclear factor of kappa light chain signaling in B cells of patients with common variable immunodeficiency. J Allergy Clin Immunol. 2017;139(1):220–31. e8
78. van de Ven AA, et al. Defective calcium signaling and disrupted CD20-B-cell receptor dissociation in patients with common variable immunodeficiency disorders. J Allergy Clin Immunol. 2012;129(3):755–61. e7
79. Schena F, et al. Dependence of immunoglobulin class switch recombination in B cells on vesicular release of ATP and CD73 ectonucleotidase activity. Cell Rep. 2013;3(6):1824–31.
80. Yu JE, et al. TLR-mediated B cell defects and IFN-alpha in common variable immunodeficiency. J Clin Immunol. 2012;32(1):50–60.
81. Clemente A, et al. B cells from common variable immunodeficiency patients fail to differentiate to antibody secreting cells in response to TLR9 ligand (CpG-ODN) or anti-CD40+IL21. Cell Immunol. 2011;268(1):9–15.
82. Barsotti NS, et al. IL-10-producing regulatory B cells are decreased in patients with common variable immunodeficiency. PLoS One. 2016;11(3):e0151761.

83. Kofod-Olsen E, et al. Altered fraction of regulatory B and T cells is correlated with autoimmune phenomena and splenomegaly in patients with CVID. Clin Immunol. 2016;162:49–57.
84. Litinsky I, et al. Sarcoidosis: TB or not TB? Ann Rheum Dis. 2002;61(5):385–6.
85. Poeck H, et al. Plasmacytoid dendritic cells, antigen, and CpG-C license human B cells for plasma cell differentiation and immunoglobulin production in the absence of T-cell help. Blood. 2004;103(8):3058–64.
86. He B, et al. The transmembrane activator TACI triggers immunoglobulin class switching by activating B cells through the adaptor MyD88. Nat Immunol. 2010;11(9):836–45.
87. Ozcan E, et al. Transmembrane activator, calcium modulator, and cyclophilin ligand interactor drives plasma cell differentiation in LPS-activated B cells. J Allergy Clin Immunol. 2009;123(6):1277–86.e5.
88. Groom JR, et al. BAFF and MyD88 signals promote a lupuslike disease independent of T cells. J Exp Med. 2007;204(8):1959–71.
89. Treml LS, et al. TLR stimulation modifies BLyS receptor expression in follicular and marginal zone B cells. J Immunol. 2007;178(12):7531–9.
90. Ng LG, et al. BAFF costimulation of Toll-like receptor-activated B-1 cells. Eur J Immunol. 2006;36(7):1837–46.
91. Bayry J, et al. Common variable immunodeficiency is associated with defective functions of dendritic cells. Blood. 2004;104(8):2441–3.
92. Cunningham-Rundles C, Radigan L. Deficient IL-12 and dendritic cell function in common variable immune deficiency. Clin Immunol. 2005;115(2):147–53.
93. Scott-Taylor TH, et al. Monocyte derived dendritic cell responses in common variable immunodeficiency. Clin Exp Immunol. 2004;138(3):484–90.
94. Viallard JF, et al. Altered dendritic cell distribution in patients with common variable immunodeficiency. Arthritis Res Ther. 2005;7(5):R1052–5.
95. Yong PF, et al. Selective deficits in blood dendritic cell subsets in common variable immunodeficiency and X-linked agammaglobulinaemia but not specific polysaccharide antibody deficiency. Clin Immunol. 2008;127(1):34–42.
96. Cunningham-Rundles C, et al. TLR9 activation is defective in common variable immune deficiency. J Immunol. 2006;176(3):1978–87.
97. Marron TU, Yu JE, Cunningham-Rundles C. Toll-like receptor function in primary B cell defects. Front Biosci (Elite Ed). 2012;4:1853–63.
98. Lanzavecchia A, et al. Understanding and making use of human memory B cells. Immunol Rev. 2006;211:303–9.
99. Ruprecht CR, Lanzavecchia A. Toll-like receptor stimulation as a third signal required for activation of human naive B cells. Eur J Immunol. 2006;36(4):810–6.
100. Bernasconi NL, Traggiai E, Lanzavecchia A. Maintenance of serological memory by polyclonal activation of human memory B cells. Science. 2002;298(5601):2199–202.
101. Taraldsrud E, et al. Common variable immunodeficiency revisited: normal generation of naturally occurring dendritic cells that respond to Toll-like receptors 7 and 9. Clin Exp Immunol. 2014;175(3):439–48.
102. Yu JE, et al. Toll-like receptor 7 and 9 defects in common variable immunodeficiency. J Allergy Clin Immunol. 2009;124(2):349–56, 356.e1–3.
103. van de Ven AA, et al. B-cell defects in common variable immunodeficiency: BCR signaling, protein clustering and hardwired gene mutations. Crit Rev Immunol. 2011;31(2):85–98.
104. Ebbo M, et al. Innate lymphoid cells: major players in inflammatory diseases. Nat Rev Immunol. 2017;17(11):665–78.
105. Vely F, et al. Evidence of innate lymphoid cell redundancy in humans. Nat Immunol. 2016;17(11):1291–9.
106. Cols M, et al. Expansion of inflammatory innate lymphoid cells in patients with common variable immune deficiency. J Allergy Clin Immunol. 2016;137(4):1206–15. e6
107. Geier CB, et al. Reduced numbers of circulating group 2 innate lymphoid cells in patients with common variable immunodeficiency. Eur J Immunol. 2017;47(11):1959–69.

108. Gao Y, et al. Common variable immunodeficiency is associated with a functional deficiency of invariant natural killer T cells. J Allergy Clin Immunol. 2014;133(5):1420–8, 1428.e1.
109. Sanchez LA, et al. Two sides of the same coin: pediatric-onset and adult-onset common variable immune deficiency. J Clin Immunol. 2017;37(6):592–602.
110. Kralickova P, et al. Cytomegalovirus disease in patients with common variable immunodeficiency: three case reports. Int Arch Allergy Immunol. 2014;163(1):69–74.
111. Wheat WH, et al. Possible role of human herpesvirus 8 in the lymphoproliferative disorders in common variable immunodeficiency. J Exp Med. 2005;202(4):479–84.
112. Morimoto Y, Routes JM. Granulomatous disease in common variable immunodeficiency. Curr Allergy Asthma Rep. 2005;5(5):370–5.
113. Bates CA, et al. Granulomatous-lymphocytic lung disease shortens survival in common variable immunodeficiency. J Allergy Clin Immunol. 2004;114(2):415–21.
114. Ardeniz O, Cunningham-Rundles C. Granulomatous disease in common variable immunodeficiency. Clin Immunol. 2009;133(2):198–207.
115. Jorgensen SF, et al. A cross-sectional study of the prevalence of gastrointestinal symptoms and pathology in patients with common variable immunodeficiency. Am J Gastroenterol. 2016;111(10):1467–75.
116. Venhoff N, et al. The role of HLA DQ2 and DQ8 in dissecting celiac-like disease in common variable immunodeficiency. J Clin Immunol. 2013;33(5):909–16.
117. Washington K, et al. Gastrointestinal pathology in patients with common variable immunodeficiency and X-linked agammaglobulinemia. Am J Surg Pathol. 1996;20(10):1240–52.
118. Daniels JA, et al. Gastrointestinal tract pathology in patients with common variable immunodeficiency (CVID): a clinicopathologic study and review. Am J Surg Pathol. 2007;31(12):1800–12.
119. Ward C, et al. Abnormal liver function in common variable immunodeficiency disorders due to nodular regenerative hyperplasia. Clin Exp Immunol. 2008;153(3):331–7.
120. Fuss IJ, et al. Nodular regenerative hyperplasia in common variable immunodeficiency. J Clin Immunol. 2013;33(4):748–58.
121. Malamut G, et al. Nodular regenerative hyperplasia: the main liver disease in patients with primary hypogammaglobulinemia and hepatic abnormalities. J Hepatol. 2008;48(1):74–82.
122. Quinti I, et al. Long-term follow-up and outcome of a large cohort of patients with common variable immunodeficiency. J Clin Immunol. 2007;27(3):308–16.
123. Seve P, et al. Autoimmune hemolytic anemia and common variable immunodeficiency: a case-control study of 18 patients. Medicine (Baltimore). 2008;87(3):177–84.
124. Guffroy A, et al. Neutropenia in patients with common variable immunodeficiency: a rare event associated with severe outcome. J Clin Immunol. 2017;37(7):715–26.
125. Boileau J, et al. Autoimmunity in common variable immunodeficiency: correlation with lymphocyte phenotype in the French DEFI study. J Autoimmun. 2011;36(1):25–32.
126. Chapel H, et al. Confirmation and improvement of criteria for clinical phenotyping in common variable immunodeficiency disorders in replicate cohorts. J Allergy Clin Immunol. 2012;130(5):1197–8. e9
127. Mouillot G, et al. B-cell and T-cell phenotypes in CVID patients correlate with the clinical phenotype of the disease. J Clin Immunol. 2010;30(5):746–55.
128. Oraei M, et al. Naive CD4+ T cells and recent thymic emigrants in common variable immunodeficiency. J Investig Allergol Clin Immunol. 2012;22(3):160–7.
129. Maglione PJ. Autoimmune and lymphoproliferative complications of common variable immunodeficiency. Curr Allergy Asthma Rep. 2016;16(3):19.
130. van de Ven AA, Warnatz K. The autoimmune conundrum in common variable immunodeficiency disorders. Curr Opin Allergy Clin Immunol. 2015;15(6):514–24.
131. Podjasek JC, Abraham RS. Autoimmune cytopenias in common variable immunodeficiency. Front Immunol. 2012;3:189.
132. Rensing-Ehl A, et al. Clinical and immunological overlap between autoimmune lymphoproliferative syndrome and common variable immunodeficiency. Clin Immunol. 2010;137(3):357–65.

133. Castigli E, et al. TACI is mutant in common variable immunodeficiency and IgA deficiency. Nat Genet. 2005;37(8):829–34.
134. Zhang L, et al. Transmembrane activator and calcium-modulating cyclophilin ligand interactor mutations in common variable immunodeficiency: clinical and immunologic outcomes in heterozygotes. J Allergy Clin Immunol. 2007;120(5):1178–85.
135. Salzer U, et al. Screening of functional and positional candidate genes in families with common variable immunodeficiency. BMC Immunol. 2008;9:3.
136. Lee JJ, et al. Transmembrane activator and calcium-modulator and cyclophilin ligand interactor mutations in common variable immunodeficiency. Curr Opin Allergy Clin Immunol. 2008;8(6):520–6.
137. Verma N, et al. Immune deficiency and autoimmunity in patients with CTLA-4 (CD152) mutations. Clin Exp Immunol. 2017;190(1):1–7.
138. Schubert D, et al. Autosomal dominant immune dysregulation syndrome in humans with CTLA4 mutations. Nat Med. 2014;20(12):1410–6.
139. Gamez-Diaz L, et al. The extended phenotype of LPS-responsive beige-like anchor protein (LRBA) deficiency. J Allergy Clin Immunol. 2016;137(1):223–30.
140. Lopez-Herrera G, et al. Deleterious mutations in LRBA are associated with a syndrome of immune deficiency and autoimmunity. Am J Hum Genet. 2012;90(6):986–1001.
141. Hou TZ, et al. Identifying functional defects in patients with immune dysregulation due to LRBA and CTLA-4 mutations. Blood. 2017;129(11):1458–68.
142. Vorechovsky I, et al. Chromosomal radiosensitivity in common variable immune deficiency. Mutat Res. 1993;290(2):255–64.
143. Chua I, Quinti I, Grimbacher B. Lymphoma in common variable immunodeficiency: interplay between immune dysregulation, infection and genetics. Curr Opin Hematol. 2008;15(4):368–74.
144. Dhalla F, et al. Review of gastric cancer risk factors in patients with common variable immunodeficiency disorders, resulting in a proposal for a surveillance programme. Clin Exp Immunol. 2011;165(1):1–7.
145. Mellemkjaer L, et al. Cancer risk among patients with IgA deficiency or common variable immunodeficiency and their relatives: a combined Danish and Swedish study. Clin Exp Immunol. 2002;130(3):495–500.
146. Seymour B, Miles J, Haeney M. Primary antibody deficiency and diagnostic delay. J Clin Pathol. 2005;58(5):546–7.
147. Roberts CA, et al. Investigation of common variable immunodeficiency patients and healthy individuals using autoimmune lymphoproliferative syndrome biomarkers. Hum Immunol. 2013;74(12):1531–5.
148. Rizzi M, et al. Outcome of allogeneic stem cell transplantation in adults with common variable immunodeficiency. J Allergy Clin Immunol. 2011;128(6):1371–4. e2
149. Wehr C, et al. Multicenter experience in hematopoietic stem cell transplantation for serious complications of common variable immunodeficiency. J Allergy Clin Immunol. 2015;135(4):988–97. e6
150. Ballow M, et al. Immunodeficiencies. Clin Exp Immunol. 2009;158(Suppl 1):14–22.
151. Orange JS, et al. Use of intravenous immunoglobulin in human disease: a review of evidence by members of the Primary Immunodeficiency Committee of the American Academy of Allergy, Asthma and Immunology. J Allergy Clin Immunol. 2006;117(4 Suppl):S525–53.
152. Gardulf A, et al. Subcutaneous immunoglobulin replacement in patients with primary antibody deficiencies: safety and costs. Lancet. 1995;345(8946):365–9.
153. Gardulf A, et al. Children and adults with primary antibody deficiencies gain quality of life by subcutaneous IgG self-infusions at home. J Allergy Clin Immunol. 2004;114(4):936–42.

Late-Onset Combined Immunodeficiencies (LOCID)

4

Eduardo López-Granados

4.1 Common Variable Immunodeficiency: B or Combined, T and B Immunodeficiency

"Common variable immunodeficiency" is a descriptive definition established in 1971 by a World Health Organization committee to identify less-well-characterized syndromes of antibody deficiency, from other primary antibody deficiencies with more homogeneous clinical description and Mendelian inheritance [1, 2]. Therefore CVID was established as a diagnosis of exclusion. First attempts to subclassify CVID patients, attending to their distinct immunological characteristics, were based on in vitro B cell activation and immunoglobulin production [3, 4].

In 1999, the European Society for Immune Deficiencies (ESID) and the Pan-American Group for Immunodeficiency (PAGID) proposed consensus criteria to harmonize the diagnosis of CVID [5]. A probable CVID was defined in a male or female patient with a marked decreased IgG and a marked decrease of at least one of the other two immunoglobulin isotypes, IgA or IgM. Poor isohemagglutinins and/or poor antibody response to vaccines had to be also demonstrated. Therefore, defective antibody production was the clue immunological defect that compiled patients under this diagnosis. Onset of immunodeficiency at a greater than 2 years of age and the exclusion of other forms of primary and secondary hypogammaglobulinemia were also required [5].

CVID was soon appreciated to be a clinically heterogeneous disease. Most patients presented increased susceptibility to infections of the respiratory tract, mostly caused by encapsulated bacteria. Some patients presented complications as splenomegaly, granulomatous lesions, autoimmune complications, and malignancy [6].

E. López-Granados
Coordinador del Servicio de Inmunología, Hospital Universitario La Paz-IdiPAZ, Madrid, Spain
e-mail: elgranados@salud.madrid.org

M. M. D'Elios, M. Rizzi (eds.), *Humoral Primary Immunodeficiencies*,
Rare Diseases of the Immune System, https://doi.org/10.1007/978-3-319-91785-6_4

These complications were used by Chapel at the Oxford Group [7], to classify patients in distinct clinical phenotypes with varying prognoses. The phenotype seems to be defined early in the follow-up of patients, and the prognosis was greatly different, with a normal life expectancy in "infections only" group and a 50% of survival at 30 years in the "disease-related complications" group. These data were confirmed in the New York and french cohorts [8].

The disturbance of T cell function in CVID and its participation in the pathogenesis and clinical course have been suggested for many years, prior and after the proposal of the 1999 CVID criteria [9, 10]. Defective thymopoiesis of naïve T cells, decreased activation and proliferation of T cells, the impairment of T cell receptor (TCR) signaling, enhanced apoptosis, and abnormal cytokine production, such as enhanced IFN-γ production with skewed Th1/Th2 responses and reduced IL-4, IL-5, and IL-10, reduced expression of CD40L (CD154), and reduced generation of antigen-specific memory T cells [9, 10, 11–24], were described in several CVID cohorts. More importantly, poor T cell function at diagnosis has been associated with death at an early age [6]. A profoundly impaired T cell function in some CVID patients had also been inferred based on the occurrence of opportunistic infections in series of patients and case reports [6, 25].

Despite growing appreciation of a component of cellular T deficiency in many CVID patients, further attempts for subclassification of CVID on the basis of immunological parameters were focused on the B cell compartment, as impaired B cell function and antibody formation still constituted the hallmark of CVID.

The identification of a subgroup of CVID patients who lack inducible co-stimulatory molecule (ICOS) in 2003 represented a first identification of a monogenic defect leading to a CVID phenotype [26]. ICOS belongs to the family of co-stimulatory T cell molecules together with CD28 and cytotoxic T-lymphocyte antigen-4 (CTLA-4) and therefore indicated the possible appearance of CVID phenotype as a consequence of a genetic T cell dysfunction [26].

Renewed attempts for a clinically useful subclassification of CVID based on pathogenesis focused on the definition of phenotypic subsets of peripheral blood B cells [27, 28]. A large pan-European multicenter trial (EUROclass trial) was carried out in 303 patients based on a consensus of 2 previous classification schemes attending to the B cell phenotyping and clinical course [29]. A severe reduction of switched memory B cells in most of the patients was associated with higher risk of splenomegaly and granulomatous disease. An expansion of $CD21^{low}$ B cells was present in patients with splenomegaly, while expansion of transitional B cells was significantly linked with lymphadenopathy. The severe reduction of switched memory B cell compartment in most CVID patients suggested impairment of the germinal center reaction [29].

Meanwhile, in a large cohort of CVID patients, diagnosed following 1999 PAGID-ESID criteria, *Giovannetti* et al. investigated several phenotypic and functional parameters of T cell-mediated immunity [30]. These included reduced thymic output, with disrupted CD4 and CD8 TCR repertoires. Activation markers and cytokine production suggested an increased T cell activation with enhanced T cell turnover and apoptosis. The severity of the defects observed in patients paralleled with a decreased in naïve CD4+ T cells. Numbers of naïve CD4+ T cells had a strong negative correlation with clinical severity of the disease. These authors proposed to include the level of naïve CD4+ T cells as a parameter for CVID classification and probable prognosis [30].

In 2009, the International Union of Immunological Societies Expert Primary Immunodeficiency Committee redefined the conditions as "common variable Immunodeficiency disorders." The acronym of the disease was maintained, while emphasizing the heterogeneous nature of these hypogammaglobulinemic states [31].

4.2 The Proposed Definition of LOCID Within CVID Cohorts

In 2009, the DEFI French national study on adults with primary immunodeficiency with hypogammaglobulinemia compiled results from 313 CVID patients, from 41 centers [32]. The median age at evaluation was 45 years. Diagnosis criteria used were consistent with ESID/PAGID 1999 criteria [5].

Clinical data were collected, including history of infections and autoimmune, lymphoproliferative, and malignant complications. At enrollment, a blood sample was collected to determine T and B cell phenotypes. In male patients, gene sequencing was performed to exclude X-linked hyper IgM syndrome, X-linked lymphoproliferative diseases, and X-linked agammaglobulinemia. Human immunodeficiency virus (HIV) infection was ruled out by viral load quantification.

Patients were considered to have a severe T cell deficiency if they had experienced infections indicative of severe defect of cell-mediated immunity and/or had a $CD4^+$ T lymphocyte count <200 × 10^6 cells/L at the time of evaluation. Infections of severe T cell defect were consistent with the classification system of manifestations in HIV infection and defined as opportunistic infections (OI) [33]. Unusual infections, as pulmonary tuberculosis of recurrent herpes virus infection, were not considered as they can occur in patients without severe immunodeficiency. The definition of late-onset combined immunodeficiency (LOCID) was proposed for this subset of patients [32].

Within the DEFI study, 17 (5, 4%) of the 313 patients with CVID had a history of OI, with a total of 22 infective events recorded. This percentage was similar to a previous large US study, in which 13 (5, 2%) of 248 CVID patients suffered OI. Median age at occurrence of the first OI was 33 years. Only 3 out of 17 patients had received prior immunosuppressive therapy. In addition, 11 patients had a CD4+ T cell count <200 × 10^6 cells/L but no previous OI. Therefore, a total of 28 patients were defined as LOCID, and clinical and analytical comparison of this LOCID subgroup to the remaining CVID patients was performed [32].

The sex ratio was comparable between the LOCID and the rest of CVIDs. A higher frequency of consanguinity was found in parents of patients with LOCID. LOCID patients presented with a high prevalence of lymphoproliferative disorders, which had been previously associated with abnormalities in the T cell phenotype [30]. The low CD4+ T cell counts in LOCID patients were associated with significantly decreased naïve CD4+ T cells, which together with the late occurrence of OI might suggest a progressive decrease in the naïve population [32].

Based on these results, the DEFI study group raised a question: if those "LOCID" patients should be diagnosed with CVID. These patients were considered to be putative variants of severe combined immune deficiency (SCID).

A previous attempt to explore a possible adenosine deaminase (ADA) deficiency in a series of 44 CVID patients revealed no apparent ADA enzymatic defect [34]. A previous description of recombination-activating gene 1 or 2 (RAG1 or RAG2) hypomorphic mutation in three girls aged 3–10 years, with clinical and immunological features, consisted in extensive granulomatous disease, hypogammaglobulinemia, splenomegaly, and mild infections as those normally seen in SCID prompted the authors to explore the possible presence of RAG hypomorphic mutations in 19 adult CVID patients without findings [35].

The final conclusion of the DEFI study group was that CVID patients with severe T cell deficiency differed from the rest in immunological and clinical presentation and could be considered a different group of patients. Because those patients might have variants of SCID, a final proposal to identify them as LOCID was made. Unfortunately, no molecular studies in SCID-related genes could be accomplished to explore such possibility in the DEFI CVID study group. A proposal to confirm those findings in prospective studies by systematic recording of T cell phenotype was made, to allow a more precise diagnosis, specific prophylactic recommendation, and tailored genetic studies [32].

However, according to other authors' commentaries [36], the identification of pure combined T and B immune defects in CVID cohorts among those patients suffering OI or presenting with severe defective T cell phenotyping would require exclusion of patient receiving immunosuppressive therapy or presenting with neoplasms, what could determine a secondary rather than primary defect. As indicated by H. Chapel, in an Oxford series of 118 patients, 4 out of 9 CVID patients with OI had received immunosuppressive therapy [36].

An association of CD4 lymphopenia with splenomegaly or gastrointestinal disease in the DEFI study and the association of gluten-resistant enteropathy with splenomegaly and such enteropathy with persistent lymphadenopathy and hepatomegaly in the Oxford group might suggest a viral or lymphoproliferative origin, in relation with the CD4 lymphopenia [36]. Therefore, longitudinal studies to monitor the stability or progression of CD4+ T cell numbers in comparison with the results at diagnosis were proposed to contribute to a better understanding of the cellular defect in some CVID patients [36].

Further studies from the Oxford group of the T cell phenotype in patients with CVID identified significant reduction in naïve T cells, with reduced total CD4+ T cells and recent thymic emigrant numbers, most prominently in those with autoimmune cytopenias or polyclonal lymphoproliferation [37].

Along the years since the proposal of the 1999 ESID/PAGID criteria for the diagnosis of common variable immunodeficiency disorders [5], accumulated evidence and clinical experience suggested the existence of the subgroups of CVID patients based on clinical and phenotypic characteristics: infection-only vs.

disease-related complications, severe reduction of switched memory B cells, opportunistic infections, and severe CD4+ T cell lymphopenia as potential LOCID patients. Therefore, a rationale for reviewing the 1999 criteria was clearly stated.

4.3 Redefinition of Diagnosis Criteria for CVID to Exclude Combined Immunodeficiencies

In 2014 the European Society for Immunodeficiencies proposed a set of revised criteria for the diagnosis of CVID that included, among others, the increase in the age of diagnosis from 2 to 4 years and the exclusion of severe T cell defects defined as two of the following: CD4 < 200 cells/μL, naïve CD4 < 10%, and T cell proliferation absent to exclude patients that could be considered as combined immunodeficiencies (CID) [38].

Further conclusions of the DEFI French national study of adults with primary hypogammaglobulinemia were obtained from 521 patients with primary hypogammaglobulinemia once exclusion criteria as lymphoma, prior lymphoma, or aggressive immunosuppressive therapy were applied [38]. Clinical data were compiled and the "infection-only" and "disease-related complication" phenotypes defined according to the classification proposed by Chapel [7, 8].

An alternative to the ESID revised criteria was proposed, the DEFI CVID 2015 definition. The major difference in terms of the exclusion of potential combined immunodeficiencies within the CVID patients was their definition of LOCID by the presence of a profound T cell defect defined as naïve CD4 < 200 cells/μL or opportunistic infection.

From 351 patients diagnosed with CVID according to the 1999 ESID/PAGID criteria, 289 were maintained under this diagnosis, whereas 6 were excluded and considered CID following the more restrictive ESID 2014 criteria. The application of the proposed DEFI 2015 criteria on the very same 351 patients resulted in 244 patients maintained on the CVID diagnosis, while 62 were excluded as considered LOCID [38].

Therefore, the more restrictive criteria of severe T cell defect from the ESID 2014 definition excluded only 2% of the initial CVID population, being considered patients with CID. Most of these patients presented severe combined T and B cell defect, but onset of disease was delayed to early adulthood (median, 26 years) in opposition to classical CID. Age at onset did not differ significantly from that in the patients with CVID. The estimated 5-year overall survival (OS) of these patients is 50% [38]. Some of these patients as children with CID might require hematopoietic stem cell transplantation (HSCT).

Based on previous results, the DEFI study group proposed a surrogate marker for T cell defects associated with poor outcome together with the occurrence of opportunistic infections. These markers defined a population that increased from 6 to 62 when compared to the ESID 2014 definition. This population exhibited a more profound B cell defect and a poor outcome. The demographics were very similar to that from the rest of CVID patients, with similar age at onset of symptoms, diagnosis, and familiar cases with only slightly increased consanguinity. In these patients, there was a higher frequency of disease-related complications [38].

A diagnosis of LOCID then might be used in patients previously diagnosed with CVID with onset of symptoms or diagnosis in late childhood or adulthood. In addition to usual care and treatment with immunoglobulin replacement therapy, LOCID patients could require special consideration, as prioritization of genetic studies. A possible unique or discrete number of gene defects leading to a diagnosis of CVID that could be reconsidered as CID applying the ESID 2014 or LOCID de DEFI 2015 criteria remain elusive.

Several recent clinical case reports identified patients with clinical and immunological characteristics resembling CVID or fulfilling CVID criteria that turned out to harbor genetic variants in genes commonly associated with SCID. CVID patients with early onset, chronic enteropathy, failure to thrive, and continuous reduction of lymphocytes could present homozygous mutations in Janus kinase 3 (*JAK3*) gene [39]. In addition, hypomorphic mutations in recombination-activating genes (*RAG*) have been associated with clinical phenotypes of leaky SCID or even resembling cases of CVID with granulomatous complications, opportunistic infections, and autoimmunity [40, 41]. Moreover, atypical SCID or late-onset combined immunodeficiency with clinical features of CVID could be in relation to leaky mutations or revertant somatic mosaicism in prototypical SCID genes such as *IL2RG* [42].

The increased age for diagnosis to >4 years and the incorporation of exclusion criteria accounting for profound T cell defects in CVID definition have rendered the inclusion of patients with these characteristics less probable.

4.4 The Advent of Next-Generation Sequencing to the Field of CID-LOCID and CVID

The clinical heterogeneity of CVID and the predominantly sporadic cases has complicated the diagnostic and the identification of the underlying genetic defect of the disease, allowing a molecular characterization of the origin in less than 20% of the patients with the advent of next-generation sequencing (NGS) approaches.

The existence of monogenic traits, usually in familiar forms of the disease which constitute only a small fraction of the CVID cases, leads to reclassification of CVID-like diseases and establishing new therapeutic approaches based on the affected pathways that have markedly improved affected patients' prognoses. Specific variants in these genes as well as in others have been reported to confer susceptibility to the disease or to originate similar phenotypes to CVID blurring even more the boundaries that define this disorder. Furthermore, some of the mutations have incomplete penetrance, and many sporadic cases remain unexplained after deep genetic analyses, suggesting that an important fraction of CVID cases might not follow a monogenic Mendelian pattern of inheritance.

In recent studies using whole-genome and exome sequencing to study CVID, 15–30% of CVID patients have been proposed to have a monogenic origin [43–46]. Clear clarification about the attempt to discard CID or LOCID by either ESID 2014 or DEFI 2015 criteria is not always easy to trace. Nevertheless, genetic results in those studies have not clearly unmasked mutations or pathogenic variants in one of a few genes previously related with combined immunodeficiencies with severe T cell defect that could have not been previously identified due to atypical phenotypic presentation. On the contrary, the application of exclusion criteria and proper statement of those according to any of the most recent proposed criteria for CVID will gradually exclude those patients from the CVID group.

On a practical basis, CVID, CVID-like monogenic disorders, and CID or LOCID are usually all present on the same immunology clinic and centers. Combined immunological, clinical, and genetic characteristics are gradually untangling this group of most prevalent symptomatic primary immunodeficiencies that previously were mostly being considered under original 1999 CVID diagnosis criteria. A better pathogenic definition will help us to improve the therapeutic approaches for some common complications of this group of patients other than infections as enteropathy, autoimmunity, and granulomatous and lymphoproliferative complications. Repurposing of current or in development immunosuppressive drugs and biologicals will be possible upon better understanding of genetic and molecular basis on their immune dysfunction.

Finally, the unfortunate clinical severity of many complications, and the growing appreciation of the relation in some cases of a severe T cell deficiency with poor outcome, has established the rationale to consider a hematopoietic stem cell transplantation (HSCT) as a putative curative option in some cases [47]. A consensus and harmonized approach for the definition of severe T cell defects would facilitate the identification of the genetic bases of these cases, whose better pathogenic understanding would reinforce critical therapeutic decisions as to accomplish a HSCT.

References

1. Fudenberg H, Good RA, Goodman HC, et al. Primary immunodeficiencies: report of a World Health Organization committee. Pediatrics. 1971;47:927–46.
2. Cooper MD, Faulk WP, Fudenberg HH, Good RA, Hitzig W, Kunkel H, et al. Classification of primary immunodeficiencies. N Engl J Med. 1973;288:966–7.
3. Saiki O, Ralph P, Cunningham-Rundles C, Good RA. Three distinct stages of B-cell defects in common varied immunodeficiency. Proc Natl Acad Sci U S A. 1982;79:6008–12.
4. Bryant A, Calver NC, Toubi E, et al. Classification of patients with common variable immunodeficiency by B cell secretion of IgM and IgG in response to anti-IgM and interleukin-2. Clin Immunol Immunopathol. 1990;56:239–48.
5. Conley ME, Notarangelo LD, Etzioni A. Diagnostic criteria for primary immunodeficiencies: representing PAGID (Pan-American Group for Immunodeficiency) and ESID (European Society for Immunodeficiencies). Clin Immunol. 1999;93:190–7.
6. Cunningham-Rundles C, Bodian C. Common variable immunodeficiency: clinical and immunological features of 248 patients. Clin Immunol. 1999;92:34–48.
7. Chapel H, Lucas M, Lee M, et al. Common variable immunodeficiency disorders: division into distinct clinical phenotypes. Blood. 2008;112:277–86.
8. Chapel H, Lucas M, Patel S, et al. Confirmation and improvement of criteria for clinical phenotyping in common variable immunodeficiency disorders in replicate cohorts. J Allergy Clin Immunol. 2012;130:1197–1198.e9.

9. Bayry J, Hermine O, Webster DA, Lévy Y, Kaveri SV. Common variable immunodeficiency: the immune system in chaos. Trends Mol Med. 2005;11:370–6.
10. Goldacker S, Warnatz K. Tackling the heterogeneity of CVID. Curr Opin Allergy Clin Immunol. 2005;5:504–9.
11. Serrano D, et al. Characterization of the T cell receptor repertoire in patients with common variable immunodeficiency: oligoclonal expansion of CD8+ T cells. Clin Immunol. 2000;97:248–58.
12. Guazzi V, et al. Assessment of thymic output in common variable immunodeficiency patients by evaluation of T cell receptor excision circles. Clin Exp Immunol. 2002;129:346–53.
13. Pirovano S, et al. Impaired thymic output and restricted T-cell repertoire in two infants with immunodeficiency and early-onset generalized dermatitis. Immunol Lett. 2003;86:93–7.
14. Isgro A, et al. Bone marrow clonogenic capability, cytokine production, and thymic output in patients with common variable immunodeficiency. J Immunol. 2005;174:5074–81.
15. Boncristiano M, et al. Defective recruitment and activation of ZAP-70 in common variable immunodeficiency patients with T cell defects. Eur J Immunol. 2000;30:2632–8.
16. Paccani SR, et al. Defective VAV expression and impaired F-actin reorganization in a subset of common variable immunodeficiency patients with T-cell defects. Blood. 2005;106(2):626–34.
17. Di Renzo M, et al. Enhanced apoptosis of T cells in common variable immunodeficiency (CVID): role of defective CD28 costimulation. Clin Exp Immunol. 2000;120:503–11.
18. Di Renzo M, et al. Enhanced T cell apoptosis in common variable immunodeficiency: negative role of the fas/fas ligand system and of the Bcl-2 family proteins and possible role of TNF-RS. Clin Exp Immunol. 2001;125:117–22.
19. Sneller MC, Strober W. Abnormalities of lymphokine gene expression in patients with common variable immunodeficiency. J Immunol. 1990;144:3762–9.
20. Farrington M, et al. CD40 ligand expression is defective in a subset of patients with common variable immunodeficiency. Proc Natl Acad Sci U S A. 1994;91:1099–103.
21. Fischer MB, et al. A defect in the early phase of T-cell receptor mediated T-cell activation in patients with common variable immunodeficiency. Blood. 1994;84:4234–41.
22. Majolini MB, et al. Uncoupling of T-cell antigen receptor and downstream protein tyrosine kinases in common variable immunodeficiency. Clin Immunol Immunopathol. 1997;84:98–102.
23. Holm AM, et al. Abnormal interleukin-7 function in common variable immunodeficiency. Blood. 2005;105(7):2887–90.
24. Farrant J, Spickett G, Matamoros N, et al. Study of B and T cell phenotypes in blood from patients with common variable immunodeficiency (CVID). Immunodeficiency. 1994;5:159–69.
25. Oksenhendler E, Gerard L, Fieschi C, et al. Infections in 252 patients with common variable immunodeficiency. Clin Infect Dis. 2008;46:1547–54.
26. Grimbacher B, Hutloff A, Schlesier M, et al. Homozygous loss of ICOS is associated with adult-onset common variable immunodeficiency. Nat Immunol. 2003;4:261–8.
27. Warnatz K, Denz A, Drager R, Braun M, Groth C, Wolff-Vorbeck G, Eibel H, Schlesier M, Peter HH. Severe deficiency of switched memory B cells (CD27_IgM_IgD_) in subgroups of patients with common variable immunodeficiency: a new approach to classify a heterogeneous disease. Blood. 2002;99:1544–51.
28. Piqueras B, Lavenu-Bombled C, Galicier L, Bergeron-van der Cruyssen F, Mouthon L, Chevret S, Debre P, Schmitt C, Oksenhendler E. Common variable immunodeficiency patient classification based on impaired B cell memory differentiation correlates with clinical aspects. J Clin Immunol. 2003;23:385–400.
29. Wehr C, Kivioja T, Schmitt C, Ferry B, Witte T, Eren E, Vlkova M, Hernandez M, Detkova D, Bos PR, Poerksen G, von Bernuth H, Baumann U, Goldacker S, Gutenberger S, Schlesier M, Bergeron-van der Cruyssen F, Le Garff M, Debré P, Jacobs R, Jones J, Bateman E, Litzman J, van Hagen PM, Plebani A, Schmidt RE, Thon V, Quinti I, Espanol T, Webster AD, Chapel H, Vihinen M, Oksenhendler E, Peter HH, Warnatz K. The EUROclass trial: defining subgroups in common variable immunodeficiency. Blood. 2008;111(1):77–85.

30. Giovannetti A, Pierdominici M, Mazzetta F, et al. Unravelling the complexity of T cell abnormalities in common variable immunodeficiency. J Immunol. 2007;178:3932–43.
31. Notarangelo LD, Fischer A, Geha RS, Casanova JL, Chapel H, Conley ME, et al. Primary immunodeficiencies: 2009 update. J Allergy Clin Immunol. 2009;124:1161–78.
32. Malphettes M, Gérard L, Carmagnat M, Mouillot G, Vince N, Boutboul D, Bérezné A, Nove-Josserand R, Lemoing V, Tetu L, Viallard JF, Bonnotte B, Pavic M, Haroche J, Larroche C, Brouet JC, Fermand JP, Rabian C, Fieschi C, Oksenhendler E, DEFI Study Group. Late-onset combined immune deficiency: a subset of common variable immunodeficiency with severe T cell defect. Clin Infect Dis. 2009;49(9):1329–38.
33. Centers for Disease Control and Prevention. 1993 revised classification system for HIV infection and expanded surveillance case definition for AIDS among adolescents and adults. JAMA. 1993;269:729–30.
34. Fleischman A, Hershfield MS, Toutain S, et al. Adenosine deaminase deficiency and purine nucleoside phosphorylase deficiency in common variable immunodeficiency. Clin Diagn Lab Immunol. 1998;5:399–400.
35. Schuetz C, Huck K, Gudowius S, et al. An immunodeficiency disease with RAG mutations and granulomas. N Engl J Med. 2008;358:2030–8.
36. Aslam A, Chapel H. Dissecting the group of common variable immunodeficiency disorders. Clin Infect Dis. 2009;49(9):1339–40.
37. Bateman EA, Ayers L, Sadler R, Lucas M, Roberts C, Woods A, Packwood K, Burden J, Harrison D, Kaenzig N, Lee M, Chapel HM, Ferry BL. T cell phenotypes in patients with common variable immunodeficiency disorders: associations with clinical phenotypes in comparison with other groups with recurrent infections. Clin Exp Immunol. 2012;170(2):202–11.
38. Bertinchamp R, Gérard L, Boutboul D, Malphettes M, Fieschi C, Oksenhendler E, DEFI Study Group. Exclusion of patients with a severe T-cell defect improves the definition of common variable immunodeficiency. J Allergy Clin Immunol Pract. 2016;4(6):1147–57.
39. Abolhassani H, Cheraghi T, Rezaei N, Aghamohammadi A, Hammarström L. Common variable immunodeficiency or late-onset combined immunodeficiency: a new hypomorphic JAK3 patient and review of the literature. J Investig Allergol Clin Immunol. 2015;25(3):218–20.
40. Abolhassani H, Wang N, Aghamohammadi A, Rezaei N, Lee YN, Frugoni F, Notarangelo LD, Pan-Hammarström Q, Hammarström L. A hypomorphic recombination-activating gene 1 (RAG1) mutation resulting in a phenotype resembling common variable immunodeficiency. J Allergy Clin Immunol. 2014;134(6):1375–80.
41. Buchbinder D, Baker R, Lee YN, Ravell J, Zhang Y, McElwee J, Nugent D, Coonrod EM, Durtschi JD, Augustine NH, Voelkerding KV, Csomos K, Rosen L, Browne S, Walter JE, Notarangelo LD, Hill HR, Kumánovics A. Identification of patients with RAG mutations previously diagnosed with common variable immunodeficiency disorders. J Clin Immunol. 2015;35(2):119–24.
42. Okuno Y, Hoshino A, Muramatsu H, Kawashima N, Wang X, Yoshida K, Wada T, Gunji M, Toma T, Kato T, Shiraishi Y, Iwata A, Hori T, Kitoh T, Chiba K, Tanaka H, Sanada M, Takahashi Y, Nonoyama S, Ito M, Miyano S, Ogawa S, Kojima S, Kanegane H. Late-onset combined immunodeficiency with a novel IL2RG mutation and probable revertant somatic mosaicism. J Clin Immunol. 2015;35(7):610–4.
43. van Schouwenburg PA, Davenport EE, Kienzler A-K, Marwah I, Wright B, Lucas M, et al. Application of whole genome and RNA sequencing to investigate the genomic landscape of common variable immunodeficiency disorders. Clin Immunol. 2015;160:301–14.
44. Maffucci P, Filion CA, Boisson B, Itan Y, Shang L, Casanova J-L, et al. Genetic diagnosis using whole exome sequencing in common variable immunodeficiency. Front Immunol. 2016;7:220.
45. Kienzler A-K, Hargreaves CE, Patel SY. The role of genomics in common variable immunodeficiency disorders. Clin Exp Immunol. 2017;188:326–32.
46. Ameratunga R, Lehnert K, Woon ST, Gillis D, Bryant VL, Slade CA, Steele R. Diagnosing common variable immunodeficiency disorder in the era of genome sequencing. Clin Rev Allergy Immunol. 2018;54(2):261–8.

47. Wehr C, Gennery AR, Lindemans C, Schulz A, Hoenig M, Marks R, Recher M, Gruhn B, Holbro A, Heijnen I, Meyer D, Grigoleit G, Einsele H, Baumann U, Witte T, Sykora KW, Goldacker S, Regairaz L, Aksoylar S, Ardeniz Ö, Zecca M, Zdziarski P, Meyts I, Matthes-Martin S, Imai K, Kamae C, Fielding A, Seneviratne S, Mahlaoui N, Slatter MA, Güngör T, Arkwright PD, van Montfrans J, Sullivan KE, Grimbacher B, Cant A, Peter HH, Finke J, Gaspar HB, Warnatz K, Rizzi M, Inborn Errors Working Party of the European Society for Blood and Marrow Transplantation and the European Society for Immunodeficiency. Multicenter experience in hematopoietic stem cell transplantation for serious complications of common variable immunodeficiency. J Allergy Clin Immunol. 2015;135(4):988–97.

Genetics of CVID

5

Vasssilios Lougaris and Alessandro Plebani

CVID is characterized by low immunoglobulin serum levels and defective antibody response. Clinical manifestations of CVID include recurrent infections, mainly of the respiratory and gastrointestinal tract, autoimmune phenomena ranging from autoimmune thyroiditis to systemic lupus erythematosus (SLE), autoimmune cytopenias, splenomegaly, granulomata, and increased susceptibility to cancer and lymphomas [1]. The age of onset is variable, and any age group may be involved, although the higher prevalence is considered during the second and third decade of life; both sexes are involved in an equal manner. The complex clinical phenotype of CVID [1] has long suggested that a common denominator, i.e., hypogammaglobulinemia with peripheral B cell maturation defects, may be related to immunological impairment due to different genetic defects, explaining this clinical heterogeneity. In the last two decades, the genetic findings in CVID have validated this hypothesis, adding significant complexity to the classical definition of CVID.

While the first description of CVID was made in the early 1950s [2], it took almost 50 years before the first genetic cause of CVID was identified [3]. In 2003, ICOS deficiency was described in four adult-onset CVID patients: the expression of ICOS (inducible T cell costimulator), a T cell receptor that binds ICOS ligand (ICOSL) expressed on B cells, was lacking due to a homozygous deletion of exons 2 and 3 from the *ICOS* encoding gene [3]. Lymph node analysis from an ICOS-deficient patient revealed an essential requirement for ICOS in the generation of an effective germinal center reaction [4].

Following the identification of human ICOS deficiency in CVID, mutations in *TNFRSF13B* encoding for TACI, expressed on B cells, were found to be associated

V. Lougaris · A. Plebani (✉)
Pediatrics Clinic and Institute for Molecular Medicine A. Nocivelli,
Department of Clinical and Experimental Sciences, University of Brescia,
ASST Spedali Civili of Brescia, Brescia, Italy
e-mail: alessandro.plebani@unibs.it

M. M. D'Elios, M. Rizzi (eds.), *Humoral Primary Immunodeficiencies*,
Rare Diseases of the Immune System, https://doi.org/10.1007/978-3-319-91785-6_5

with CVID in humans [5, 6]. In a cohort of 162 unrelated CVID patients, Salzer et al. [6] identified homozygous (C104R, S144X) and heterozygous (C104R, A181E, S194X, and R202H) mutations in TACI. Patients carrying the homozygous S144X and C104R mutations lacked B cell TACI expression and showed defective binding to APRIL but not to BAFF, since the expression of the BAFF receptor (BAFF-R) was unaltered. In addition, in vitro experiments for the same patients showed that APRIL and BAFF failed to induce class-switch recombination in TACI-mutated B cells. The heterozygous variants C104R, A181E, S194X, and R202H were reported to be associated with defective antibody production [6]. In parallel, a second group [5] identified *TNFRSF13B* mutations in a small number of patients affected with CVID and SIgAD supporting the hypothesis that CVID and SIgAD may share similar pathogenetic mechanisms. In both studies, B cell evaluation did not coincide with the mouse model [7], confirming the existence of important differences between the animal and the human immune systems.

After the first description of TACI mutations in CVID, screening of larger cohorts of patients for TACI mutations underlined the great genetic variability of this gene, thus rendering difficult the definition of the pathogenetic role of these genetic findings. Several novel mutations have been reported [5, 6, 8–11]. In the largest cohort of CVID patients ($N = 564$) studied to date [11], the C104R monoallelic TACI mutation, present in 4.6% of included patients and in 0.9% of 675 healthy controls analyzed for this study, resulted associated with an elevated risk for the development of hypogammaglobulinemia, lymphoproliferation, and autoimmunity [11]. Thus, available data suggest that while biallelic *TNFRSF13B* variants that abrogate TACI on B cells are responsible for CVID, the role of heterozygous variants is still in debate and should be probably considered as associated with rather than causative of CVID.

Since TACI is a member of a TNF receptor superfamily, including BAFFR and BCMA that bind to BAFF and APRIL (BAFFR binds only BAFF), and based also on available knockout animal data, the candidate gene approach led to further investigation of the above mentioned genes. Analysis of the *TNFRSF13C* gene encoding for BAFFR in 48 patients [12] revealed the presence of three novel variants, all at the heterozygous state, P21R, G64V, and H159Y, that are considered as single nucleotide polymorphisms (SNPs). Of interest, the P21R variant was recently shown to alter the polymerization of BAFFR on the surface of B cells, contributing therefore to the pathogenesis of CVID [13].

Recently, mutations in *TNFRSF13C,* the gene encoding for BAFFR, were found to be associated with adult-onset CVID in two siblings with low peripheral B cell counts [14]. They both carried a homozygous 24 bp in-frame deletion (del89-96) located in exon 2 of the *TNFRSF13C* gene leading to the lack of BAFFR on B cell surface. Both patients presented hypogammaglobulinemia (low IgG and IgM, normal IgA serum levels). They also did not mount a T-independent immune response against pneumococcal cell wall polysaccharides, but only one BAFF R-deficient sibling developed recurrent infections and was put on replacement treatment with immunoglobulins.

Analysis of the *TNFSF13B* gene encoding for BAFF showed the presence of a single novel synonymous variant, V63V, in a single patient in the heterozygous state

[15]. Analysis of the genes encoding for BCMA and APRIL in CVID patients revealed the presence of the S81N, T159T, T175T, K179Q (BCMA) and G67R, N96S (APRIL) variants, at the same frequency as observed in healthy individuals, thus suggesting the lack of an association between these variants with the pathogenesis of CVID [16].

After the description of mutations in TACI and BAFFR, CD19 deficiency was identified in four patients [17]. Three patients harbored the homozygous deletion 1384del(ga), while one harbored the homozygous insertion 972ins(a). Both mutations led to a premature stop codon and thus lack of CD19 expression on the B cell surface. CD27+ memory B cells were decreased in affected patients, as typically observed in CVID. BCR cross-linking failed to induce a vigorous B cell activation, and recall response to vaccinations was poor [17]. Another patient with CD19 deficiency was identified after the initial description, carrying a compound heterozygous mutation in the gene encoding for CD19 [18]. More in detail, mutation analysis of *CD19* revealed a mutation in the splice acceptor site of intron 5 (IVS5-1G>T) of the maternal allele, resulting in skipping of exon 6, and a truncated protein product. The paternal allele was disrupted by a gross deletion encompassing at least the *ATP2A1*, *CD19*, and *NFATC2IP* genes [18].

Upon CD19 deficiency, CD20 deficiency due to a compound mutation of the noncanonical splice donor sequence of exon 5 of the *CD20* gene was identified in a single patient with hypogammaglobulinemia [19]. The patient showed defective antibody formation upon T-independent antigen stimulation, similarly to what observed in the CD20 knockout mice [19].

A patient with hypogammaglobulinemia, severe nephropathy, and lack of CD19 expression on B cells was recently described [20]. However, the lack of CD19 was not due to CD19 deficiency but to CD81 deficiency, a member of the tetraspanin family that interacts with CD19 and CD21 on the B cell surface, due to a homozygous c.561+1G>A mutation in the *CD81* gene resulting in a complete lack of CD81 expression. Memory B cells were reduced. As observed in CD19 deficiency, BCR cross-linking failed to activate properly B cells; on the contrary, T cell defects were not observed [20].

Immunological evaluation of an adult patient with recurrent infections and hypogammaglobulinemia revealed lack of CD21 expression on B cells [21]. Sequence analysis revealed a compound heterozygous deleterious mutation in the *CR2* gene (encoding CD21) (c.1225+1G>C/W766X). B cell maturation evaluation showed reduced class-switched memory B cells. In vitro experiments revealed absent co-stimulatory activity of C3d in enhancing suboptimal B cell receptor stimulation. Vaccination responses to protein antigens were normal, but the response to pneumococcal polysaccharide vaccination was moderately impaired [21].

Until this point, all the genetic defects described to be associated or causative of CVID were related to receptors expressed on the cell surface. However, novel genetic defects affecting cytoplasmic proteins have been reported in patients with clinical and immunological phenotype compatible with CVID. Salzer et al. [22] reported on a single patient from consanguineous family, with progressive B cell lymphopenia, hypogammaglobulinemia, and severe autoimmunity, affected with

PRKCD deficiency due to a homozygous (c.1352+1G>A) mutation affecting a splice site leading to absent expression of the encoded protein. PRKCD deficiency due to a R614W homozygous deleterious mutation was also reported in a single patient with chronic, low-grade Epstein-Barr virus (EBV) infection [23]. The patient had chronic lymphadenopathy, splenomegaly, autoantibodies, elevated immunoglobulins, and natural killer dysfunction. Interestingly, the homozygous G510S mutation in PRKCD was identified in three patients affected with systemic lupus erytematosous, with B cell defective apoptosis and hyperproliferation [24].

The essential role of the PI3K pathway in the human immune system was underlined by the identification of dominant-activating germline mutations in the gene encoding the PI(3)K catalytic subunit p110δ in patients with CVID-like phenotype (currently named as APDS-1, activated phosphoinositide 3-kinase δ syndrome) [25, 26]. Affected patients presented variable features, such as lymphopenia, hypogammaglobulinemia, variable B and T cell maturational defects, and, of note, T cell senescence [25, 26]. A comprehensive study of a large cohort of affected patients revealed an increased prevalence of B cell lymphomas in patients carrying activating p110δ mutations [27].

Besides the identification of dominant mutations in the p110δ catalytic subunit of PI3K in patients with APDS-1, monoallelic mutations in PIK3R1, the gene encoding for the regulatory subunit p85α of PI3K, were identified [28–30], causing APDS-2. Affected patients presented recurrent respiratory infections, gut involvement, enlarged lymph nodes and tonsils, normal to elevated IgM serum levels, low IgG and IgA, and variable lymphopenia [28–30] recalling a CVID-like phenotype. Of interest, evaluation of NK cells in both APDS-1 and APDS-2 revealed important functional NK cell defects [31, 32], a rather uncommon feature for CVID.

Considering that in APDS, both types 1 and 2, the genetic defect leads to hyperactivation of the PI3K pathway, and thus of mTOR and AKT, targeted inhibition of this cascade with rapamycin, an mTOR inhibitor, or specific PI3K inhibitors, is under clinical consideration [25, 26, 28, 29].

A rare genetic variant in the gene encoding for TWEAK leading to TWEAK deficiency was identified in a single family with three affected family members (father, daughter, and son) presenting with antibody deficiency, recurrent infections, and defective vaccine response [33], compatible with CVID. All patients carried a rare mutation in the sixth exon of TWEAK resulting in the amino acid substitution R145C within the conserved TNF-homology domain of the full-length protein. Functional in vitro experiments showed that the mutant protein caused inhibition of BAFF-dependent B cell survival and proliferation, suggesting thus a causative pathogenetic role of this mutant for CVID in this family [33].

The identification of LRBA (lipopolysaccharide-responsive beige-like anchor protein) deficiency in patients with CVID and/or autoimmune disorders added another important piece in the puzzle of CVID genetics [34, 35]. Lopez-Herrera et al. identified five CVID patients harboring homozygous mutations (I2657S, R1683X, E59X, and homozygous deletion including exons 1 and 2) in the gene encoding for LRBA that resulted in the loss of protein expression. All patients had early-onset hypogammaglobulinemia and severe autoimmune manifestations.

Immunological evaluation revealed disturbed B cell development, defective in vitro B cell activation, immunoglobulin secretion and proliferation, and defects in B cell autophagy [34]. LRBA deficiency due to a homozygous deletion from exon 1 to exon 30 was recently reported in a single patient with autoimmunity but without hypogammaglobulinemia, underlying that LRBA defects may present with variable immunological phenotypes [35]. Considering the complicated clinical course of LRBA deficiency, as underlined by long-term follow-up of relatively numerous affected patients [36], HSCT has been implemented in a small number of cases, with variable results [36, 37].

An important role for components of the NF-kB pathway in the pathogenesis of CVID has recently been described. Regarding the noncanonical NF-kB pathway, germline mutations in NFKB2 were described in a small number of patients affected with early-onset hypogammaglobulinemia, recurrent infections, autoimmune features, and adrenal insufficiency [38]. The NFKB2 mutations identified lead to altered processing of p100 and therefore affect p52 nuclear translocation. Upon the initial description of NFKB2 deficiency, additional CVID patients with NFKB2 mutations have been described [39–41]. Of interest, evaluation of NK cells from affected patients revealed defective cytotoxic activity, a rather unusual feature for CVID [41].

Regarding the canonical NF-kB pathway, monoallelic mutations in NFKB1 were recently identified in adult-onset CVID patients [42]. Affected patients presented with hypogammaglobulinemia, recurrent infections, and variable autoimmune features. The identified mutations altered the normal processing of p105 and the nuclear localization of p50 [42]. Evaluation of B cell maturation showed both early and late B cell developmental alterations in NFKB1 mutated patients [43]. Following the identification of this genetic defect, additional cases have been described, broadening the clinical and immunological phenotype, that now also includes EBV-driven lymphoproliferation and autoinflammatory manifestations [44, 45]. Of interest, as observed in NFKB2 deficiency, NK cell evaluation in affected patients revealed functional alterations as well as maturation perturbations [46], suggesting a more complex form and not a "simple" humoral defect.

In the context of more complex forms of CVID, a novel genetic form was recently identified caused by monoallelic mutations in Cytotoxic T lymphocyte antigen 4 (CTLA-4) [47, 48]. CTLA-4 is expressed in regulatory T cells upon activation and exhibits an inhibitory function on T cell biology. Affected patients present a complex syndrome of immune dysregulation characterized by variable features such hypogammaglobulinemia, lymphopenia, autoimmune cytopenias, lymphoproliferation, and granulomas [47, 48], resembling LRBA deficiency [34, 36]. Of note, affected patients seem to present an increased risk of gastric cancer, which has been experimentally confirmed in animal models [49]. Considering the available knowledge on the biology of CTLA-4, targeted treatments such as CTLA4-Ig may become promising tools in the treatment of patients affected with CTLA-4 or LRBA deficiency, since LRBA regulates CTLA-4 expression [50, 51].

Genes involved in the DNA repair process have also been implicated in the pathogenesis of CVID. This is the case of *Msh5*, a gene encoded in the central MHC class III region, and of its obligate heterodimerization partner *Msh4* that have a critical role in regulating meiotic homologous recombination. Sekine et al. [52] presented evidence that the human *MSH5* alleles containing two nonsynonymous polymorphisms (L85F/P786S) may be involved in the pathogenesis of selective IgA deficiency and common variable immunodeficiency (CVID).

Finally, and while mutations in RAG1/2 are normally associated with severe combined immunodeficiency [53], hypomorphic mutations in these genes have been described in a limited number of patients affected with a CVID-like phenotype [54–56].

In conclusion, during the last decades, the great advances in the field of genetics by means of candidate gene approach, linkage analysis, and next-generation sequencing have allowed to identify the defective genes responsible for several forms of primary immunodeficiencies, including CVID. Until recently the diagnosis of CVID was based mainly on the combination of hypogammaglobulinemia and B cell maturational defects. However the extreme clinical variability of CVID had indirectly suggested that CVID was not a single disease, but a group of different disorders sharing a common immunological phenotype and variable clinical features. The genetic findings in CVID have now confirmed this hypothesis. Thus a more precise classification of CVID should group patients according to the underlying genetic defects.

References

1. Cunningham-Rundles C. The many faces of common variable immunodeficiency. Hematology Am Soc Hematol Educ Program. 2012;2012:301–5.
2. Bruton OC, Apt L, Gitlin D, Janeway AC. Absence of serum gamma globulins. AMA Am J Dis Child. 1952;84(5):632–6.
3. Grimbacher B, Hutloff A, Schlesier M, Glocker E, Warnatz K, Dräger R, Eibel H, Fischer B, Schäffer AA, Mages HW, Kroczek RA, Peter HH. Homozygous loss of ICOS is associated with adult-onset common variable immunodeficiency. Nat Immunol. 2003;4(3):261–8.
4. Warnatz K, Bossaller L, Salzer U, Skrabl-Baumgartner A, Schwinger W, van der Burg M, van Dongen JJ, Orlowska-Volk M, Knoth R, Durandy A, Draeger R, Schlesier M, Peter HH, Grimbacher B. Human ICOS deficiency abrogates the germinal center reaction and provides a monogenic model for common variable immunodeficiency. Blood. 2006;107(8):3045–52.
5. Castigli E, Wilson SA, Garibyan L, Rachid R, Bonilla F, Schneider L, Geha RS. TACI is mutant in common variable immunodeficiency and IgA deficiency. Nat Genet. 2005;37:829–34.
6. Salzer U, Chapel HM, Webster ADB, Pan-Hammarstrom Q, Schmitt-Graeff A, Schlesier M, Peter HH, Rockstroh JK, Schneider P, Schaffer AA, Hammarstrom L, Grimbacher B. Mutations in TNFRSF13B encoding TACI are associated with common variable immunodeficiency in humans. Nat Genet. 2005;37:820–8.
7. Yan M, Wang H, Chan B, Roose-Girma M, Erickson S, Baker T, Tumas D, Grewal IS, Dixit VM. Activation and accumulation of B cells in TACI-deficient mice. Nat Immun. 2001;2:638–43.
8. Pan-Hammarstrom Q, Salzer U, Du L, Bjorkander J, Cunningham-Rundles C, Nelson DL, Bacchelli C, Gaspar HB, Offer S, Behrens TW, Grimbacher B, Hammarstrom L. Reexamining the role of TACI coding variants in common variable immunodeficiency and selective IgA deficiency. Nat Genet. 2007;39:429–30.

9. Castigli E, Wilson S, Garibyan L, Rachid R, Bonilla F, Schneider L, Morra M, Curran J, Geha R. Reexamining the role of TACI coding variants in common variable immunodeficiency and selective IgA deficiency. Nat Genet. 2007;39:430–1.
10. Lougaris V, Gallizzi R, Vitali M, Baronio M, Salpietro A, Bergbreiter A, Salzer U, Badolato R, Plebani A. A novel compound heterozygous TACI mutation in an autosomal recessive common variable immunodeficiency (CVID) family. Hum Immunol. 2012;73(8):836–9.
11. Salzer U, Bacchelli C, Buckridge S, Pan-Hammarstrom Q, Jennings S, Lougaris V, Bergbreiter A, Hagena T, Birmelin J, Plebani A, Webster ADB, Peter H-H, et al. Relevance of biallelic versus monoallelic TNFRSF13B mutations in distinguishing disease-causing from risk-increasing TNFRSF13B variants in antibody deficiency syndromes. Blood. 2009;113:1967–76.
12. Losi CG, Silini A, Fiorini C, Soresina A, Meini A, Ferrari S, Notarangelo LD, Lougaris V, Plebani A. Mutational analysis of human BAFF receptor TNFRSF13C (BAFF-R) in patients with common variable immunodeficiency. J Clin Immunol. 2005;25(5):496–502.
13. Pieper K, Rizzi M, Speletas M, Smulski CR, Sic H, Kraus H, Salzer U, Fiala GJ, Schamel WW, Lougaris V, Plebani A, Hammarstrom L, Recher M, Germenis AE, Grimbacher B, Warnatz K, Rolink AG, Schneider P, Notarangelo LD, Eibel H. A common single nucleotide polymorphism impairs B-cell activating factor receptor's multimerization, contributing to common variable immunodeficiency. J Allergy Clin Immunol. 2014;133:1222–5.
14. Warnatz K, Salzer U, Rizzi M, Fischer B, Gutenberger S, Böhm J, Kienzler AK, Pan-Hammarström Q, Hammarström L, Rakhmanov M, Schlesier M, Grimbacher B, Peter HH, Eibel H. B-cell activating factor receptor deficiency is associated with an adult-onset antibody deficiency syndrome in humans. Proc Natl Acad Sci U S A. 2009;106(33):13945–50.
15. Losi CG, Salzer U, Gatta R, Lougaris V, Cattaneo G, Meini A, Soresina A, Grimbacher B, Plebani A. Mutational analysis of human BLyS in patients with common variable immunodeficiency. J Clin Immunol. 2006;26(4):396–9.
16. Salzer U, Neumann C, Thiel J, Woellner C, Pan-Hammarström Q, Lougaris V, Hagena T, Jung J, Birmelin J, Du L, Metin A, Webster DA, Plebani A, Moschese V, Hammarström L, Schäffer AA, Grimbacher B. Screening of functional and positional candidate genes in families with common variable immunodeficiency. BMC Immunol. 2008;7(9):3.
17. van Zelm MC, Reisli I, van der Burg M, Castaño D, van Noesel CJ, van Tol MJ, Woellner C, Grimbacher B, Patiño PJ, van Dongen JJ, Franco JL. An antibody-deficiency syndrome due to mutations in the CD19 gene. N Engl J Med. 2006;354(18):1901–12.
18. Kanegane H, Agematsu K, Futatani T, Sira MM, Suga K, Sekiguchi T, van Zelm MC, Miyawaki T. Novel mutations in a Japanese patient with CD19 deficiency. Genes Immun. 2007;8(8):663–70.
19. Kuijpers TW, Bende RJ, Baars PA, Grummels A, Derks IA, Dolman KM, Beaumont T, Tedder TF, van Noesel CJ, Eldering E, van Lier RA. CD20 deficiency in humans results in impaired T cell-independent antibody responses. J Clin Invest. 2010;120(1):214–22.
20. van Zelm MC, Smet J, Adams B, Mascart F, Schandené L, Janssen F, Ferster A, Kuo CC, Levy S, van Dongen JJ, van der Burg M. CD81 gene defect in humans disrupts CD19 complex formation and leads to antibody deficiency. J Clin Invest. 2010;120(4):1265–74.
21. Thiel J, Kimmig L, Salzer U, Grudzien M, Lebrecht D, Hagena T, Draeger R, Völxen N, Bergbreiter A, Jennings S, Gutenberger S, Aichem A, Illges H, Hannan JP, Kienzler AK, Rizzi M, Eibel H, Peter HH, Warnatz K, Grimbacher B, Rump JA, Schlesier M. Genetic CD21 deficiency is associated with hypogammaglobulinemia. J Allergy Clin Immunol. 2012;129(3):801–10.
22. Salzer E, Santos-Valente E, Klaver S, Ban SA, Emminger W, Prengemann NK, Garncarz W, Müllauer L, Kain R, Boztug H, Heitger A, Arbeiter K, Eitelberger F, Seidel MG, Holter W, Pollak A, Pickl WF, Förster-Waldl E, Boztug K. B-cell deficiency and severe autoimmunity caused by deficiency of protein kinase C δ. Blood. 2013;121(16):3112–6.
23. Kuehn HS, Niemela JE, Rangel-Santos A, Zhang M, Pittaluga S, Stoddard JL, Hussey AA, Evbuomwan MO, Priel DA, Kuhns DB, Park CL, Fleisher TA, Uzel G, Oliveira JB. Loss-of-function of the protein kinase C δ (PKCδ) causes a B-cell lymphoproliferative syndrome in humans. Blood. 2013;121(16):3117–25.

24. Belot A, Kasher PR, Trotter EW, Foray AP, Debaud AL, Rice GI, Szynkiewicz M, Zabot MT, Rouvet I, Bhaskar SS, Daly SB, Dickerson JE, Mayer J, O'Sullivan J, Juillard L, Urquhart JE, Fawdar S, Marusiak AA, Stephenson N, Waszkowycz B, Beresford MW, Biesecker LG, Black GCM, René C, Eliaou JF, Fabien N, Ranchin B, Cochat P, Gaffney PM, Rozenberg F, Lebon P, Malcus C, Crow YJ, Brognard J, Bonnefoy N. Protein kinase cδ deficiency causes mendelian systemic lupus erythematosus with B cell-defective apoptosis and hyperproliferation. Arthritis Rheum. 2013;65(8):2161–71.
25. Angulo I, Vadas O, Garçon F, Banham-Hall E, Plagnol V, Leahy TR, et al. Phosphoinositide 3-kinase δ gene mutation predisposes to respiratory infection and airway damage. Science. 2013;342(6160):866–71.
26. Lucas CL, Kuehn HS, Zhao F, Niemela JE, Deenick EK, Palendira U, Avery DT, Moens L, Cannons JL, Biancalana M, Stoddard J, Ouyang W, Frucht DM, Rao VK, Atkinson TP, Agharahimi A, Hussey AA, Folio LR, Olivier KN, Fleisher TA, Pittaluga S, Holland SM, Cohen JI, Oliveira JB, Tangye SG, Schwartzberg PL, Lenardo MJ, Uzel G. Dominant-activating germline mutations in the gene encoding the PI(3)K catalytic subunit p110d result in T cell senescence and human immunodeficiency. Nat Immunol. 2014;15(1):88–97.
27. Kracker S, Curtis J, Ibrahim MA, Sediva A, Salisbury J, Campr V, Debré M, Edgar JD, Imai K, Picard C, Casanova JL, Fischer A, Nejentsev S, Durandy A. Occurrence of B-cell lymphomas in patients with activated phosphoinositide 3-kinase δ syndrome. J Allergy Clin Immunol. 2014;134(1):233–6.
28. Deau MC, Heurtier L, Frange P, Suarez F, Bole-Feysot C, Nitschke P, et al. A human immunodeficiency caused by mutations in the PIK3R1 gene. J Clin Invest. 2014;124(9):3923–8.
29. Lucas CL, Zhang Y, Venida A, Wang Y, Hughes J, McElwee J, et al. Heterozygous splice mutation in PIK3R1 causes human immunodeficiency with lymphoproliferation due to dominant activation of PI3K. J Exp Med. 2014;211(13):2537–47.
30. Lougaris V, Faletra F, Lanzi G, Vozzi D, Marcuzzi A, Valencic E, Piscianz E, Bianco A, Girardelli M, Baronio M, Loganes C, Fasth A, Salvini F, Trizzino A, Moratto D, Facchetti F, Giliani S, Plebani A, Tommasini A. Altered germinal center reaction and abnormal B cell peripheral maturation in PI3KR1-mutated patients presenting with HIGM-like phenotype. Clin Immunol. 2015;159(1):33–6.
31. Lougaris V, Patrizi O, Baronio M, Tabellini G, Tampella G, Lanzi G, Salvini F, Trizzino A, Parolini S, Plebani A. p85[a] is an intrinsic regulator of human natural killer effector functions. J Allergy Clin Immunol. 2016;138(2):605–608.e3. https://doi.org/10.1016/j.jaci.2016.01.026.
32. Ruiz-Garcia R, Vargas-Hernandez A, Chinn IK, Angelo LS, Cao TN, Coban-Akdemir Z, Jhangiani SN, Meng Q, Forbes LR, Muzny DM, Allende LM, Ehlayel MS, Gibbs RA, Lupski JR, Uzel G, Orange JS, Mace EM. Mutations in PI3K110D cause impaired natural killer cell function partially rescued by rapamycin treatment. J Allergy Clin Immunol. 2018;142:605–617.e7. https://doi.org/10.1016/j.jaci.2017.11.042.
33. Wang HY, Ma CA, Zhao Y, Fan X, Zhou Q, Edmonds P, Uzel G, Oliveira JB, Orange J, Jain A. Antibody deficiency associated with an inherited autosomal dominat mutation in TWEAK. Proc Natl Acad Sci U S A. 2013;110(13):5127–32.
34. Lopez-Herrera G, Tampella G, Pan-Hammarström Q, Herholz P, Trujillo-Vargas CM, Phadwal K, Simon AK, Moutschen M, Etzioni A, Mory A, Srugo I, Melamed D, Hultenby K, Liu C, Baronio M, Vitali M, Philippet P, Dideberg V, Aghamohammadi A, Rezaei N, Enright V, Du L, Salzer U, Eibel H, Pfeifer D, Veelken H, Stauss H, Lougaris V, Plebani A, Gertz EM, Schäffer AA, Hammarström L, Grimbacher B. Deleterious mutations in LRBA are associated with a syndrome of immune deficiency and autoimmunity. Am J Hum Genet. 2012;90(6):986–1001.
35. Burns SO, Zenner HL, Plagnol V, Curtis J, Mok K, Eisenhut M, Kumararatne D, Doffinger R, Thrasher AJ, Nejentsev S. LRBA gene deletion in a patient presenting with autoimmunity without hypogammaglobulinemia. J Allergy Clin Immunol. 2012;130(6):1428–32.
36. Gamez-Diaz L, August D, Stepensky P, Revel-Vilk S, Seidel MG, Noriko M, Morio T, AJJ W, Blessing J, Van de Veerdonk F, Feuchtinger T, Kanariou M, Schmitt-Graeff A, Jung S, Seneviratne S, Burns S, Belohradsky BH, Rezaei N, Bakthiar S, Speckmann C, Jordan M,

Grimbacher B. The extended phenotype of LPS-responsive beige-like anchor protein (LRBA) deficiency. J Allergy Clin Immunol. 2016;137(1):223–30.
37. Backthiar S, Gamez-Diaz L, Jarish A, Soerensen J, Grimbacher B, Belohradsky B, Keller KM, Rietschel C, Klingebiel T, Koletzko S, Albert MH, Bader P. Treatment of infantile inflammatory bowel disease and autoimmunity by allogeneic stem cell transplantation in LPS-responsive beige-like anchor deficiency. Front Immunol. 2017;8:52.
38. Chen K, Coonrod EM, Kumanovics A, Franks ZF, Durtschi JD, Margraf RL, Wu W, Heikal NM, Augustine NH, Ridge PG, Hill HR, Jorde LB, Weyrich AS, Zimmerman GA, Gundlapalli AV, Bohnsack JF, Voelkerding KV. Germline mutations in NFKB2 implicate the noncanonical NF-kB pathway in the pathogenesis of common variable immunodeficiency. Am J Hum Genet. 2013;93(5):812–24.
39. Lindsley AW, Qian Y, Valencia CA, Shah K, Zhang K, Assasd A. Combined immune deficiency in a patient with a novel NFKB2 mutation. J Clin Immunol. 2014;34(8):910–5.
40. Lee CE, Fulcher DA, Whittle B, Chand R, Fewings N, Field M, Andrews D, Goodnow CC, Cook MC. Autosomal dominant B cell deficiency with alopecia due to a mutation in NFKB2 that results in non processable p100. Blood. 2014;124(19):2964–72.
41. Lougaris V, Tabellini G, Vitali M, Baronio M, Patrizi O, Tampella G, Biasini A, Moratto D, Parolini S, Plebani A. Defective natural killer-cell cytotoxic activity in NFKB2-mutated CVID-like disease. J Allergy Clin Immunol. 2015;135:1641–3.
42. Fliegauf M, Bryant VL, Frede N, Slade C, Woon ST, Lehnert K, Winzer S, Bulashevska A, Scerri T, Leung E, Jordan A, Keller B, de Vries E, Cao H, Yang F, Schäffer AA, Warnatz K, Browett P, Douglass J, Ameratunga RV, van der Meer JW, Grimbacher B. Haploinsufficiency of the NF-kB1 subunit p50 in common variable immunodeficiency. Am J Hum Genet. 2015;97(3):389–403.
43. Lougaris V, Moratto D, Baronio M, Tampella G, van der Meer JW, Badolato R, Fliegauf M, Plebani A. Early and late B-cell developmental impairment in nuclear factor kappa B, subunit 1-mutated common variable immunodeficiency disease. J Allergy Clin Immunol. 2017;139:349–352.e1. https://doi.org/10.1016/j.jaci.2016.05.045.
44. Schipp C, Nabhani S, Bienemann K, Simanovsky N, Kfir-Erenfeld S, Assayag-Asherie N, Oommen PT, Revel-Vilk S, Honscheid A, Gombert M, Ginzel S, Schaffer D, Laws HJ, Yenenof E, Fleckenstein B, Borkhardt A, Stepensky P, Fischer U. Specific antibody deficiency and autoinflammatory disease extend the clinical and immunological spectrum of NFKB1 loss-of-function mutations in humans. Haematologica. 2016;101(10):e392–6.
45. Boztug H, Hirschmugl T, Holter W, Lakatos K, Kager L, Trapin D, Pickl W, Forster-Wadl E, Boztug K. Nf-kB1 haploinsufficiency causing immunodeficiency and EBV-driven lymphoproliferation. J Clin Immunol. 2016;36(6):533–40.
46. Lougaris V, Patrizi O, Baronio M, Tabellini G, Tampella G, Damiati E, Frede N, van der Meer JW, Fliegauf M, Grimbacher B, Parolini S, Plebani A. NFKB1 regulates human NK cell maturation and effector functions. Clin Immunol. 2017;175:99–108. https://doi.org/10.1016/j.clim.2016.11.012.
47. Schubert D, Bode C, Kenefeck R, Hou TZ, Wing JB, Kennedy A, Bulashevska A, Petersen BS, Schäffer AA, Grüning BA, Unger S, Frede N, Baumann U, Witte T, Schmidt RE, Dueckers G, Niehues T, Seneviratne S, Kanariou M, Speckmann C, Ehl S, Rensing-Ehl A, Warnatz K, Rakhmanov M, Thimme R, Hasselblatt P, Emmerich F, Cathomen T, Backofen R, Fisch P, Seidl M, May A, Schmitt-Graeff A, Ikemizu S, Salzer U, Franke A, Sakaguchi S, Walker LSK, Sansom DM, Grimbacher B. Autosomal dominant immune dysregulation in humans with CTLA4 mutations. Nat Med. 2014;20(12):1410–6. https://doi.org/10.1038/nm.3746.
48. Kuehn HS, Ouyang W, Lo B, Deenick EK, Niemela JE, Avery DT, Schickel JN, Tran DQ, Stoddard J, Zhang Y, Frucht DM, Dumitriu B, Scheinberg P, Folio LR, Frein CA, Price S, Koh C, Heller T, Seroogy CM, Huttenlocher A, Rao VK, Su HC, Kleiner D, Notarangelo LD, Rampertaap Y, Olivier KN, McElwee J, Hughes J, Pittaluga S, Oliveira JB, Meffre E, Fleisher TA, Holland SM, Lenardo MJ, Tangye SG, Uzel G. Immune dysregulation in human subjects with heterozygous germline mutations in CTLA-4. Science. 2014;345(6204):1623–7. https://doi.org/10.1126/science.1255904.

49. Miska J, Lui JB, Toomer KH, Devarajan P, Cai X, Houghton J, Lopez DM, Abreu MT, Wang G, Chen Z. Initiation of inflammatory tumorigenesis by CTLA4 insufficiency due to type 2 cytokines. J Exp Med. 2018;215:841–58.
50. Lo B, Zhang K, Lu W, Zheng L, Zhang Q, Kanellopoulou C, Zhang Y, Liu Z, Fritz JM, Marsh R, Husami A, Kissell D, Nortman S, Chaturvedi V, Haines H, Young LR, Mo J, Filipovich AH, Bleesing JJ, Mustillo P, Stephens M, Rueda CM, Chougnet CA, Hoebe K, McElwee J, Hughes JD, Karakoc-Aydiner E, Matthews HF, Price S, Su HC, Rao VK, Lenardo MJ, Jordan MD. Autoimmune disease: patients with LRBA deficiency show CTLA4 loss and immune dysregulation responsive to abatacept therapy. Science. 2015;349(6246):436–40.
51. Alroqi FJ, Charbonnier LM, Baris S, Kiykim A, Chou J, Platt CD, Algassim A, Keles S, Al Saud BK, Alkuraya FS, Jordan M, Geha RS, Chatila TA. Exaggerated follicular helper T cell responses in patients with LRBA deficiency caused by failure of CTLA4-mediated regulation. J Allergy Clin Immunol. 2018;141:1050–1059.e10. https://doi.org/10.1016/j.jaci.2017.05.022.
52. Sekine H, Ferreira RC, Pan-Hammarström Q, Graham RR, Ziemba B, de Vries SS, Liu J, Hippen K, Koeuth T, Ortmann W, Iwahori A, Elliott MK, Offer S, Skon C, Du L, Novitzke J, Lee AT, Zhao N, Tompkins JD, Altshuler D, Gregersen PK, Cunningham-Rundles C, Harris RS, Her C, Nelson DL, Hammarström L, Gilkeson GS, Behrens TW. Role for Msh5 in the regulation of Ig class switch recombination. Proc Natl Acad Sci U S A. 2007;104(17):7193–8.
53. Sobacchi C, Marrella V, Rucci F, Vezzoni P, Villa A. RAG-dependent primary immunodeficiencies. Hum Mutat. 2006;27(12):1174–84. Review
54. Abolhassani H, Wang N, Aghamohammadi A, Rezaei N, Lee YN, Frugoni F, Notarangelo LD, Pan-Hammarström Q, Hammarström L. A hypomorphic recombination-activating gene 1 (RAG1) mutation resulting in a phenotype resembling common variable immunodeficiency. J Allergy Clin Immunol. 2014;134(6):1375–80. https://doi.org/10.1016/j.jaci.2014.04.042.
55. Buchbinder D, Baker R, Lee YN, Ravell J, Zhang Y, McElwee J, Nugent D, Coonrod EM, Durtschi JD, Augustine NH, Voelkerding KV, Csomos K, Rosen L, Browne S, Walter JE, Notarangelo LD, Hill HR, Kumánovics A. Identification of patients with RAG mutations previously diagnosed with common variable immunodeficiency disorders. J Clin Immunol. 2015;35(2):119–24. https://doi.org/10.1007/s10875-014-0121-5.
56. Schröder C, Baerlecken NT, Pannicke U, Dörk T, Witte T, Jacobs R, Stoll M, Schwarz K, Grimbacher B, Schmidt RE, Atschekzei F. Evaluation of RAG1 mutations in an adult with combined immunodeficiency and progressive multifocal leukoencephalopathy. Clin Immunol. 2017;179:1–7. https://doi.org/10.1016/j.clim.2016.12.013.

ICOS Deficiency

6

Ulrich Salzer

6.1 Definition

ICOS deficiency is an autosomal recessive inherited primary immunodeficiency and was the first monogenetic defect described in CVID. Although originally described in two families presenting mainly with an antibody deficiency and bacterial infections, additional patients broadened the phenotype to a combined immunodeficiency including frequent autoimmune manifestations.

6.2 Etiology

ICOS (inducible costimulator) belongs to the B7 family of ligands and receptors which are expressed on the surface of immune cells. Its closest relatives are CD28, cytotoxic T-lymphocyte antigen-4 (CTLA-4; CD152), and programmed cell death-1 (PD-1) (reviewed in [1–3]). ICOS and CD28 mediate costimulatory signals when engaged by their respective ligands. In contrast, CTLA-4 and PD-1 counteract the costimulation induced by ICOS and CD28. CD28 is readily expressed on resting T cells, whereas CTLA-4, PD-1, and ICOS are expressed only after T-cell activation. ICOS binds its unique ligand, ICOS-L [synonyms: CD275, ligand of ICOS (LICOS), hGL50, B7h, B7RP-1, and B7-H2] [4]. ICOS-L is expressed in a variety of tissues by both lymphoid and non-lymphoid cells. Proinflammatory stimuli promote its

U. Salzer (✉)
Faculty of Medicine, Department of Rheumatology and Clinical Immunology, Medical Center—University of Freiburg, Freiburg im Breisgau, Germany

Faculty of Medicine, Center for Chronic Immunodeficiency (CCI), Medical Center—University of Freiburg, Freiburg im Breisgau, Germany
e-mail: ulrich.salzer@uniklinik-freiburg.de

M. M. D'Elios, M. Rizzi (eds.), *Humoral Primary Immunodeficiencies*, Rare Diseases of the Immune System, https://doi.org/10.1007/978-3-319-91785-6_6

upregulation [5]. The human ICOS gene is located on the chromosomal region 2q33–34 together with the genes for CTLA-4 and CD28, clustering within a tight 300 kb region [6, 7]. The ICOS gene has five exons encoding a 2620-nucleotide-long mRNA which translates into a 199 amino acid protein expressed as a 55–60 kDa disulfide-linked homodimer (Fig. 6.1a) [4, 8]. Whereas constitutive expression is usually very low or absent, expression of ICOS is rapidly induced on T cells after activation by both T-cell receptor and CD28 signaling [6, 8–10]. In addition, ICOS can be upregulated by IL-4 in mice [11], and ICOS is expressed at higher levels on Th2 cells [6]. In contrast, IL-12 and IL-23 but not IL-4 enhance ICOS expression on human T cells [12]. ICOS expression is highly regulated, and its deregulated expression leads to an SLE-like phenotype in mice [13]. This regulation is initiated by the ubiquitin ligase Roquin [14] and mediated at the posttranscriptional level by micro-RNAs [15].

The intracellular domain of ICOS carries a YMFM motif capable of binding to the p85a subunit of phosphatidylinositol-3-kinase (PI3K) (Fig. 6.1a), showing similarity to the YMNM motif found in CD28 [6]. In addition CD28 and ICOS share other signaling pathways like Erk1/2, protein kinase B, and phosphoinositide-dependent kinase-1, p38 [16]. Signaling through ICOS (and CD28) induces proliferation, T-cell survival, and differentiation. ICOS is a co-inducer of IL-4, IL-5, IL-6, granulocyte-macrophage colony-stimulating factor, TNF-α, and interferon gamma (IFN-γ). More importantly ICOS superinduces IL-10 [8]. Both CD28 and ICOS are involved in the development and homeostasis of regulatory T cells (Tregs) [17, 18].

ICOS plays a distinct role in germinal center (GC) formation in lymphatic tissues, where ICOS controls the generation of C–C chemokine receptor type 5 (CXCR5)-positive follicular T-helper cells (TFH) [19], on which it is highly

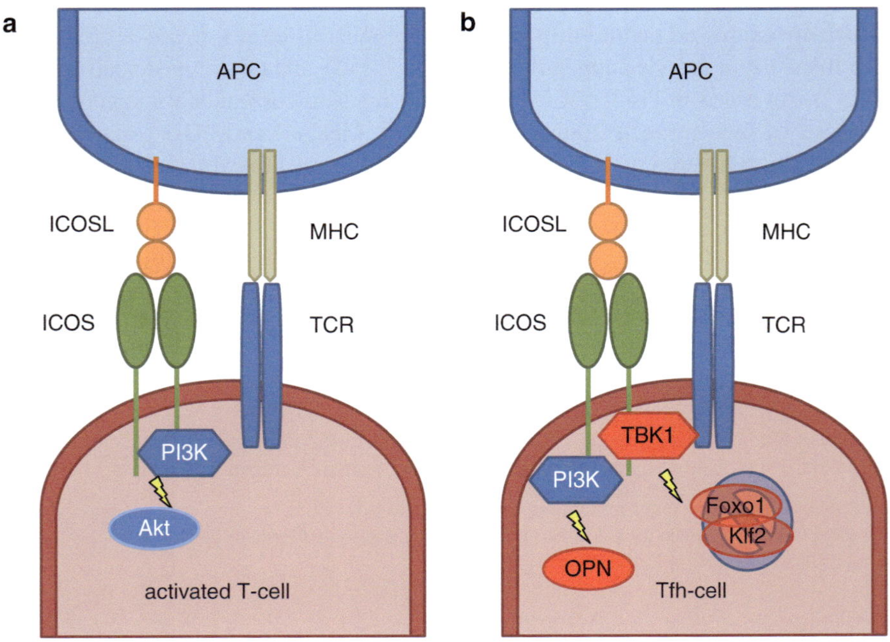

Fig. 6.1 ICOS signaling pathways in T cells (**a**) and follicular T-helper cells (**b**)

expressed within the light zone of the GC [20]. ICOS signaling drives the migration of TFH cells from the T–B cell margin region into the follicles via two pathways: ICOS-dependent upregulation of CXCR5 (reviewed in [21]) attracts T cells into the B-cell follicle guided by the chemokine ligand chemokine (C–X–C motif) ligand 13, which is produced by follicular dendritic cells. Secondly, ICOS induces IL-10 [22] and IL-21 in TFH [23], which help to maintain GCs and support the differentiation of B cells into class-switched memory cells and long-lived plasma cells [24]. CD8α dendritic cells expressing ICOSL initiate the program of TFH differentiation [25], whereas B cells are required for their maintenance [26].

The ICOS intracellular domain was recently shown to be exclusively able to bind the signaling adaptor TBK1, which is a member of the inhibitor of NF-kB kinase family (Fig. 6.1b) [27]. The signaling via TBK1 was shown to be essential for the generation of TFH cells. The interaction of ICOS with TBK1 leads to inactivation of FOXO1, which in turn downregulates Klf2, thereby derepressing the TFH transcriptional program [28, 29]. In addition, ICOS promotes nuclear localization of osteopontin (OPN) via PI3K signaling, which stabilizes Bcl6, the major TFH transcription factor, by repressing its ubiquitination (Fig. 6.1b) [30].

6.3 Clinical Manifestations

A total of 16 patients from 7 families have been reported with ICOS deficiency [31]. All observed mutations were deleterious leading to absent ICOS protein expression (Fig. 6.2). In four families with a large genomic deletion covering ICOS exons 2 and 3, a common ancestor is assumed [32, 33]. The other three families all showed mutations in ICOS exon 2, two were single-nucleotide deletions [34, 35] and one a 10 bp deletion [36]. Both childhood and adult onset of symptoms were observed [31]. Recurrent bacterial infections of the respiratory tract were the most common manifestation, but patients also suffered from infections caused by herpes simplex virus and cytomegalovirus, and one patient developed a *Pneumocystis jirovecii* infection [34]. Infections of the gastrointestinal tract, which were mostly of bacterial origin, occurred in several ICOS-deficient patients [31].

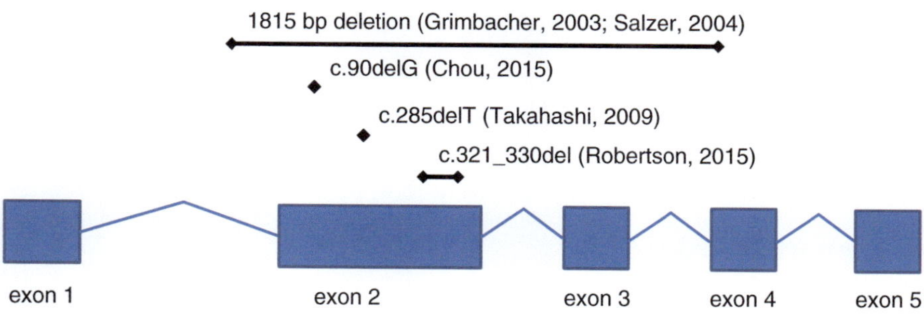

Fig. 6.2 Structure of the ICOS gene and schematic representation of known mutations

Disorders of autoimmunity and immune dysregulation were noted in about three quarter of the patients. These included enteropathy, arthritis, psoriasis, splenomegaly, cytopenias, and granulomas [31]. Two patients developed malignancy, one HPV-associated vulvar carcinoma and one T-cell derived large granular lymphocyte lymphoma [31].

All but one ICOS-deficient patient had hypogammaglobulinemia, and vaccination responses usually were negative. In all patients TFH cells and switched memory B cells were reduced, reflecting the disturbed GC reaction [31]. Total B-cell numbers were normal in children but declined in adults. This may be due to reduced bone marrow B-cell output caused by a partial block in bone marrow B-cell development at the pre-BI stage, which was observed in some ICOS-deficient patients [37]. Overall the T-cell and B-cell phenotypes varied considerably between the different families [31].

6.4 Diagnosis

Since all currently known mutations in ICOS are deleterious and result in absent protein expression, analysis of ICOS on activated T cells by flow cytometry may be used as a diagnostic screening test in suspected patients. The final diagnosis, however, requires genetic analysis by DNA sequencing.

6.5 Management

Immunoglobulin substitution and antibiotic treatment of breakthrough infections are the mainstays of treatment for ICOS deficiency, like for CVID in general [31]. In the planning of monitoring, the high rates of autoimmune and immunedysregulatory complications should be taken into account. In addition, because of the occurrence of viral and opportunistic infections in some ICOS-deficient patients, the disorder may be regarded as combined immunodeficiency and consequently also treated and followed up as such a disease. In cases of conventional treatment failure, hematopoietic stem cell transplantation may be considered [31].

References

1. Carreno BM, Collins M. The B7 family of ligands and its receptors: new pathways for costimulation and inhibition of immune responses. Annu Rev Immunol. 2002;20:29–53.
2. Greenwald RJ, Freeman GJ, Sharpe AH. The B7 family revisited. Annu Rev Immunol. 2005;23:515–48.
3. Sharpe AH, Freeman GJ. The B7-CD28 superfamily. Nat Rev Immunol. 2002;2:116–26.
4. Hutloff A, Dittrich AM, Beier KC, Eljaschewitsch B, Kraft R, Anagnostopoulos I, Kroczek RA. ICOS is an inducible T-cell co-stimulator structurally and functionally related to CD28. Nature. 1999;397:263–6.

5. Swallow MM, Wallin JJ, Sha WC. B7h, a novel costimulatory homolog of B7.1 and B7.2, is induced by TNFalpha. Immunity. 1999;11:423–32.
6. Coyle AJ, Lehar S, Lloyd C, Tian J, Delaney T, Manning S, Nguyen T, Burwell T, Schneider H, Gonzalo JA, Gosselin M, Owen LR, Rudd CE, Gutierrez-Ramos JC. The CD28-related molecule ICOS is required for effective T cell-dependent immune responses. Immunity. 2000;13:95–105.
7. Ling V, Wu PW, Finnerty HF, Agostino MJ, Graham JR, Chen S, Jussiff JM, Fisk GJ, Miller CP, Collins M. Assembly and annotation of human chromosome 2q33 sequence containing the CD28, CTLA4, and ICOS gene cluster: analysis by computational, comparative, and microarray approaches. Genomics. 2001;78:155–68.
8. Beier KC, Hutloff A, Dittrich AM, Heuck C, Rauch A, Büchner K, Ludewig B, Ochs HD, Mages HW, Kroczek RA. Induction, binding specificity and function of human ICOS. Eur J Immunol. 2000;30:3707–17.
9. Okamoto N, Tezuka K, Kato M, Abe R, Tsuji T. PI3-kinase and MAP-kinase signaling cascades in AILIM/ICOS- and CD28-costimulated T-cells have distinct functions between cell proliferation and IL-10 production. Biochem Biophys Res Commun. 2003;310:691–702.
10. Parry RV, Rumbley CA, Vandenberghe LH, June CH, Riley JL. CD28 and inducible costimulatory protein Src homology 2 binding domains show distinct regulation of phosphatidylinositol 3-kinase, Bcl-xL, and IL-2 expression in primary human CD4 T lymphocytes. J Immunol. 2003;171:166–74.
11. Yagi J, Arimura Y, Dianzani U, Uede T, Okamoto T, Uchiyama T. Regulatory roles of IL-2 and IL-4 in H4/inducible costimulator expression on activated CD4+ T cells during Th cell development. J Immunol. 2003;171:783–94.
12. Wassink L, Vieira PL, Smits HH, Kingsbury GA, Coyle AJ, Kapsenberg ML, Wierenga EA. ICOS expression by activated human Th cells is enhanced by IL-12 and IL-23: increased ICOS expression enhances the effector function of both Th1 and Th2 cells. J Immunol. 2004;173:1779–86.
13. Vinuesa CG, Cook MC, Angelucci C, Athanasopoulos V, Rui L, Hill KM, Yu D, Domaschenz H, Whittle B, Lambe T, Roberts IS, Copley RR, Bell JI, Cornall RJ, Goodnow CC. A RING-type ubiquitin ligase family member required to repress follicular helper T cells and autoimmunity. Nature. 2005a;435:452–8.
14. Yu D, Tan AH, Hu X, Athanasopoulos V, Simpson N, Silva DG, Hutloff A, Giles KM, Leedman PJ, Lam KP, Goodnow CC, Vinuesa CG. Roquin represses autoimmunity by limiting inducible T-cell co-stimulator messenger RNA. Nature. 2007;450:299–303.
15. Glasmacher E, Hoefig KP, Vogel KU, Rath N, Du L, Wolf C, Kremmer E, Wang X, Heissmeyer V. Roquin binds inducible costimulator mRNA and effectors of mRNA decay to induce microRNA-independent post-transcriptional repression. Nat Immunol. 2010;11:725–33.
16. Arimura Y, Kato H, Dianzani U, Okamoto T, Kamekura S, Buonfiglio D, Miyoshi-Akiyama T, Uchiyama T, Yagi J. A co-stimulatory molecule on activated T cells, H4/ICOS, delivers specific signals in T(h) cells and regulates their responses. Int Immunol. 2002;14:555–66.
17. Herman AE, Freeman GJ, Mathis D, Benoist C. CD4+CD25+ T regulatory cells dependent on ICOS promote regulation of effector cells in the prediabetic lesion. J Exp Med. 2004;199:1479–89.
18. Salomon B, Lenschow DJ, Rhee L, Ashourian N, Singh B, Sharpe A, Bluestone JA. B7/CD28 costimulation is essential for the homeostasis of the CD4+CD25+ immunoregulatory T cells that control autoimmune diabetes. Immunity. 2000;12:431–40.
19. Bossaller L, Burger J, Draeger R, Grimbacher B, Knoth R, Plebani A, Durandy A, Baumann U, Schlesier M, Welcher AA, Peter HH, Warnatz K. ICOS deficiency is associated with a severe reduction of CXCR5+CD4 germinal center Th cells. J Immunol. 2006;177:4927–32.
20. Kim CH, Rott LS, Clark-Lewis I, Campbell DJ, Wu L, Butcher EC. Subspecialization of CXCR5+ T cells: B helper activity is focused in a germinal center-localized subset of CXCR5+ T cells. J Exp Med. 2001;193:1373–81.
21. Vinuesa CG, Tangye SG, Moser B, Mackay CR. Follicular B helper T cells in antibody responses and autoimmunity. Nat Rev Immunol. 2005b;5:853–65.

22. Witsch EJ, Peiser M, Hutloff A, Büchner K, Dorner BG, Jonuleit H, Mages HW, Kroczek RA. ICOS and CD28 reversely regulate IL-10 on re-activation of human effector T cells with mature dendritic cells. Eur J Immunol. 2002;32:2680–6.
23. Bauquet AT, Jin H, Paterson AM, Mitsdoerffer M, Ho IC, Sharpe AH, Kuchroo VK. The costimulatory molecule ICOS regulates the expression of c-Maf and IL-21 in the development of follicular T helper cells and TH-17 cells. Nat Immunol. 2009;10:167–75.
24. Ozaki K, Spolski R, Ettinger R, Kim HP, Wang G, Qi CF, Hwu P, Shaffer DJ, Akilesh S, Roopenian DC, Morse HC 3rd, Lipsky PE, Leonard WJ. Regulation of B cell differentiation and plasma cell generation by IL-21, a novel inducer of Blimp-1 and Bcl-6. J Immunol. 2004;173:5361–71.
25. Shin C, Han JA, Koh H, Choi B, Cho Y, Jeong H, Ra JS, Sung PS, Shin EC, Ryu S, Do Y. CD8α(−) dendritic cells induce antigen-specific T follicular helper cells generating efficient humoral immune responses. Cell Rep. 2015;11:1929–40.
26. Choi YS, Kageyama R, Eto D, Escobar TC, Johnston RJ, Monticelli L, Lao C, Crotty S. ICOS receptor instructs T follicular helper cell versus effector cell differentiation via induction of the transcriptional repressor Bcl6. Immunity. 2011;34:932–46.
27. Pedros C, Zhang Y, Hu JK, Choi YS, Canonigo-Balancio AJ, Yates JR 3rd, Altman A, Crotty S, Kong KF. A TRAF-like motif of the inducible costimulator ICOS controls development of germinal center TFH cells via the kinase TBK1. Nat Immunol. 2016;17:825–33.
28. Stone EL, Pepper M, Katayama CD, Kerdiles YM, Lai CY, Emslie E, Lin YC, Yang E, Goldrath AW, Li MO, Cantrell DA, Hedrick SM. ICOS coreceptor signaling inactivates the transcription factor FOXO1 to promote Tfh cell differentiation. Immunity. 2015;42:239–51.
29. Weber JP, Fuhrmann F, Feist RK, Lahmann A, Al Baz MS, Gentz LJ, Vu Van D, Mages HW, Haftmann C, Riedel R, Grün JR, Schuh W, Kroczek RA, Radbruch A, Mashreghi MF, Hutloff A. ICOS maintains the T follicular helper cell phenotype by down-regulating Krüppel-like factor 2. J Exp Med. 2015;212:217–33.
30. Leavenworth JW, Verbinnen B, Yin J, Huang H, Cantor H. A p85α-osteopontin axis couples the receptor ICOS to sustained Bcl-6 expression by follicular helper and regulatory T cells. Nat Immunol. 2015;16:96–106.
31. Schepp J, Chou J, Skrabl-Baumgartner A, Arkwright PD, Engelhardt KR, Hambleton S, Morio T, Röther E, Warnatz K, Geha R, Grimbacher B. 14 years after discovery: clinical follow-up on 15 patients with inducible co-stimulator deficiency. Front Immunol. 2017;8:964.
32. Grimbacher B, Hutloff A, Schlesier M, Glocker E, Warnatz K, Dräger R, Eibel H, Fischer B, Schäffer AA, Mages HW, Kroczek RA, Peter HH. Homozygous loss of ICOS is associated with adult-onset common variable immunodeficiency. Nat Immunol. 2003;4:261–8.
33. Salzer U, Maul-Pavicic A, Cunningham-Rundles C, Urschel S, Belohradsky BH, Litzman J, Holm A, Franco JL, Plebani A, Hammarstrom L, Skrabl A, Schwinger W, Grimbacher B. ICOS deficiency in patients with common variable immunodeficiency. Clin Immunol. 2004;113:234–40.
34. Chou J, Massaad MJ, Cangemi B, Bainter W, Platt C, Badran YR, Raphael BP, Kamin DS, Goldsmith JD, Pai SY, Al-Herz W, Geha RS. A novel mutation in ICOS presenting as hypogammaglobulinemia with susceptibility to opportunistic pathogens. J Allergy Clin Immunol. 2015;136:794–797.e1.
35. Takahashi N, Matsumoto K, Saito H, Nanki T, Miyasaka N, Kobata T, Azuma M, Lee SK, Mizutani S, Morio T. Impaired CD4 and CD8 effector function and decreased memory T cell populations in ICOS-deficient patients. J Immunol. 2009;182:5515–27.
36. Robertson N, Engelhardt KR, Morgan NV, Barge D, Cant AJ, Hughes SM, Abinun M, Xu Y, Koref MS, Arkwright PD, Hambleton S. Astute clinician report: a novel 10 bp frameshift deletion in exon 2 of ICOS causes a combined immunodeficiency associated with an enteritis and hepatitis. J Clin Immunol. 2015;35:598–603.
37. Warnatz K, Bossaller L, Salzer U, Skrabl-Baumgartner A, Schwinger W, van der Burg M, van Dongen JJ, Orlowska-Volk M, Knoth R, Durandy A, Draeger R, Schlesier M, Peter HH, Grimbacher B. Human ICOS deficiency abrogates the germinal center reaction and provides a monogenic model for common variable immunodeficiency. Blood. 2006;107:3045–52.

CD19 Deficiency due to Genetic Defects in the *CD19* and *CD81* Genes

7

Menno C. van Zelm and Ismail Reisli

7.1 Identification and Characterization of CD19 and Complex Members CD21, CD81, and CD225

In 1983, CD19 was first described to be a membrane marker specifically expressed on B cells [1]. Importantly, it was expressed on mature B cells as well as early progenitors, even prior to surface immunoglobulin (Ig) and two previously characterized markers that are now known as CD20 [2] and CD21 [3] (Fig. 7.1).

Several years later, the *CD19* gene was cloned and turned out to encode a single transmembrane protein with an N-terminal extracellular domain containing two Ig-like domains and a C-terminal intracellular tail with conserved tyrosine residues necessary for intracellular signaling [4, 5] (Fig. 7.1). CD19 was found to directly bind to CD21 (complement receptor 2; CR2) [6], which binds to complement fragment C3d and is the receptor for Epstein-Barr virus (EBV) [7–9]. Two other components of the same complex were found to be CD81 (TAPA-1) and CD225 (encoded by the *IFITM1* gene) [10]. CD81 and CD225 had been identified before [11, 12] and were found to bind each other [13]. The proteins are not lineage-restricted and bind each other independent of CD19 or CD21. Conversely, CD19 expression does require the presence of CD81 [14–16], and in turn CD19 directly

As part of: "Humoral Primary Immunodeficiencies" by Springer press, edited by Mario D'Elios and Martha Rizzi

M. C. van Zelm (✉)
Department of Immunology and Pathology, Central Clinical School, Monash University and The Alfred Hospital, Melbourne, VIC, Australia
e-mail: menno.vanzelm@monash.edu

I. Reisli
Division of Pediatric Allergy and Immunology, Department of Pediatrics, Meram Medical Faculty, Necmettin Erbakan University, Konya, Turkey

M. M. D'Elios, M. Rizzi (eds.), *Humoral Primary Immunodeficiencies*, Rare Diseases of the Immune System, https://doi.org/10.1007/978-3-319-91785-6_7

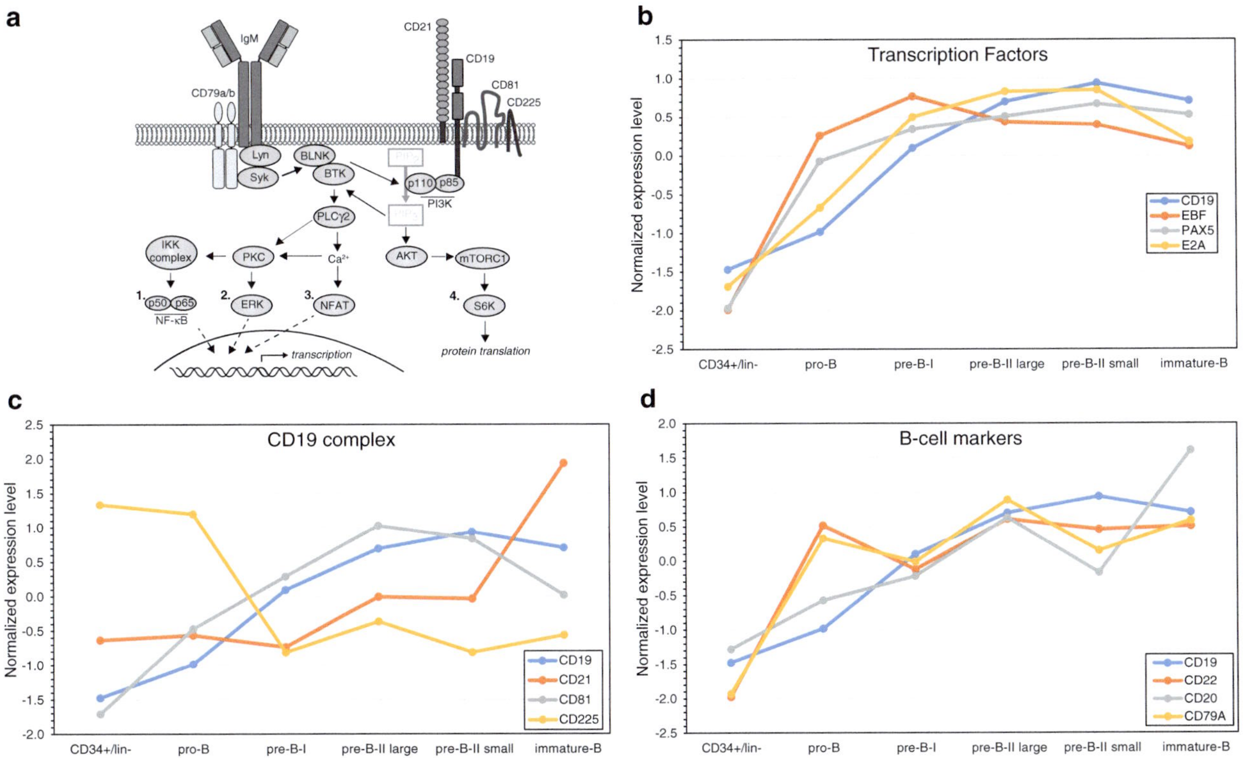

Fig. 7.1 CD19 complex function and gene expression levels in B-cell precursors. (**a**) Upon antigen recognition, the BCR induces a signaling cascade. The CD19 complex acts to lower the threshold for activation through recruitment of phosphoinositide 3-kinase (PI3K). Together, these signals induce nuclear translocation of at least three transcription factors (NF-kB, ERK, and NFAT) and stimulate protein translation. (**b–d**) Gene expression levels of CD19 complex members (**b**), other B-cell markers (**c**), and transcription factors (**d**). Data are derived from purified B-cell precursors using Affymetrix HG-U133A/B Gene Chips, and data were normalized into zero mean and unit standard deviation (z-score) [47]

binds CD21 [6]. The complex of CD19/CD21/CD81/CD225 is fully formed on immature and mature B cells (Fig. 7.1) and functions to augment signaling through surface immunoglobulins (B-cell antigen receptor; BCR) [10, 17].

B-cell lineage commitment from hematopoietic stem cells is a stepwise process and critically depends on several transcription factors, including E2A, EBF, and Pax5 [18–20]. In addition to functioning as B-cell commitment factor, Pax5 directly regulates CD19 gene expression [21]. As a result, CD19 membrane expression is a direct marker of committed B cells and is reflective of the expression of Pax5 (Fig. 7.1).

7.2 Antibody Deficiency due to CD19 Defects

As CD19 is reliable marker for B cells and good antibodies have been available since the early 1980s, it is generally included in diagnostic work-up of immunological and hematological diseases. Thus, defective CD19 expression can be readily assessed from peripheral blood lymphocytes, and this has formed the basis of the first description of CD19-deficient individuals [22]. Until that time, genetic defects underlying predominantly antibody deficiencies (PAD) had only been identified in patients with agammaglobulinemia and a complete lack of B cells and in patients with a defect in germinal center responses and Ig class-switch recombination [23]. CD19-deficient patients differed from both groups in regard to the presence of B cells in blood and normal architecture of germinal centers in lymphoid tissue despite hypogammaglobulinemia [22, 24–29].

In total, 11 patients from 8 families have been described with a CD19 deficiency (Table 7.1). Ten patients have biallelic genetic defects in *CD19* (Fig. 7.2), and all but one were homozygous. Although not all parents from patients with homozygous defects were confirmed to be relatives, taking into account the rarity of the mutant alleles, CD19 deficiency is most likely to be found in children from consanguineous parents. Remarkably, the heterozygous splice site mutation c.947-1G>T from Japanese patient C1 was also found in homozygous state in French patient G1. Considering the different genetic backgrounds, it is likely that these events occurred independently and that to date eight unique genetic lesions in *CD19* have been described. These concerned four small insertions and/or deletions, one large deletion, and two splice site mutations that all resulted in complete absence of truncated CD19 proteins. In only one case, a missense mutation concerning a conserved tryptophan resulted in the complete absence of membrane CD19 [27]. The complete absence of CD19 membrane expression resulted in reduced CD21 expression levels, but did not affect CD81 or CD225 expression (Fig. 7.3).

The 11th patient (H1) did not carry mutations in her *CD19* alleles (Fig. 7.2). Instead, a homozygous splice site mutation was identified in the *CD81* gene that disrupted membrane expression of both CD19 and CD81 (Fig. 7.3) [26]. CD21 was only slightly reduced and CD225 normally expressed on the patient's B cells. Using in vitro complementation experiments, it was demonstrated that the defective CD81 expression resulted in the absence of CD19 on the patient's B cells. These results confirmed and extended previous observations of the dependence of CD19 membrane expression in CD81 [14–16].

Table 7.1 Epidemiological, genetic, and clinical characteristics of all CD19 deficiency cases that have been reported to date

Patient	Descent	Gene	Gender	Age at onset	Age at diagnosis	Presenting manifestations	Clinical manifestations before diagnosis	Clinical manifestations at diagnosis	Treatment	Outcome	Reference
A1	Turkish	CD19	F	1	10	LRI	Recurrent LRI and meningitis	COPD, postinfectious GN	IVIG	Mild SLE, good	[22, 25]
A2			M	0.5	12	Recurrent URI/LRI	Recurrent LRI and otitis	Recurrent URI/LRI	IVIG	Good	
B1	Colombian	CD19	M	7	35	URI	Recurrent LRI, chronic sinusitis	LRI, bacterial conjunctivitis, gastritis	IVIG, sinus surgery	Good	[22]
B2			F	6	33	URI	LRI, herpes zoster, chronic sinusitis	Recurrent bacterial conjunctivitis/dacryocystitis, diarrhea	IVIG, sinus surgery	Good	
B3			F	5	49	URI	Recurrent LRI, recurrent skin abscesses, chronic sinusitis	LRI, recurrent bacterial conjunctivitis, chronic diarrhea	IVIG, sinus surgery	Good	
C1	Japanese	CD19	M	5	8[a]	Pyelonephritis, bronchitis, gastritis, thrombocytopenia	NR	Pyelonephritis, bronchitis, gastritis, thrombocytopenia	IVIGs	Good	[24]
D1	Moroccan	CD19	M	NR	6	URI/LRI	Recurrent URI/LRI, *S. pneumoniae* septicemia	Recurrent URI/LRI	IVIG, SCIG	Good	[27]

E1	Kurdish	CD19	F	5	11	URI, giardiasis	Recurrent URI	Pneumococcal meningitis	NR	Good	[28]
F1	Moroccan	CD19	F	13	31	Failure to thrive, microscopic hematuria, proteinuria	Chronic sinusitis, pneumococcal pneumonia	IgA nephropathy, nephrotic syndrome	Sinus surgery	Nephrotic syndrome/ESRD	[28]
G1	French	CD19	M	3mo	11[b]	RSV bronchiolitis, asthma mimicking symptoms	Asthma resembling symptoms Recurrent URI/ LRI	Bronchiectasis, lobar atelectasis, COPD	IVIG, lobectomy	Chronic lung disease	[29]
H1	Moroccan	CD81	F	2	6[c]	NR	IgA nephropathy, Henoch-Schönlein purpura	Thrombocytopenia, hypogammaglobulinemia	IVIG, immune suppression	Nephrotic syndrome/ESRD	[26]

Table adapted from [29]

COPD chronic obstructive pulmonary disease, *ESRD* end-stage renal disease, *F* female, *GN* glomerulonephritis, *IVIGs* intravenous immunoglobulins, *LRI* lower respiratory infection, *M* male, *NR* non-reported, *RSV* respiratory syncytial virus, *SCIGs* subcutaneous immunoglobulins, *URI* upper respiratory infection

[a]Diagnosis of CVID and IVIG therapy at age of 5 year, genetic diagnosis of CD19 deficiency at age of 8 year

[b]Diagnosis of hypogammaglobulinemia and IVIG therapy at age of 7 year, genetic diagnosis of CD19 deficiency at age of 11 year

[c]Diagnosis of IgA nephropathy and Henoch-Schönlein purpura at age of 3.5 year, genetic diagnosis of CD19 deficiency and start IVIG at age of 6 year

a

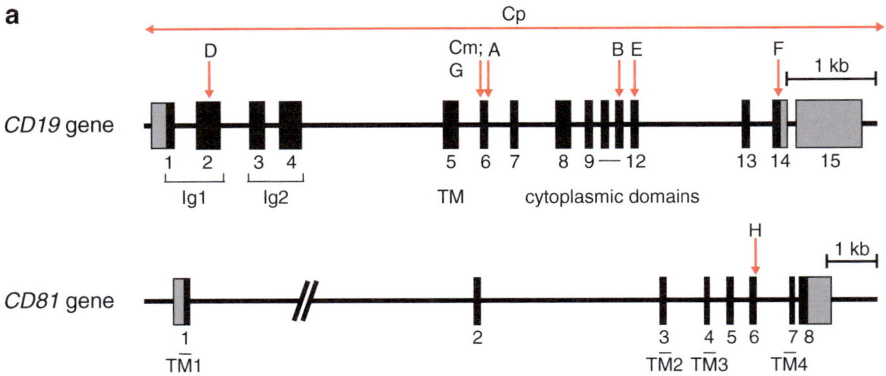

b

family	descent	patients	gene	allele	mutation	effect on protein	reference
A	Turkish	2	*CD19*	both	c.972insA	p.R325A fsX4	22, 25
B	Colombian	3	*CD19*	both	c.1384delGA	p.N463R fsX3	22
C	Japanese	1	*CD19*	maternal paternal	c.947-1G>T deletion of entire gene	p.A316D fsX5 p.X	24
D	Moroccan	1	*CD19*	both	c.156G>C	p.W52C	27
E	Kurdish	1	*CD19*	both	c.1464delC	p.P488P fsX15	28
F	Moroccan	1	*CD19*	both	c.1653_1671+9del28ins23	G551G fsX25	28
G	French	1	*CD19*	both	c.947-1G>T *	p.A316D fsX5	29
H	Moroccan	1	*CD81*	both	c.561+1G>A	p.E188M fsX13	26

* same mutation as maternal allele of patient from Fam C

Fig. 7.2 Overview genetic defects in CD19-deficient patients. (**a**) Schematic depiction of the human *CD19* and *CD81* genes with the positions of the identified genetic defects. (**b**) Overview of mutant alleles in 11 patients from 8 unrelated families

7.3 Clinical and Immunological Characteristics

All 11 patients presented during childhood, predominantly with recurrent upper and/or lower respiratory infections (Table 7.1). In several cases, bacterial septicemia, meningitis, and conjunctivitis have been observed, as well as gastrointestinal problems. The severity of infections is highly variable between patients, and the benign disease course in four patients was likely the cause of delayed diagnosis in adulthood, 18–44 years after onset of infections (patients B1-3 and F1).

In addition to bacterial infections, several patients experienced complications due to viral infections (herpes zoster, RSV) or parasites (giardiasis). Furthermore, noninfectious complications have been observed as well. These are mostly restricted

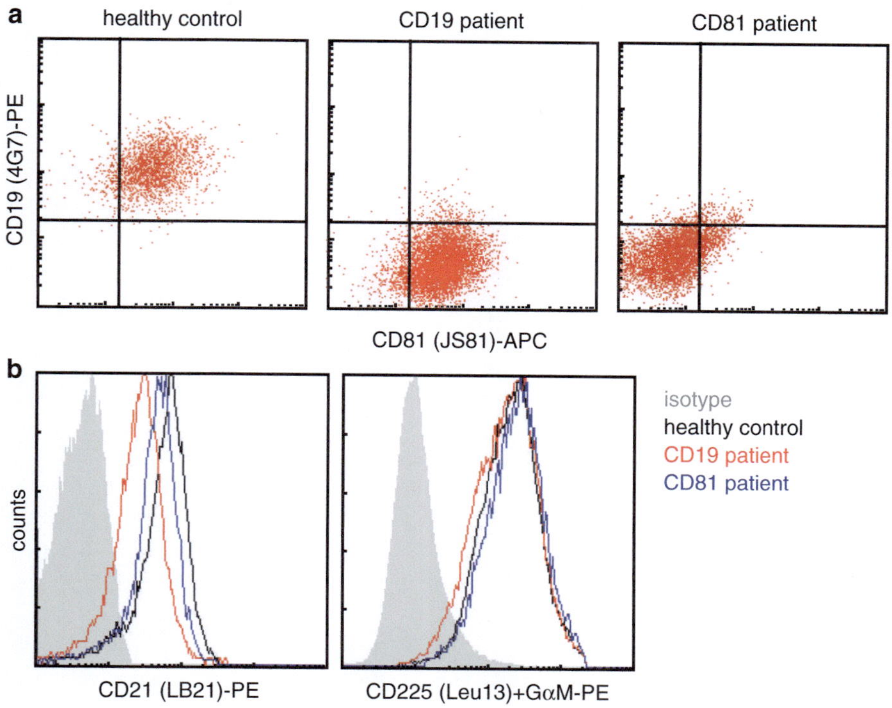

Fig. 7.3 Expression of CD19 complex members on B cells. (**a**) Dot plots showing CD19 and CD81 expression on B cells from a healthy control, patient D1 with a CD19 gene defect, and patient H1 with a CD81 gene defect. (**b**) CD21 and CD225 expression levels on B cells from the same individuals as in A (Adapted from [26, 27])

to autoimmunity, especially thrombocytopenia and systemic lupus erythematosus (SLE). Finally, two patients, one with CD19 and one with CD81 gene defects, suffered from IgA nephropathy.

Immunologically, all patients show typical features of antibody deficiency with low IgG in combination with reduced serum IgA and/or IgM levels (Tables 7.2 and 7.3) and impaired responses to vaccinations (Tables 7.2 and 7.3). Only patient F1 was specifically deficient in IgG1 with normal to high levels of other IgG subclasses, IgM and IgA, and normal responses to previous vaccinations (Table 7.3). Thus, with the exception of patient F1, CD19-deficient patients fit the criteria of common variable immunodeficiency (CVID) [30, 31].

Leukocyte and lymphocyte subsets were normally present in all patients, with the exception of low total B-cell numbers in one child and one adult with *CD19* gene defects. The reduced IgG serum levels were accompanied by low memory B-cell numbers, again with the exception of patient F1. Interestingly, most patients showed reduced numbers of transitional B cells. On the other hand, the patients did not display an expansion of $CD21^{low}$ B cells that is frequently found in patients with CVID [32, 33]. This was irrespective of the generally lower expression levels of CD21 on patient's B cells as a result of the absence of CD19 (Fig. 7.3b) [22, 27].

Table 7.2 Immunological characteristics of pediatric CD19-deficient patients

	A1	A2	C1	D1	E1	G1	H1	Normal values
Gender	F	M	M	M	F	M	F	
Age (year)	10	12	8	6	11	11	4	
Blood cells (cells/μL)								
Lymphocytes	4480	1900	ND	1630	2745	ND	2195	2906 ± 1081[a]
CD3+ T cells	3270	1700	1775	1107	2141	ND	1385	2000 ± 766
CD4+ T cells	1792	669	1064	637	1125	ND	956	1247 ± 601
CD8+ T cells	1478	1031	781	353	796	ND	345	547 ± 184
CD20+ B cells	806	60	538	321	300	ND	426	453 ± 265
CD16/CD56+ NK cells	313	100	ND	156	184	ND	292	266 ± 170
B-cell subsets (% of CD20)								
Transitional	ND	8	ND	3	**0**	5	**1**	6 ± 3
Naive mature	91	87	67.5	90	89	91	90	66 ± 9
CD27+IgM+IgD+ memory	**3**	**2**	5.4	**3**	8	**2**	4	7 ± 3
CD27+IgD− memory	**2**	**1**	7.6	**3**	**2**	**1**	**3**	11 ± 5
Ig serum levels (g/L)								
IgG	**3.25**	**0.91**	**2.49**	**3.00**	**2.30**	**4.4**	**2.40**	5.04–14.64
IgG1	ND	ND	ND	ND	**0.66**	**1.7**	ND	2.92–8.16
IgG2	ND	ND	ND	ND	**1.44**	3.4	ND	0.83–5.13
IgG3	ND	ND	ND	ND	36	0.4	ND	0.08–1.11
IgG4	ND	ND	ND	ND	**<0.01**	0.002	ND	0.01–1.21
IgA	2.92	**0.01**	**0.10**	0.50	1.25	Normal	0.71	0.27–1.95
IgM	**0.25**	0.59	**0.18**	**0.40**	**0.35**	**0.4**	**0.35**	0.24–2.10
IgE (IU/mL)	37	ND	9	ND	ND	ND	ND	0–100
Isohemagglutinins	**Absent**	ND	ND	**Low**	ND	ND	ND	
Vaccination responses	**Impaired**	**Impaired**	**Impaired**	**Impaired**	**Impaired**	**Impaired**	**Impaired**	
Autoantibodies	SS-A, ANA	–	ND	ND	ND	ND	Anti-platelet	

M male, *F* female, *ND* not determined. Only positive tests for autoantibodies are indicated. Bold font indicates subnormal values
[a]Mean ± SD from [27]

Table 7.3 Immunological characteristics of adult CD19-deficient patients

	B1	B2	B3	F1	Normal values
Gender	M	F	F	F	
Age (year)	35	33	49	31	
Blood cells (cells/μL)					
Lymphocytes	2182	2508	2059	1440	1000–2800
CD3+ T cells	1520	1855	1384	1152	700–2100
CD4+ T cells	713	1070	620	590	300–1400
CD8+ T cells	720	692	696	533	200–900
CD19+ B cells	286	521	268	**61**	100–500
CD16/CD56+ NK cells	277	348	288	**23**	90–600
B-cell subsets (% of CD20)					
Transitional	ND	ND	ND	**0**	2 (1–3)[a]
Naive mature	92	96	92	59	67 (54–76)[a]
CD27+IgM+IgD+ memory	**5**	**1**	**3**	22	15 (11–23)[a]
CD27+IgD− memory	**1**	**0**	**2**	12	15 (10–20)[a]
Ig serum levels (g/L)					
IgG	**2.04**	**1.98**	**2.56**	**4.93**	7.51–15.6
IgG1	ND	ND	ND	**1.70**	4.9–11.4
IgG2	ND	ND	ND	3.06	1.5–6.4
IgG3	ND	ND	ND	2.11	0.2–1.1
IgG4	ND	ND	ND	2	0.08–1.4
IgA	**0.18**	**0.07**	**0.19**	3.50	0.82–4.53
IgM	**0.47**	**0.30**	0.60	1.35	0.46–3.04
IgE (IU/mL)	ND	ND	ND	ND	0–100
Isohemagglutinins	**Low**	**Low**	**Low**	Present	
Vaccination responses	**Impaired**	**Impaired**	**Impaired**	Normal	
Autoantibodies	–	–	Anti-DNA	ANA	

M male, *F* female, *ND* not determined. Only positive tests for autoantibodies are indicated. Bold font indicates subnormal values and underlined supranormal
[a]Median (IQR) from [46]

Heterozygous carriers of *CD19* or *CD81* gene defects have reduced expression of surface CD19 on their B cells [22, 25–27, 34]. In carriers with CD19 gene defects, this is accompanied by reduced CD21 expression levels. Despite these phenotypical changes, extensive analysis of 30 carriers revealed that these were not more susceptible to infections and had normal total serum IgG, IgA, and IgM levels, as well as normal responses to vaccinations and circulating memory B cells [25].

7.4 CD19 Function

The impaired antibody responses in CD19-deficient patients seemed to result from defective activation of B cells via their BCRs. B cells from all tested patients showed impaired fluxes of intracellular Ca2+ upon stimulation with anti-IgM [22, 26, 27]. CD19 is already expressed in precursor B cells in the bone marrow at the stage where the pre-BCR is expressed. Signaling via the pre-BCR is crucial for developmental progression of progenitor B cells. As a result, genetic defects in genes encoding components of this pre-BCR (Igμ, CD79a, CD79b, and λ14.1) and directly downstream signaling molecules (BTK, BLNK, PLCγ2) result in a complete absence of mature B cells and hypogammaglobulinemia [23]. As CD19-deficient patients do not lack mature B cells, it can be concluded that CD19 does not have a critical role in pre-BCR signaling. However, 2/11 patients presented with low total B-cell numbers (Tables 7.2 and 7.3). Thus, in line with mouse models [35, 36], it is possible that human progenitor B-cell differentiation is less efficient in the absence of CD19.

Importantly, in vitro stimulation of B cells was dependent on CD19 even in the absence of complement, suggesting that the CD19-complex can be recruited to the BCR in the absence of crosslinking via C3d and CD21. Indeed, CD21 is not required for B-cell activation via the BCR with large amounts of antigen [37, 38]. Only with limiting amounts of IgM, crosslinking the BCR via complement and CD21 to the CD19 complex is needed to induce a Ca2+ flux [37]. The potential of CD19 to signal independently of CD21 likely underlies the relatively mild phenotype of CD21-deficient individuals. Their B cells express normal to high levels of CD19 and are capable of mounting specific antibody responses [37, 38].

Complement-independent recruitment of the CD19 complex to the BCR is thought to be regulated via the CD81-tetraspanin network [39]. Upon antigen binding, the BCR triggers signaling and reorganization of the cytoskeleton [40]. This increases BCR mobility and diffusion [41] to allow interactions with CD19 that is immobilized on the membrane by the CD81-tetraspanin network. Specifically, CD19-mediated recruitment of Vav, PLCγ2, and PI3K enhances BCR-induced signaling.

In addition to enhancing BCR signaling, CD19-mediated recruitment has been shown to enhance Toll-like receptor (TLR)9 and BAFFR signaling [42, 43]. Rather than a co-receptor complex that is recruited, it might be more appropriate to view the CD19 complex as a generic hub used by receptors in and on B cells to induce PI3K signaling.

7.5 Prospects for Diagnosis and Prognosis of CD19 Deficiency

CD19 deficiency is a rare autosomal cause of an antibody disorder with childhood onset. To date, only 11 cases have been described from 8 unrelated families. However, they were caused by nine unique genetic events in the *CD19* and *CD81* genes. Thus, it is important to consider during the diagnostic work-up. The use of a CD19 antibody in combination with another broadly B-cell reactive antibody such as CD20, CD22, IgM, or IgD is preferred to prevent misdiagnosis of agammaglobulinemia.

Currently, all identified mutations result in absence of membrane CD19 expression. This could be due to selective reporting as absence of CD19 provides the best clue for a CD19 deficiency. The conserved tyrosines in the C-terminal cytoplasmic tail of CD19 are critical for its function [44, 45]. Hence, mutations that affect these residues or that result in truncated forms could potentially be expressed while still lack functional properties. It is therefore suggested to perform functional analysis of BCR signaling, e.g., Ca2+ flux, for selected cases with B-cell intrinsic cause of autosomal recessive antibody deficiency.

The predominant clinical complications of CD19-deficient patients are recurrent respiratory infections (Table 7.1). However, despite the low IgG levels, several patients have autoantibodies and have developed an autoimmune disease. The mechanisms by which absence of CD19 expression contributes to autoimmunity remain unclear. CD19 functions as a generic hub to modulate PI3K signaling downstream of the BCR, TLR, and BAFFR. It can be envisaged that lack of CD19 alters the threshold and changes the Ig gene repertoire and functional properties of newly developing B cells making these more prone to autoreactivity. Therefore, it is advised to carefully monitor patients clinically and serologically to enable early treatment prior to irreversible organ damage.

References

1. Nadler LM, Anderson KC, Marti G, Bates M, Park E, Daley JF, Schlossman SF. B4, a human B lymphocyte-associated antigen expressed on normal, mitogen-activated, and malignant B lymphocytes. J Immunol. 1983;131:244.
2. Stashenko P, Nadler LM, Hardy R, Schlossman SF. Characterization of a human B lymphocyte-specific antigen. J Immunol. 1980;125:1678.
3. Nadler LM, Stashenko P, Hardy R, van Agthoven A, Terhorst C, Schlossman SF. Characterization of a human B cell-specific antigen (B2) distinct from B1. J Immunol. 1981;126:1941.
4. Stamenkovic I, Seed B. CD19, the earliest differentiation antigen of the B cell lineage, bears three extracellular immunoglobulin-like domains and an Epstein-Barr virus-related cytoplasmic tail. J Exp Med. 1988;168:1205.
5. Tedder TF, Isaacs CM. Isolation of cDNAs encoding the CD19 antigen of human and mouse B lymphocytes. A new member of the immunoglobulin superfamily. J Immunol. 1989;143:712.
6. Matsumoto AK, Kopicky-Burd J, Carter RH, Tuveson DA, Tedder TF, Fearon DT. Intersection of the complement and immune systems: a signal transduction complex of the B lymphocyte-containing complement receptor type 2 and CD19. J Exp Med. 1991;173:55.
7. Tedder TF, Clement LT, Cooper MD. Expression of C3d receptors during human B cell differentiation: immunofluorescence analysis with the HB-5 monoclonal antibody. J Immunol. 1984;133:678.
8. Moore MD, Cooper NR, Tack BF, Nemerow GR. Molecular cloning of the cDNA encoding the Epstein-Barr virus/C3d receptor (complement receptor type 2) of human B lymphocytes. Proc Natl Acad Sci U S A. 1987;84:9194.
9. Weis JH, Morton CC, Bruns GA, Weis JJ, Klickstein LB, Wong WW, Fearon DT. A complement receptor locus: genes encoding C3b/C4b receptor and C3d/Epstein-Barr virus receptor map to 1q32. J Immunol. 1987;138:312.
10. Bradbury LE, Kansas GS, Levy S, Evans RL, Tedder TF. The CD19/CD21 signal transducing complex of human B lymphocytes includes the target of antiproliferative antibody-1 and Leu-13 molecules. J Immunol. 1992;149:2841.
11. Chen YX, Welte K, Gebhard DH, Evans RL. Induction of T cell aggregation by antibody to a 16kd human leukocyte surface antigen. J Immunol. 1984;133:2496.
12. Oren R, Takahashi S, Doss C, Levy R, Levy S. TAPA-1, the target of an antiproliferative antibody, defines a new family of transmembrane proteins. Mol Cell Biol. 1990;10:4007.

13. Takahashi S, Doss C, Levy S, Levy R. TAPA-1, the target of an antiproliferative antibody, is associated on the cell surface with the Leu-13 antigen. J Immunol. 1990;145:2207.
14. Maecker HT, Levy S. Normal lymphocyte development but delayed humoral immune response in CD81-null mice. J Exp Med. 1997;185:1505.
15. Miyazaki T, Muller U, Campbell KS. Normal development but differentially altered proliferative responses of lymphocytes in mice lacking CD81. EMBO J. 1997;16:4217.
16. Tsitsikov EN, Gutierrez-Ramos JC, Geha RS. Impaired CD19 expression and signaling, enhanced antibody response to type II T independent antigen and reduction of B-1 cells in CD81-deficient mice. Proc Natl Acad Sci U S A. 1997;94:10844.
17. Matsumoto AK, Martin DR, Carter RH, Klickstein LB, Ahearn JM, Fearon DT. Functional dissection of the CD21/CD19/TAPA-1/Leu-13 complex of B lymphocytes. J Exp Med. 1993;178:1407.
18. Zhuang Y, Soriano P, Weintraub H. The helix-loop-helix gene E2A is required for B cell formation. Cell. 1994;79:875.
19. Urbanek P, Wang ZQ, Fetka I, Wagner EF, Busslinger M. Complete block of early B cell differentiation and altered patterning of the posterior midbrain in mice lacking Pax5/BSAP. Cell. 1994;79:901.
20. Lin H, Grosschedl R. Failure of B-cell differentiation in mice lacking the transcription factor EBF. Nature. 1995;376:263.
21. Kozmik Z, Wang S, Dorfler P, Adams B, Busslinger M. The promoter of the CD19 gene is a target for the B-cell-specific transcription factor BSAP. Mol Cell Biol. 1992;12:2662.
22. van Zelm MC, Reisli I, van der Burg M, Castaño D, van Noesel CJM, van Tol MJD, Woellner C, Grimbacher B, Patiño PJ, van Dongen JJM, Franco JL. An antibody-deficiency syndrome due to mutations in the CD19 gene. N Engl J Med. 2006;354:1901.
23. Conley ME, Dobbs AK, Farmer DM, Kilic S, Paris K, Grigoriadou S, Coustan-Smith E, Howard V, Campana D. Primary B cell immunodeficiencies: comparisons and contrasts. Annu Rev Immunol. 2009;27:199.
24. Kanegane H, Agematsu K, Futatani T, Sira MM, Suga K, Sekiguchi T, van Zelm MC, Miyawaki T. Novel mutations in a Japanese patient with CD19 deficiency. Genes Immun. 2007;8:663.
25. Artac H, Reisli I, Kara R, Pico-Knijnenburg I, Adin-Cinar S, Pekcan S, Jol-van der Zijde CM, van Tol MJ, Bakker-Jonges LE, van Dongen JJ, van der Burg M, van Zelm MC. B-cell maturation and antibody responses in individuals carrying a mutated CD19 allele. Genes Immun. 2010;11:523.
26. van Zelm MC, Smet J, Adams B, Mascart F, Schandene L, Janssen F, Ferster A, Kuo CC, Levy S, van Dongen JJ, van der Burg M. CD81 gene defect in humans disrupts CD19 complex formation and leads to antibody deficiency. J Clin Invest. 2010;120:1265.
27. van Zelm MC, Smet J, van der Burg M, Ferster A, Le PQ, Schandene L, van Dongen JJ, Mascart F. Antibody deficiency due to a missense mutation in CD19 demonstrates the importance of the conserved tryptophan 41 in immunoglobulin superfamily domain formation. Hum Mol Genet. 2011;20:1854.
28. Vince N, Boutboul D, Mouillot G, Just N, Peralta M, Casanova JL, Conley ME, Bories JC, Oksenhendler E, Malphettes M, Fieschi C, D. S. Group. Defects in the CD19 complex predispose to glomerulonephritis, as well as IgG1 subclass deficiency. J Allergy Clin Immunol. 2011;127:538.
29. Skendros P, Rondeau S, Chateil JF, Bui S, Bocly V, Moreau JF, Theodorou I, Aladjidi N. Misdiagnosed CD19 deficiency leads to severe lung disease. Pediatr Allergy Immunol. 2014;25:603.
30. Conley ME, Notarangelo LD, Etzioni A. Diagnostic criteria for primary immunodeficiencies. Representing PAGID (Pan-American Group for Immunodeficiency) and ESID (European Society for Immunodeficiencies). Clin Immunol. 1999;93:190.
31. Bousfiha A, Jeddane L, Al-Herz W, Ailal F, Casanova JL, Chatila T, Conley ME, Cunningham-Rundles C, Etzioni A, Franco JL, Gaspar HB, Holland SM, Klein C, Nonoyama S, Ochs HD, Oksenhendler E, Picard C, Puck JM, Sullivan KE, Tang ML. The 2015 IUIS phenotypic classification for primary immunodeficiencies. J Clin Immunol. 2015;35:727.

32. Warnatz K, Wehr C, Drager R, Schmidt S, Eibel H, Schlesier M, Peter HH. Expansion of CD19(hi)CD21(lo/neg) B cells in common variable immunodeficiency (CVID) patients with autoimmune cytopenia. Immunobiology. 2002;206:502.
33. Wehr C, Kivioja T, Schmitt C, Ferry B, Witte T, Eren E, Vlkova M, Hernandez M, Detkova D, Bos PR, Poerksen G, von Bernuth H, Baumann U, Goldacker S, Gutenberger S, Schlesier M, Bergeron-van der Cruyssen F, Le Garff M, Debre P, Jacobs R, Jones J, Bateman E, Litzman J, van Hagen PM, Plebani A, Schmidt RE, Thon V, Quinti I, Espanol T, Webster AD, Chapel H, Vihinen M, Oksenhendler E, Peter HH, Warnatz K. The EUROclass trial: defining subgroups in common variable immunodeficiency. Blood. 2008;111:77.
34. Reisli I, Artac H, Pekcan S, Kara R, Yumiu K, Karagol C, Cimen O, Sen M, Artac M. CD19 deficiency: a village screening study. Turk Arch Ped. 2009;44:127.
35. Otero DC, Rickert RC. CD19 function in early and late B cell development. II. CD19 facilitates the pro-B/pre-B transition. J Immunol. 2003;171:5921.
36. Diamant E, Keren Z, Melamed D. CD19 regulates positive selection and maturation in B lymphopoiesis: lack of CD19 imposes developmental arrest of immature B cells and consequential stimulation of receptor editing. Blood. 2005;105:3247.
37. Thiel J, Kimmig L, Salzer U, Grudzien M, Lebrecht D, Hagena T, Draeger R, Voelxen N, Bergbreiter A, Jennings S, Gutenberger S, Aichem A, Illges H, Hannan JP, Kienzler AK, Rizzi M, Eibel H, Peter HH, Warnatz K, Grimbacher B, Rump JA, Schlesier M. Genetic CD21 deficiency is associated with hypogammaglobulinemia. J Allergy Clin Immunol. 2012;129:801.
38. Wentink MW, Lambeck AJ, van Zelm MC, Simons E, van Dongen JJ, IJspeert H, Scholvinck EH, van der Burg M. CD21 and CD19 deficiency: two defects in the same complex leading to different disease modalities. Clin Immunol. 2015;161:120.
39. Mattila PK, Feest C, Depoil D, Treanor B, Montaner B, Otipoby KL, Carter R, Justement LB, Bruckbauer A, Batista FD. The actin and tetraspanin networks organize receptor nanoclusters to regulate B cell receptor-mediated signaling. Immunity. 2013;38:461.
40. Freeman SA, Jaumouille V, Choi K, Hsu BE, Wong HS, Abraham L, Graves ML, Coombs D, Roskelley CD, Das R, Grinstein S, Gold MR. Toll-like receptor ligands sensitize B-cell receptor signalling by reducing actin-dependent spatial confinement of the receptor. Nat Commun. 2015;6:6168.
41. Treanor B, Depoil D, Gonzalez-Granja A, Barral P, Weber M, Dushek O, Bruckbauer A, Batista FD. The membrane skeleton controls diffusion dynamics and signaling through the B cell receptor. Immunity. 2010;32:187.
42. Keppler SJ, Gasparrini F, Burbage M, Aggarwal S, Frederico B, Geha RS, Way M, Bruckbauer A, Batista FD. Wiskott-Aldrich syndrome interacting protein deficiency uncovers the role of the co-receptor CD19 as a generic hub for PI3 kinase signaling in B cells. Immunity. 2015;43:660.
43. Morbach H, Schickel JN, Cunningham-Rundles C, Conley ME, Reisli I, Franco JL, Meffre E. CD19 controls Toll-like receptor 9 responses in human B cells. J Allergy Clin Immunol. 2016;137:889.
44. Sato S, Miller AS, Howard MC, Tedder TF. Regulation of B lymphocyte development and activation by the CD19/CD21/CD81/Leu 13 complex requires the cytoplasmic domain of CD19. J Immunol. 1997;159:3278.
45. Wang Y, Brooks SR, Li X, Anzelon AN, Rickert RC, Carter RH. The physiologic role of CD19 cytoplasmic tyrosines. Immunity. 2002;17:501.
46. Mouillot G, Carmagnat M, Gerard L, Garnier JL, Fieschi C, Vince N, Karlin L, Viallard JF, Jaussaud R, Boileau J, Donadieu J, Gardembas M, Schleinitz N, Suarez F, Hachulla E, Delavigne K, Morisset M, Jacquot S, Just N, Galicier L, Charron D, Debre P, Oksenhendler E, Rabian C, D. S. Group. B-cell and T-cell phenotypes in CVID patients correlate with the clinical phenotype of the disease. J Clin Immunol. 2010;30:746.
47. van Zelm MC, van der Burg M, de Ridder D, Barendregt BH, de Haas EF, Reinders MJ, Lankester AC, Revesz T, Staal FJ, van Dongen JJ. Ig gene rearrangement steps are initiated in early human precursor B cell subsets and correlate with specific transcription factor expression. J Immunol. 2005;175:5912.

Genetic CD21 Deficiency

8

Jens Thiel

8.1 Definition

CD21 (complement receptor 2, CR2) deficiency has been first described in 2012 by Thiel et al. in a single patient [1]. To date, three further patients have been reported [2, 3]. CD21 deficiency is caused by compound heterozygous or homozygous mutations in the *CD21* gene.

8.2 Etiology

Genetic CD21 deficiency is a very rare disorder leading to recurrent infections and hypogammaglobulinemia. CD21 is the complement receptor 2, and together with CD19, CD81, and CD225, it is part of the B-cell coreceptor complex. The B-cell coreceptor complex lowers the activation threshold of the B-cell antigen receptor, meaning that the coligation of C3d-decorated antigen to the B-cell receptor and CD21 increases activating signaling into B cells [4]. CD21 is mainly expressed on follicular dendritic cells and mature B lymphocytes, and it consists of 15 to 16 short consensus repeats, a transmembrane domain, and a short intracytoplasmatic tail [1, 5]. CD21 binds C3d-opsonized immune complexes and enhances the immune response to low-dose antigens [2, 6, 7]. CD21 is crucial for antigen uptake and presentation and involved in the clearance of immune complexes [2, 8]. In mice, complement receptor type 1 (CD35) and type 2 (CD21) are encoded by the same locus (*CR2*), and *CR2* knockout mice do therefore not exactly reflect the human phenotype of CD21 deficiency. In *CR2* knockout mice, the formation of

J. Thiel
Faculty of Medicine, Department of Internal Medicine, Clinic for Rheumatology and Clinical Immunology, Medical Center - University of Freiburg, Freiburg im Breisgau, Germany
e-mail: jens.thiel@uniklinik-freiburg.de

M. M. D'Elios, M. Rizzi (eds.), *Humoral Primary Immunodeficiencies*,
Rare Diseases of the Immune System, https://doi.org/10.1007/978-3-319-91785-6_8

long-term memory and specific antibody production are impaired [9]. Defects in human CD19 and CD81 lead to impaired B-cell receptor activation upon antigenic stimulation and result in a humoral immunodeficiency with first manifestation early in life [10, 11].

8.3 Clinical Manifestations

The patients described by Thiel et al. [1] and Wentink et al. [2] had a relatively mild clinical phenotype with recurrent bacterial infections in one patient and possibly autoimmune-mediated myalgia in the second patient. The two siblings recently reported by Rosain et al. [3] had a more severe phenotype with recurrent upper and lower respiratory tract infections first presenting in early childhood. These two siblings were born to consanguineous parents. Therefore, other pathogenic gene variants with an influence on the clinical and immunological phenotype could not be completely ruled out by the authors.

8.4 Immunological Phenotype

The hallmark of CD21 deficiency is a decrease in the formation of class-switched memory B cells that has been reported in all CD21-deficient patients [1–3]. Absolute numbers of B, T, and NK cells are normal. Thiel et al. demonstrated that binding of C3d-containing immune complexes is severely reduced in CD21 deficiency leading to a complete loss of costimulatory activity of C3d in enhancing suboptimal B-cell receptor stimulation [1]. Therefore, in CD21 deficiency the impaired memory B-cell formation is likely a consequence of suboptimal B-cell stimulation and not an intrinsic defect of memory formation [2]. Accordingly, Wentink et al. report a close to normal frequency of somatic hypermutation and class-switch recombination in CD21 deficiency [2]. Hypogammaglobulinemia has been reported in all CD21-deficient patients, with low IgG and IgA in the patient described first; hypogammaglobulinemia affecting IgG, IgA, and IgM in the patient reported by Wentink et al.; and low to normal IgG but normal IgM in the two siblings [3]. Except for the patient of Wentink et al., all patients had an impaired vaccination response.

8.5 Diagnosis

CD21 deficiency should be ruled out in patients with clinical signs of humoral immunodeficiency, hypogammaglobulinemia, and a decrease in class-switched memory B cells. The absence of CD21 expression on peripheral B cells can easily be detected by immunophenotyping.

References

1. Thiel J, Kimmig L, Salzer U, Grudzien M, Lebrecht D, Hagena T, Draeger R, Voelxen N, Bergbreiter A, Jennings S, Gutenberger S, Aichem A, Illges H, Hannan JP, Kienzler AK, Rizzi M, Eibel H, Peter HH, Warnatz K, Grimbacher B, Rump JA, Schlesier M. Genetic CD21 deficiency is associated with hypogammaglobulinemia. J Allergy Clin Immunol. 2012;129(3):801–810.e6. https://doi.org/10.1016/j.jaci.2011.09.027.
2. Wentink MW, Lambeck AJ, van Zelm MC, Simons E, van Dongen JJ, IJspeert H, Schölvinck EH, van der Burg M. CD21 and CD19 deficiency: two defects in the same complex leading to different disease modalities. Clin Immunol. 2015;161(2):120–7. https://doi.org/10.1016/j.clim.2015.08.010.
3. Rosain J, Miot C, Lambert N, Rousselet MC, Pellier I, Picard C. CD21 deficiency in 2 siblings with recurrent respiratory infections and hypogammaglobulinemia. J Allergy Clin Immunol Pract. 2017;5(6):1765–1767.e3. https://doi.org/10.1016/j.jaip.2017.04.011.
4. Carter RH, Fearon DT. CD19: lowering the threshold for antigen receptor stimulation of B lymphocytes. Science. 1992;256(5053):105–7.
5. Szakonyi G, Guthridge JM, Li D, Young K, Holers VM, Chen XS. Structure of complement receptor 2 in complex with its C3d ligand. Science. 2001 Jun 1;292(5522):1725–8.
6. Aegerter-Shaw M, Cole JL, Klickstein LB, Wong WW, Fearon DT, Lalley PA, Weis JH. Expansion of the complement receptor gene family. Identification in the mouse of two new genes related to the CR1 and CR2 gene family. J Immunol. 1987;138(10):3488–94.
7. Iida K, Nadler L, Nussenzweig V. Identification of the membrane receptor for the complement fragment C3d by means of a monoclonal antibody. J Exp Med. 1983;158(4):1021–33.
8. Erdei A, Isaák A, Török K, Sándor N, Kremlitzka M, Prechl J, Bajtay Z. Expression and role of CR1 and CR2 on B and T lymphocytes under physiological and autoimmune conditions. Mol Immunol. 2009;46(14):2767–73. https://doi.org/10.1016/j.molimm.2009.05.181.
9. Molina H, Holers VM, Li B, Fung Y, Mariathasan S, Goellner J, Strauss-Schoenberger J, Karr RW, Chaplin DD. Markedly impaired humoral immune response in mice deficient in complement receptors 1 and 2. Proc Natl Acad Sci U S A. 1996;93(8):3357–61.
10. van Zelm MC, Reisli I, van der Burg M, Castaño D, van Noesel CJ, van Tol MJ, Woellner C, Grimbacher B, Patiño PJ, van Dongen JJ, Franco JL. An antibody-deficiency syndrome due to mutations in the CD19 gene. N Engl J Med. 2006;354(18):1901–12.
11. van Zelm MC, Smet J, Adams B, Mascart F, Schandené L, Janssen F, Ferster A, Kuo CC, Levy S, van Dongen JJ, van der Burg M. CD81 gene defect in humans disrupts CD19 complex formation and leads to antibody deficiency. J Clin Invest. 2010;120(4):1265–74. https://doi.org/10.1172/JCI39748.

TACI Deficiency

9

Astrid Bergbreiter and Ulrich Salzer

9.1 Definition

Heterozygous, compound heterozygous, or homozygous alterations in the TNFRSF13B gene are associated with various forms of antibody deficiency including IgA deficiency and common variable immunodeficiency (CVID). These genetic alterations have a low penetrance and are generally not regarded as disease causing, but may be important genetic cofactors affecting especially the T cell-independent antibody responses and increasing risks for autoimmunity and lymphoproliferation. Therefore TACI deficiency is currently viewed as a disease-modifying factor in various forms of antibody deficiency.

9.2 Etiology

The tumor necrosis factor (TNF) superfamily member transmembrane activator and CAML interactor (TACI, encoded by TNFRSF13B) belongs to a group of molecules which regulate B cell homeostasis, differentiation, and function. Its ligands are BAFF (B cell-activating factor, synonyms BLyS, THANK, TALL-1, and zTNF4, encoded by TNFSF13B) and APRIL (a proliferation-inducing ligand, synonyms

A. Bergbreiter
Department of Dermatology, University Hospital Regensburg, Regensburg, Germany
e-mail: Astrid.Bergbreiter@klinik.uni-regensburg.de

U. Salzer (✉)
Department of Rheumatology and Clinical Immunology, Faculty of Medicine, Medical Center—University of Freiburg, Freiburg im Breisgau, Germany

Center for Chronic Immunodeficiency (CCI), Faculty of Medicine, Medical Center—University of Freiburg, Freiburg im Breisgau, Germany
e-mail: ulrich.salzer@uniklinik-freiburg.de

M. M. D'Elios, M. Rizzi (eds.), *Humoral Primary Immunodeficiencies*,
Rare Diseases of the Immune System, https://doi.org/10.1007/978-3-319-91785-6_9

TALL-2 and TRDL-1, protein A, encoded by TNFRSF17), both of which are able to bind to TACI and BCMA (TNFRSF17), whereas BAFFR (BAFF receptor, encoded by TNFRSF13C) is exclusively bound by BAFF only. TACI is able to bind APRIL and BAFF with equally high affinity [1] and serves as the only receptor for BAFF/APRIL heterotrimers [2]. Additionally, both APRIL and its receptor TACI were shown to be capable of interacting with proteoglycans [3, 4]. TACI is a type III transmembrane protein, which contains two cysteine-rich extracellular ligand-binding domains characteristic of members of the TNFR superfamily and shows an expression pattern restricted to lymphocytes (Fig. 9.1).

BAFFR binds BAFF with highest affinity and is expressed on all peripheral B cells from the transitional stage onward except plasmablasts and plasma cells [5]. By interacting with BAFFR, BAFF mediates survival of BAFFR expressing peripheral B cell subsets. In both BAFF and BAFFR knockout mice, severe B cell lymphopenia and humoral immunodeficiency are observed [6, 7]. BCMA expression is confined to terminally differentiated B cells [8, 9] and ensures the survival of long-lived plasma cells in the bone marrow [10]. TACI shows some unique structural features distinct from its closest relatives BCMA and BAFFR. TACI expression varies on distinct B cell subpopulations. In humans, a pronounced expression is found on marginal zone B cells and on CD27+ memory B cell subsets [5, 8, 9]. TACI expression is also more regulated and strongly induced after in vitro treatment with various B cell stimulation agents [11, 12]. TACI has two additional 5′ exons allowing the receptor to be expressed as two splice variants containing either one or

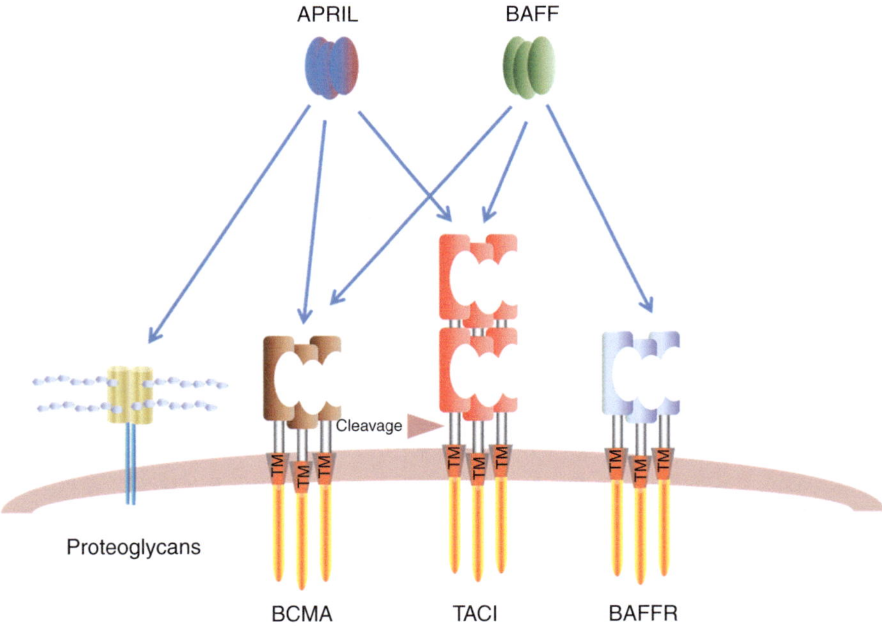

Fig. 9.1 Overview of the family of BAFF/APRIL ligands and receptors

two cysteine-rich extracellular domains, of which only one seems to be functionally relevant [13]. The alternative mRNA splicing of the human TACI gene results in two different main isoforms, the short and long TACI isoforms. Murine B cells and human pre-B cells transduced with the long TACI isoform expressed CD19 and IgG. These cells had less XBP-1 and BLIMP-1 mRNA. Cells transduced with the short TACI isoform became larger and CD138 positive and had more BLIMP-1 and XBP-1 mRNA and morphologically resembled plasma cells. These cells also showed an activation of the classical NFκB pathway and the short TACI protein co-localized with MyD88 and calcium-modulating cyclophilin ligand [14].

Single BAFF or APRIL homotrimers are able to bind TACI, but for efficient signaling ligand multimers are necessary. Soluble BAFF was shown to form 60mers, which are very potent activators of TACI. APRIL can build multimers by binding to heparan sulfate proteoglycans (reviewed in [15]). It was shown that in BAFF and APRIL heteromers, the number of BAFF and APRIL proteins forming the heteromers influences receptor-binding specificities and activities. Trimers consisting of one BAFF and two APRIL proteins bound to TACI and BCMA but not to BAFF receptor, thereby showing similarity to APRIL. Heteromers which consist of two BAFF and one APRIL protein only weakly bind to BAFF-R but preferably bind to TACI and to BCMA. Since heteromers were shown to be less active than BAFF, it was hypothesized that they might reduce BAFF activity in vivo [16]. It was also reported that an endogenous soluble form of the TACI protein was detected in vivo. The soluble protein is released by a disintegrin and metalloproteinase 10 (ADAM 10). The remaining membrane fragment of the protein is cleaved by a gamma-secretase. Soluble TACI can assemble homotypically. By binding BAFF and APRIL, soluble TACI can inhibit B cell survival and NFκB activation. Interestingly, soluble TACI was found in the sera of patients with SLE. The amount of soluble TACI in the serum correlated with disease activity [1]. Similar to TACI, there also exists a soluble form of the BAFF receptor. It is cleaved from the cell surface by ADAM 10 in circulating B cells or by ADAM 17 in germinal center B cells. Shedding of the BAFFR is BAFF dependent and only occurs in cells which co-express TACI [17].

Inside the cell, a binding site for MyD88 is located within the cytoplasmic domain of TACI. Signaling via TACI-MyD88-IRAK1-IRAK4-TRAF6-TAK1 leads to activation of the canonical NFκB pathway [18]. Finally, TACI was originally identified as a CAML interacting receptor [19, 20] and thus is able to signal both via the NFκB and NFAT/AP-1 signaling pathways (Fig. 9.2).

TACI interacts in a ligand-dependent way with activated TLR7 and TLR9 [21]. In vitro studies established APRIL and BAFF as T cell-independent inducers of immunoglobulin class-switch recombination in B cells via TACI [22–24]. In response to APRIL and BAFF, murine naive B cells secrete switched isotypes IgG1 and IgA and switch to IgE with addition of IL-4. This was mediated through both BAFFR and TACI [24]. In this respect the APRIL-TACI interaction is critical for the induction of IgA as APRIL−/− mice show a selective deficiency of this isotype and BAFFR does not bind APRIL [25]. Similarly in humans, BAFF and APRIL mediate class switching toward IgG and IgA in the presence of IL-10 or TGF-β and IgE in the presence of IL-4 [23].

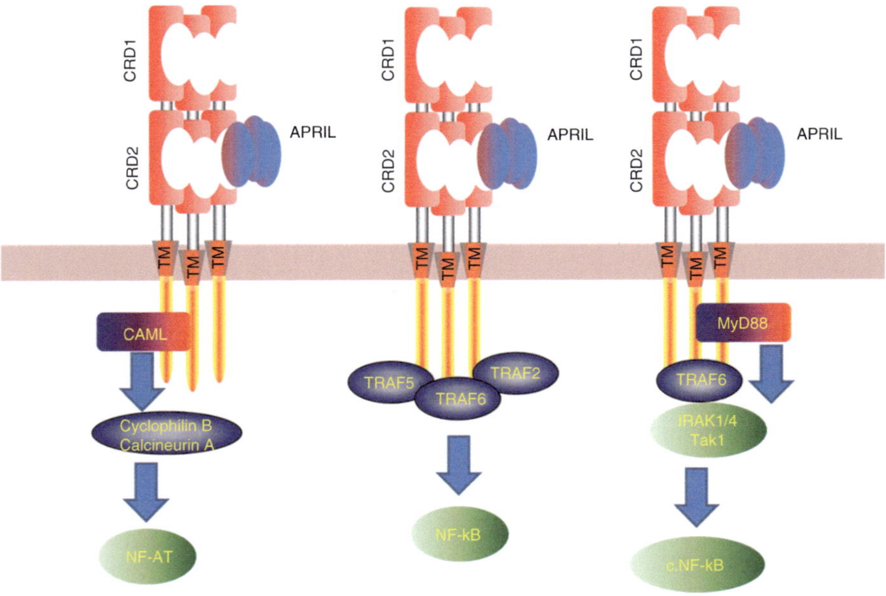

Fig. 9.2 TACI structure, downstream interaction partners, and signaling

The in vivo role of TACI in immune responses has been addressed by several mouse models. Three *tnfrs13b*-deficient mouse strains have been initially generated, which show considerable diversity in their immunological phenotypes [26–28]. Von Bülow et al. demonstrated impaired generation and maintenance of T cell-independent type II responses directed against polysaccharide antigens of encapsulated bacteria like *Streptococcus pneumoniae* in their TACI-deficient mice. Total B cell numbers were elevated, but otherwise B cells developed normally. The architecture of secondary lymphoid organs was normal with intact germinal centers reflecting the unimpaired T cell-dependent antibody responses in the mice [27]. A second TACI knockout mouse reported by Yan et al. [28] confirmed the findings of expansion of peripheral B cells and the impaired T cell-independent type II response; in addition, these second strains of TACI knockout mice had an altered splenic architecture with prominent germinal centers and an increased cellularity of B cell follicles. In vitro B cells were hyperresponsive to mitogenic stimuli resulting in enhanced proliferation and immunoglobulin (Ig) production supporting a role of TACI as a negative regulator [28]. This observation was further confirmed by a third report [26] on a TACI-deficient mouse strain developing a fatal SLE-like disorder. In addition, lymphoma occurred in up to 15% of these TACI−/− mice. Thus in conclusion, the early knockout studies in mice suggested predominantly an inhibitory role for TACI in immune responses. However, the complete knockout of TACI in mice probably does not reflect the human situation, where usually heterozygous point mutations are found. To address this issue, several mouse models carrying the murine equivalents C76R and A144E of the two most frequent amino acid alterations in humans, C104R and A181E, have been generated [29–32]. Interestingly, these four different mouse strains show again considerable phenotypic differences, which might be attributed to the type of genetic manipulation (transgenic mice on a TACI knockout background versus point mutation knock-in mice) or the different genetic backgrounds. The first two reported mouse strains, expressing either the C76R or the A144E variant in a TACI−/− background, showed reduced serum IgA or IgA and IgM levels as well as impaired type II T cell-independent antibody responses but lacked signs of lymphoproliferation and autoimmunity [30, 31]. The third reported mouse strain, a C76R knock-in mutant expressed under the endogenous TACI promoter, showed hypogammaglobulinemia affecting IgM and IgG1, impaired T cell-independent vaccination responses, and elevated B cell numbers and splenomegaly [32]. The recently reported second A144E mouse model had low IgG, IgA, and IgM and impaired antipneumococcal antibody responses [29], but did not show signs of lymphoproliferation.

9.3 Immunological and Clinical Manifestations of Human TACI Deficiency

Further evidence that TACI positively regulates terminal B cell differentiation came from the discovery that mutations in the TNFRSF13b/TACI gene were associated with CVID in humans [23, 33]. Single nucleotide changes, either missense or nonsense or frameshift, are most common. According to their location and type of mutation, three major groups can be identified (Fig. 9.3). The first group (type I) are missense mutations affecting the ligand-binding domains of TACI. These mutations usually lead to an impairment of ligand binding to the mutated receptor [33, 34]. The

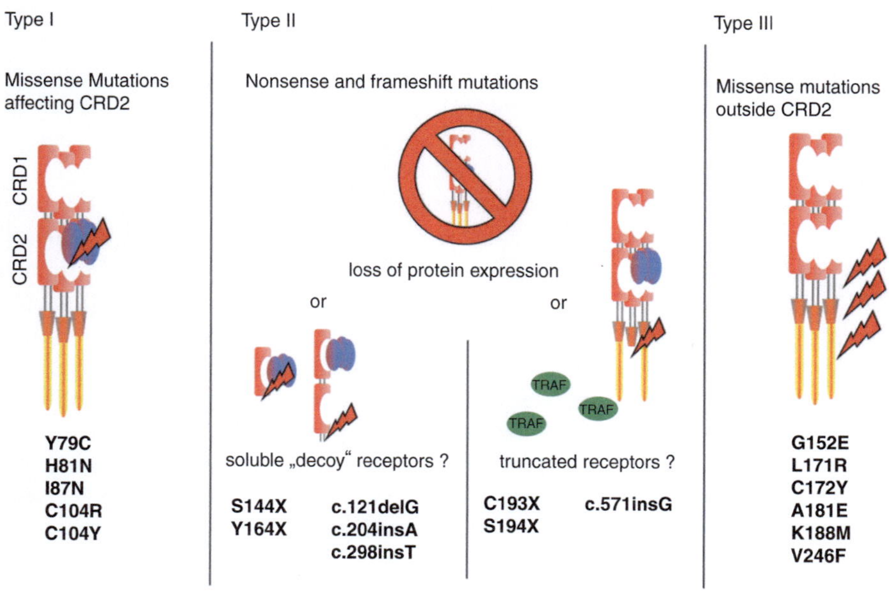

Fig. 9.3 TACI mutation types

most common TACI variant found, C104R, is the prototypical member of this group. The disruption of a disulfide bridge by this mutation causes a complete loss of binding activity in homozygous mutated patients and a 50% loss in heterozygotes [33, 34]. Although an early in vitro study suggested possible dominant-negative effects driven by the mutant C104R allele [35], this could not be confirmed in vivo and by other studies. The type II mutations are frameshift or nonsense mutations, which most likely lead to loss of protein expression, thereby causing haploinsufficiency in the heterozygous state. Interestingly, many patients with Smith-Magenis syndrome (SMS) show a microdeletion at chromosome 17 p11.2. Since the TACI gene is located within this chromosomal region, the effect of only one remaining TACI allele can be studied in these patients. SMS patients with only one TACI allele showed indeed a reduced expression of TACI and impaired B cell activation. These findings support the view that the loss of one TACI allele results in haploinsufficiency [36, 37]. The third group of TACI mutations are missense mutations located outside the ligand-binding domain. The prototypic member of this group is A181E. These mutations cluster around the transmembrane region, and only few mutations are found in the intracellular TACI domain. The exact mutation mechanism for each of these mutations is currently unknown, but for the murine A144E equivalent, it could be recently demonstrated that the mutated protein is unstable resulting in deficient expression, thus causing haploinsufficiency [29].

Contrasting with the expanded and hyperactive B cell phenotype in TACI-deficient mice, peripheral B cells in human TACI deficiency tend to be normal or slightly reduced, with reduced CD27+ memory B cells numbers in most of the patients. Although TACI shows predominant expression on CD27+ memory B cells, the reductions of these cells are not specific for TACI deficiency but are common in CVID [38]. Many TACI-deficient patients show an enlargement of the secondary lymphoid organs, including the spleen, lymph nodes, and tonsils [33, 34]. Some patients with TACI mutations developed non-Hodgkin lymphoma [23, 34]. In this respect human TACI deficiency mirrors the phenotypes of TACI-deficient mouse models as described above. Furthermore, several lines of evidence from studies on human lymphomas point toward an important role of BAFF and its receptors in lymphomagenesis. TACI, BCMA, and BAFF-R are expressed on multiple myeloma cell lines. BAFF is also expressed by multiple myeloma cells and is also found in the bone marrow of patients with multiple myeloma [9]. CLL B cells also express BAFF, BCMA, and TACI. Triggering of the BAFF receptor activates the noncanonical NFκB pathway, and triggering of BCMA and TACI activates the canonical NFκB pathway. Blocking of the canonical NFκB pathway, but not the alternative NFκB pathway, inhibited the proliferation of CLL cells stimulated by BAFF and APRIL [39]. TACI mutations were also found in a limited number of patients with Good's syndrome, which is characterized by a combined immunodeficiency and thymoma. Saenz-Cuesta found one patient in a cohort of six patients with Good's syndrome with a E117G mutation in TACI, and Margraf et al. reported one patient with a potentially disease-causing heterozygous nonsense mutation (p.Lys154Ter), leading to a premature stop codon before the transmembrane domain and therefore probably to a truncated protein [40, 41]. In a Greek study, patients with sarcoidosis were analyzed for TACI variants. Two patients out of

71 patients screened showed TACI variants, R202H and E36L. In patients displaying tonsillar hypertrophy without an infectious cause, the TACI variants I87N and c.204insA were detected [42].

Autoimmune manifestations occur frequently in patients with TACI deficiency. Most common are autoimmune cytopenias, which occur at similar high frequencies as in other primary immunodeficiencies [43]. Some insights regarding the pathomechanism behind the increased rates of autoimmunity come from studies of the BAFF ligand and receptor system in human autoimmune disease and mouse models. Transgenic mice overexpressing BAFF show signs of an SLE-like disease when they age [44, 45]. The fact that elevated BAFF and APRIL levels were found in SLE patients also suggested a role for TACI in autoimmune manifestations in patients with rheumatic diseases [46–47]. One report, however, showed an inverse correlation between the activity of SLE in patients and APRIL serum levels [49]. In the serum of patients with rheumatic diseases—SLE, rheumatic arthritis, polymyositis, and ankylosing spondylitis—elevated levels of APRIL/BAFF heterotrimers were found in comparison with healthy controls, suggesting an influence of ligand oligomers in disease pathology [2, 50]. Since the BAFF/APRIL-TACI axis seemed to be involved in the pathogenesis of SLE, the coding region of TACI was analyzed in 119 patients with SLE, but no disease-associated mutations were detected [51]. It was assumed that survival signals via BAFF-R in the presence of high BAFF levels would lead to survival of autoreactive B cells. High BAFF levels, however, were not found to impair negative B cell selection. They lead to expansion of autoreactive B cells with low affinity from the normal B cell repertoire. Obviously, autoantibody production from innate B cells is the basic mechanism for the development of autoimmunity and uncontrolled B cell survival. On the one hand, TLR7 can upregulate TACI expression [52]; on the other hand, upregulation of TLR7 via BAFF is TACI dependent [53]. TACI activation can lead to autoantibody production. In mice, loss of TACI expression inhibited class-switched autoantibody production [54]. In a SLE mouse model (Nba2.Yaa), TACI deficiency resulted in a reduced disease activity and a reduced development of glomerulonephritis. Mortality of TACI−/− mice was lower compared to the control group, whereas it was higher than within the control in BCMA−/− mice. In mice with TACI and BCMA deficiency, mortality was comparable to TACI−/− mice. APRIL and TACI−/− mice showed a reduced reaction to T cell-independent type II antigens [55]. If only one TACI allele is carrying a mutation, there is an increased risk of developing autoimmune phenomena. Patients carrying one mutated TACI C104R allele showed, compared to individuals carrying two mutated TACI C104R alleles, high serum levels of antinuclear antibodies. Remarkably, central B cell tolerance is disturbed both in individuals with one mutated and with two mutated TACI C104R alleles. In CVID patients, however, peripheral B cell tolerance is impaired, too. Therefore, the defects in central B cell tolerance cannot be compensated [21].

TACI-deficient patients show impaired antibody responses against polysaccharides after vaccination with pneumovax [23], which is similar in TACI-deficient mice [27]. The extent of hypogammaglobulinemia in humans with TACI deficiency is more variable as compared to TACI-deficient mice, which usually show only mild hypogammaglobulinemia. In humans all the immunoglobulin isotypes may be affected ranging from hypogammaglobulinemia in the majority of affected to agammaglobulinemia [33, 34] and to IgG subclass deficiencies [42] as well as to IgA deficiency [23, 33] in some. Mutations in the TACI gene were also detected in 1–2% of healthy individuals [56], who usually show normal immunoglobulin levels. This led to the assumption that there might be also an advantage for individuals carrying a TACI mutation. TACI-deficient mice produced IgD antibodies for certain antigens. Infections with *Citrobacter rodentium*, being a murine model for human *E. coli* infections, was cleared with higher efficacy in TACI KO mice than in TACI WT mice [57]. It was suggested that TACI deficiency gives an advantage in younger individuals when it is of great importance to deal with enteritis. In our Western lifestyle and with people reaching higher age under good hygienic conditions, the disadvantages of carrying a TACI mutation including the development of CVID, malignancies, or autoimmunity prevails [57]. TACI variants were also found in Swedish patients with wheeze and asthma. It is unknown, however, in which way TACI variants might increase the risk for asthma [58]. TACI also seems to play a role in the pathogenesis of COPD. The synthesis of IgA1 was elevated in COPD lung tissue. TACI, BAFF, APRIL, and IL-6 were stronger expressed in lung tissue and epithelia of COPD patients than in healthy individuals. IgA is upregulated via the IL-6/IL-6 receptor or the BAFF/APRIL/TACI pathway [59].

9.4 Diagnosis and Management

Since TACI mutations are not disease causing, their verification is currently not considered clinically relevant and is reserved to research studies. Expression analysis of TACI protein (e.g., by flow cytometry) is, however, usually not sufficient to diagnose a TACI defect, since many mutations leave protein expression unimpaired and TACI expressing CD27+ memory B cells may only be detected in low numbers in antibody-deficient patients irrespective of their TACI mutation status. Thus confirmation of a TACI mutation should be done by genetic analysis.

The management of CVID patients carrying a TACI mutation does not differ from conventional CVID. However, one should take into account the higher rates of autoimmune and lymphoproliferative complications seen in these individuals.

References

1. Hoffmann FS, Kuhn PH, Laurent SA, Hauck SM, Berer K, Wendlinger SA, Krumbholz M, Khademi M, Olsson T, Dreyling M, Pfister HW, Alexander T, Hiepe F, Kümpfel T, Crawford HC, Wekerle H, Hohlfeld R, Lichtenthaler SF, Meinl E. The immunoregulator soluble TACI is released by ADAM10 and reflects B cell activation in autoimmunity. J Immunol. 2015;194:542–52.
2. Roschke V, Sosnovtseva S, Ward CD, Hong JS, Smith R, Albert V, Stohl W, Baker KP, Ullrich S, Nardelli B, Hilbert DM, Migone TS. BLyS and APRIL form biologically active heterotrimers that are expressed in patients with systemic immune-based rheumatic diseases. J Immunol. 2002;169:4314–21.

3. Bischof D, Elsawa SF, Mantchev G, Yoon J, Michels GE, Nilson A, Sutor SL, Platt JL, Ansell SM, von Bulow G, Bram RJ. Selective activation of TACI by syndecan-2. Blood. 2006;107:3235–42.
4. Ingold K, Zumsteg A, Tardivel A, Huard B, Steiner QG, Cachero TG, Qiang F, Gorelik L, Kalled SL, Acha-Orbea H, Rennert PD, Tschopp J, Schneider P. Identification of proteoglycans as the APRIL-specific binding partners. J Exp Med. 2005;201:1375–83.
5. Ng LG, Sutherland AP, Newton R, Qian F, Cachero TG, Scott ML, Thompson JS, Wheway J, Chtanova T, Groom J, Sutton IJ, Xin C, Tangye SG, Kalled SL, Mackay F, Mackay CR. B cell-activating factor belonging to the TNF family (BAFF)-R is the principal BAFF receptor facilitating BAFF costimulation of circulating T and B cells. J Immunol. 2004;173: 807–17.
6. Sasaki Y, Casola S, Kutok JL, Rajewsky K, Schmidt-Supprian M. TNF family member B cell-activating factor (BAFF) receptor-dependent and -independent roles for BAFF in B cell physiology. J Immunol. 2004;173:2245–52.
7. Schneider P, Takatsuka H, Wilson A, Mackay F, Tardivel A, Lens S, Cachero TG, Finke D, Beermann F, Tschopp J. Maturation of marginal zone and follicular B cells requires B cell activating factor of the tumor necrosis factor family and is independent of B cell maturation antigen. J Exp Med. 2001;194:1691–7.
8. Avery DT, Kalled SL, Ellyard JI, Ambrose C, Bixler SA, Thien M, Brink R, Mackay F, Hodgkin PD, Tangye SG. BAFF selectively enhances the survival of plasmablasts generated from human memory B cells. J Clin Invest. 2003;112:286–97.
9. Novak AJ, Darce JR, Arendt BK, Harder B, Henderson K, Kindsvogel W, Gross JA, Greipp PR, Jelinek DF. Expression of BCMA, TACI, and BAFF-R in multiple myeloma: a mechanism for growth and survival. Blood. 2004;103:689–94.
10. O'Connor BP, Raman VS, Erickson LD, Cook WJ, Weaver LK, Ahonen C, Lin LL, Mantchev GT, Bram RJ, Noelle RJ. BCMA is essential for the survival of long-lived bone marrow plasma cells. J Exp Med. 2004;199:91–8.
11. Batten M, Fletcher C, Ng LG, Groom J, Wheway J, Laabi Y, Xin X, Schneider P, Tschopp J, Mackay CR, Mackay F. TNF deficiency fails to protect BAFF transgenic mice against autoimmunity and reveals a predisposition to B cell lymphoma. J Immunol. 2004;172:812–22.
12. Sakurai D, Kanno Y, Hase H, Kojima H, Okumura K, Kobata T. TACI attenuates antibody production costimulated by BAFF-R and CD40. Eur J Immunol. 2007;37:110–8.
13. Hymowitz SG, Patel DR, Wallweber HJ, Runyon S, Yan M, Yin J, Shriver SK, Gordon NC, Pan B, Skelton NJ, Kelley RF, Starovasnik MA. Structures of APRIL-receptor complexes: like BCMA, TACI employs only a single cysteine-rich domain for high affinity ligand binding. J Biol Chem. 2005;280:7218–27.
14. Garcia-Carmona Y, Cols M, Ting AT, Radigan L, Yuk FJ, Zhang L, Cerutti A, Cunningham-Rundles C. Differential induction of plasma cells by isoforms of human TACI. Blood. 2015;125:1749–58.
15. Mackay F, Schneider P. Cracking the BAFF code. Nat Rev Immunol. 2009;9:491–502.
16. Schuepbach-Mallepell S, Das D, Willen L, Vigolo M, Tardivel A, Lebon L, Kowalczyk-Quintas C, Nys J, Smulski C, Zheng TS, Maskos K, Lammens A, Jiang X, Hess H, Tan SL, Schneider P. Stoichiometry of heteromeric BAFF and APRIL cytokines dictates their receptor binding and signaling properties. J Biol Chem. 2015;290:16330–42.
17. Smulski CR, Kury P, Seidel LM, Staiger HS, Edinger AK, Willen L, Seidl M, Hess H, Salzer U, Rolink AG, Rizzi M, Schneider P, Eibel H. BAFF- and TACI-dependent processing of BAFFR by ADAM proteases regulates the survival of B cells. Cell Rep. 2017;18:2189–202.
18. He B, Santamaria R, Xu W, Cols M, Chen K, Puga I, Shan M, Xiong H, Bussel JB, Chiu A, Puel A, Reichenbach J, Marodi L, Döffinger R, Vasconcelos J, Issekutz A, Krause J, Davies G, Li X, Grimbacher B, Plebani A, Meffre E, Picard C, Cunningham-Rundles C, Casanova JL, Cerutti A. The transmembrane activator TACI triggers immunoglobulin class switching by activating B cells through the adaptor MyD88. Nat Immunol. 2010;11:836–45.
19. von Bulow GU, Bram RJ. NF-AT activation induced by a CAML-interacting member of the tumor necrosis factor receptor superfamily. Science. 1997;278:138–41.

20. von Bulow GU, Russell H, Copeland NG, Gilbert DJ, Jenkins NA, Bram RJ. Molecular cloning and functional characterization of murine transmembrane activator and CAML interactor (TACI) with chromosomal localization in human and mouse. Mamm Genome. 2000;11:628–32.
21. Romberg N, Chamberlain N, Saadoun D, Gentile M, Kinnunen T, Ng YS, Virdee M, Menard L, Cantaert T, Morbach H, Rachid R, Martinez-Pomar N, Matamoros N, Geha R, Grimbacher B, Cerutti A, Cunningham-Rundles C, Meffre E. CVID-associated TACI mutations affect autoreactive B cell selection and activation. J Clin Invest. 2013;123:4283–93.
22. Castigli E, Wilson SA, Scott S, Dedeoglu F, Xu S, Lam KP, Bram RJ, Jabara H, Geha RS. TACI and BAFF-R mediate isotype switching in B cells. J Exp Med. 2005;201:35–9.
23. Castigli E, Wilson SA, Garibyan L, Rachid R, Bonilla F, Schneider L, Geha RS. TACI is mutant in common variable immunodeficiency and IgA deficiency. Nat Genet. 2005;37:829–34.
24. Litinskiy MB, Nardelli B, Hilbert DM, He B, Schaffer A, Casali P, Cerutti A. DCs induce CD40-independent immunoglobulin class switching through BLyS and APRIL. Nat Immunol. 2002;3:822–9.
25. Castigli E, Scott S, Dedeoglu F, Bryce P, Jabara H, Bhan AK, Mizoguchi E, Geha RS. Impaired IgA class switching in APRIL-deficient mice. PNAS. 2004;101:3903–8.
26. Seshasayee D, Valdez P, Yan M, Dixit VM, Tumas D, Grewal IS. Loss of TACI causes fatal lymphoproliferation and autoimmunity, establishing TACI as an inhibitory BLyS receptor. Immunity. 2003;18:279–88.
27. von Bulow GU, van Deursen JM, Bram RJ. Regulation of the T-independent humoral response by TACI. Immunity. 2001;14:573–82.
28. Yan M, Wang H, Chan B, Roose-Girma M, Erickson S, Baker T, Tumas D, Grewal IS, Dixit VM. Activation and accumulation of B cells in TACI-deficient mice. Nat Immunol. 2001;2:638–43.
29. Jabara HH, Lee JJ, Janssen E, Ullas S, Liadaki K, Garibyan L, Benson H, Sannikova T, Bram R, Hammarstrom L, Cruz AC, Siegel R, Manis J, Malley R, Geha RS. Heterozygosity for transmembrane activator and calcium modulator ligand interactor A144E causes haploinsufficiency and pneumococcal susceptibility in mice. J Allergy Clin Immunol. 2017;139:1293–1301.e4.
30. Lee JJ, Jabara HH, Garibyan L, Rauter I, Sannikova T, Dillon SR, Bram R, Geha RS. The C104R mutant impairs the function of transmembrane activator and calcium modulator and cyclophilin ligand interactor (TACI) through haploinsufficiency. J Allergy Clin Immunol. 2010;126:1234–41.e2.
31. Lee JJ, Rauter I, Garibyan L, Ozcan E, Sannikova T, Dillon SR, Cruz AC, Siegel RM, Bram R, Jabara H, Geha RS. The murine equivalent of the A181E TACI mutation associated with common variable immunodeficiency severely impairs B-cell function. Blood. 2009;114:2254–62.
32. Bacchelli C, Buckland KF, Buckridge S, Salzer U, Schneider P, Thrasher AJ, Gaspar HB. The C76R transmembrane activator and calcium modulator cyclophilin ligand interactor mutation disrupts antibody production and B-cell homeostasis in heterozygous and homozygous mice. J Allergy Clin Immunol. 2011;127:1253–9.e13.
33. Salzer U, Chapel HM, Webster AD, Pan-Hammarstrom Q, Schmitt-Graeff A, Schlesier M, Peter HH, Rockstroh JK, Schneider P, Schaffer AA, Hammarstrom L, Grimbacher B. Mutations in TNFRSF13B encoding TACI are associated with common variable immunodeficiency in humans. Nat Genet. 2005;37:820–8.
34. Salzer U, Bacchelli C, Buckridge S, Pan-Hammarström Q, Jennings S, Lougaris V, Bergbreiter A, Hagena T, Birmelin J, Plebani A, Webster AD, Peter HH, Suez D, Chapel H, McLean-Tooke A, Spickett GP, Anover-Sombke S, Ochs HD, Urschel S, Belohradsky BH, Ugrinovic S, Kumararatne DS, Lawrence TC, Holm AM, Franco JL, Schulze I, Schneider P, Gertz EM, Schäffer AA, Hammarström L, Thrasher AJ, Gaspar HB, Grimbacher B. Relevance of biallelic versus monoallelic TNFRSF13B mutations in distinguishing disease-causing from risk-increasing TNFRSF13B variants in antibody deficiency syndromes. Blood. 2009;113:1967–76.
35. Garibyan L, Lobito AA, Siegel RM, Call ME, Wucherpfennig KW, Geha RS. Dominant-negative effect of the heterozygous C104R TACI mutation in common variable immunodeficiency (CVID). J Clin Invest. 2007;117:1550–7.

36. Chinen J, Martinez-Gallo M, Gu W, Cols M, Cerutti A, Radigan L, Zhang L, Potocki L, Withers M, Lupski JR, Cunningham-Rundles C. Transmembrane activator and CAML interactor (TACI) haploinsufficiency results in B-cell dysfunction in patients with Smith-Magenis syndrome. J Allergy Clin Immunol. 2011;127:1579–86.
37. Romberg N, Virdee M, Chamberlain N, Oe T, Schickel JN, Perkins T, Cantaert T, Rachid R, Rosengren S, Palazzo R, Geha R, Cunningham-Rundles C, Meffre E. TNF receptor superfamily member 13b (TNFRSF13B) hemizygosity reveals transmembrane activator and CAML interactor haploinsufficiency at later stages of B-cell development. J Allergy Clin Immunol. 2015;136:1315–25.
38. Warnatz K, Denz A, Dräger R, Braun M, Groth C, Wolff-Vorbeck G, Eibel H, Schlesier M, Peter HH. Severe deficiency of switched memory B cells (CD27(+)IgM(−)IgD(−)) in subgroups of patients with common variable immunodeficiency: a new approach to classify a heterogeneous disease. Blood. 2002;99:1544–51.
39. Endo T, Nishio M, Enzler T, Cottam HB, Fukuda T, James DF, Karin M, Kipps TJ. BAFF and APRIL support chronic lymphocytic leukemia B-cell survival through activation of the canonical NF-kappaB pathway. Blood. 2007;109:703–10.
40. Margraf RL, Coonrod EM, Durtschi JD, Augustine NH, Voelkerding KV, Hill HR, Kumánovics A. TACI mutation p.Lys154Ter identified in Good Syndrome. Clin Immunol. 2013;146:10–2.
41. Sáenz-Cuesta M, Martínez-Pomar N, de Gracia J, Echaniz P, Villegas E, Prada A, Otaegui D, Matamoros N, Cuadrado E. TACI mutation in Good's Syndrome: in search of a genetic basis. Clin Immunol. 2012;145:27–30.
42. Speletas M, Salzer U, Florou Z, Petinaki E, Daniil Z, Bardaka F, Gourgoulianis KI, Skoulakis C, Germenis AE. Heterozygous alterations of TNFRSF13B/TACI in tonsillar hypertrophy and sarcoidosis. Clin Dev Immunol. 2013;2013:532437.
43. Fischer A, Provot J, Jais JP, Alcais A, Mahlaoui N, Members of the CEREDIH French PID Study Group. Autoimmune and inflammatory manifestations occur frequently in patients with primary immunodeficiencies. J Allergy Clin Immunol. 2017;140:1388–1393.e8.
44. Mackay F, Woodcock SA, Lawton P, Ambrose C, Baetscher M, Schneider P, Tschopp J, Browning JL. Mice transgenic for BAFF develop lymphocytic disorders along with autoimmune manifestations. J Exp Med. 1999;190:1697–710.
45. Khare SD, Sarosi I, Xia XZ, McCabe S, Miner K, Solovyev I, Hawkins N, Kelley M, Chang D, Van G, Ross L, Delaney J, Wang L, Lacey D, Boyle WJ, Hsu H. Severe B cell hyperplasia and autoimmune disease in TALL-1 transgenic mice. Proc Natl Acad Sci U S A. 2000;97:3370–5.
46. Chu VT, Enghard P, Schürer S, Steinhauser G, Rudolph B, Riemekasten G, Berek C. Systemic activation of the immune system induces aberrant BAFF and APRIL expression in B cells in patients with systemic lupus erythematosus. Arthritis Rheum. 2009;60:2083–93.
47. Treamtrakanpon W, Tantivitayakul P, Benjachat T, Somparn P, Kittikowit W, Eiam-ong S, Leelahavanichkul A, Hirankarn N, Avihingsanon Y. APRIL, a proliferation-inducing ligand, as a potential marker of lupus nephritis. Arthritis Res Ther. 2012;14:R252.
48. Becker-Merok A, Nikolaisen C, Nossent HC. B-lymphocyte activating factor in systemic lupus erythematosus and rheumatoid arthritis in relation to autoantibody levels, disease measures and time. Lupus. 2006;15:570–6.
49. Stohl W, Metyas S, Tan SM, Cheema GS, Oamar B, Roschke V, Wu Y, Baker KP, Hilbert DM. Inverse association between circulating APRIL levels and serological and clinical disease activity in patients with systemic lupus erythematosus. Ann Rheum Dis. 2004;63:1096–103.
50. Dillon SR, Harder B, Lewis KB, Moore MD, Liu H, Bukowski TR, Hamacher NB, Lantry MM, Maurer M, Krejsa CM, Ellsworth JL, Pederson S, Elkon KB, Wener MH, Dall'Era M, Gross JA. B-lymphocyte stimulator/a proliferation-inducing ligand heterotrimers are elevated in the sera of patients with autoimmune disease and are neutralized by atacicept and B-cell maturation antigen-immunoglobulin. Arthritis Res Ther. 2010;12:R48.
51. Salzer U, Birmelin J, Bacchelli C, Witte T, Buchegger-Podbielski U, Buckridge S, Rzepka R, Gaspar HB, Thrasher AJ, Schmidt RE, Melchers I, Grimbacher B. Sequence analysis of TNFRSF13b, encoding TACI, in patients with systemic lupus erythematosus. J Clin Immunol. 2007;27:372–7.

52. Groom JR, Fletcher CA, Walters SN, Grey ST, Watt SV, Sweet MJ, Smyth MJ, Mackay CR, Mackay F. BAFF and MyD88 signals promote a lupuslike disease independent of T cells. J Exp Med. 2007;204:1959–71.
53. Figgett WA, Fairfax K, Vincent FB, Le Page MA, Katik I, Deliyanti D, Quah PS, Verma P, Grumont R, Gerondakis S, Hertzog P, O'Reilly LA, Strasser A, Mackay F. The TACI receptor regulates T-cell-independent marginal zone B cell responses through innate activation-induced cell death. Immunity. 2013;39:573–83.
54. Figgett WA, Deliyanti D, Fairfax KA, Quah PS, Wilkinson-Berka JL, Mackay F. Deleting the BAFF receptor TACI protects against systemic lupus erythematosus without extensive reduction of B cell numbers. J Autoimmun. 2015;61:9–16.
55. Tran NL, Schneider P, Santiago-Raber ML. TACI-dependent APRIL signaling maintains autoreactive B cells in a mouse model of systemic lupus erythematosus. Eur J Immunol. 2017;47:713–23.
56. Pan-Hammarström Q, Salzer U, Du L, Björkander J, Cunningham-Rundles C, Nelson DL, Bacchelli C, Gaspar HB, Offer S, Behrens TW, Grimbacher B, Hammarström L. Reexamining the role of TACI coding variants in common variable immunodeficiency and selective IgA deficiency. Nat Genet. 2007;39:429–30.
57. Tsuji S, Stein L, Kamada N, Nuñez G, Bram R, Vallance BA, Sousa AE, Platt JL, Cascalho M. TACI deficiency enhances antibody avidity and clearance of an intestinal pathogen. J Clin Invest. 2014;124:4857–66.
58. Janzi M, Melén E, Kull I, Wickman M, Hammarström L. Rare mutations in TNFRSF13B increase the risk of asthma symptoms in Swedish children. Genes Immun. 2012;13:59–65.
59. Ladjemi MZ, Lecocq M, Weynand B, Bowen H, Gould HJ, Van Snick J, Detry B, Pilette C. Increased IgA production by B-cells in COPD via lung epithelial interleukin-6 and TACI pathways. Eur Respir J. 2015;45:980–93.

LRBA Deficiency

10

Laura Gámez-Díaz

10.1 Introduction

Among the syndromes associated to immune dysregulation and antibody deficiency, we find a rare autosomal recessive disease known as lipopolysaccharide-responsive beige-like anchor (LRBA) deficiency. This syndrome was first described in 2012 in five children harboring four different homozygous mutations in *LRBA*, all of which abolished the LRBA protein expression [1]. LRBA deficiency presents early in life and is characterized by a wide spectrum of clinical manifestations ranging from autoimmunity, enteropathy, and organomegaly, to hypogammaglobulinemia, recurrent respiratory infections, polyendocrinopathy, growth retardation, and neurologic diseases [2–5]. Initially, LRBA deficiency was described as a monogenetic cause of common variable immunodeficiency (CVID) with autoimmune complications, as the first LRBA-deficient patients suffered mostly from recurrent infections and abnormalities in the B-cell compartment accompanied by autoimmune cytopenias [1]. However, further description from additional patients places LRBA deficiency into the expanding group of immunodysregulation syndromes due to the high frequency of different autoimmune manifestations that are observed in more than 90 affected patients described up to date worldwide.

L. Gámez-Díaz
Center for Chronic Immunodeficiency, University Medical Center of Freiburg, University of Freiburg, Freiburg im Breisgau, Germany
e-mail: laura.gamez@uniklinik-freiburg.de

M. M. D'Elios, M. Rizzi (eds.), *Humoral Primary Immunodeficiencies*, Rare Diseases of the Immune System, https://doi.org/10.1007/978-3-319-91785-6_10

10.2 Etiology

LRBA deficiency is caused by loss-of-protein biallelic mutations in *LRBA*. To date, around 50 different homozygous or compound heterozygous mutations in *LRBA* have been reported in the literature without showing any evident genotype-phenotype correlation [2, 3, 5]. These mutations include missense mutations, nonsense mutations, splice site mutations, deletions, and duplications, which are distributed throughout all LRBA protein domains affecting equally the protein stability [2, 3, 5]. However, residual LRBA expression has been detected in some patients harboring homozygous missense mutations at the c-terminus of the LRBA protein. One of them remains healthy at the age of 7 years, whereas the other patients present with a less severe clinical and immune phenotype [2, 6, 7]. In addition, LRBA deficiency affects similarly females and males, and there is no ethnical susceptibility reported so far.

10.3 Clinical Manifestations

Patients with LRBA deficiency manifest with a heterogeneous group of clinical symptoms and immunological findings, including:

- *Immune dysregulation* is the main clinical feature of LRBA deficiency, since more than 90% of LRBA-deficient patients suffer from at least one autoimmune disorder. Inflammatory bowel disease-like (IBD-like) (Fig. 10.1), autoimmune hemolytic anemia (AIHA), and autoimmune thrombocytopenia (ITP) are the most frequent autoimmune entities affecting 62–76%, 57–70%, and 30–50% of the patients, respectively [2–5]. Chronic diarrhea and unresponsiveness to treatment have been related to growth failure observed in about 25% of LRBA-deficient patients. Juvenile idiopathic arthritis (JIA), neutropenia, chronic autoimmune hepatitis, eczema, type 1 diabetes (T1D), autoimmune thyroiditis, arthritis, uveitis, psoriasis, vitiligo, and alopecia can also occur but are less frequent [2–5]. Chronic erosive and nonerosive arthritis and polyendocrinopathy disorder have also been reported in three patients [8, 9]. Moreover, a history of atopic disorders has been documented in LRBA deficiency, such as food allergy, insect sting allergies, allergic dermatitis, urticaria, and asthma [5].
- *Organomegaly* or lymphoproliferative disorders are observed in 76–86% of LRBA-deficient patients, including splenomegaly, lymphadenopathy, and hepatomegaly [2–5] (Fig. 10.1).
- *Recurrent infections* are mostly affecting the upper and lower respiratory tract (70–76% of patients), including pneumonia, sinusitis, and otitis media [2–5]. These infections frequently caused parenchymal lung abnormalities such as lymphocytic infiltrates and bronchiectasis in the context of LRBA deficiency (Fig. 10.1). Bronchiolitis obliterans organizing pneumonia (BOOP) has been reported in one patient [10]. Up to date, LRBA-deficient patients do not show susceptibility to any particular pathogen, but all of them have presented at least

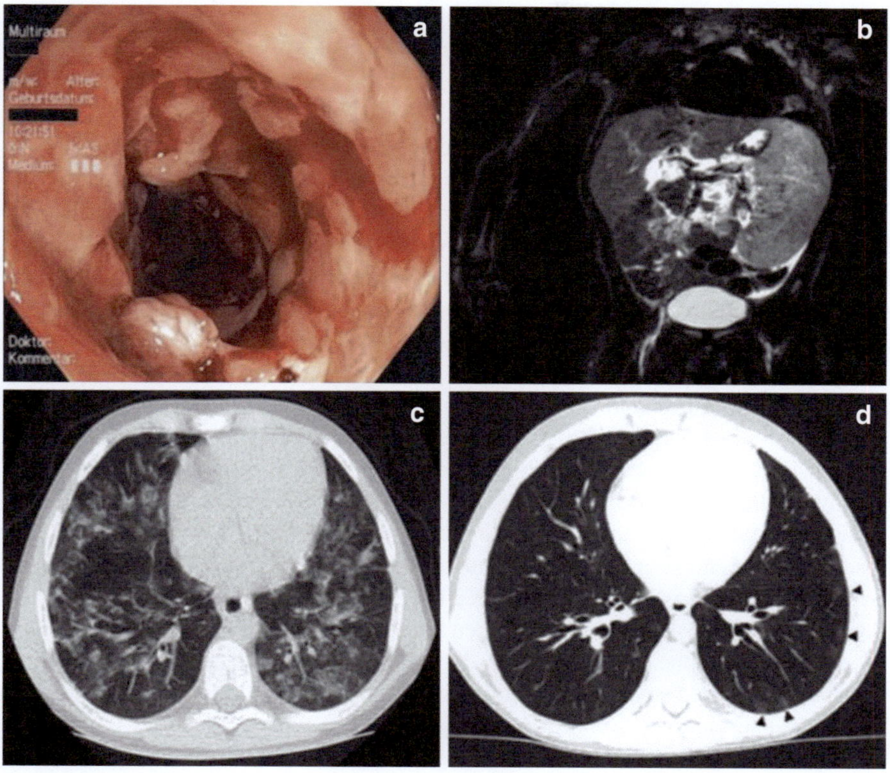

Fig. 10.1 Intestinal, pulmonary, and splenic alterations in LRBA-deficient patients. (**a**) Colonoscopy revealing severe circular inflammation in the rectum, numerous ulcerations, and mucosal edema and erythema. (**b**) Magnetic resonance image of marked splenomegaly. (**c**) High-resolution chest-computed tomographic scan showing atypical, partly conflating patchy alveolar consolidations in both lungs. (**d**) Marked regression of alveolar consolidation 2 years after therapy and slight bilateral ground-glass infiltrates (Obtained from *Gámez-Diaz et al. JACI, 2017*)

one documented infection mostly associated to opportunistic microorganisms including, *Campylobacter jejuni*, *Morganella morganii*, *Proteus mirabilis*, *Yersinia enterocolitica*, *Cryptosporidium parvum*, *Giardia lamblia*, *Legionella pneumophila*, aspergillosis, and chronic mucocutaneous candidiasis (CMC) [2–5]. Infections caused by *Staphylococcus aureus* have also been reported [4].

- *Hypogammaglobulinemia* is observed in 50–80% of LRBA-deficient patients, presenting with reduction of one, two, or three immunoglobulin isotypes. Reductions of IgG alone, or in combination with low IgM and/or IgA, are the most frequently observed entities in LRBA deficiency [2]. Specific antibody response after vaccination is however variable.
- *Neurologic complications* are reported in about 20% of patients with diagnosis of LRBA deficiency [3, 5]. They include unilateral optic nerve atrophy, granuloma-like lesions coupled with a demyelinating process, and cerebral

granuloma associated with strabismus, hemiplegia, and seizures. Optic neuritis, brain abscess, cerebral and cerebellar atrophy, as well as parietal lobe lesion have also been reported [3, 5].

LRBA deficiency resembles the overall picture of patients with cytotoxic T-lymphocyte antigen 4 (CTLA-4) insufficiency, which is caused by autosomal heterozygous mutations in *CTLA-4* [11]. Both syndromes are characterized by the presence of autoantibody-mediated cytopenias, organomegaly, hypogammaglobulinemia, organ-specific autoimmunity, and lymphocytic infiltration of nonlymphoid organs [12]. However, the clinical onset of LRBA deficiency is characteristically in childhood (mean age of 5 year), whereas most CTLA-4-insufficient patients developed their first symptoms in adolescence or early adulthood [12, 13]. Although CTLA-4-insufficient patients are more prone to develop malignancies, several types of tumors have also been observed in patients with LRBA deficiency, including Burkitt lymphoma [7], Epstein-Barr virus lymphoma, lymphomatous central nervous system pseudotumor [1], dysplastic tubular adenoma and polyps [14], multifocal gastric cancer, and malignant melanoma [15]. Lower mortality and morbidity are reported in CTLA-4-insufficient patients suggesting additional roles of LRBA that are CTLA-4 independent. Disease penetrance is approximately 60% in CTLA-4 mutation carriers, while LRBA deficiency presents nearly complete penetrance [11–13]. Furthermore, the heterogeneity of the clinical phenotype in LRBA-deficient patients is also observed in affected members from the same family carrying an identical mutation in *LRBA*, as demonstrated in one child harboring a homozygous mutation in *LRBA* who is currently healthy despite having two affected siblings with the same mutation, suggesting the existence and influence of modifier genes and microbial/environmental triggers that are still unknown [2]. In addition, LRBA deficiency should also be considered as a clinical differential diagnosis of autoimmune lymphoproliferative syndrome (ALPS), immune dysregulation, polyendocrinopathy, enteropathy, X-linked syndrome (IPEX), and signal transducer and activator of transcription 3 (STAT3) gain-of-function (GOF) [16]. These syndromes share several clinical similarities including autoimmune cytopenias, multi-organ autoimmunity, organomegaly, and lymphoproliferation. However, ALPS is caused by mutations in *FAS*, *FASL*, *CASP10* that lead to a defective lymphocyte apoptosis mediated through the Fas/Fas ligand (FASL) pathway [17], IPEX is caused by defective suppression capacity of regulatory T cells due to mutations in the transcription factor *FOXP3* [18], and somatic GOF mutations in *STAT3* confer increased STAT3 transcriptional activity, impair cytokine signaling, and diminish Treg compartment [16]. A comparison of the main characteristics of these PIDs is summarized (Table 10.1).

Absence of LRBA protein expression causes LRBA deficiency, but overexpression of LRBA is associated with cancer cell growth, particularly in the kidney, pancreas, colon, rectum, and lung [19]. However, the expression levels of LRBA varied greatly depending on the tumor type and developmental stage. These results indicate that LRBA might play a role in the suppression of apoptosis, thereby facilitating cell proliferation and cell survival [19]. Additionally, increased expression of LRBA has been observed in erythroid progenitor cells suggesting the possible involvement of LRBA in hematopoietic disorders [20]. Further analysis should focus on determining the potential role of LRBA in cancer development as anticancer therapeutic target.

Table 10.1 Differential diagnosis of LRBA deficiency with other immune dysregulation syndromes

PID	LRBA deficiency	CTLA-4 insufficiency	ALPS	IPEX
Characteristic				
Gene affected	*LRBA*	*CTLA-4*	*TNFRSF6* (FAS) *FAS-L, CASP10*	*FOXP3*
Hereditary pattern	Germinal, autosomal recessive	Germinal, autosomal dominant	Germinal or somatic, mostly autosomal dominant and recessive in few cases	X-linked
Penetrance	Complete (only one individual remain healthy)	Incomplete Around 60%	Missense mutations in intracellular domain: 90% Truncated mutations in intracellular domain: 70% Any mutation in extracellular domain: 30%	Complete
Genotype-phenotype correlation	No (heterogeneous syndrome)	No (heterogeneous syndrome)	Yes (heterogeneous syndrome)	No (heterogeneous syndrome)
Gender predominance	No	No	Male (75%)	Male
Onset	Childhood	Early adulthood	Neonatal	Neonatal
Autoimmune cytopenias	Yes	Yes	Yes	Yes
Enteropathy	Yes	Yes	Not frequent	Yes
Organomegaly	Yes	Yes	Yes	Yes
Hypogammaglobulinemia	Yes (around 60%)	Yes (around 80%)	Few cases. Mostly, hyper-IgG and hyper-IgA	No. Elevated IgE
Recurrent infections	Yes	Yes	Not frequent	Rare
Lymphoproliferation	Yes	Yes	Yes	Yes
Endocrinopathy	T1DM, thyroiditis	Yes	No	T1DM, thyroiditis

(continued)

Table 10.1 (continued)

PID	LRBA deficiency	CTLA-4 insufficiency	ALPS	IPEX
Main laboratory findings	Decrease of: • Tregs (controversial) • $CD27^{+}IgD^{-}$ B cells • $CD138^{+}$ B cells • CTLA-4 expression • CTLA-4 trans-endocytosis • LRBA expression (complete absence in most cases)	Decrease of: • CTLA-4 expression • CTLA-4 ligand binding • CTLA-4 trans-endocytosis • $CD27^{+}IgD^{-}$ B cells Increase of: • $CD21^{low}$ B cells	Increase of: • Circulating $TCR\alpha\beta^{+}$ T cells • $CD4^{-}CD8^{-}$ T lymphocytes • Plasma levels of FasL • Plasma levels of IL-10 • T-cell apoptosis	Reduce of: • Foxp3 expression • Tregs suppression capacity Increase of: • Eosinophils • Th2 cytokine production
Mimics murine model	No	No	Yes	Yes

10.4 Pathophysiology of LRBA Deficiency

Although the exact biological role of LRBA is not fully understood, a recent study has shown that LRBA is required for the post-translational expression and trafficking of CTLA-4 [7]. CTLA-4 is a protein receptor expressed in activated conventional T cells and in regulatory T cells (Tregs). Upon stimulation of the T-cell receptor (TCR), CTLA-4 is mobilized in vesicles to the cell surface where it captures the co-stimulatory molecules CD80 and CD86 from antigen-presenting cells (APC) by a mechanism called trans-endocytosis, thereby downregulating the proinflammatory response [21]. Several negative response elements or proteins that modulate the transcriptional or the post-translational expression of CTLA-4 have been identified. Among those, the AP-1 protein complex binds to a four-amino acid (YVKM) motif of the cytoplasmic tail of CTLA-4, allowing the trafficking of CTLA-4 to AP-1 containing vesicles to lysosomes for degradation [21]. In contrast, LRBA allows the recycling of CTLA-4 to AP-1containing vesicles to the cell membrane of Tregs by binding the YVKM motif of CTLA-4, thereby blocking the AP-1-binding site and controlling the T cell activation proinflammatory response [7]. In the absence of LRBA (as seen in LRBA deficiency), diminished CTLA-4 protein levels are observed due to increased CTLA-4 lysosomal degradation due to enhanced AP-1 binding. Low CTLA-4 levels might contribute to a defective regulation of the immune response and to the development of autoimmune manifestations and lymphoproliferation that are frequently observed in LRBA-deficient patients [7, 12] (Fig. 10.2).

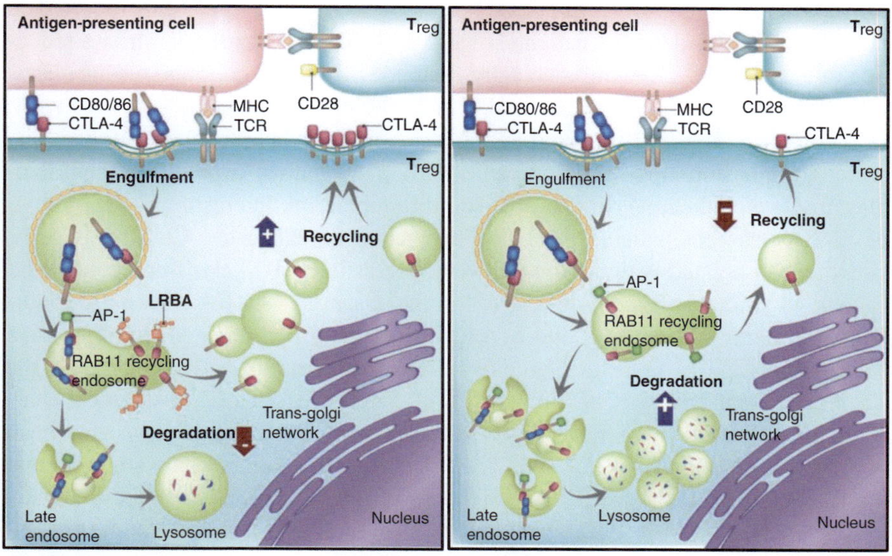

Fig. 10.2 LRBA regulates CTLA-4 trafficking in Tregs. Upon activation of T cells, LRBA competes with higher affinity against AP-1 for binding the YVKM motif of the CTLA-4 tail. LRBA-CTLA-4 interaction is required to guide CTLA-4-containing vesicles to the cell surface in order to capture and engulf the co-stimulatory molecules CD80 and CD86 from the antigen-presenting cells (APC), thereby effectively controlling T-cell activation. In the absence of LRBA, the adaptor protein AP-1 binds to CTLA-4 leading to its lysosomal degradation (Modified from *Sansom D. Science. 2015*)

The mechanisms underlying the B-cell abnormalities and the antibody deficiency observed in patients with LRBA deficiency, have been attributed to the high apoptosis rate observed in LRBA-deficient B cells as a consequence of defective autophagy after serum deprivation [1]. Autophagy is a catabolic process that degrades long-lived proteins and organelles to guarantee protein homeostasis and protein quality control at steady state or especially during starvation or stress conditions, thereby supporting cell survival [22]. Interestingly, short- and long-lived plasma cells need to reshape and expand their endoplasmic reticulum (ER) in order to produce a high number of immunoglobulins after encountering an antigen [22]. This process causes severe oxidative, proteasome, and ER stress that can be counterbalanced by enhancing autophagy, thereby limiting the ER capacity and the immunoglobulin production, as well as promoting energy production and cell survival. However, when autophagy is defective, like in atg5-deficient cells, reduced B-cell survival and reduced ATP levels are observed [22], evidencing an essential role of autophagy during plasma cell differentiation. Therefore, defective autophagy in the absence of LRBA might explain the low numbers of switched memory B cells and plasmablasts.

10.5 Laboratory Findings

Immunologic abnormalities on the humoral response include decreased serum titers of IgG in 57–84% of the affected patients, solely or in combination with reduced IgM and IgA [2, 3]. Defective specific antibody response has been reported in 50–70% of LRBA-deficient patients. In addition, 40–60% of patients show a reduction of total B cells, affecting especially switched memory B cells and plasmablasts, which are detected in low counts in 80% and 90% of affected patients, respectively. In accordance, *in vitro* stimulated LRBA-deficient B cells failed to proliferate, differentiate into antibody-secreting cells (ASC), and induce expression of plasmablast markers, indicating defects in B-cell differentiation. Interestingly, nearly 80% of LRBA-deficient patients presented expansion of exhausted $CD21^{low}$ B cells, which are associated with autoimmune cytopenias in CVID [23]. T-cell counts and CD4:CD8 ratio are typically unaffected in the absence of LRBA. However, abnormal T-cell activation and *in vitro* hyperproliferation (upon CD3 stimulation) have been observed [7]. Aberrant regulatory T-cell functionality and reduction of the Tregs' canonical markers, including CTLA-4, Helios, and CD25, are typical characteristics of LRBA deficiency [24]. Reduced numbers of Tregs have also been observed in about 70% of the cases [2, 24]. However, a recent study suggests that the frequency of Tregs in LRBA deficiency might be underestimated due to low CD25 expression levels, IL-2 consumption, CD4 lymphopenia, or immunosuppressive treatments that reduce FOXP3 expression [25]. Additionally, Tregs exist in human blood as $FOXP3^{high}$ or $FOXP3^{low}$ cells; therefore, low FOXP3 expression might not be indicative of low Treg numbers in LRBA deficiency [25]. In addition, elevated circulating T-follicular helper (TFH) cells biased toward a Th1-like phenotype have been observed in affected patients, reflecting the impaired control of TFH due to aberrant CTLA-4 expression in Tregs [24]. Finally, increased frequencies of of Th1-like, Th17 and Th22 cells along with increased expression of T-box transcription factor (TBET), runt-related transcription factor 1 (RUNX1) and T-cell memory phenotype (CD45RO) have also been reported [7, 26, 27].

10.6 Diagnosis

Due to the wide spectrum of clinical manifestations, LRBA deficiency should be suspected in patients presenting with hypogammaglobulinemia only (and be classified as an antibody-disorder disease), and/or autoimmune cytopenias (and be classified as an immune dysregulation syndrome), and/or inflammatory bowel disease (and be classified as enteropathy), or with a combination of all three. In addition, patients with clinical phenotypes of ALPS-Ph, IPEX-like, CTLA-4 insufficiency, and STAT3 GOF with *FAS, FASL, CASP10*, *FOXP3*, *CTLA-4*, and *STAT3* wild-type sequences should be tested for LRBA deficiency. Currently, the diagnosis of LRBA deficiency relies on the identification of biallelic mutations in *LRBA* that are usually found by whole exome sequencing or targeted sequencing [2–5]. However, increased levels of LRBA protein in immune cells after stimulation can be detected by Western blotting or by flow cytometry and can be used to screen for LRBA deficiency when comparing with a healthy donor, since *LRBA*-biallelic mutation carriers, present complete absence or severely reduced LRBA protein. In fact, a flow cytometry-based test for LRBA deficiency has been recently pusblished. This test allows to discriminate with 94% sensitivity and 80% specificity LRBA-mutation carriers from LRBA-wild type patients [28]. Thus, LRBA protein detection might be useful as initial screening tool of suspected LRBA-deficient patients, narrowing down the amount of patients that need *LRBA* sequencing, thereby facilitating early diagnosis and accelerating treatment implementation [2]. Moreover, impaired CTLA-4 expression in Tregs can help to strengthen the diagnosis when suspecting LRBA deficiency. Interestingly, two functional assays allow discrimination of CTLA-4 from LRBA mutation carriers [25]. The first assay is based on the expression of CTLA-4 by memory Tregs (mTregs), in which mTregs of healthy donors express ten-fold more CTLA-4 than naïve conventional Tregs (nTcon). In contrast, mTregs from CTLA-4-insufficient and LRBA-deficient patients present only a five-fold and three-fold higher expression, respectively [25]. However, upon stimulation with CD3/CD28 beads, LRBA-deficient Tregs increase their CTLA-4 expression 20 to 30 times compared to baseline levels and even more when Tregs are treated with a lysosomal inhibitor such as bafilomycin [25]. Tregs from CTLA-4-insufficient patients on the other hand, keep a low CTLA-4 expression after stimulation, indicating that in LRBA deficiency the CTLA-4 translation is not affected. The second discriminating assay is based on the CTLA-4 trafficking in Tregs. Specifically, patients with *CTLA-4* mutations present with severely reduced trans-endocytosis of CD80–CD86 molecules in Tregs, whereas this process is unaffected in LRBA-deficient patients [25]. Therefore, after clinical suspicion of LRBA deficiency, detection of LRBA protein, evaluation of CTLA-4 levels in mTregs, or measurement of CD80–CD86 trans-endocytosis depending on CTLA-4, might contribute to the diagnosis of LRBA deficiency and/or to monitor the efficacy of therapies such as in patients that underwent HSCT. The final diagnosis of LRBA deficiency relies however, on the identification of biallelic mutations in *LRBA*.

10.7 Management and Treatment

The clinical management of patients with LRBA deficiency is mainly focused on controlling the hypogammaglobulinemia, infections, lymphoproliferation, and autoimmunity. Hypogammaglobulinemia is treated with subcutaneous or intravenous immunoglobulin replacement, in addition to antimicrobial treatment used to control the infectious trigger [2, 3]. Immunosuppressive therapy is used to control lymphoproliferation and autoimmunity and includes steroids, rituximab, hydroxychloroquine, mycophenolate mofetil, and azathioprine among other immunosuppressant agents that are not preventing the long-term deterioration of LRBA-deficient patients [2–5, 29, 30]. Therapy with sirolimus, however, was reported to improve completely the frequency and severity of diarrhea, allowing LRBA-deficient patients to recover weight [2, 3]. In addition, based on the recent knowledge of the contribution of CTLA-4 in the pathogenesis of LRBA deficiency, therapy with abatacept (a fusion protein composed of the Fc region of human IgG1 and the extracellular part of CTLA-4 that inhibits T-cell responses by competing for costimulatory ligands) has been included as a therapeutic option. In fact, a 5–8-year follow-up of two LRBA-deficient patients treated with abatacept showed improvement of the patient's general clinical status such as their pulmonary function. In addition, reduction of soluble CD25, which is a marker for T-cell-mediated inflammation, increase of memory T cells, reduction of T follicular helper cells, and improvement of specific antibody response to polysaccharides were observed in LRBA-deficient patients under abatacept treatment [7]. At present, 12 LRBA-deficient patients with severe clinical courses of disease that were mostly unresponsive to immunosuppression treatment underwent hematopoietic stem cell transplantation (HSCT). Four out of the 12 patients died within 3 months after HSCT due to preexisting infections, graft failure, multi-organ failure, and thrombotic microangiopathy [31]. In contrast, the remaining eight patients presented with complete, good, or partial remission. Particularly, five of those patients showed full chimerism after HSCT, presenting a significant reduction of numbers and intensity of LRBA-related symptoms without relapse and without the necessity for immunosuppressants and immunoglobulin replacement, being therefore in complete or good remission [31]. The three remaining patients are in partial remission, presenting a chimerism of less than 90% and undergoing current immunosuppressive treatment [31]. Although HSCT treatment for LRBA-deficient patients needs to be evaluated in a bigger cohort to prove its efficacy, HSCT is currently recommended, if a suitable donor is present, before the patient presents long-term organ damage that may negatively affect the results of the HSCT.

10.8 Biological Characteristics of LRBA

LRBA is a member of the BEACH domain-containing protein (BDCP) family along with eight other human proteins (Fig. 10.3). Among them are the lysosomal trafficking regulator (LYST), neurobeachin (NBEA), neurobeachin-like 1 (NBEAL1), neurobeachin-like 2 (NBEAL2), WD and FYVE zinc finger domain-containing protein 3 (WDFY3), WD and FYVE zinc finger domain-containing protein 4 (WDFY4), neutral sphingomyelinase activation-associated factor (NSMAF) also known as FAN, and WD repeat domain 81 (WDR81). In BDCPs, BEACH domains are located at the C-terminal end of the protein, usually preceded by a pleckstrin homology (PH) domain and followed by 4–16 repeats of WD dipeptide [32]. WD domain-containing proteins have been implicated in a wide range of cellular functions including cell cycle control, transcriptional regulation, signal transduction, autophagy, apoptosis, and vesicle trafficking [33, 34], whereas BEACH domain-containing proteins are mostly associated to act as scaffolding proteins. The N-terminal part of the BDCPs is weakly conserved, and only few domains have been identified so far. BDCPs are widely expressed in tissues, but little is known about their specific function and the molecular mechanisms through which they act. It has been suggested that they occupy individual and distinct physiological roles mainly involved in vesicle trafficking, cytokinesis, as well as receptor signaling, and that they might work as facilitators of protein-protein interactions [33, 34]. Mutations in genes encoding for BDCP members have been associated with different clinical entities, including a primary immunodeficiency known as Chediak-Higashi syndrome (CHS) and a megakaryocyte lineage disorder known as the gray platelet syndrome (GPS) [35, 36]. CHS is caused by biallelic mutations in *LYST* and it is characterized by hypopigmentation of the skin, eyes, and hair, prolonged bleeding times, recurrent infections, and abnormal natural killer and neutrophil function, since LYST has been suggested to be essential for sorting of cytotoxic granules [35]. On the other hand, patients with homozygous mutations in *NBEAL-2* suffer from GPS, which is characterized by thrombocytopenia and enlarged platelets due to specific absence of alpha-granules [37].

In humans, LRBA is located in the region 31.3 of chromosome 4, and it shares 90% homology with its murine counterpart. According to the Ensembl (www.ensembl.org) and NCBI (National Center for Biotechnology Information: www.ncbi.nlm.nih.gov) databases, human LRBA encodes two protein transcripts, LRBA-001 (ENST00000510413; NP_001186211) and LRBA-002 (ENST00000357115; NP_006717), that are translated into proteins of 2851 aa and 2863 aa, respectively. The two isoforms differ in exon 39, which is absent in isoform 1. The biological relevance of the human isoforms and their expression in the different human tissues have not yet been evaluated. However, LRBA mRNA has been detected in several human tissues including the spleen, lymph node, thymus, tonsil, bone marrow, fetal liver, heart, placenta, lung, liver, skeletal muscle, kidney, and pancreas [1]. Finally, a homology analysis revealed that LRBA is highly conserved among species.

Computational predictions suggest that human LRBA is located in the cytosol, at the plasma membrane, in the endoplasmic reticulum, and in the Golgi apparatus. In accordance, *in vitro* analysis of plasmids containing BEACH-WD domains of LRBA fused to green fluorescent protein (GFP), localized predominately in the cytosol of murine macrophages at steady state [38]. However, upon LPS stimulation, LRBA associated with the endoplasmic reticulum (ER), Golgi complex, plasma membrane, and within lysosomes [38]. Furthermore, studies using

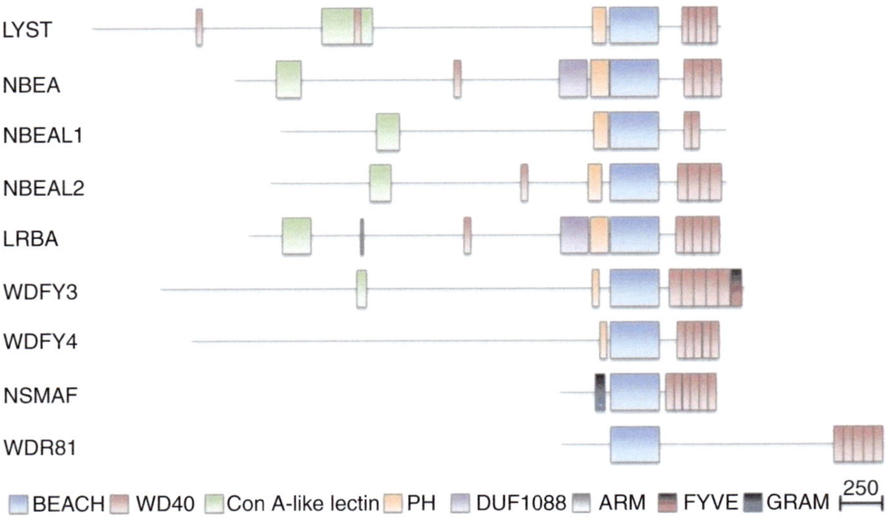

Fig. 10.3 BEACH domain-containing protein family. Representative diagram of all protein domains of human members of the BEACH domain-containing family (Obtained from *Cullinane A, Traffic, 2013*)

ImageStream showed localization of LRBA within recycling endosomes and the trans-Golgi network in normal human T cells, suggesting a role of LRBA in vesicle trafficking [7]. In fact, trafficking of transferring receptor (CD71) and CTLA-4 was found reduced in the absence of LRBA despite normal trafficking of CD28, ICOS, PD-1, and CD154-containing vesicles, indicating a role of LRBA in specific trafficking routes [7].

10.9 LRBA Deficiency Mouse Model

Human and murine LRBA share 90% of protein homology indicating an essential role of LRBA during evolution. Similar to humans, LRBA is broadly expressed in murine tissues and it is upregulated two to four folds in immune cells after LPS stimulation [1, 38]. The immune phenotype of LRBA knockout (KO) mice has been recently described [39, 40]. Remarkably, mice lacking LRBA remain healthy after 2-year follow-up under specific pathogenic conditions (SPF) without developing overt disease or increased disease severity after antigenic challenging [39, 40]. Human and murine LRBA deficiencies are similar in terms of a trend towards growth retardation and abnormalities in the regulatory T-cell compartment, including severely diminished CTLA-4 expression and, in less extent, reduction of CD25 and Helios. Frequencies and functionality of Tregs are, however, different. Reduced numbers of Tregs and poor Treg suppression capacity have been observed in

LRBA-deficient patients, whereas LRBA KO mice showed comparable numbers to their wild-type littermates [2, 24, 40]. In addition, LRBA KO mice presented normal development and repartition of T-cell subsets in the thymus and spleen, correlating with normal frequencies of $CD4^+$ and $CD8^+$ cells in the blood of LRBA-deficient patients. However, a skewing of peripheral T cells towards a memory phenotype ($CD45RO^+$) is observed in the absence of human or murine LRBA [2, 7]. Memory T cells play a critical role in host defense, but increased numbers are frequently associated with dysregulated Treg functionality, as found in patients with colorectal and gastric cancers [41, 42]. Moreover, an increased frequency of T follicular helper cells that is associated with an ineffective regulation of antibody response has been recently observed in the peripheral blood of LRBA-deficient patients [24], as well as in the Peyer's patches of LRBA KO mice after acute infection with *Salmonella typhimurium* despite normal findings on intestinal histological analysis [40].

The findings on NK cells in humans and mice lacking LRBA are controversial. In humans, normal counts of $CD16^+$ $CD56^+$ cells are observed as normal in most LRBA-deficient patients as well as in LRBA KO mice [2, 3, 39, 40]. Using a CD107a translocation assay, the NK cell cytotoxic activity was found regular in LRBA-deficient patients despite LRBA being associated with endosomal trafficking [1]. In contrast, murine LRBA-deficient NK cells impaired granzyme B secretion and activation of NKG2D and NKp46 signaling, suggesting a pivotal role of LRBA in antiviral and antitumoral responses [43]. However, LRBA KO mice mounted normal response against lymphocytic choriomeningitis virus (LCMV) in an acute and chronic infection setting [39, 40], and none of the LRBA patients' cohorts reported so far showed any predisposition to viral infections and/or to malignancies [2, 3, 5]. In addition, the defective NK cell functionality in LRBA KO mice was associated with resistance to lethal graft-versus-host disease (GvHD), encouraging physicians to treat LRBA-deficient patients with HSCT [43]. However, up to date, 12 patients with LRBA deficiency have been treated with HSCT resulting in 5 complete/good remissions, 3 partial remissions, and 4 deaths [31], confirming the complexity of LRBA deficiency and the need to further analyze the role of LRBA not only in human NK cells but also in other relevant immune actors involved in the GvHD response. This information will help clinicians to decide on the benefits of treating LRBA-deficient patients with HSCT.

The main differences between human and mice lacking LRBA were observed in the B-cell compartment, since total serum IgG and IgM and specific T-dependent and T-independent antibodies and antibody-secreting cells (ASCs) were found to be normal in LRBA KO mice, whereas 60–80% of LRBA-deficient patients suffer from hypogammaglobulinemia and present with poor specific antibody response [2, 40].

Moreover, serum and secretory IgA levels were surprisingly increased in LRBA KO mice regardless of age or treatment of the mice [40]. In addition, and contrary to what has been observed in LRBA-deficient patients, B-cell subsets from LRBA KO mice were found to be normal in terms of frequency and distribution in the bone marrow (pro-, pre-, and immature and mature B cells) and in the spleen (transitional, follicular and marginal zone B cells). Only B-1a cells were severely reduced in the peritoneum of LRBA KO mice in comparison with their WT littermates [40]. B-1 cells secrete spontaneously natural antibodies against either self-antigens or against pathogen-expressed molecules [44]. In addition, peritoneal B-1 cells are considered as the major source of IL-10 production in the B-cell lineage that is implicated in the regulation of tissue homeostasis [45]. Interestingly, IgA-secreting B-1 cells existing in the intestinal lamina propria are derived from peritoneal B-1 cells in an IL-5 and microbiota-dependent manner [46, 47]. This indicates that early exposure to commensal microbiota might be crucial for the development of local IgA-producing B-1 cells and therefore the maintenance of intestinal homeostasis. These observations reveal a possible role of LRBA in the development and/or maintenance of B-1a cells and in the production or regulation of IgA.

10.10 Summary and Outlook

Biallelic loss-of-protein mutations in *LRBA* cause an early-onset syndrome presenting with immunodeficiency and immune dysregulation, known as LRBA deficiency. Affected patients suffer mostly from autoimmune cytopenias, enteropathy, and lymphoproliferation, resembling the clinical picture of patients with CTLA-4 insufficiency, ALPS, IPEX, and STAT-3 GOF. Although the genetic diagnosis is required for any of the above syndromes, screening diagnostic tests based on the detection of LRBA protein in immune cells after stimulation might be useful to reduce the diagnostic delay, allowing timely clinical interventions. Moreover, a follow-up of bigger LRBA deficiency patients' cohorts would provide definitive evidence on the efficacy of HSCT and CTLA-4-Ig fusion protein for the treatment of LRBA deficiency.

Although the biological role of LRBA in immunity is not completely understood, autoimmune manifestations are explained by reduced CTLA-4 expression on Tregs and activated Tcon cells as consequence of high CTLA-4 lysosomal degradation in the absence of LRBA. In addition, patients with LRBA deficiency present recurrent infections and hypogammaglobulinemia due to the low numbers of switched memory B cells and plasmablasts due to defective autophagy and increased apoptosis of B cells after encountering an antigen. These findings on T- and B-cell compartments demonstrate an essential role of LRBA in immune tolerance and in the maintenance of humoral immunity. However, the underlying molecular mechanisms involved in the regulation of CTLA-4 as well as in autophagy/apoptosis processes need further evaluation. Contrary to human LRBA deficiency, LRBA KO mice do not present evident signs of disease despite low levels of CTLA-4, reduced frequency of IL-10-producing B cells, and increased numbers of T follicular helper cells. Interestingly, increased levels of IgA were found in mice lacking LRBA. Future studies to elucidate the role of LRBA in the regulation of IgA, and its involvement on mucosal immunity, and on B-1 cell migration are needed. Finally, investigations on clarifying the discrepancies between human and murine LRBA deficiency should be addressed.

References

1. Lopez-Herrera G, Tampella G, Pan-Hammarstrom Q, Herholz P, Trujillo-Vargas CM, Phadwal K, et al. Deleterious mutations in LRBA are associated with a syndrome of immune deficiency and autoimmunity. Am J Hum Genet. 2012;90(6):986–1001.
2. Gamez-Diaz L, August D, Stepensky P, Revel-Vilk S, Seidel MG, Noriko M, et al. The extended phenotype of LPS-responsive beige-like anchor protein (LRBA) deficiency. J Allergy Clin Immunol. 2016;137(1):223–30.
3. Alkhairy OK, Abolhassani H, Rezaei N, Fang M, Andersen KK, Chavoshzadeh Z, et al. Spectrum of phenotypes associated with mutations in LRBA. J Clin Immunol. 2016;36(1):33–45.
4. Kostel Bal S, Haskologlu S, Serwas NK, Islamoglu C, Aytekin C, Kendirli T, et al. Multiple presentations of LRBA deficiency: a single-center experience. J Clin Immunol. 2017;37:790–800.
5. Azizi G, Abolhassani H, Mahdaviani SA, Chavoshzadeh Z, Eshghi P, Yazdani R, et al. Clinical, immunologic, molecular analyses and outcomes of iranian patients with LRBA deficiency: a longitudinal study. Pediatr Allergy Immunol. 2017;28(5):478–84.
6. Serwas NK, Kansu A, Santos-Valente E, Kuloglu Z, Demir A, Yaman A, et al. Atypical manifestation of LRBA deficiency with predominant IBD-like phenotype. Inflamm Bowel Dis. 2015;21(1):40–7.
7. Lo B, Zhang K, Lu W, Zheng L, Zhang Q, Kanellopoulou C, et al. AUTOIMMUNE DISEASE. Patients with LRBA deficiency show CTLA4 loss and immune dysregulation responsive to abatacept therapy. Science. 2015;349(6246):436–40.
8. Levy E, Stolzenberg MC, Bruneau J, Breton S, Neven B, Sauvion S, et al. LRBA deficiency with autoimmunity and early onset chronic erosive polyarthritis. Clin Immunol. 2016;168:88–93.
9. Bakhtiar S, Ruemmele F, Charbit-Henrion F, Levy E, Rieux-Laucat F, Cerf-Bensussan N, et al. Atypical manifestation of LPS-responsive beige-like anchor deficiency syndrome as an autoimmune endocrine disorder without enteropathy and immunodeficiency. Front Pediatr. 2016;4:98.
10. Shokri S, Nabavi M, Hirschmugl T, Aghamohammadi A, Arshi S, Bemanian MH, et al. LPS-responsive beige-like anchor gene mutation associated with possible bronchiolitis obliterans organizing pneumonia associated with hypogammaglobulinemia and normal IgM phenotype and low number of B cells. Acta Med Iran. 2016;54(10):620–3.
11. Schubert D, Bode C, Kenefeck R, Hou TZ, Wing JB, Kennedy A, et al. Autosomal dominant immune dysregulation syndrome in humans with CTLA4 mutations. Nat Med. 2014;20(12):1410–6.
12. Lo B, Fritz JM, Su HC, Uzel G, Jordan MB, Lenardo MJ. CHAI and LATAIE: new genetic diseases of CTLA-4 checkpoint insufficiency. Blood. 2016;128(8):1037–42.
13. Schwab C, Gabrysch A, Olbrich P, Patiño V, Warnatz K, Wolff D, Hoshino A, Kobayashi M, Imai K, Takagi M, Dybedal I, Haddock JA, Sansom DM, Lucena JM, Seidl M, Schmitt-Graeff A, Reiser V, Emmerich F, Frede N, Bulashevska A, Salzer U, Schubert D, Hayakawa S, Okada S, Kanariou M, Kucuk ZY, Chapdelaine H, Petruzelkova L, Sumnik Z, Sediva A, Slatter M, Arkwright PD, Cant A, Lorenz HM, Giese T, Lougaris V, Plebani A, Price C, Sullivan KE, Moutschen M, Litzman J, Freiberger T, van de Veerdonk FL, Recher M, Albert MH, Hauck F, Seneviratne S, Pachlopnik Schmid J, Kolios A, Unglik G, Klemann C, Speckmann C, Ehl S, Leichtner A, Blumberg R, Franke A, Snapper S, Zeissig S, Cunningham-Rundles C, Giulino-Roth L, Elemento O, Dückers G, Niehues T, Fronkova E, Kanderová V, Platt CD, Chou J, Chatila TA, Geha R, McDermott E, Bunn S, Kurzai M, Schulz A, Alsina L, Casals F, Deyà-Martinez A, Hambleton S, Kanegane H, Taskén K, Neth O, Grimbacher B. Phenotype, penetrance, and treatment of 133 cytotoxic T-lymphocyte antigen 4-insufficient subjects. J Allergy

Clin Immunol. 2018; https://doi.org/10.1016/j.jaci.2018.02.055. [pii: S0091-6749(18)30630-4. Epub ahead of print. PubMed PMID: 29729943; PubMed Central PMCID: PMC6215742].
14. Tesi B, Priftakis P, Lindgren F, Chiang SC, Kartalis N, Lofstedt A, et al. Successful hematopoietic stem cell transplantation in a patient with LPS-responsive beige-like anchor (LRBA) gene mutation. J Clin Immunol. 2016;36(5):480–9.
15. Bratanic N, Kovac J, Pohar K, Trebusak Podkrajsek K, Ihan A, Battelino T, et al. Multifocal gastric adenocarcinoma in a patient with LRBA deficiency. Orphanet J Rare Dis. 2017;12(1):131.
16. Milner JD, Vogel TP, Forbes L, Ma CA, Stray-Pedersen A, Niemela JE, et al. Early-onset lymphoproliferation and autoimmunity caused by germline STAT3 gain-of-function mutations. Blood. 2015;125(4):591–9.
17. Neven B, Magerus-Chatinet A, Florkin B, Gobert D, Lambotte O, De Somer L, et al. A survey of 90 patients with autoimmune lymphoproliferative syndrome related to TNFRSF6 mutation. Blood. 2011;118(18):4798–807.
18. Barzaghi F, Passerini L, Bacchetta R. Immune dysregulation, polyendocrinopathy, enteropathy, x-linked syndrome: a paradigm of immunodeficiency with autoimmunity. Front Immunol. 2012;3:211.
19. Wang JW, Gamsby JJ, Highfill SL, Mora LB, Bloom GC, Yeatman TJ, et al. Deregulated expression of LRBA facilitates cancer cell growth. Oncogene. 2004;23(23):4089–97.
20. Fujishima N, Hirokawa M, Aiba N, Ichikawa Y, Fujishima M, Komatsuda A, et al. Gene expression profiling of human erythroid progenitors by micro-serial analysis of gene expression. Int J Hematol. 2004;80(3):239–45.
21. Sansom DM. IMMUNOLOGY. Moving CTLA-4 from the trash to recycling. Science. 2015;349(6246):377–8.
22. Pengo N, Scolari M, Oliva L, Milan E, Mainoldi F, Raimondi A, et al. Plasma cells require autophagy for sustainable immunoglobulin production. Nat Immunol. 2013;14(3):298–305.
23. Warnatz K, Wehr C, Drager R, Schmidt S, Eibel H, Schlesier M, et al. Expansion of CD19(hi) CD21(lo/neg) B cells in common variable immunodeficiency (CVID) patients with autoimmune cytopenia. Immunobiology. 2002;206(5):502–13.
24. Charbonnier LM, Janssen E, Chou J, Ohsumi TK, Keles S, Hsu JT, et al. Regulatory T-cell deficiency and immune dysregulation, polyendocrinopathy, enteropathy, X-linked-like disorder caused by loss-of-function mutations in LRBA. J Allergy Clin Immunol. 2015;135(1):217–27.
25. Hou TZ, Verma N, Wanders J, Kennedy A, Soskic B, Janman D, et al. Identifying functional defects in patients with immune dysregulation due to LRBA and CTLA-4 mutations. Blood. 2017;129(11):1458–68.
26. Azizi G, Mirshafiey A, Abolhassani H, Yazdani R, Ghanavatinejad A, Noorbakhsh F, Rezaei N, Aghamohammadi A. The imbalance of circulating T helper subsets and regulatory T cells in patients with LRBA deficiency: correlation with disease severity. J Cell Physiol. 2018;233(11):8767–77. https://doi.org/10.1002/jcp.26772. [Epub 2018 May 28. PubMed PMID: 29806698].
27. De Bruyne M, Bogaert DJ, Venken K, Van den Bossche L, Bonroy C, Roels L, Tavernier SJ, van de Vijver E, Driessen A, van Gijn M, Gámez-Diaz L, Elewaut D, Grimbacher B, Haerynck F, Moes N, Dullaers M. A novel LPS-responsive beige-like anchor protein (LRBA) mutation presents with normal cytotoxic T lymphocyte-associated protein 4 (CTLA-4) and overactive T_H17 immunity. J Allergy Clin Immunol. 2018. pii: S0091-6749(18)31270-3. doi: https://doi.org/10.1016/j.jaci.2018.08.026. [Epub ahead of print. PubMed PMID: 30193839].
28. Gámez-Díaz L, Sigmund EC, Reiser V, Vach W, Jung S, Grimbacher B. Rapid flow cytometry-based test for the diagnosis of lipopolysaccharide responsive beige-like anchor (LRBA) deficiency. Front Immunol. 2018;9:720. https://doi.org/10.3389/fimmu.2018.00720. [eCollection 2018. PubMed PMID: 29740429; PubMed Central PMCID: PMC5925005].
29. Azizi G, Abolhassani H, Yazdani R, Mohammadikhajehdehi S, Parvaneh N, Negahdari B, et al. New therapeutic approach by sirolimus for enteropathy treatment in patients with LRBA deficiency. Eur Ann Allergy Clin Immunol. 2017;49(5):235–9.
30. Seidel MG, Hirschmugl T, Gamez-Diaz L, Schwinger W, Serwas N, Deutschmann A, et al. Long-term remission after allogeneic hematopoietic stem cell transplantation in LPS-

responsive beige-like anchor (LRBA) deficiency. J Allergy Clin Immunol. 2015;135(5):1384–90.e1–8.
31. Seidel MG, Bohm K, Dogu F, Worth A, Thrasher A, Florkin B, et al. Treatment of severe forms of LPS-responsive beige-like anchor protein deficiency with allogeneic hematopoietic stem cell transplantation. J Allergy Clin Immunol. 2018;141:770–775.e1.
32. Cullinane AR, Schaffer AA, Huizing M. The BEACH is hot: a LYST of emerging roles for BEACH-domain containing proteins in human disease. Traffic. 2013;14(7):749–66.
33. Smith TF, Gaitatzes C, Saxena K, Neer EJ. The WD repeat: a common architecture for diverse functions. Trends Biochem Sci. 1999;24(5):181–5.
34. Li D, Roberts R. WD-repeat proteins: structure characteristics, biological function, and their involvement in human diseases. Cell Mol Life Sci. 2001;58(14):2085–97.
35. Introne W, Boissy RE, Gahl WA. Clinical, molecular, and cell biological aspects of Chediak-Higashi syndrome. Mol Genet Metab. 1999;68(2):283–303.
36. Nurden A et al. Blood Reviews. 2007.
37. Kerr WG, Heller M, Herzenberg LA. Analysis of lipopolysaccharide-response genes in B-lineage cells demonstrates that they can have differentiation stage-restricted expression and contain SH2 domains. Proc Natl Acad Sci U S A. 1996;93(9):3947–52.
38. Wang JW, Howson J, Haller E, Kerr WG. Identification of a novel lipopolysaccharide-inducible gene with key features of both A kinase anchor proteins and chs1/beige proteins. J Immunol. 2001;166(7):4586–95.
39. Burnett DL, Parish IA, Masle-Farquhar E, Brink R, Goodnow CC. Murine LRBA deficiency causes CTLA-4 deficiency in Tregs without progression to immune dysregulation. Immunol Cell Biol. 2017;95(9):775–88.
40. Gamez-Diaz L, Neumann J, Jager F, Proietti M, Felber F, Soulas-Sprauel P, et al. Immunological phenotype of the murine Lrba knockout. Immunol Cell Biol. 2017;95:789–802.
41. Perrone G, Ruffini PA, Catalano V, Spino C, Santini D, Muretto P, et al. Intratumoural FOXP3-positive regulatory T cells are associated with adverse prognosis in radically resected gastric cancer. Eur J Cancer. 2008;44(13):1875–82.
42. Galon J, Costes A, Sanchez-Cabo F, Kirilovsky A, Mlecnik B, Lagorce-Pages C, et al. Type, density, and location of immune cells within human colorectal tumors predict clinical outcome. Science. 2006;313(5795):1960–4.
43. Park MY, Sudan R, Srivastava N, Neelam S, Youngs C, Wang JW, et al. LRBA is essential for allogeneic responses in bone marrow transplantation. Sci Rep. 2016;6:36568.
44. Martin F, Oliver AM, Kearney JF. Marginal zone and B1 B cells unite in the early response against T-independent blood-borne particulate antigens. Immunity. 2001;14(5):617–29.
45. Baumgarth N. The double life of a B-1 cell: self-reactivity selects for protective effector functions. Nat Rev Immunol. 2011;11(1):34–46.
46. Beagley KW, Murray AM, McGhee JR, Eldridge JH. Peritoneal cavity CD5 (Bla) B cells: cytokine induced IgA secretion and homing to intestinal lamina propria in SCID mice. Immunol Cell Biol. 1995;73(5):425–32.
47. Kroese FG, Ammerlaan WA, Kantor AB. Evidence that intestinal IgA plasma cells in mu, kappa transgenic mice are derived from B-1 (Ly-1 B) cells. Int Immunol. 1993;5(10):1317–27.

11 BAFF Receptor Deficiency

Cristian R. Smulski, Patricia Odermatt, and Hermann Eibel

11.1 BAFFR Expression

Starting from hematopoietic stem cells, B lymphocytes develop in human bone marrow through successive developmental stages. Progression through these stages is mainly regulated by the rearrangement of the variable parts of the immunoglobulin heavy (H) and light (L) chains. After the successful rearrangement of H- and L-chain loci, functional IgM molecules are assembled and expressed together with the signal-transducing components Ig-α and Ig-β in the form of B cell antigen receptors on the cell surface of immature IgM^+ B cells. Since the rearrangement of immunoglobulin gene segments allows the generation of autoreactive receptors, the self-reactivity of IgM molecules expressed is tested and eventually corrected by receptor editing in immature B cells. Then, only those cells with low avidity to self-antigens can leave the bone marrow and migrate as so-called transitional B cells to the spleen where they conclude their early, antigen-independent steps of B cell development (reviewed in [1]).

During this last phase, B lymphocytes start to express BAFF receptor (BAFFR), a member of the TNF receptor superfamily [2, 3]. TNF-R family members are characterized by extracellular cysteine-rich domains (CRDs), which serve for ligand binding as well as for ligand-independent assembly of receptor monomers into dimers, trimers, or multimers [1, 4, 5]. Receptors of this family contain one to five CRDs; however BAFFR is an atypical representative of this family since it contains only a partial CRD which functions as ligand binding and self-assembly domain at the same time [1]. It is expressed on the surface of all peripheral B cell subsets except for plasma cells and for centroblasts of the dark zone of germinal centers [6] (Fig. 11.1).

C. R. Smulski · P. Odermatt · H. Eibel (✉)
Faculty of Medicine, Center for Chronic Immunodeficiency, Medical Center—University of Freiburg, University of Freiburg, Freiburg, Germany
e-mail: hermann.eibel@uniklinik-freiburg.de

M. M. D'Elios, M. Rizzi (eds.), *Humoral Primary Immunodeficiencies*, Rare Diseases of the Immune System, https://doi.org/10.1007/978-3-319-91785-6_11

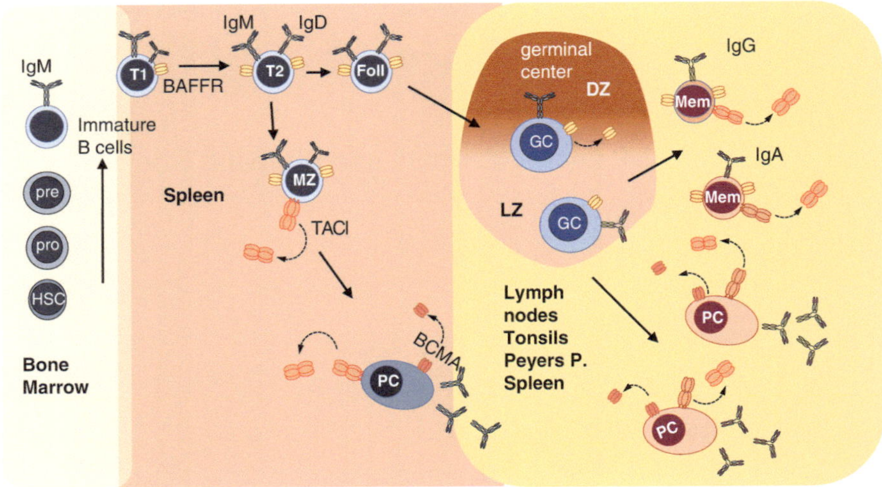

Fig. 11.1 B lymphocyte development. B cell precursors develop in the bone marrow from hematopoietic stem cells (HSC) until they reach the stage of IgM+ immature B cells. These immature B cells migrate from the bone marrow to the spleen where they differentiate via the transitional 1 (T1) and transitional 2 (T2) stages into mature, naïve, follicular B cells (Foll) or into marginal zone B cells (MZ). Both subsets express IgM and IgD on their surface. Naïve follicular B cells express more IgD than IgM and MZ B cells more IgM than IgD. MZ B cells recognizing bacterial cell wall antigens develop rapidly into short-lived plasma cells secreting IgM antibodies. Follicular B cells differentiate in response to antigen and interactions with T-follicular helper cells in germinal centers into proliferating centroblasts located in the dark zone (DZ), where centroblasts undergo somatic hypermutation and class-switch recombination. Centroblasts shuttle to the light zone (LZ), where they turn into centrocytes which can be selected by interactions with follicular dendritic cells and T-follicular helper cells into the pool of long-lived memory B cells and plasma cells expressing high-affinity class-switched immunoglobulins. BAFFR expression starts when IgM$^+$ immature B cells leave the bone marrow. It increases on T1 and T2 B cells. The development of BAFFR-deficient B cells stops at this stage. Naïve follicular B cells express only BAFFR but not TACI, which is expressed by MZ B cells, switched memory B cells, and plasma cells. DZ B cells are in contact with BAFF resulting in shedding of BAFFR. Centrocytes express low levels of BAFFR, which is then upregulated again by switched memory B cells. Short- and long-lived plasma cells express TACI and BCMA. Both receptors are shedded constitutively. **Alternative figure legend:** For explanation see text. *HSC* hematopoietic stem cell, *T1, T2* transitional B cells, *DZ* dark zone, *LZ* light zone, *Mem* switched memory B cells

BAFFR has two close relatives termed TACI (encoded by *TNFRSF13B*) and BCMA (encoded by *TNFRSF17*) sharing BAFF as a common ligand. Different from BAFFR, TACI is expressed by activated B cells, marginal zone B cells, memory B cells, and plasma cells, in which it acts as pro-survival receptor [7–10]. BCMA is upregulated in activated B cells and expressed constitutively by plasma cells supporting the survival of long-lived bone marrow plasma cells [11].

Experiments performed in mice demonstrated that the expression of functional B cell antigen receptors (BCR) and tonic BCR signaling enhances BAFFR expression by immature and transitional B cells [12, 13], although functional BAFFR is expressed in the absence of SYK-dependent BCR signaling [14] or in cells lacking Ig-α (CD79A), which is an essential component of B cell receptors. In these cells, BAFFR expression is needed for survival [15].

11.2 Ligand Binding

BAFFR and the two closely related receptors TACI and BCMA bind to the TNF family ligand BAFF, but different from these two relatives, BAFFR cannot bind the cytokine APRIL in spite of its similarity to BAFF. Therefore, APRIL binds only to TACI and BCMA and supports the survival of plasma cells [16].

BAFF [17–19] and APRIL [20] are homotrimeric type II transmembrane proteins and exist as membrane-bound forms and soluble trimers. While shedding of BAFF occurs at the plasma membrane, APRIL is proteolytically processed in the Golgi apparatus by furine proteases [16]. BAFF can also oligomerize into 20 homotrimers, creating a 60mer unit resembling a virus capsid-like structure [21–23]. The formation of BAFF 60mer is pH dependent, and oligomerization is facilitated under basic conditions [22]. In addition to its transmembrane domain, to the furine processing site, and to the TNF homology domain, which is responsible for receptor binding, BAFF has an extended D-E loop, called the "flap." This region supports trimer-trimer interactions which are needed for the assembly of the 60mer [22, 24]. Although BAFF trimers have sufficient biological activity to activate BAFFR, its higher-order oligomeric forms are by far more active, most likely because they engage multiple BAFF receptors at the same time leading to signal amplification [22, 23] (Fig. 11.2).

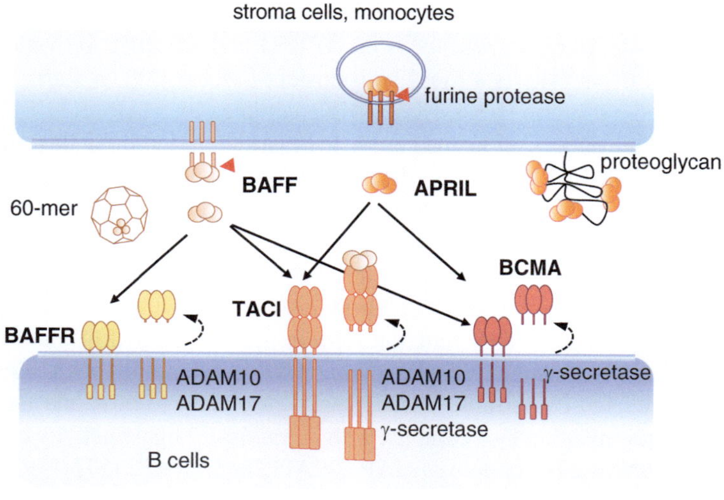

Fig. 11.2 The BAFF/BAFFR family. BAFFR, TACI, and BCMA are expressed by cells of the B cell lineage, whereas their ligands are expressed by cells of the monocyte lineage and by stroma cells. BAFF and APRIL are cleaved by furine proteases. BAFF can assemble into trimers or into higher oligomeric complexes containing up to 60 BAFF molecules (60-mers). Binding of APRIL to proteoglycans increases the local concentration of APRIL and promotes binding to TACI and BCMA and signaling. After BAFF binding, BAFFR is proteolytically cleaved in TACI+ cells by ADAM10 and/or ADAM17, whereas TACI is shed constitutively by ADAM proteases and γ-secretase. Since it is a small protein, BCMA is only processed by γ-secretase

In contrast to BAFF, APRIL has close to the N-terminus of the soluble form a stretch of basic amino acids which allow binding to heparan sulfate proteoglycans (HSPG) found on the surface of many cell types. HSPG binding of APRIL induces ligand multimerization [25, 26], which strongly enhances APRIL-induced signaling under physiological concentrations of APRIL [26]. Additionally, heteromers of BAFF and APRIL have been found in patients with autoimmune diseases, and they seem to downregulate BAFF activity [27].

BAFF (encoded by the *TNFSF13B* gene) and APRIL (encoded by *TNFSF13*) exhibit similar expression patterns. Both can be produced by monocytes, macrophages, and dendritic cells but also by stromal cells of the bone marrow [17, 18, 28]. In addition, there is also evidence for T cells to express the ligands [18, 29]. Expression levels and concentrations of soluble BAFF and APRIL increase in response to pro-inflammatory cytokines [30] and correlate inversely to the expression of BAFFR and TACI [31].

11.3 Activation of the Noncanonical NF-κB Pathway

BAFF binding to BAFFR extends the half-life of immature, transitional, and mature B cells by activating a series of different pathways, which significantly boost basic survival functions including protein synthesis and energy metabolism. Similar to the TNF receptor family members CD40, LTβR, and RANK, BAFFR triggers the noncanonical NF-κB2-dependent pathway [32, 33].

NF-kB proteins comprise several members of the Rel transcription factor family (reviewed in [34]). Here, we will focus on NF-κB1 and NF-κB2. Activation of the canonical NF-κB pathway is a rapid but transient process [35]. It starts by phosphorylation of the trimeric IKKα, IKKβ, IKKγ complex by MAP 3K7 (TAK1) and the subsequent phosphorylation and complete or partial proteasomal degradation of IκBa and NF-κB1/p105 releasing p50/relA and p50-c-rel heterodimers into the nucleus where they act as transcriptional activators. Compared to NF-κB1, the activation of the noncanonical NF-κB pathway is a slow process as it fully depends on the cytoplasmic accumulation and activation of the NF-κB-inducing kinase NIK (MAP 3K14). Its essential role in the NF-κB2 signaling pathway is underlined by genetic defects abrogating NIK function [36]. In the case of BAFFR, activation of NIK and more downstream of NF-κB2 starts with BAFF binding to BAFFR. Under resting, unstimulated conditions, TRAF3 binds efficiently to NIK and targets the kinase for ubiquitinylation by a complex with ubiquitin-E3 ligase activity composed from cellular inhibitors of apoptosis cIAP1, cIAP2, and TRAF2 [37] (Fig. 11.3).

Proteasomal degradation of NIK keeps the active kinase concentrations very low and prevents the phosphorylation and activation of NF-κB2 by IKKα (IKK1), which is activated through phosphorylation by NIK. When BAFF binds to BAFFR, the receptor most likely undergoes a conformational change allowing the recruitment of TRAF3. Its association with BAFFR leads to the dissociation of the NIK-TRAF2/3-cIAP1/2 complex, exposes the lysine residue K46 of TRAF3 to ubiquitin ligases, and initiates TRAF3 degradation by the proteasome. This reduces the concentrations of

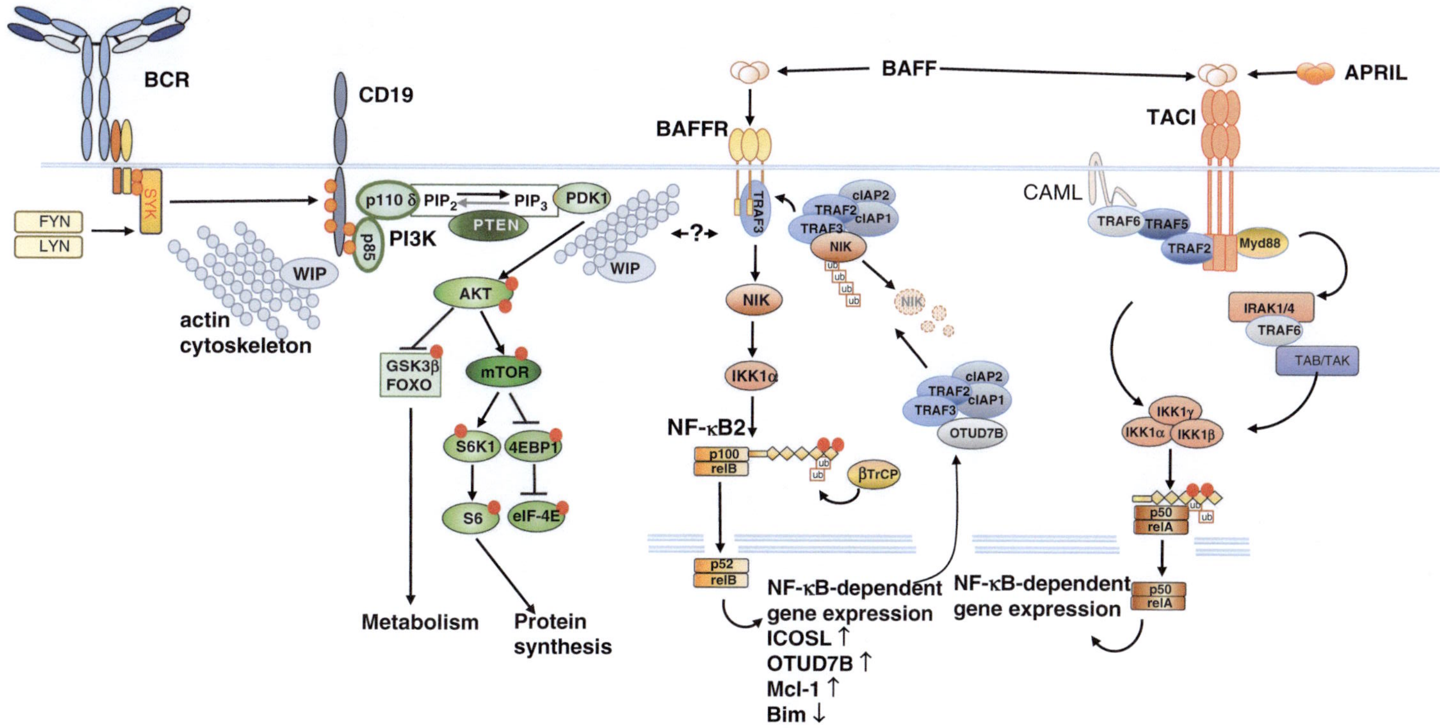

Fig. 11.3 BAFF-induced signaling pathways and cellular responses. BAFF binding to BAFFR induces the noncanonical NF-κB pathway and a PI3K-dependent signaling cascade which requires interactions with the cytoskeleton and components also involved in BCR signaling. TACI activates the classical NF-κB pathway. Details are explained in the text

active TRAF3 and promotes the accumulation of NIK. Since most of the NIK protein has to be newly produced by protein synthesis requiring newly transcribed mRNA as template, the activation of IKK1 downstream of BAFFR is a slow process which takes several hours to be detected. NIK starts to phosphorylate IKK1 [38], and the activated form of IKK1 phosphorylates NF-κB2 p100 at its C-terminal serine residues 866 and 870 [39]. The phosphorylated form of NF-κB2 now becomes a target of the E3 ubiquitin ligase βTrCP, which adds ubiquitins to lysine residue K856. Ubiquitinylated NF-κB2 then binds to the regulatory subunit of the proteasome [40] allowing cleavage of the p100 precursor into its active form p52 which translocates together with RelB into the nucleus to regulate the transcription of NF-κB2 target genes.

11.4 Target Genes

Activation of the noncanonical NF-κB2 pathway is to some extent also regulated by the canonical pathway since NF-κB1 positively regulates the transcription of NF-κB2 [41]. However, in the absence of NF-κB2-inducing signals, increased levels of NF-κB2 p100 function as inhibitor (IkB) of RelB and RelA [42–44]. In addition, if RelB concentrations are low, dimeric forms of processed NF-κB2 p52 may also act as inhibitor of NF-κB2 target genes [45]. Several downstream target genes of NF-κB2 p52/RelB induced by BAFF binding to BAFFR have been identified. Among these genes is ICOSL, which is upregulated in response to BAFF. Its interactions with ICOS expressed on activated T cells provide costimulatory signals and promote the development of follicular T helper cells [46]. This role of NIK and NF-κB2 in activating ICOSL expression is further supported by the analysis of B cells from NIK-deficient patients as they fail to upregulate ICOSL expression in response to CD40L [36]. The anti-apoptotic Bcl-2 family member Mcl-1 is another target of BAFFR signaling. Recently it has been shown that TRAF3 can enter the nucleus, where it binds to a transcriptional regulator termed cAMP response element binding protein (CREB). This leads to CREB ubiquitinylation and degradation. Similar to NIK, decreased TRAF concentrations allow the accumulation of Mcl-1, which then acts as pro-survival factor by stabilizing the mitochondrial outer membrane [47].

In addition to the activation of NF-κB2, phosphorylation of IKK1 by NIK also induces a negative feedback loop which prevents the accumulation of NIK. The reaction starts with the phosphorylation of NIK by IKK1 followed by the cIAP/TRAF2/3-independent degradation of NIK [48]. A second negative feedback loop is activated by OTUD7B which is a NF-κB2 target gene [49]. Activation of BAFFR, LTβR, or CD40 increases the expression of OTUD7B. The deubiquitinase then rapidly binds to TRAF3 and promotes the formation of a larger protein complex composed of OTUD7B, TRAF3, TRAF2, and cIAP1/2, which interacts with the signaling receptor. By deubiquitinating TRAF3, OTUD7B therefore acts as negative regulator of the NF-κB2 and limits BAFFR-dependent cellular activation (Fig. 11.3).

11.5 Activation of PI3-Kinase

In addition to the noncanonical NF-κB2 pathway, binding of BAFF to BAFFR can activate the phosphoinositide-3-kinase-dependent signaling cascade. The precise mechanism of BAFFR-induced PI3K activation is still not well understood. However, experiments performed in mice showed that BAFFR-dependent activation of PI3K relies on borrowing components and factors which were shown to be part of the B cell antigen receptor pathway [50, 51]. Similar to the B cell receptor [52], BAFFR-induced signals require the remodeling of the cytoskeleton via interactions between the tetraspanin network, CD19, and the Wiskott-Aldrich syndrome interacting protein (WIP) [53]. This suggests that BAFFR is part of a larger complex of transmembrane and membrane-associated proteins which share common signaling components that are activated in a context-dependent manner.

In B cells, heteromeric PI3K is composed from the regulatory p85β and the p110δ subunits and catalyzes the synthesis of membrane phosphatidylinositol phospholipids with phosphatidylinositol 3,4 bis-phosphate (PIP_2) and phosphatidylinositol 3,4,5 tris-phosphate (PIP_3) as main products [54]. Its direct opponent is the phosphatase PTEN, which dephosphorylates PIP_2 and PIP_3. Both membrane phospholipids serve as anchors for several kinases containing pleckstrin homology (PH) domains such as AKT (or PKB), PDK1, and BTK as well as for the phospholipase Cγ (reviewed in [54]). Phosphorylation of phosphatidylinositol requires membrane recruitment of PI3K, which is best studied for BCR-induced activation. In this case, antigen binding leads to the phosphorylation of tyrosine residues in tandem YXXM motifs in the cytoplasmic tail of the BCR-associated co-receptor molecule CD19. Phosphorylated YXXM serves as docking site for the p85β subunit of PI3K, which now can start to exert its activity at the plasma membrane. The cytoplasmic adapter molecule BCAP (PIK3AP1) has a similar function [55], and interestingly Bcap−/− Cd19−/− double knockout mice [56] have a similar phenotype like Baffr−/− mice [57] hallmarked by arrested B cell development at the stage of transitional B cell. Downstream of PI3K, PDK1 activates the AKT/mTOR axis leading to metabolic reprogramming of B cells, which increases their fitness and life span (reviewed in [58]). BAFFR-dependent activation of the PI3K/AKT/mTOR axis has been best described in mice. There it was shown that the treatment of splenic B cells with BAFF leads to the phosphorylation of AKT at both Ser437 and T308 in a PI3K-dependent manner [59, 60] and more downstream, in the phosphorylation of the small ribosomal protein S6 and of the translation inhibitor 4EBP1. Since phosphorylated S6 serves as activator and non-phosphorylated 4EBP1 as inhibitor of protein synthesis, engagement of BAFFR by BAFF directly upregulates protein synthesis. In parallel, by phosphorylating GSK3β and PIM2, BAFFR-dependent activation of the AKT/mTOR pathway stabilizes MCL-1 [47, 59, 60], which improves mitochondrial function and ATP production (Fig. 11.3).

11.6 BAFFR Processing

We recently found that BAFF binding to BAFFR triggers shedding of the extracellular part of BAFFR in the presence of co-expressed TACI [6]. The in-depth analysis of the BAFFR shedding process revealed that BAFFR processing is catalyzed by the metalloprotease ADAM10 in TACI$^+$ resting marginal zone and switched memory B cells. The released extracellular domain was not found to function as a soluble decoy receptor for BAFF, and its other leftovers, the transmembrane part and the cytoplasmic domain, are internalized and translocated to lysosomes where they are most likely degraded. Therefore, BAFFR processing differs from the shedding of TACI, which is cleaved constitutively by ADAM10 releasing its extracellular domain in the form of a decoy receptor for BAFF and possible also for APRIL [61]. Similar to TACI, BCMA is also processed constitutively by γ-secretase [61], which also cleaves the part of TACI remaining in the plasma membrane after the extracellular part has been shed by the activity of ADAM10 [61].

As it will be discussed below, this difference between processed BAFFR and TACI molecules may be an important factor in explaining the differences between BAFFR and TACI deficiency. As pointed out above, the processing of BAFFR in resting primary B cells is a tightly regulated process, which requires both ligand binding and expression of TACI. Since in contrast to TACI BAFFR does not associate with ADAM10 in resting cells, the protein is out of reach of the metalloprotease. BAFF binding, however, can enhance the clustering of BAFFR and TACI and decrease the distance between BAFFR and ADAM10 [6]. In addition, it may also change the conformation of BAFFR and expose the cleavage site to ADAM10. B cells responding to TLR and BCR signals induce TACI expression. BAFF-induced processing of BAFFR by ADAM10 plays an important physiological role in these cells since it limits BAFFR signaling and, as a consequence, their survival and differentiation into antibody-secreted cells.

Different from the cleavage by ADAM10, BAFFR expressed by germinal center B cells is mainly processed by ADAM17. In the germinal center (GC), activated B cells commute between the dark zone and the light zone. Proliferation, somatic hypermutation, and class-switch recombination take place in the dark zone, whereas the affinity-based selection of class-switched memory B cells and plasma cells expressing highly specific antibodies occurs in the light zone [62]. Different from the BAFFR-positive light zone GC B cells (centrocytes), dark zone B cells (centroblasts) are heavily loaded with BAFF, which induces BAFFR processing by ADAM17 [6]. Thus, BAFFR seems to provide limited survival signals to dark zone B cells, whereas the survival of light zone B cells is secured by BCR signals induced by the binding of surface immunoglobulin molecules which have increased their affinity to their cognate antigen above the threshold which is set by interactions with T-follicular helper cells and by the competing IgG and IgA antibodies secreted by plasma cells located in the periphery of the germinal center [63].

11.7 Selection and Autoimmunity

With the previously described mechanisms regulating the expression pattern, signaling, and processing of BAFFR, TACI, and BCMA, many of the earlier observations made by studying mouse models and human samples can be explained. As it has been demonstrated by mouse models and by studying human BAFFR deficiency, BAFFR signaling is essential for the survival of transitional and naïve B cells [64], for the development of transitional B cells into marginal zone B cells, and for the differentiation of naïve and marginal zone B cells into short-lived IgM-secreting plasma cells [1]. The fine-tuned balance between BAFF-induced survival of dark zone B cells and affinity-based selection of centrocytes in the light zone is disturbed when BAFF is present in excess, as it is modeled by BAFF-transgenic mice [65]. In humans, the fatal role of increased BAFF levels is impressively documented by genome-wide association studies of case-control samples from Sardegna, which revealed that an insertion-deletion variant of the BAFF-encoding TNFSF13B gene is associated with the risk of developing multiple sclerosis or systemic lupus erythematodes. This variant results in a shorter version of BAFF mRNA, which is no longer targeted by miRNA-15a and other micro-RNAs for repression or degradation. The increased stability of BAFF mRNA leads to an increase in BAFF levels in a gene dosage-dependent manner resulting in 1.5–2-fold higher BAFF levels and therefore to more circulating B cells as well as increased serum IgG and IgM concentrations in homozygous carriers of this *TNFSF13B* variant [66].

The TACI variants, C104R or C104Y, which are linked to the development of CVID/antibody deficiency, destroy the ligand binding domain of TACI without disturbing the expression of the receptor on the cell surface. In C104R carrying individuals ADAM10-mediated shedding of TACI therefore releases soluble forms of TACI, which are incapable of acting as decoy receptors neutralizing excess BAFF and APRIL. This results in increases BAFF levels in TACI-deficient patients [31] and enhances their risk of developing autoimmunity and lymphoproliferation, which are two characteristic manifestations found in TACI deficiency [67, 68] and Taci−/− mice [69, 70]. Thus, TACI deficiency shares some common features with autoimmune diseases linked to increased BAFF levels [66]. In addition, its immunodeficient component can be best explained by the role of TACI in supporting T-independent immune responses [71–74] and the survival of plasma cells [8, 10].

11.8 BAFFR Deficiency in Humans

Several missense mutations changing base pairs encoding amino acid residues in the extra- or intracellular part of BAFFR have been found in humans [75–77]. None of these mutations disturbs B cell maturation, and therefore—except for the frequent polymorphism changing proline residue 21 into arginine (P21R)—their contribution to primary immunodeficiency remains to be shown. The P21R BAFFR variant is encoded by a frequent single nucleotide polymorphism (rs77874543). The affected proline residue is located in a small loop directly preceding the BAFF binding domain. Biochemical and functional analyses revealed that this region is essential for ligand-independent association of BAFFR polypeptide chains into multimeric nanoclusters resembling the pre-ligand assembly domain of BAFFR [1]. Our study also demonstrated that BAFFR clustering is not a prerequisite for the development of naïve mature B cells from immature/transitional B cells, but it strongly enhances BAFF binding and supports BAFF-dependent differentiation of naïve and marginal zone B cells into IgM-secreting plasmablasts. Since the P21R variant is completely resistant against BAFF-induced processing of BAFFR by ADAM10, the mutation seems to compensate its reduced capacity to bind BAFF. This feature may mask in part the impaired differentiation of P21R+ B cells into IgM-secreting plasmablasts and prevent the development of overt immunodeficiency.

Different from these point mutations, the homozygous 24 bp in-frame deletion within the TNFRSF13C gene removing the codons of eight amino acids from the transmembrane part of BAFFR blocks B cell development at the transition from $CD10^+$ immature/transitional 1 B cells to transitional 2/naïve and marginal zone B cells [64]. We found this autosomal recessive mutation in two siblings of a consanguineous family. In its homozygous form, it has 100% penetrance due to the lack of BAFFR expression, whereas the heterozygous form is indistinguishable from healthy donors with wild-type BAFFR. The immunological phenotype of human BAFFR deficiency mainly resembles the phenotype of *Baffr−/−* mice and is characterized by very low numbers of circulating B cells, low IgM, and IgG antibody titers but increased levels of serum IgA. However, some aspects differ between humans and mice. First, deletion of *Baffr* in mice does not affect the development of B1 B cells. In the BAFFR-deficient humans, B1 B cells or any other B cell subsets, which would resemble the B1 B cell subset of mice, were not found. However, since the BAFFR deficiency was diagnosed in two individuals who both were older than 60, the lack of B1 B cells might have been due to a characteristic feature of B1 B cells made in mice, namely, that these cells form a separate lineage, which develops during embryonic life and disappears in aging mice [78–80]. However, an impaired output of immature B cells from bone marrow precursor cells is unlikely to account for the absence of B1 B cells because both BAFFR-deficient individuals had similar numbers or even more transitional B cells than younger adults. The second major difference between BAFFR-deficient humans and mice is the severe lymphopenia observed in humans, which is stronger than in *Baffr−/−* mice and manifests as an almost complete lack of circulating naïve B cells, marginal zone B cells, and switched memory B cells. Again, this difference may be age-related, but it may also reflect differences in the half-life of transitional B cells between mice and humans or differences in TACI expression, which has been described to be expressed by transitional B cells in mice [2, 81]. The absence of marginal zone B cells correlated well with defective T-independent vaccination responses against Pneumovax, which contains a mixture of 23 different cell wall polysaccharides from *S. pneumoniae* strains. The low but detectable IgG response to the T-dependent antigen tetanus toxoid, the high IgA serum concentrations, and the presence of IgA^+ plasma cells in the *lamina propria* of the small intestine showed that human B cells can differentiate into plasma cells without BAFFR. This correlates with experiments performed in *Baffr−/−* mice, which demonstrated that BAFFR-deficient B cells can successfully complete the germinal center reaction [82] and develop into switched memory B cells and plasma cells which then survive without BAFFR [83, 84]. BAFFR-independent long-term survival of memory B cells in humans is also supported by the analysis of SLE patients treated with the BAFF-neutralizing antibody belimumab. These clinical studies documented the strong (>75%) decrease in naïve B cells within one and a half years of treatment, which was in sharp contrast to the increase in switched memory B cells [85, 86]. Similar to the numbers of switched memory B cells, IgG antibody concentrations, which were build up before starting the BAFF-neutralizing therapy, remained constant, whereas the increase of antibody titers against neoantigens from influenza virus was significantly lower in belimumab-treated patients than in controls [87]. In a similar study, the population of switched memory B cells did also not decrease within a half year treatment of rheumatoid arthritis patients with TACI-Ig fusion protein (atacicept) [88].

In summary, switched memory B cells can perfectly survive without receiving BAFFR- or TACI-dependent pro-survival signals and develop into IgA-secreting plasma cells. Different from switched memory B cells, the survival of transitional, naïve, and marginal zone B cells as well as the differentiation of transitional B cells into marginal zone B cells depends essentially on BAFF-induced survival signals, which increase the life span of these cells by stabilizing mitochondria and by enhancing protein synthesis. Since transitional B cells are to some extent able to develop into plasma cells even in the absence of BAFFR, BAFFR deficiency does not become manifest as dramatically as NIK or NF-kB2 deficiency, which strongly impair more B and T cell responses than the deletion of BAFFR. Although switched memory B cells express high levels of BAFFR and of TACI, they do not seem to require neither BAFFR nor TACI for long-term survival. Therefore, the function of both BAFF receptors in these cells remains an open question which has to be solved in the future.

References

1. Pieper K, Rizzi M, Speletas M, Smulski CR, Sic H, Kraus H, Salzer U, Fiala GJ, Schamel WW, Lougaris V, Plebani A, Hammarstrom L, Recher M, Germenis AE, Grimbacher B, Warnatz K, Rolink AG, Schneider P, Notarangelo LD, Eibel H. A common single nucleotide polymorphism impairs B-cell activating factor receptor's multimerization, contributing to common variable immunodeficiency. J Allergy Clin Immunol. 2014;133:1222–5.
2. Ng LG, Sutherland AP, Newton R, Qian F, Cachero TG, Scott ML, Thompson JS, Wheway J, Chtanova T, Groom J, Sutton IJ, Xin C, Tangye SG, Kalled SL, Mackay F, Mackay CR. B cell-activating factor belonging to the TNF family (BAFF)-R is the principal BAFF receptor facilitating BAFF costimulation of circulating T and B cells. J Immunol. 2004;173:807–17.
3. Rodig SJ, Shahsafaei A, Li B, Mackay CR, Dorfman DM. BAFF-R, the major B cell-activating factor receptor, is expressed on most mature B cells and B-cell lymphoproliferative disorders. Hum Pathol. 2005;36:1113–9.
4. Naismith JH, Sprang SR. Modularity in the TNF-receptor family. Trends Biochem Sci. 1998;23:74–9.

5. Do RK, Hatada E, Lee H, Tourigny MR, Hilbert D, Chen-Kiang S. Attenuation of apoptosis underlies B lymphocyte stimulator enhancement of humoral immune response. J Exp Med. 2000;192:953–64.
6. Smulski CR, Kury P, Seidel LM, Staiger HS, Edinger AK, Willen L, Seidl M, Hess H, Salzer U, Rolink AG, Rizzi M, Schneider P, Eibel H. BAFF- and TACI-dependent processing of BAFFR by ADAM proteases regulates the survival of B cells. Cell Rep. 2017;18:2189–202.
7. Gross JA, Johnston J, Mudri S, Enselman R, Dillon SR, Madden K, Xu W, Parrish-Novak J, Foster D, Lofton-Day C, Moore M, Littau A, Grossman A, Haugen H, Foley K, Blumberg H, Harrison K, Kindsvogel W, Clegg CH. TACI and BCMA are receptors for a TNF homologue implicated in B-cell autoimmune disease. Nature. 2000;404:995–9.
8. Mantchev GT, Cortesao CS, Rebrovich M, Cascalho M, Bram RJ. TACI is required for efficient plasma cell differentiation in response to T-independent Type 2 antigens. J Immunol. 2007;179:2282–8.
9. Ozcan E, Garibyan L, Lee JJ, Bram RJ, Lam KP, Geha RS. Transmembrane activator, calcium modulator, and cyclophilin ligand interactor drives plasma cell differentiation in LPS-activated B cells. J Allergy Clin Immunol. 2009;123:1277–86.e5.
10. Tsuji S, Cortesao C, Bram RJ, Platt JL, Cascalho M. TACI deficiency impairs sustained Blimp-1 expression in B cells decreasing long-lived plasma cells in the bone marrow. Blood. 2011;118:5832–9.
11. O'Connor BP, Raman VS, Erickson LD, Cook WJ, Weaver LK, Ahonen C, Lin LL, Mantchev GT, Bram RJ, Noelle RJ. BCMA is essential for the survival of long-lived bone marrow plasma cells. J Exp Med. 2004;199:91–8.
12. Rowland SL, Leahy KF, Halverson R, Torres RM, Pelanda R. BAFF receptor signaling aids the differentiation of immature B cells into transitional B cells following tonic BCR signaling. J Immunol. 2010;185:4570–81.
13. Smith SH, Cancro MP. Cutting edge: B cell receptor signals regulate BLyS receptor levels in mature B cells and their immediate progenitors. J Immunol. 2003;170:5820–3.
14. Hobeika E, Levit-Zerdoun E, Anastasopoulou V, Pohlmeyer R, Altmeier S, Alsadeq A, Dobenecker MW, Pelanda R, Reth M. CD19 and BAFF-R can signal to promote B-cell survival in the absence of Syk. EMBO J. 2015;34:925–39.
15. Levit-Zerdoun E, Becker M, Pohlmeyer R, Wilhelm I, Maity PC, Rajewsky K, Reth M, Hobeika E. Survival of Igalpha-deficient mature B cells requires BAFF-R function. J Immunol. 2016;196:2348–60.
16. Bossen C, Cachero TG, Tardivel A, Ingold K, Willen L, Dobles M, Scott ML, Maquelin A, Belnoue E, Siegrist CA, Chevrier S, Acha-Orbea H, Leung H, Mackay F, Tschopp J, Schneider P. TACI, unlike BAFF-R, is solely activated by oligomeric BAFF and APRIL to support survival of activated B cells and plasmablasts. Blood. 2008;111:1004–12.
17. Shu HB, Hu WH, Johnson H. TALL-1 is a novel member of the TNF family that is down-regulated by mitogens. J Leukoc Biol. 1999;65:680.
18. Schneider P, Mackay CR, Steiner V, Hofmann K, Bodmer JL, Holler N, Ambrose C, Lawton P, Bixler S, Acha-Orbea H, Valmori D, Romero P, Werner-Favre C, Zubler RH, Browning JL, Tschopp J. BAFF, a novel ligand of the tumor necrosis factor family, stimulates B cell growth. J Exp Med. 1999;189:1747–56.
19. Moore PA, Belvedere O, Orr A, Pieri K, LaFleur DW, Feng P, Soppet D, Charters M, Gentz R, Parmelee D, Li Y, Galperina O, Giri J, Roschke V, Nardelli B, Carrell J, Sosnovtseva S, Greenfield W, Ruben SM, Olsen HS, Fikes J, Hilbert DM. BLyS: member of the tumor necrosis factor family and B lymphocyte stimulator. Science. 1999;285:260–3.
20. Hahne M, Kataoka T, Schröter M, Hofmann K, Irmler M, Bodmer JL, Schneider P, Bornand T, Holler N, French LE, Sordat B, Rimoldi D, Tschopp J. APRIL, a new ligand of the tumor necrosis factor family stimulates tumor cell growth. J Exp Med. 1998;188:1185–90.
21. Liu Y, Hong X, Kappler J, Jiang L, Zhang R, Xu L, Pan C, Martin WE, Murphy RC, Shu HB, Dai S, Zhang G. Ligand–receptor binding revealed by the TNF family member TALL-1. Nature. 2003;423:49–56.

22. Liu Y, Xu L, Opalka N, Kappler J, Shu HB, Zhang B. Crystal structure of sTALL-1 reveals a virus-like assembly of TNF family ligands. Cell Press. 2002;108:383–94.
23. Cachero TG, Schwartz IM, Qian F, Day ES, Bossen C, Ingold K, Tardivel A, Krushinskie D, Eldredge J, Silvian L, Lugovskoy A, Farrington GK, Strauch K, Schneider P, Whitty A. Formation of virus-like clusters is an intrinsic property of the tumor necrosis factor family member BAFF (B cell activating factor). Biochemistry. 2005;45:2006–13.
24. Karpusas M, Cachero TG, Qian F, Sjodin AB, Mullen C, Strauch K, Hsu YM, Kalled SL. Crystal structure of extracellular human BAFF, a TNF family member that stimulates B lymphocytes. J Mol Biol. 2002;315:1145–54.
25. Ingold K, Zumsteg A, Tardivel A, Huard B, Steiner QG, Cachero TG, Qiang F, Gorelik L, Kalled SL, Acha-Orbea H, Rennert PD, Tschopp J, Schneider P. Identification of proteoglycans as the APRIL-specific binding partners. J Exp Med. 2005;201:1375–83.
26. Kimberley FC, van Bostelen L, Cameron K, Hardenberg G, Marquart JA, Hahne M, Medema JP. The proteoglycan (heparan sulfate proteoglycan) binding domain of APRIL serves as a platform for ligand multimerization and cross-linking. FASEB J. 2009;23:1584–95.
27. Schuepbach-Mallepell S, Das D, Willen L, Vigolo M, Tardivel A, Lebon L, Kowalczyk-Quintas C, Nys J, Smulski C, Zheng TS, Maskos K, Lammens A, Jiang X, Hess H, Tan SL, Schneider P. Stoichiometry of heteromeric BAFF and APRIL cytokines dictates their receptor binding and signaling properties. J Biol Chem. 2015;290:16330–42.
28. Nardelli B, Belvedere O, Roschke V, Moore PA, Olsen HS, Migone TS, Sosnovtseva S, Carrell J, Feng P, Giri J, Hilbert DM. Synthesis and release of B-lymphocyte stimulator from myeloid cells. Blood J. 2001;97:198–204.
29. Thangarajh M, Masterman T, Helgeland L, Rot U, Jonsson MV, Eide GE, Pirskanen R, Hillert J, Jonsson R. The thymus is a source of B-cell-survival factors-APRIL and BAFF-in myasthenia gravis. J Neuroimmunol. 2006;178:161–6.
30. Litinskiy MB, Nardelli B, Hilbert DM, He B, Schaffer A, Casali P, Cerutti A. DCs induce CD40-independent immunoglobulin class switching through BLyS and APRIL. Nat Immunol. 2002;3:822–9.
31. Kreuzaler M, Rauch M, Salzer U, Birmelin J, Rizzi M, Grimbacher B, Plebani A, Lougaris V, Quinti I, Thon V, Litzman J, Schlesier M, Warnatz K, Thiel J, Rolink AG, Eibel H. Soluble BAFF levels inversely correlate with peripheral B cell numbers and the expression of BAFF receptors. J Immunol. 2012;188:497–503.
32. Claudio E, Brown K, Park S, Wang H, Siebenlist U. BAFF-induced NEMO-independent processing of NF-kappa B2 in maturing B cells. Nat Immunol. 2002;3:958–65.
33. Kayagaki N, Yan M, Seshasayee D, Wang H, Lee W, French DM, Grewal IS, Cochran AG, Gordon NC, Yin J, Starovasnik MA, Dixit VM. BAFF/BLyS receptor 3 binds the B cell survival factor BAFF ligand through a discrete surface loop and promotes processing of NF-kappaB2. Immunity. 2002;17:515–24.
34. Zhang Q, Lenardo MJ, Baltimore D. 30 Years of NF-kappaB: a blossoming of relevance to human pathobiology. Cell. 2017;168:37–57.
35. Vallabhapurapu S, Karin M. Regulation and function of NF-kappaB transcription factors in the immune system. Annu Rev Immunol. 2009;27:693–733.
36. Willmann KL, Klaver S, Dogu F, Santos-Valente E, Garncarz W, Bilic I, Mace E, Salzer E, Conde CD, Sic H, Majek P, Banerjee PP, Vladimer GI, Haskologlu S, Bolkent MG, Kupesiz A, Condino-Neto A, Colinge J, Superti-Furga G, Pickl WF, van Zelm MC, Eibel H, Orange JS, Ikinciogullari A, Boztug K. Biallelic loss-of-function mutation in NIK causes a primary immunodeficiency with multifaceted aberrant lymphoid immunity. Nat Commun. 2014;5:5360.
37. Liao G, Zhang M, Harhaj EW, Sun SC. Regulation of the NF-kappaB-inducing kinase by tumor necrosis factor receptor-associated factor 3-induced degradation. J Biol Chem. 2004;279:26243–50.
38. Ling L, Cao Z, Goeddel DV. NF-kappaB-inducing kinase activates IKK-alpha by phosphorylation of Ser-176. Proc Natl Acad Sci U S A. 1998;95:3792–7.
39. Xiao G, Harhaj EW, Sun SC. NF-kappaB-inducing kinase regulates the processing of NF-kappaB2 p100. Mol Cell. 2001;7:401–9.

40. Amir RE, Haecker H, Karin M, Ciechanover A. Mechanism of processing of the NF-kappa B2 p100 precursor: identification of the specific polyubiquitin chain-anchoring lysine residue and analysis of the role of NEDD8-modification on the SCF(beta-TrCP) ubiquitin ligase. Oncogene. 2004;23:2540–7.
41. Dejardin E, Droin NM, Delhase M, Haas E, Cao Y, Makris C, Li ZW, Karin M, Ware CF, Green DR. The lymphotoxin-beta receptor induces different patterns of gene expression via two NF-kappaB pathways. Immunity. 2002;17:525–35.
42. Sun SC, Ganchi PA, Beraud C, Ballard DW, Greene WC. Autoregulation of the NF-kappa B transactivator RelA (p65) by multiple cytoplasmic inhibitors containing ankyrin motifs. Proc Natl Acad Sci U S A. 1994;91:1346–50.
43. Derudder E, Dejardin E, Pritchard LL, Green DR, Korner M, Baud V. RelB/p50 dimers are differentially regulated by tumor necrosis factor-alpha and lymphotoxin-beta receptor activation: critical roles for p100. J Biol Chem. 2003;278:23278–84.
44. Yilmaz ZB, Weih DS, Sivakumar V, Weih F. RelB is required for Peyer's patch development: differential regulation of p52-RelB by lymphotoxin and TNF. EMBO J. 2003;22:121–30.
45. Li T, Morgan MJ, Choksi S, Zhang Y, Kim YS, Liu ZG. MicroRNAs modulate the noncanonical transcription factor NF-kappaB pathway by regulating expression of the kinase IKKalpha during macrophage differentiation. Nat Immunol. 2010;11:799–805.
46. Hu H, Wu X, Jin W, Chang M, Cheng X, Sun SC. Noncanonical NF-kappaB regulates inducible costimulator (ICOS) ligand expression and T follicular helper cell development. Proc Natl Acad Sci U S A. 2011;108:12827–32.
47. Maurer U, Charvet C, Wagman AS, Dejardin E, Green DR. Glycogen synthase kinase-3 regulates mitochondrial outer membrane permeabilization and apoptosis by destabilization of MCL-1. Mol Cell. 2006;21:749–60.
48. Razani B, Zarnegar B, Ytterberg AJ, Shiba T, Dempsey PW, Ware CF, Loo JA, Cheng G. Negative feedback in noncanonical NF-kappaB signaling modulates NIK stability through IKKalpha-mediated phosphorylation. Sci Signal. 2010;3:ra41.
49. Hu H, Brittain GC, Chang JH, Puebla-Osorio N, Jin J, Zal A, Xiao Y, Cheng X, Chang M, Fu YX, Zal T, Zhu C, Sun SC. OTUD7B controls non-canonical NF-kappaB activation through deubiquitination of TRAF3. Nature. 2013;494:371–4.
50. Schweighoffer E, Vanes L, Nys J, Cantrell D, McCleary S, Smithers N, Tybulewicz VL. The BAFF receptor transduces survival signals by co-opting the B cell receptor signaling pathway. Immunity. 2013;38:475–88.
51. Jellusova J, Miletic AV, Cato MH, Lin WW, Hu Y, Bishop GA, Shlomchik MJ, Rickert RC. Context-specific BAFF-R signaling by the NF-kappaB and PI3K pathways. Cell Rep. 2013;5:1022–35.
52. Mattila PK, Feest C, Depoil D, Treanor B, Montaner B, Otipoby KL, Carter R, Justement LB, Bruckbauer A, Batista FD. The actin and tetraspanin networks organize receptor nanoclusters to regulate B cell receptor-mediated signaling. Immunity. 2013;38:461–74.
53. Keppler SJ, Gasparrini F, Burbage M, Aggarwal S, Frederico B, Geha RS, Way M, Bruckbauer A, Batista FD. Wiskott-Aldrich syndrome interacting protein deficiency uncovers the role of the co-receptor CD19 as a generic Hub for PI3 kinase signaling in B cells. Immunity. 2015;43:660–73.
54. Fruman DA, Cantley LC. Phosphoinositide 3-kinase in immunological systems. Semin Immunol. 2002;14:7–18.
55. Okada T, Maeda A, Iwamatsu A, Gotoh K, Kurosaki T. BCAP: the tyrosine kinase substrate that connects B cell receptor to phosphoinositide 3-kinase activation. Immunity. 2000;13:817–27.
56. Aiba Y, Kameyama M, Yamazaki T, Tedder TF, Kurosaki T. Regulation of B-cell development by BCAP and CD19 through their binding to phosphoinositide 3-kinase. Blood. 2008;111:1497–503.
57. Thompson JS, Bixler SA, Qian F, Vora K, Scott ML, Cachero TG, Hession C, Schneider P, Sizing ID, Mullen C, Strauch K, Zafari M, Benjamin CD, Tschopp J, Browning JL, Ambrose C. BAFF-R, a newly identified TNF receptor that specifically interacts with BAFF. Science. 2001;293:2108–11.

58. Jellusova J, Rickert RC. The PI3K pathway in B cell metabolism. Crit Rev Biochem Mol Biol. 2016;51:359–78.
59. Patke A, Mecklenbrauker I, Erdjument-Bromage H, Tempst P, Tarakhovsky A. BAFF controls B cell metabolic fitness through a PKC beta- and Akt-dependent mechanism. J Exp Med. 2006;203:2551–62.
60. Woodland RT, Fox CJ, Schmidt MR, Hammerman PS, Opferman JT, Korsmeyer SJ, Hilbert DM, Thompson CB. Multiple signaling pathways promote B lymphocyte stimulator dependent B-cell growth and survival. Blood. 2008;111:750–60.
61. Hoffmann FS, Kuhn PH, Laurent SA, Hauck SM, Berer K, Wendlinger SA, Krumbholz M, Khademi M, Olsson T, Dreyling M, Pfister HW, Alexander T, Hiepe F, Kumpfel T, Crawford HC, Wekerle H, Hohlfeld R, Lichtenthaler SF, Meinl E. The immunoregulator soluble TACI is released by ADAM10 and reflects B cell activation in autoimmunity. J Immunol. 2015;194:542–52.
62. Mesin L, Ersching J, Victora GD. Germinal center B cell dynamics. Immunity. 2016;45:471–82.
63. Kräutler NJ, Suan D, Butt D, Bourne K, Hermes JR, Chan TD, Sundling C, Kaplan W, Schofield P, Jackson J, Basten A, Christ D, Brink R. Differentiation of germinal center B cells into plasma cells is initiated by high-affinity antigen and completed by Tfh cells. J Exp Med. 2017;214:1259.
64. Warnatz K, Salzer U, Rizzi M, Fischer B, Gutenberger S, Bohm J, Kienzler AK, Pan-Hammarstrom Q, Hammarstrom L, Rakhmanov M, Schlesier M, Grimbacher B, Peter HH, Eibel H. B-cell activating factor receptor deficiency is associated with an adult-onset antibody deficiency syndrome in humans. Proc Natl Acad Sci U S A. 2009;106:13945–50.
65. Mackay F, Woodcock SA, Lawton P, Ambrose C, Baetscher M, Schneider P, Tschopp J, Browning JL. Mice transgenic for BAFF develop lymphocytic disorders along with autoimmune manifestations. J Exp Med. 1999;190:1697–710.
66. Steri M, Orru V, Idda ML, Pitzalis M, Pala M, Zara I, Sidore C, Faa V, Floris M, Deiana M, Asunis I, Porcu E, Mulas A, Piras MG, Lobina M, Lai S, Marongiu M, Serra V, Marongiu M, Sole G, Busonero F, Maschio A, Cusano R, Cuccuru G, Deidda F, Poddie F, Farina G, Dei M, Virdis F, Olla S, Satta MA, Pani M, Delitala A, Cocco E, Frau J, Coghe G, Lorefice L, Fenu G, Ferrigno P, Ban M, Barizzone N, Leone M, Guerini FR, Piga M, Firinu D, Kockum I, Lima Bomfim I, Olsson T, Alfredsson L, Suarez A, Carreira PE, Castillo-Palma MJ, Marcus JH, Congia M, Angius A, Melis M, Gonzalez A, Alarcon Riquelme ME, da Silva BM, Marchini M, Danieli MG, Del Giacco S, Mathieu A, Pani A, Montgomery SB, Rosati G, Hillert J, Sawcer S, D'Alfonso S, Todd JA, Novembre J, Abecasis GR, Whalen MB, Marrosu MG, Meloni A, Sanna S, Gorospe M, Schlessinger D, Fiorillo E, Zoledziewska M, Cucca F. Overexpression of the cytokine BAFF and autoimmunity risk. N Engl J Med. 2017;376:1615–26.
67. Castigli E, Wilson SA, Garibyan L, Rachid R, Bonilla F, Schneider L, Geha RS. TACI is mutant in common variable immunodeficiency and IgA deficiency. Nat Genet. 2005;37:829–34.
68. Salzer U, Chapel HM, Webster AD, Pan-Hammarstrom Q, Schmitt-Graeff A, Schlesier M, Peter HH, Rockstroh JK, Schneider P, Schaffer AA, Hammarstrom L, Grimbacher B. Mutations in TNFRSF13B encoding TACI are associated with common variable immunodeficiency in humans. Nat Genet. 2005;37:820–8.
69. Seshasayee D, Valdez P, Yan M, Dixit VM, Tumas D, Grewal IS. Loss of TACI causes fatal lymphoproliferation and autoimmunity, establishing TACI as an inhibitory BLyS receptor. Immunity. 2003;18:279–88.
70. Yan M, Brady JR, Chan B, Lee WP, Hsu B, Harless S, Cancro M, Grewal IS, Dixit VM. Identification of a novel receptor for B lymphocyte stimulator that is mutated in a mouse strain with severe B cell deficiency. Curr Biol. 2001b;11:1547–52.
71. von Bülow G, van Deursen JM, Bram RJ. Regulation of the T-independent humoral response by TACI. Immunity. 2001;14:573–82.
72. Batten M, Fletcher C, Ng LG, Groom J, Wheway J, Laabi Y, Xin X, Schneider P, Tschopp J, Mackay CR, Mackay F. TNF deficiency fails to protect BAFF transgenic mice against autoimmunity and reveals a predisposition to B cell lymphoma. J Immunol. 2004;172:812–22.

73. Puga I, Cols M, Barra CM, He B, Cassis L, Gentile M, Comerma L, Chorny A, Shan M, Xu W, Magri G, Knowles DM, Tam W, Chiu A, Bussel JB, Serrano S, Lorente JA, Bellosillo B, Lloreta J, Juanpere N, Alameda F, Baro T, de Heredia CD, Toran N, Catala A, Torrebadell M, Fortuny C, Cusi V, Carreras C, Diaz GA, Blander JM, Farber CM, Silvestri G, Cunningham-Rundles C, Calvillo M, Dufour C, Notarangelo LD, Lougaris V, Plebani A, Casanova JL, Ganal SC, Diefenbach A, Arostegui JI, Juan M, Yague J, Mahlaoui N, Donadieu J, Chen K, Cerutti A. B cell-helper neutrophils stimulate the diversification and production of immunoglobulin in the marginal zone of the spleen. Nat Immunol. 2011;13:170–80.
74. Magri G, Miyajima M, Bascones S, Mortha A, Puga I, Cassis L, Barra CM, Comerma L, Chudnovskiy A, Gentile M, Llige D, Cols M, Serrano S, Arostegui JI, Juan M, Yague J, Merad M, Fagarasan S, Cerutti A. Innate lymphoid cells integrate stromal and immunological signals to enhance antibody production by splenic marginal zone B cells. Nat Immunol. 2014;15:354–64.
75. Losi CG, Silini A, Fiorini C, Soresina A, Meini A, Ferrari S, Notarangelo LD, Lougaris V, Plebani A. Mutational analysis of human BAFF receptor TNFRSF13C (BAFF-R) in patients with common variable immunodeficiency. J Clin Immunol. 2005;25:496–502.
76. Hildebrand JM, Luo Z, Manske MK, Price-Troska T, Ziesmer SC, Lin W, Hostager BS, Slager SL, Witzig TE, Ansell SM, Cerhan JR, Bishop GA, Novak AJ. A BAFF-R mutation associated with non-Hodgkin lymphoma alters TRAF recruitment and reveals new insights into BAFF-R signaling. J Exp Med. 2010;207:2569–79.
77. Kutukculer N, Gulez N, Karaca NE, Aksu G, Berdeli A. Three different classifications, B lymphocyte subpopulations, TNFRSF13B (TACI), TNFRSF13C (BAFF-R), TNFSF13 (APRIL) gene mutations, CTLA-4 and ICOS gene polymorphisms in Turkish patients with common variable immunodeficiency. J Clin Immunol. 2012;32:1165–79.
78. Martin F, Kearney JF. B1 cell: similarities and differences with other B cell subsets. Curr Opin Immunol. 2001;13:195–201.
79. Pillai S, Cariappa A, Moran ST. Positive selection and lineage commitment during peripheral B-lymphocyte development. Immunol Rev. 2004;197:206–18.
80. Hardy RR, Hayakawa K. Perspectives on fetal derived CD5+ B1 B cells. Eur J Immunol. 2015;45:2978–84.
81. Jacobs HM, Thouvenel CD, Leach S, Arkatkar T, Metzler G, Scharping NE, Kolhatkar NS, Rawlings DJ, Jackson SW. Cutting edge: BAFF promotes autoantibody production via TACI-dependent activation of transitional B cells. J Immunol. 2016;196:3525–31.
82. Rahman ZS, Rao SP, Kalled SL, Manser T. Normal induction but attenuated progression of germinal center responses in BAFF and BAFF-R signaling-deficient mice. J Exp Med. 2003;198:1157–69.
83. Benson MJ, Dillon SR, Castigli E, Geha RS, Xu S, Lam KP, Noelle RJ. Cutting edge: the dependence of plasma cell and independence of memory B cell on BAFF and APRIL. J Immunol. 2008;180:3655–9.
84. Rauch M, Tussiwand R, Bosco N, Rolink AG. Crucial role for BAFF-BAFF-R signaling in the survival and maintenance of mature B cells. PLoS One. 2009;4:e5456.
85. Furie R, Petri M, Zamani O, Cervera R, Wallace DJ, Tegzova D, Sanchez-Guerrero J, Schwarting A, Merrill JT, Chatham WW, Stohl W, Ginzler EM, Hough DR, Zhong ZJ, Freimuth W, van Vollenhoven RF. A phase III, randomized, placebo-controlled study of belimumab, a monoclonal antibody that inhibits B lymphocyte stimulator, in patients with systemic lupus erythematosus. Arthritis Rheum. 2011;63:3918–30.
86. Stohl W, Hiepe F, Latinis KM, Thomas M, Scheinberg MA, Clarke A, Aranow C, Wellborne FR, Abud-Mendoza C, Hough DR, Pineda L, Migone TS, Zhong ZJ, Freimuth WW, Chatham WW. Belimumab reduces autoantibodies, normalizes low complement levels, and reduces select B cell populations in patients with systemic lupus erythematosus. Arthritis Rheum. 2012;64:2328–37.

87. Chatham WW, Wallace DJ, Stohl W, Latinis KM, Manzi S, McCune WJ, Tegzova D, McKay JD, Avila-Armengol HE, Utset TO, Zhong ZJ, Hough DR, Freimuth WW, Migone TS. Effect of belimumab on vaccine antigen antibodies to influenza, pneumococcal, and tetanus vaccines in patients with systemic lupus erythematosus in the BLISS-76 trial. J Rheumatol. 2012;39:1632–40.
88. van Vollenhoven RF, Kinnman N, Vincent E, Wax S, Bathon J. Atacicept in patients with rheumatoid arthritis and an inadequate response to methotrexate: results of a phase II, randomized, placebo-controlled trial. Arthritis Rheum. 2011;63:1782–92.

TWEAK Deficiency

12

Ulrich Salzer

12.1 Definition

TWEAK (TNF-like weak inducer of apoptosis) deficiency has been first described by Wang et al. in 2013 in a single family [1]. It is caused by heterozygous mutations in the TNFSF12/WEAK gene.

12.2 Etiology

TWEAK (synonyms: TNFSF12, APO3L, DR3LG) is a member of the TNF ligand superfamily and is highly conserved between mice and man [2]. The TNFSF12/TWEAK gene is encoded by 7 exons and located on human chromosome 17 in direct neighborhood to the TNFSF13 gene, which encodes APRIL, another important TNF superfamily member. By alternative splicing the membrane-bound fusion protein TWEPRIL is formed [3].

The 249-amino acid long TWEAK protein contains a C-terminal TNF homology domain, a stalk region, a transmembrane part, and a short N-terminal intracellular tail. It is synthesized as a type II transmembrane protein, from which a soluble ligand is released by furin protease-mediated cleavage at amino acid site 94. Soluble TWEAK is released from different leucocytes [2, 4] and acts mainly as a proinflammatory cytokine in response to acute or chronic tissues damage.

U. Salzer
Faculty of Medicine, Department of Rheumatology and Clinical Immunology, Medical Center—University of Freiburg, Freiburg im Breisgau, Germany

Faculty of Medicine, Center for Chronic Immunodeficiency (CCI), Medical Center—University of Freiburg, Freiburg im Breisgau, Germany
e-mail: ulrich.salzer@uniklinik-freiburg.de

M. M. D'Elios, M. Rizzi (eds.), *Humoral Primary Immunodeficiencies*,
Rare Diseases of the Immune System, https://doi.org/10.1007/978-3-319-91785-6_12

The murine and human TWEAK receptors, designated as Fn14 (fibroblast growth factor-inducible-14), were originally discovered in 1999 [5] and 2000 [6] as an immediate early response gene, which is induced by growth factors. Wiley demonstrated that Fn14 is the sole TWEAK receptor [7]. Upon binding of TWEAK, the TNFR-associated factors 1, 2, 3, and 5 are recruited to the Fn14 intracellular domain [7, 8], and NFk-B signaling is induced [8, 9]. In addition the MAPK signaling pathway is induced [10]. The expression of Fn14 is inducible and regulated [5, 6]. The TWEAK-Fn14 pathway is primarily implicated in wound healing processes, angiogenesis [5, 7, 11], and stimulates progenitor cells in various tissues [12, 13] to proliferate while inhibiting their differentiation. Thus, in case of acute injury, the physiological role of the TWEAK-Fn14 axis seems to stimulate angiogenesis, progenitor cell proliferation, and local inflammation to initiate and direct tissue repair processes [14]. However in states of chronic inflammation and continued tissue damage, as observed in many autoimmune diseases, TWEAK via Fn14 perpetuates the pathological processes by stimulating proliferation, fibrosis, neo-angiogenesis, and chronic inflammation in disorders like rheumatoid arthritis [15], lupus nephritis [16], and inflammatory skin diseases [17].

In summary the TWEAK/Fn14 interaction links acute inflammation to tissue repair in health and chronic inflammation to pathological tissue remodeling processes in disease. However, both TWEAK- [18, 19] and Fn14-deficient mice [12] did not show any overt immunological or especially immunodeficient phenotype. Thus, although mutations in many of the TNF family of ligands and receptors cause primary immunodeficiency in humans, the first description of human TWEAK mutations in a family with CVID like antibody deficiency may at first glance be somewhat surprising, but is clearly linked to the inherent propensity of these cysteine-rich protein families to multimerize [1]. Indeed the mutation R145C described in the affected individuals forms both intramolecular complexes of TWEAK and together with the related TNF ligand BAFF large hybrid TWEAK/BAFF protein complexes via intermolecular disulfide bridges. The R145C TWEAK mutant thereby acts like a scavenger for BAFF. The formation of trimeric or larger monomeric or heteromeric protein complexes is typical for members of the TNF superfamily of ligand and receptors [20–22], and their correct formation is often essential for the initiation of downstream signaling events. However heteromeric complexes may also be observed in disease states like BAFF/APRIL heterotrimers in rheumatic diseases [23]. Indeed, the mutated R145C TWEAK molecule by itself is capable of binding to its receptor Fn14, but signaling is impaired [1]. And even though the heteromers formed by the mutant TWEAK and BAFF proteins showed slightly enhanced binding to BAFFR, the signaling was impaired. The mutant also inhibited BAFF-dependent survival and Ig class switching in primary cells [1]. In line with these observations, the phenotype of TWEAK deficiency partly resembles that of patients with BAFF-R defects [24, 25].

12.3 Clinical Manifestations

All three affected individuals in the index family had a history of bacterial ear and sinus infections. Other infectious manifestations were pneumonia, osteomyelitis, pneumococcal meningitis, and multiple warts caused by HPV. Noninfectious manifestations included thrombocytopenia and neutropenia [1]. IgA and IgM were low in all three, total IgG was low in two family members, and IgG2/IgG4 subclass deficiency was found in one. All affected individuals had impaired or absent antibody responses against T-dependent (diphtheria and tetanus toxoid) and independent antigens (pneumococcal polysaccharides). Total B-cell numbers were reduced with a selective deficiency in CD27+ memory B cells. CD8+ T cells and TCR a/b+ double-negative T cells (DNTs) were increased in numbers [1].

12.4 Diagnosis

The new antibody deficiency-causing mutations in TWEAK are very rare, considering the unique mutation mechanism, which seems to be specific to the R145C TWEAK mutation. Nevertheless, based on the observed immunological phenotype, TWEAK deficiency may be suspected in antibody deficiency patients with elevated DNTs and co-occurring warts and should be confirmed by genetic testing.

References

1. Wang HY, Ma CA, Zhao Y, Fan X, Zhou Q, Edmonds P, Uzel G, Oliveira JB, Orange J, Jain A. Antibody deficiency associated with an inherited autosomal dominant mutation in TWEAK. Proc Natl Acad Sci U S A. 2013;110:5127–32.
2. Chicheportiche Y, Bourdon PR, Xu H, Hsu YM, Scott H, Hession C, Garcia I, Browning JL. TWEAK, a new secreted ligand in the tumor necrosis factor family that weakly induces apoptosis. J Biol Chem. 1997;272:32401–10.
3. Pradet-Balade B, Medema JP, López-Fraga M, Lozano JC, Kolfschoten GM, Picard A, Martínez-A C, Garcia-Sanz JA, Hahne M. An endogenous hybrid mRNA encodes TWE-PRIL, a functional cell surface TWEAK-APRIL fusion protein. EMBO J. 2002;21:5711–20.
4. Kaplan MJ, Lewis EE, Shelden EA, Somers E, Pavlic R, McCune WJ, Richardson BC. The apoptotic ligands TRAIL, TWEAK, and Fas ligand mediate monocyte death induced by autologous lupus T cells. J Immunol. 2002;169:6020–9.
5. Meighan-Mantha RL, Hsu DK, Guo Y, Brown SA, Feng SL, Peifley KA, Alberts GF, Copeland NG, Gilbert DJ, Jenkins NA, Richards CM, Winkles JA. The mitogen-inducible Fn14 gene encodes a type I transmembrane protein that modulates fibroblast adhesion and migration. J Biol Chem. 1999;274:33166–76.
6. Feng SL, Guo Y, Factor VM, Thorgeirsson SS, Bell DW, Testa JR, Peifley KA, Winkles JA. The Fn14 immediate-early response gene is induced during liver regeneration and highly expressed in both human and murine hepatocellular carcinomas. Am J Pathol. 2000;156:1253–61.
7. Wiley SR, Cassiano L, Lofton T, Davis-Smith T, Winkles JA, Lindner V, Liu H, Daniel TO, Smith CA, Fanslow WC. A novel TNF receptor family member binds TWEAK and is implicated in angiogenesis. Immunity. 2001;15:837–46.
8. Brown SA, Richards CM, Hanscom HN, Feng SL, Winkles JA. The Fn14 cytoplasmic tail binds tumour-necrosis-factor-receptor-associated factors 1, 2, 3 and 5 and mediates nuclear factor-kappa B activation. Biochem J. 2003;371:395–403.
9. Saitoh T, Nakayama M, Nakano H, Yagita H, Yamamoto N, Yamaoka S. TWEAK induces NF-kappaB2 p100 processing and long lasting NF-kappaB activation. J Biol Chem. 2003;278:36005–12.
10. Ando T, Ichikawa J, Wako M, Hatsushika K, Watanabe Y, Sakuma M, Tasaka K, Ogawa H, Hamada Y, Yagita H, Nakao A. TWEAK/Fn14 interaction regulates RANTES production,

BMP-2-induced differentiation, and RANKL expression in mouse osteoblastic MC3T3-E1 cells. Arthritis Res Ther. 2006;8:R146.
11. Lynch CN, Wang YC, Lund JK, Chen YW, Leal JA, Wiley SR. TWEAK induces angiogenesis and proliferation of endothelial cells. J Biol Chem. 1999;274:8455–9.
12. Girgenrath M, Weng S, Kostek CA, Browning B, Wang M, Brown SA, Winkles JA, Michaelson JS, Allaire N, Schneider P, Scott ML, Hsu YM, Yagita H, Flavell RA, Miller JB, Burkly LC, Zheng TS. TWEAK, via its receptor Fn14, is a novel regulator of mesenchymal progenitor cells and skeletal muscle regeneration. EMBO J. 2006;25:5826–39.
13. Jakubowski A, Ambrose C, Parr M, Lincecum JM, Wang MZ, Zheng TS, Browning B, Michaelson JS, Baetscher M, Wang B, Bissell DM, Burkly LC. TWEAK induces liver progenitor cell proliferation. J Clin Invest. 2005;115:2330–40.
14. Burkly LC, Michaelson JS, Zheng TS. TWEAK/Fn14 pathway: an immunological switch for shaping tissue responses. Immunol Rev. 2011;244:99–114.
15. Perper SJ, Browning B, Burkly LC, Weng S, Gao C, Giza K, Su L, Tarilonte L, Crowell T, Rajman L, Runkel L, Scott M, Atkins GJ, Findlay DM, Zheng TS, Hess H. TWEAK is a novel arthritogenic mediator. J Immunol. 2006;177:2610–20.
16. Schwartz N, Su L, Burkly LC, Mackay M, Aranow C, Kollaros M, Michaelson JS, Rovin B, Putterman C. Urinary TWEAK and the activity of lupus nephritis. J Autoimmun. 2006;27:242–50.
17. Sidler D, Wu P, Herro R, Claus M, Wolf D, Kawakami Y, Kawakami T, Burkly L, Croft M. TWEAK mediates inflammation in experimental atopic dermatitis and psoriasis. Nat Commun. 2017;8:15395.
18. Campbell S, Burkly LC, Gao HX, Berman JW, Su L, Browning B, Zheng T, Schiffer L, Michaelson JS, Putterman C. Proinflammatory effects of TWEAK/Fn14 interactions in glomerular mesangial cells. J Immunol. 2006;176:1889–98.
19. Maecker H, Varfolomeev E, Kischkel F, Lawrence D, LeBlanc H, Lee W, Hurst S, Danilenko D, Li J, Filvaroff E, Yang B, Daniel D, Ashkenazi A. TWEAK attenuates the transition from innate to adaptive immunity. Cell. 2005;123:931–44.
20. Bossen C, Cachero TG, Tardivel A, Ingold K, Willen L, Dobles M, Scott ML, Maquelin A, Belnoue E, Siegrist CA, Chevrier S, Acha-Orbea H, Leung H, Mackay F, Tschopp J, Schneider P. TACI, unlike BAFF-R, is solely activated by oligomeric BAFF and APRIL to support survival of activated B cells and plasmablasts. Blood. 2008;111:1004–12.
21. Cachero TG, Schwartz IM, Qian F, Day ES, Bossen C, Ingold K, Tardivel A, Krushinskie D, Eldredge J, Silvian L, Lugovskoy A, Farrington GK, Strauch K, Schneider P, Whitty A. Formation of virus-like clusters is an intrinsic property of the tumor necrosis factor family member BAFF (B cell activating factor). Biochemistry. 2006;45:2006–13.
22. Smulski CR, Kury P, Seidel LM, Staiger HS, Edinger AK, Willen L, Seidl M, Hess H, Salzer U, Rolink AG, Rizzi M, Schneider P, Eibel H. BAFF- and TACI-dependent processing of BAFFR by ADAM proteases regulates the survival of B cells. Cell Rep. 2017;18:2189–202.
23. Roschke V, Sosnovtseva S, Ward CD, Hong JS, Smith R, Albert V, Stohl W, Baker KP, Ullrich S, Nardelli B, Hilbert DM, Migone TS. BLyS and APRIL form biologically active heterotrimers that are expressed in patients with systemic immune-based rheumatic diseases. J Immunol. 2002;169:4314–21.
24. Kreuzaler M, Rauch M, Salzer U, Birmelin J, Rizzi M, Grimbacher B, Plebani A, Lougaris V, Quinti I, Thon V, Litzman J, Schlesier M, Warnatz K, Thiel J, Rolink AG, Eibel H. Soluble BAFF levels inversely correlate with peripheral B cell numbers and the expression of BAFF receptors. J Immunol. 2012;188:497–503.
25. Warnatz K, Salzer U, Rizzi M, Fischer B, Gutenberger S, Böhm J, Kienzler AK, Pan-Hammarström Q, Hammarström L, Rakhmanov M, Schlesier M, Grimbacher B, Peter HH, Eibel H. B-cell activating factor receptor deficiency is associated with an adult-onset antibody deficiency syndrome in humans. Proc Natl Acad Sci U S A. 2009;106:13945–50.

NFKB2 Defects

13

Shancy P. Jacob, Julie E. Feusier, and Karin Chen

13.1 NF-κB2 Signaling Pathway

The NF-κB family of transcription factors comprises two subfamilies: "NF-κB" proteins NF-κB1 (p105/p50) and NF-κB2 (p100/p52) and "Rel" proteins RelA (p65), RelB, and c-Rel. These structurally related proteins form homo-/heterodimers to transactivate genes involved in various biological processes, including immune responses, inflammation, apoptosis, cell growth, cell survival, and cell development [1]. All members in this family have a highly conserved 300-amino acid N-terminal Rel homology domain (RHD) conferring dimerization, nuclear localization, and binding to DNA motifs, termed "κB elements." The activity of NF-κB proteins is tightly regulated where, in quiescent cells, these proteins are normally inactive and sequestered in the cytoplasm through association with inhibitory κB-like activity or proteins (IκB, inhibitor of κB proteins). While the Rel members are inhibited by ankyrin repeat-containing inhibitors, masking DNA binding, and nuclear localization domains (NLD), NF-κB1 and NF-κB2 are synthesized as inactive preforms (p105 and p100) with a long C-terminal domain containing the inhibitory multiple ankyrin repeats. The NF-κB1/p105 and NF-κB2/p100 proteins are proteolytically activated by two important pathways: (1) the canonical, or classical, pathway which processes p105 to the active p50 form, and (2) the noncanonical pathway involving processing of p100 to the active p52 (Fig. 13.1) [2, 3].

S. P. Jacob · K. Chen (✉)
Division of Allergy and Immunology, Department of Pediatrics,
University of Utah School of Medicine, Salt Lake City, UT, USA
e-mail: karin.chen@hsc.utah.edu

J. E. Feusier
Department of Human Genetics, University of Utah School of Medicine,
Salt Lake City, UT, USA

M. M. D'Elios, M. Rizzi (eds.), *Humoral Primary Immunodeficiencies*,
Rare Diseases of the Immune System, https://doi.org/10.1007/978-3-319-91785-6_13

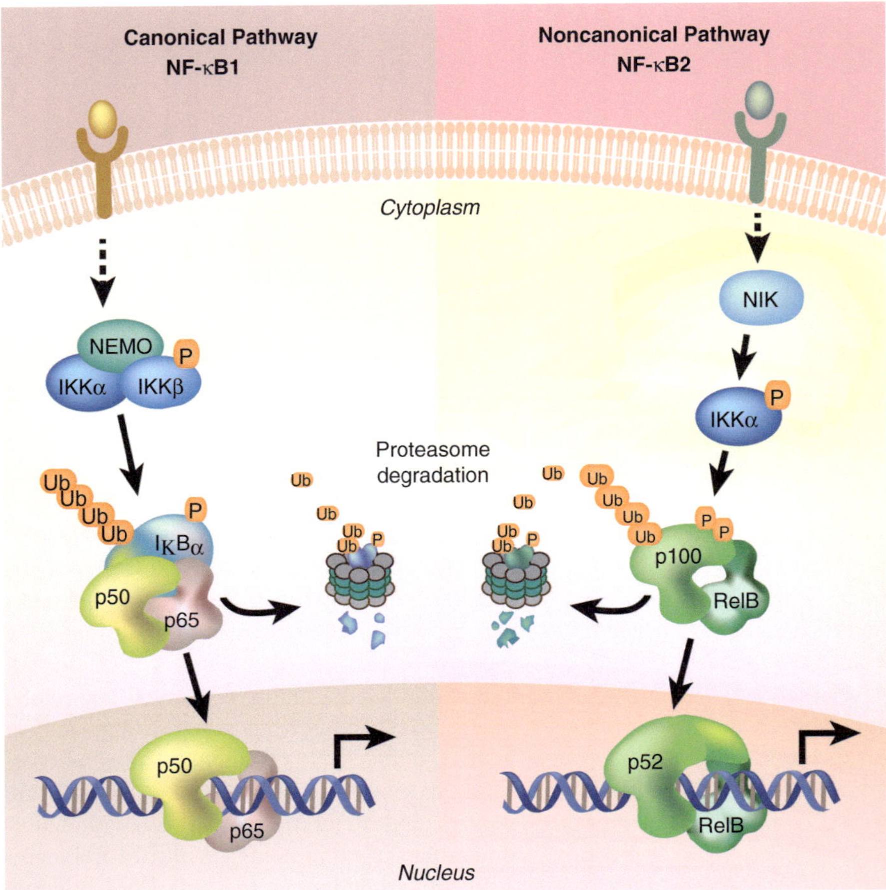

Fig. 13.1 Canonical and noncanonical NF-κB pathways. Ligand-mediated receptor activation on the cell surface leads to activation and nuclear translocation of NF-κB proteins into the nucleus where they bind their respective gene targets to initiate gene transcription and downstream cellular responses. Activation of the canonical pathway (left) leads to stimulation of a kinase cascade that phosphorylates the IκB kinase (IKK) complex that consists of IKKα, IKKβ, and NF-κB essential modulator (NEMO). The IKKβ kinase phosphorylates the inhibitor IκBα, which normally sequesters NF-κB1 in the cytoplasm. Phosphorylation stimulates ubiquitination and subsequent proteasomal degradation of IκBα, resulting in the release and nuclear localization of the p50/p65 dimer. In the noncanonical pathway (right), ligand-activated receptor stimulation results in accumulation of the NF-κB-inducing kinase (NIK), which, under nonactivating conditions, is rapidly turned over in the cytoplasm. Upon cytoplasmic accumulation, NIK subsequently phosphorylates IKKα. Activation of this kinase leads to phosphorylation of p100 at serines 866 and 870 and subsequent ubiquitination of lysine 855. The p100 protein is the inactive form of NF-κB2 that resides in the cytoplasm in complex with RelB. Ubiquitination of p100 signals its processing by the proteosome to remove the C-terminus and form p52. RelB and p52 then move as a dimer into the nucleus where they bind their genomic targets to initiate downstream responses including peripheral lymphoid organogenesis, B-cell maturation, and thymic development (Reprinted from Am J Hum Genet 93 (5):812–824; Chen K, Coonrod EM, Kumanovics A, Franks ZF, Durtschi JD, Margraf RL, Wu W, Heikal NM, Augustine NH, Ridge PG, Hill HR, Jorde LB, Weyrich AS, Zimmerman GA, Gundlapalli AV, Bohnsack JF, Voelkerding KV; Germline mutations in NFKB2 implicate the noncanonical NF-kappaB pathway in the pathogenesis of common variable immunodeficiency; Supplemental Data, Page No. 2, with permission from Elsevier)

13.1.1 Roles of the Noncanonical NF-κB Pathway

Unlike the constitutive canonical NF-κB pathway that is triggered rapidly and transiently by diverse physiological stimuli, the noncanonical pathway is induced gradually and persistently by specific members of the TNF (tumor necrosis factor) cytokine superfamily, including CD40L (CD40 ligand), BAFF (B-cell-activating factor), and lymphotoxin-β that signal via CD40, BAFF-R (BAFF receptor), and LT-βR (Lymphotoxin-β receptor) [3]. Upon activation of the noncanonical pathway, NIK (NF-κB-inducing kinase; *MAP3K14*) activates a downstream kinase IKKα that in turn phosphorylates p100 specifically at C-terminal serine residues at amino acid positions 866 and 870 [4, 5]. Phosphorylation triggers the recruitment of E3 ubiquitin ligase βTrCP which then catalyzes the ubiquitination of lysine 855 that signals the proteasomal removal of the p100 C-terminus to form p52. This allows for nuclear translocation of p52-RelB heterodimers, though homodimers and other NF-κB heterodimers can also form, to activate target genes.

As evident from studies with murine models, the noncanonical NF-κB pathway is instrumental in multiple biological processes that include (1) development and architectural organization of secondary lymphoid organs, (2) B-cell maturation and survival, (3) B-cell-mediated immune responses and antibody production [6, 7], (4) formation of germinal centers (GC), (5) dendritic cell (DC) maturation, (6) differentiation of osteoclasts, and (7) various roles in T cell responses as well as thymic epithelial cell development [3, 8, 9]. Stromal cells play a key role in mediating peripheral lymphoid organ development through expression of chemokines, via the noncanonical NF-κB pathway, which allow for chemotaxis of immune cells [10]. These chemokines are also required for the homing of antigen-loaded DC and antigen-specific T cells in the secondary lymphoid organs [11].

The noncanonical NF-κB pathway is required for survival and differentiation of naive B cell and immunoglobulin class switching in mature B cells. The combined deletion of *Nfkb2* and *Relb* in murine models [12] results in severe B-cell defects and hypogammaglobulinemia, highlighting the critical role of this pathway in B-cell maturation and differentiation. In addition, the pathway regulates T cell differentiation and maintenance of effector and memory T cells [13]. Another important role of the noncanonical NF-κB pathway is to regulate the expression of *AIRE* (autoimmune regulator), a transcription factor required for induction of central tolerance to self-antigens in the thymus, thereby ensuring removal of autoreactive T cells [14].

13.1.2 Murine Models of the Noncanonical NF-κB Pathway

The functional and developmental roles of NF-κB2 are evident from a number of murine models in which various components of the noncanonical pathway are compromised (Table 13.1). Mice lacking both p100 and p52 ($Nfkb2^{-/-}$) lack or have small peripheral lymph nodes and reduced mature B-cell numbers with severely impaired B-cell function and reduced numbers [15]. $Nfkb2^{Lym1}$ mice carry a nonsense mutation in the *Nfkb2* gene (c.2854T>A, p.Tyr868*), which encodes a

Table 13.1 Selected mouse model phenotypes of the noncanonical NF-κB pathway

Mouse model		Lymphoid organs	B cell	Other	Ref.
Nfkb2$^{-/-}$	p100$^{-/-}$ p52$^{-/-}$	Absent/disrupted architecture of secondary lymphoid organs	↓ Proliferation to agonists ↓ Antigen-specific antibodies		[30, 32]
Nfkb2$^{Lym1/Lym1}$ (c.2854T>A, p.Tyr868)	p100^{Lym1} p52$^{-/-}$	Absent/disrupted architecture of secondary lymphoid organs	↓ Proliferation to agonists ↓ Mature B-cells ↓ Antibody levels	Inflammatory lung and liver infiltrates Nfkb2$^{Lym1/+}$ with intermediate phenotype Reduced *Aire* expression Defective osteoclast differentiation	[16]
Nik$^{-/-}$		Absent/disrupted architecture of secondary lymphoid organs	↓ Antigen-specific antibodies ↓ NF-κB activation		[13, 33]
Relb$^{-/-}$		Absent/disrupted architecture of secondary lymphoid organs	↓ Proliferation to agonists	Multi-organ inflammation Thymic atrophy	[34–36]

non-processable p100. *Lym1* mice exhibit defects in B-cell maturation, decreased serum immunoglobulin levels, and defects in osteoclastogenesis [16]. *Lym1* mice also have disorganized medullary thymic epithelial cell networks and reduced expression of *Aire*. Notably, murine *Nfkb2*$^{-/-}$ models have reduced *Aire* expression and demonstrate increased autoantibodies to peripheral tissue antigens, similar to that seen in *Aire*-deficient mice [17].

13.2 Genetic and Molecular Basis of Human *NFKB2* Disease

In 2012, Quentien et al. reported four patients from three families with DAVID syndrome (deficient anterior pituitary with variable immune deficiency) that were unique among the larger cohort of subjects with ACTH deficiency in a multicenter center study. These four patients had an additional diagnosis of common variable immunodeficiency (CVID) [18]. Sequencing of several candidate genes involved in corticotrope differentiation and humoral immunity did not yield a pathogenic mutation. Nevertheless, the authors recognized that these subjects likely had a unique genetic syndrome. The following year, mutations in *NFKB2* were identified in two pedigrees affected by diagnosis of CVID in addition to central adrenal insufficiency and nail dystrophy [19]. Subsequently, the original three pedigrees with DAVID syndrome were also identified to have mutations in *NFKB2* [20].

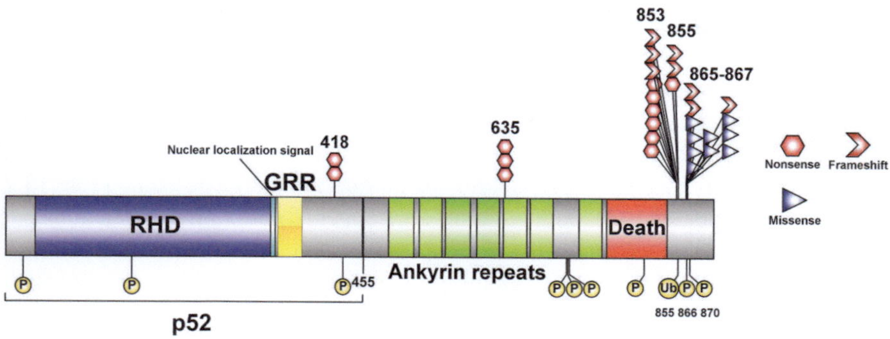

Fig. 13.2 Schematic diagram of the *NFKB2* gene and reported mutations. Each mutation symbol (nonsense, frameshift, missense) represents a single patient. Produced using the Illustrator for Biological Sequences tool. IBS, an illustrator for the presentation and visualization of biological sequences (Wenzhong Liu, Yubin Xie, Jiyong Ma, Xiaotong Luo, Peng Nie, Zhixiang Zuo, Urs Lahrmann, Qi Zhao, Yueyuan Zheng, Yong Zhao, Yu Xue and Jian Ren. *Bioinformatics* (2015) 31(20):3359–3361)

NFKB2 defects have an autosomal dominant mode of inheritance, with all reported cases thus far identified to have heterozygous mutations [19–29]. Loss-of-function mutations appear to be highly penetrant (24 of 25 reported have disease manifestations), though with variable expressivity. Of the loss-of-function mutations, the majority of mutations have been identified in the C-terminal region of the protein (Fig. 13.2), affecting critical serine phosphorylation sites at amino acid positions 866/870 and/or a lysine acceptor ubiquitination site at position 855. These result in a non-processable p100 protein with reduction of p52 nuclear translocation along with RelB heterodimers.

NFKB2 gain-of-function mutations [21] noted in Fig. 13.2 are located upstream in comparison to the loss-of-function mutations, after the glycine-rich region (p.418X) and within the ankyrin repeat domain (p.R635X). The gain-of-function mutations in particular confer an incomplete penetrance with variable expressivity, as three affected individuals were identified within two families; two related individuals who carried the same heterozygous mutations were essentially asymptomatic. In mutant constructs, the gain-of-function mutations result in increased nuclear translocation of p52 along with RelB, as well as increased *CXCL13* gene transcription. Further, the gain-of-function constructs also demonstrated increased canonical NF-κB activity, consistent with the growing understanding of the delicate balance between cytoplasmic NF-κB homo- and heterodimers which affect crosstalk between the canonical and noncanonical NF-κB pathways.

No cases of homozygous or compound heterozygous *NFKB2* mutations, nor *NFKB2* deletions/duplications, have yet been reported. Notably, neither the $Nfkb2^{-/-}$ nor $Nfkb^{lym1/lym1}$ mouse models are embryonic lethal, but it is possible that mutation(s) involving both alleles could result in more severe human disease.

13.3 Clinical Manifestations

At least 25 patients have been described in the literature with loss-of-function mutations, as well as a case series of five involving gain-of-function mutations. Patients with *NFKB2* deficiency due to loss-of-function mutations most often have an initial primary diagnosis of CVID. Clinical manifestations are summarized in Table 13.2 and include hypogammaglobulinemia, endocrinopathy, autoimmune phenomena, and ectodermal manifestations. B-cell deficiency is common. Patients are prone to recurrent respiratory infections. The onset of disease is in childhood, though with relatively few reports of life-threatening infections early in life.

The two families with reported gain-of-function mutations appear to have a more severe infectious phenotype with incomplete penetrance, described by the authors as having a combined immunodeficiency rather than first presenting with a common variable immunodeficiency-like diagnosis [21]. Affected individuals have recurrent respiratory infections including pneumonias, systemic and skin viral infections, and mucocutaneous candidiasis beyond onychomycosis. *Pneumocystis jirovecii* pneumonia presented in one adult patient.

A relatively unique feature in loss-of-function *NFKB2*-related disease, when compared to other CVID phenotypes, is the development of endocrinopathy in nearly two-thirds of patients. The endocrinopathy is an acquired condition (without reports of congenital hypoadrenalism), typically in the form of ACTH deficiency (central adrenal insufficiency). Quentien et al. described in 2010 a small population of patients with adrenal insufficiency, part of the larger adrenal insufficiency GENHYPOPIT cohort, who also had hypogammaglobulinemia [18].

Table 13.2 Percentage of loss-of-function (LOF) and gain-of-function (GOF) NFKB2 patients with clinical manifestations (noninfectious manifestations, unless otherwise noted)

	Total number of patients (*N* = 30) (%)	LOF patients (*N* = 25) (%)	GOF patients (*N* = 5) (%)
Prior diagnosis of CVID	73	88	0
Prior diagnosis of CID	10	4	60
Recurrent or unusual infection	70	72	60
Endocrinologic	53	64	0
Ectodermal	47	56	0
Respiratory tract	43	48	20
Neurologic	20	24	0
Lymphocytic organ infiltration	20	12	60
Gastrointestinal tract	17	16	20
Nephrologic	10	12	0
Hematologic	10	4	40
Malignancy	7	4	20

CVID common variable immunodeficiency; *CID* combined immunodeficiency

These patients were all subsequently found to have *NFKB2* loss-of-function mutations. A further analysis in murine models with similar mutations in the C-terminus did not yield evidence of adrenal insufficiency [20]. Thus, the pathogenesis of development of endocrinopathy and, in particular, ACTH deficiency is not known. However, as NF-κB2 regulates *AIRE* expression, it is possible that defective expression of self-antigens, in a mechanism similar to autoimmune polyglandular syndrome type 1 (APS1, also known as autoimmune polyendocrinopathy-candidiasis-ectodermal dystrophy, APECED) caused by *AIRE* mutations, leads to autoimmune endocrinopathy. The majority of NF-κB2-deficient patients who are diagnosed with central adrenal insufficiency typically present with severe hypoglycemia, in some cases leading to hypoglycemic seizures, as the initial sign of endocrine disease. Other patients develop additional endocrine issues including growth hormone deficiency, hypothyroidism, or diabetes insipidus (published cases and unpublished data).

More than half of loss-of-function patients develop ectodermal disease manifestations, including alopecia areata, alopecia totalis, vitiligo, and trachyonychia. A key distinction between the loss-of-function and gain-of-function *NFKB2*-related disease is that the gain-of-function disease manifestations reported thus far do *not* include endocrinopathies or autoimmune ectodermal disease.

13.3.1 Infectious Disease

13.3.1.1 Respiratory Infections

A large proportion of individuals with *NFKB2* mutations has increased susceptibility to upper and lower respiratory infections from various respiratory bacteria, including *Streptococcus pneumoniae* and *Haemophilus influenzae*. Specific sites of respiratory disease include otitis media, sinusitis, and pneumonia. One loss-of-function *NFKB2* patient with CVID-like disease developed an atypical mycobacterium infection [25]. *Pneumocystis jirovecii* pneumonia was diagnosed in an adult gain-of-function NFKB2 patient [21].

13.3.1.2 Viral Infections

In the original report of *NFKB2* defects, susceptibility to herpes simplex virus (HSV) was noted due to the presence of herpes labialis in all three affected individuals within one family. In addition to skin susceptibility to HSV, severe varicella and shingles/herpes zoster have been reported [20, 25], as well as severe molluscum infection of the skin [28]. Brue et al. [20] also reported a case of acute respiratory distress syndrome after influenza infection. One *NFKB2* gain-of-function patient with combined immunodeficiency had significant viral susceptibility and developed cytomegalovirus (CMV) enteritis and severe Epstein-Barr virus (EBV) in addition to warts and herpes labialis. Maccari et al. [27] reported a family with not only *NFKB2* loss-of-function mutations but also STAT5a deficiency [27]. The index patient in this report developed persistent EBV and CMV viremia. The functional immune defects due to the *STAT5A* mutation are not yet delineated; other loss-of-function NFKB2 mutations have not been associated with severe EBV or CMV.

13.3.1.3 Bacterial and Parasitic Infections

Aside from more common bacterial respiratory infections noted above, a 5-month-old boy developed meningococcal meningitis, was diagnosed with CVID at 7 years, and eventually found to have a loss-of-function mutation in *NFKB2* [25]. A proband with both an NFKB2 p.Arg853* mutation and STAT5A defect (p.R770Q) was found to have *Toxoplasma gondii* encephalitis resulting in optic neuritis and infectious foci in the brain that ultimately resolved with antimicrobial and steroid treatment [27]. Notably, the *Nfkb2*$^{-/-}$ knockout mouse is susceptible to toxoplasma encephalitis [30], though the role of the STAT5a defect in human immunity in the human case was not fully understood.

13.3.1.4 Candidiasis

Mucocutaneous candidiasis has been described in both loss-of-function as well as gain-of-function defects. Sites involve oral mucosa as well as the nails (onychomycosis). To date, no invasive candidal infections have been described.

13.3.2 Autoimmune Phenomena

Despite the relatively high incidence of ACTH deficiency/central adrenal insufficiency in loss-of-function *NFKB2* defects, no pituitary autoantibodies have been detected in this group of patients. However, given the clinical similarities between loss-of-function NF-κB2 disease and autoimmune polyglandular syndrome type 1 due to *AIRE* mutations, the possibility of a T-cell-mediated defect of thymic tolerance cannot be excluded. Conversely, though patients with NF-κB2 defects can have antithyroid autoantibodies, not all cases result in clinical hypothyroidism. However, interval screening for endocrinopathies involving acquired adrenal insufficiency, hypothyroidism, and growth hormone deficiency is reasonable. Adrenal insufficiency, whether central or peripheral, can result in life-threatening episodes of hypoglycemia and seizure. Given how easily the condition is corrected with preventive and stress dosing of steroids such as hydrocortisone, regular screening for development of adrenal insufficiency in *NFKB2* defects is well-advised. In the report of a boy with loss of function at *NFKB2* p.A867Cfs*19, no adrenal insufficiency was noted [24]. However, less than 3 years later, the child developed ACTH deficiency at 4 years of age, in addition to a partial diabetes insipidus (personal communication).

Surprisingly, autoimmune cytopenias are not a common occurrence, with only one case of immune thrombocytopenia reported [25]. Ectodermal autoimmune disease is quite common in the loss-of-function cases, as described above.

13.3.3 Other Organ Disease Manifestations

In addition to being a site of recurrent infections, lung disease manifestations can include the development of bronchiectasis, asthma, and lymphocytic interstitial lung disease, with or without granulomata. Bronchiolitis obliterans was reported by Kuehn et al. [21] in one patient with gain-of-function *NFKB2* mutation. A less common feature, gastrointestinal disease is primarily reported as a noninfectious diarrhea, without overt inflammatory bowel disease. Splenomegaly has only been reported thus far in the gain-of-function mutations, with at least one case due to EBV infection.

A few cases of autoimmune CNS disease, including aseptic meningitis and autoimmune encephalitis, have been reported. Despite the frequent diagnosis of ACTH deficiency, only one patient has been identified to have clinically significant abnormal brain MRI findings near the pituitary gland [20]. Lastly, autoimmune renal disease has been described and includes minimal change nephropathy and autoimmune proximal tubular acidosis [28, 29].

13.4 Laboratory Features

Regardless of gain-of-function or loss-of-function *NFKB2* defects, the majority of patients that have been described have hypogammaglobulinemia; most of these have defective antibody responses to antigens. All three reported gain-of-function affecteds had severe B-cell lymphopenia, whereas B-cell numbers are more highly variable in the loss-of-function patients. Many have significantly reduced memory B-cell numbers, further supporting the importance of the noncanonical NF-kB pathway in B-cell development as well as B-cell survival. In a patient with a CVID-like phenotype due to *NFKB2* p.Asp865Valfs*17 frameshift mutation, Liu et al. [25] found that T follicular helper (Tfh) cell numbers were reduced compared to controls. This finding supports that NF-κB2 is also important in development or maintenance of Tfh cells in the peripheral lymphoid organs, which further interact with B-cells to allow for development of high-affinity antibodies as well as memory B-cells.

Defective lymphocyte proliferation to mitogens (phytohemagglutinin, concanavalin A, and pokeweed mitogen) has been reported in the *NKFB2* gain-of-function cases, though with some degree of variability. Lymphocyte mitogen and antigen proliferation were normal in an adult combined immunodeficiency patient who developed *Pneumocystis jirovecii* pneumonia [21]. Defective natural killer cell cytotoxicity was described by Lougaris et al. [26], which likely contributes to patients' increased susceptibility to viral infections. In addition, anti-cytokine autoantibodies to IL12p40, IL-23, interferon-alpha (IFN-α), IFN-β, and IFN-ϖ have been reported in a patient with severe recurrent bacterial and viral infections that resolved after rituximab treatment [28]. Neutralizing anti-IFN-ϖ antibodies have also been measured in one family in our original report [19] (unpublished data).

13.5 Diagnosis

Due to the recognition of early-onset hypogammaglobulinemia, ectodermal defects, and/or ACTH deficiency in association with monogenic *NFKB2* disease, reported cases have been identified through next-generation sequencing modalities, including exome sequencing or targeted gene panels, and then confirmed through traditional gene sequencing methods. Family members can then be tested through direct sequencing at the specific *NFKB2* locus. Commercial gene sequencing of *NFKB2* is readily available in the United States and Europe either through direct sequencing or as part of next-generation sequencing gene panels.

13.6 Management

Overall, the most prevalent treatment used for patients with NF-κB2 immune defects involves gammaglobulin replacement to prevent infections. For patients with hypogammaglobulinemia and recurrent infections, intravenous or subcutaneous immunoglobulin replacement is needed. In cases of recurrent herpes labialis, antiviral prophylaxis with valacyclovir can help prevent recurrences. As *Pneumocystis jirovecii* pneumonia (PJP) has been described in an *NFKB2* gain-of-function patient with surprisingly normal lymphocyte proliferation to mitogens and antigens, PJP prophylaxis should be considered in patients who exhibit a combined immunodeficiency phenotype. Antibiotic prophylaxis can be used, though does not appear to be necessary in all cases. In the case reported by Ramakrishnan et al. [28], a child with multiple anti-cytokine antibodies, recurrent viral infections, and recurrent bacterial osteomyelitis/septic arthritis was treated with four courses of rituximab. Remarkably, this led to clinical improvement as well as cessation of the recurrent deep-seated infections. Thus, for patients with high titer or neutralizing levels of anti-cytokine antibodies, rituximab and similar anti-B-cell biologics can be considered to reduce biologically relevant recurrent infections.

No patients with *NFKB2* defects to date have been reported to have undergone hematopoietic stem cell transplantation (HSCT). If human *NFKB2* mutations do result in reduced expression of *AIRE* in thymic epithelial cells, it is unclear if a complete correction of autoimmune features, due to aberrant T cell tolerance, is possible. However, a patient with autosomal recessive NIK deficiency (caused by mutations in *MAP 3K14*) had improvement in combined immunodeficiency features after allogeneic HSCT [31]. NIK is the protein upstream of NF-κB2 which initiates the noncanonical NF-kB pathway phosphorylation cascade. This suggests that despite the presence of aberrant secondary lymphoid architecture seen in noncanonical NF-κB defects and aberrant *AIRE* expression noted in murine models, HSCT may at least partially correct the immune disorder which occurs in dysfunctional noncanonical NF-κB pathway signaling due to *NFKB2* mutations.

References

1. Sun SC. Non-canonical NF-kappaB signaling pathway. Cell Res. 2011;21(1):71–85. https://doi.org/10.1038/cr.2010.177.
2. Hayden MS, Ghosh S. Shared principles in NF-kappaB signaling. Cell. 2008;132(3):344–62. https://doi.org/10.1016/j.cell.2008.01.020.
3. Sun SC. The non-canonical NF-kappaB pathway in immunity and inflammation. Nat Rev Immunol. 2017;17(9):545–58. https://doi.org/10.1038/nri.2017.52.
4. Senftleben U, Cao Y, Xiao G, Greten FR, Krahn G, Bonizzi G, Chen Y, Hu Y, Fong A, Sun SC, Karin M. Activation by IKKalpha of a second, evolutionary conserved, NF-kappa B signaling pathway. Science. 2001;293(5534):1495–9. https://doi.org/10.1126/science.1062677.
5. Xiao G, Harhaj EW, Sun SC. NF-kappaB-inducing kinase regulates the processing of NF-kappaB2 p100. Mol Cell. 2001;7(2):401–9.
6. Pone EJ, Zan H, Zhang J, Al-Qahtani A, Xu Z, Casali P. Toll-like receptors and B-cell receptors synergize to induce immunoglobulin class-switch DNA recombination: relevance to microbial antibody responses. Crit Rev Immunol. 2010;30(1):1–29.
7. Pone EJ, Zhang J, Mai T, White CA, Li G, Sakakura JK, Patel PJ, Al-Qahtani A, Zan H, Xu Z, Casali P. BCR-signalling synergizes with TLR-signalling for induction of AID and immunoglobulin class-switching through the non-canonical NF-kappaB pathway. Nat Commun. 2012;3:767. https://doi.org/10.1038/ncomms1769.
8. Gerondakis S, Siebenlist U. Roles of the NF-kappaB pathway in lymphocyte development and function. Cold Spring Harb Perspect Biol. 2010;2(5):a000182. https://doi.org/10.1101/cshperspect.a000182.
9. Weih F, Caamano J. Regulation of secondary lymphoid organ development by the nuclear factor-kappaB signal transduction pathway. Immunol Rev. 2003;195:91–105.
10. van de Pavert SA, Mebius RE. New insights into the development of lymphoid tissues. Nat Rev Immunol. 2010;10(9):664–74. https://doi.org/10.1038/nri2832.
11. Lawrence T. The nuclear factor NF-kappaB pathway in inflammation. Cold Spring Harb Perspect Biol. 2009;1(6):a001651. https://doi.org/10.1101/cshperspect.a001651.
12. De Silva NS, Silva K, Anderson MM, Bhagat G, Klein U. Impairment of mature B cell maintenance upon combined deletion of the alternative NF-kappaB transcription factors RELB and NF-kappaB2 in B cells. J Immunol. 2016;196(6):2591–601. https://doi.org/10.4049/jimmunol.1501120.
13. Li Y, Wang H, Zhou X, Xie X, Chen X, Jie Z, Zou Q, Hu H, Zhu L, Cheng X, Brightbill HD, Wu LC, Wang L, Sun SC. Cell intrinsic role of NF-kappaB-inducing kinase in regulating T cell-mediated immune and autoimmune responses. Sci Rep. 2016;6:22115. https://doi.org/10.1038/srep22115.
14. Chin RK, Lo JC, Kim O, Blink SE, Christiansen PA, Peterson P, Wang Y, Ware C, Fu YX. Lymphotoxin pathway directs thymic Aire expression. Nat Immunol. 2003;4(11):1121–7. https://doi.org/10.1038/ni982.
15. Shinkura R, Kitada K, Matsuda F, Tashiro K, Ikuta K, Suzuki M, Kogishi K, Serikawa T, Honjo T. Alymphoplasia is caused by a point mutation in the mouse gene encoding Nf-kappa b-inducing kinase. Nat Genet. 1999;22(1):74–7. https://doi.org/10.1038/8780.
16. Tucker E, O'Donnell K, Fuchsberger M, Hilton AA, Metcalf D, Greig K, Sims NA, Quinn JM, Alexander WS, Hilton DJ, Kile BT, Tarlinton DM, Starr R. A novel mutation in the Nfkb2 gene generates an NF-kappa B2 "super repressor". J Immunol. 2007;179(11):7514–22.
17. Zhu M, Chin RK, Christiansen PA, Lo JC, Liu X, Ware C, Siebenlist U, Fu YX. NF-kappaB2 is required for the establishment of central tolerance through an Aire-dependent pathway. J Clin Invest. 2006;116(11):2964–71. https://doi.org/10.1172/JCI28326.
18. Quentien MH, Delemer B, Papadimitriou DT, Souchon PF, Jaussaud R, Pagnier A, Munzer M, Jullien N, Reynaud R, Galon-Faure N, Enjalbert A, Barlier A, Brue T. Deficit in anterior pituitary function and variable immune deficiency (DAVID) in children presenting with adrenocorticotropin deficiency and severe infections. J Clin Endocrinol Metab. 2012;97(1):E121–8. https://doi.org/10.1210/jc.2011-0407.

19. Chen K, Coonrod EM, Kumanovics A, Franks ZF, Durtschi JD, Margraf RL, Wu W, Heikal NM, Augustine NH, Ridge PG, Hill HR, Jorde LB, Weyrich AS, Zimmerman GA, Gundlapalli AV, Bohnsack JF, Voelkerding KV. Germline mutations in NFKB2 implicate the noncanonical NF-kappaB pathway in the pathogenesis of common variable immunodeficiency. Am J Hum Genet. 2013;93(5):812–24. https://doi.org/10.1016/j.ajhg.2013.09.009.
20. Brue T, Quentien MH, Khetchoumian K, Bensa M, Capo-Chichi JM, Delemer B, Balsalobre A, Nassif C, Papadimitriou DT, Pagnier A, Hasselmann C, Patry L, Schwartzentruber J, Souchon PF, Takayasu S, Enjalbert A, Van Vliet G, Majewski J, Drouin J, Samuels ME. Mutations in NFKB2 and potential genetic heterogeneity in patients with DAVID syndrome, having variable endocrine and immune deficiencies. BMC Med Genet. 2014;15:139. https://doi.org/10.1186/s12881-014-0139-9.
21. Kuehn HS, Niemela JE, Sreedhara K, Stoddard JL, Grossman J, Wysocki CA, de la Morena MT, Garofalo M, Inlora J, Snyder MP, Lewis DB, Stratakis CA, Fleisher TA, Rosenzweig SD. Novel nonsense gain-of-function NFKB2 mutations associated with a combined immunodeficiency phenotype. Blood. 2017;130(13):1553–64. https://doi.org/10.1182/blood-2017-05-782177.
22. Lal RA, Bachrach LK, Hoffman AR, Inlora J, Rego S, Snyder MP, Lewis DB. A case report of hypoglycemia and hypogammaglobulinemia: DAVID syndrome in a patient with a novel NFKB2 mutation. J Clin Endocrinol Metab. 2017;102(7):2127–30. https://doi.org/10.1210/jc.2017-00341.
23. Lee CE, Fulcher DA, Whittle B, Chand R, Fewings N, Field M, Andrews D, Goodnow CC, Cook MC. Autosomal-dominant B-cell deficiency with alopecia due to a mutation in NFKB2 that results in nonprocessable p100. Blood. 2014;124(19):2964–72. https://doi.org/10.1182/blood-2014-06-578542.
24. Lindsley AW, Qian Y, Valencia CA, Shah K, Zhang K, Assa'ad A. Combined immune deficiency in a patient with a novel NFKB2 mutation. J Clin Immunol. 2014;34(8):910–5. https://doi.org/10.1007/s10875-014-0095-3.
25. Liu Y, Hanson S, Gurugama P, Jones A, Clark B, Ibrahim MA. Novel NFKB2 mutation in early-onset CVID. J Clin Immunol. 2014;34(6):686–90. https://doi.org/10.1007/s10875-014-0064-x.
26. Lougaris V, Tabellini G, Vitali M, Baronio M, Patrizi O, Tampella G, Biasini A, Moratto D, Parolini S, Plebani A. Defective natural killer-cell cytotoxic activity in NFKB2-mutated CVID-like disease. J Allergy Clin Immunol. 2015;135(6):1641–3. https://doi.org/10.1016/j.jaci.2014.11.038.
27. Maccari ME, Scarselli A, Di Cesare S, Floris M, Angius A, Deodati A, Chiriaco M, Cambiaso P, Corrente S, Colafati GS, Utz PJ, Angelini F, Fierabracci A, Aiuti A, Carsetti R, Rosenberg JM, Cappa M, Rossi P, Bacchetta R, Cancrini C. Severe Toxoplasma gondii infection in a member of a NFKB2-deficient family with T and B cell dysfunction. Clin Immunol. 2017;183:273–7. https://doi.org/10.1016/j.clim.2017.09.011.
28. Ramakrishnan KA, Rae W, Barcenas-Morales G, Gao Y, Pengelly RJ, Patel SV, Kumararatne DS, Ennis S, Doffinger R, Faust SN, Williams AP. Anticytokine autoantibodies in a patient with a heterozygous NFKB2 mutation. J Allergy Clin Immunol. 2017;141:1479–82. https://doi.org/10.1016/j.jaci.2017.11.014.
29. Shi C, Wang F, Tong A, Zhang XQ, Song HM, Liu ZY, Lyu W, Liu YH, Xia WB. NFKB2 mutation in common variable immunodeficiency and isolated adrenocorticotropic hormone deficiency: a case report and review of literature. Medicine (Baltimore). 2016;95(40):e5081. https://doi.org/10.1097/MD.0000000000005081.
30. Caamano J, Tato C, Cai G, Villegas EN, Speirs K, Craig L, Alexander J, Hunter CA. Identification of a role for NF-kappa B2 in the regulation of apoptosis and in maintenance of T cell-mediated immunity to Toxoplasma gondii. J Immunol. 2000;165(10):5720–8.
31. Willmann KL, Klaver S, Dogu F, Santos-Valente E, Garncarz W, Bilic I, Mace E, Salzer E, Conde CD, Sic H, Majek P, Banerjee PP, Vladimer GI, Haskologlu S, Bolkent MG, Kupesiz A, Condino-Neto A, Colinge J, Superti-Furga G, Pickl WF, van Zelm MC, Eibel H, Orange JS, Ikinciogullari A, Boztug K. Biallelic loss-of-function mutation in NIK causes a primary immunodeficiency with multifaceted aberrant lymphoid immunity. Nat Commun. 2014;5:5360. https://doi.org/10.1038/ncomms6360.

32. Caamano JH, Rizzo CA, Durham SK, Barton DS, Raventos-Suarez C, Snapper CM, Bravo R. Nuclear factor (NF)-kappa B2 (p100/p52) is required for normal splenic microarchitecture and B cell-mediated immune responses. J Exp Med. 1998;187(2):185–96.
33. Yin L, Wu L, Wesche H, Arthur CD, White JM, Goeddel DV, Schreiber RD. Defective lymphotoxin-beta receptor-induced NF-kappaB transcriptional activity in NIK-deficient mice. Science. 2001;291(5511):2162–5. https://doi.org/10.1126/science.1058453.
34. Weih F, Carrasco D, Durham SK, Barton DS, Rizzo CA, Ryseck RP, Lira SA, Bravo R. Multiorgan inflammation and hematopoietic abnormalities in mice with a targeted disruption of RelB, a member of the NF-kappa B/Rel family. Cell. 1995;80(2):331–40.
35. Weih F, Durham SK, Barton DS, Sha WC, Baltimore D, Bravo R. Both multiorgan inflammation and myeloid hyperplasia in RelB-deficient mice are T cell dependent. J Immunol. 1996;157(9):3974–9.
36. Beinke S, Ley SC. Functions of NF-κB1 and NF-κB2 in immune cell biology. Biochem. J. 2004;382(2):393–409.

The WHIM Syndrome

14

Giuliana Roselli, Marinos Kallikourdis, and Antonella Viola

14.1 Introduction and Definition

The WHIM syndrome is a rare immunodeficiency characterized by **W**arts, **H**ypogammaglobulinemia, recurrent respiratory bacterial **I**nfections, and **M**yelokathexis. The latter is defined as an increased retention of mature myeloid cells in the bone marrow. Early studies identified that neutrophils in WHIM patients are retained in the bone marrow; further, they displayed an aberrant morphology with hyper-segmented nuclei [1]. Possibly as a result of the myelokathexis, severe peripheral neutropenia [2] and lymphocytopenia [3] were also observed.

We now know that the WHIM syndrome is mostly caused by heterozygous mutations on chromosome 2q21, usually inherited as autosomal dominant trait. The mutations truncate the C-terminal tail of the chemokine receptor CXCR4. CXCR4 is the cognate receptor to chemokine CXCL12, which is the receptor's unique ligand. Chemokines are small chemotactic cytokines, utilized by innate and adaptive immune cells to direct their localization, recruitment, and retention [4]. Interestingly, work in more recent years has also uncovered that chemokines and their receptors are also able to affect immune cell function, in similarity to ligands and receptors promoting immune cell activation [5].

G. Roselli
Adaptive Immunity Laboratory, Humanitas Clinical and Research Center, Rozzano, Italy

M. Kallikourdis
Adaptive Immunity Laboratory, Humanitas Clinical and Research Center, Rozzano, Italy

Department of Biomedical Sciences, Humanitas University, Rozzano, Italy

A. Viola (✉)
Department of Biomedical Sciences, University of Padova, Padova, Italy

Pediatric Research Institute "Citta della Speranza", Padova, Italy
e-mail: antonella.viola@unipd.it

M. M. D'Elios, M. Rizzi (eds.), *Humoral Primary Immunodeficiencies*,
Rare Diseases of the Immune System, https://doi.org/10.1007/978-3-319-91785-6_14

The chemokine CXCL12 is constitutively produced by stromal and endothelial cells. The CXCR4-CXCL12 interaction plays a key role in the recruitment of hematopoietic progenitors into the bone marrow and in the regulation of lymphocyte trafficking within secondary lymphoid organs such as the lymph nodes [6]. Further, it has been shown that CXCR4, together with the chemokine receptor CXCR2, are essential for controlling neutrophil homeostasis within the bone marrow. CXCR4 promotes their retention in the bone marrow, while CXCR2 promotes their egress from the bone marrow [7]. As a consequence, neutropenia in WHIM was primarily considered a problem of neutrophil egress. Similarly, lymphocytopenia may be due to aberrant trafficking of lymphocytes caused by their retention in the bone marrow and other lymphoid tissues; definitive demonstration of this may require further investigation [8].

In the WHIM syndrome, hypogammaglobulinemia mostly refers to decreased IgG antibody concentration in the serum but may also affect IgM [9]. Possibly linked to the reduced antibody titers, the number of circulating B and T lymphocytes is commonly reduced in WHIM patients, with a particular reduction of circulating $CD27^+$ memory B cells [3]. As a possible consequence of the defective B cell and antibody responses, infections of the upper respiratory tracts are common [9]. Although WHIM patients do not show an increased susceptibility to viral infections, most of them do report lesions due to human papillomavirus (HPV). Studies have suggested a role of CXCR4 in HPV-mediated keratinocyte transformation [10]. However, the mechanism underlying the specific susceptibility to HPV is still unknown [11].

It should be noted that not all the above symptoms are always simultaneously observed in the same WHIM patient [12], though indeed almost all WHIM syndrome patients feature mutations in CXCR4 and a majority of the above symptoms.

14.2 WHIM-Associated Mutations in Cxcr4

Most WHIM patients harbor somatic mutations in the C-terminal domain of the Cxcr4 gene that extend from amino acid position 308–352 [6, 3]. Most of these mutations were found to result in a premature stop codon, causing loss of the last 10–19 amino acids of the receptor. The deletion of the C-terminus has been associated with defective internalization of CXCR4 after the receptor has bound the ligand, CXCL12. Physiologically, this acts as a down-modulator of CXCR4 signaling induced by ligand binding. It is thought that the defective internalization is explained by the inability of molecules involved in the promotion of the internalization process, such as G protein-coupled receptor 6 (GRK6) and β-arrestin 2, to interact with the receptor itself [13, 14]. As a consequence of the lost negative feedback loop, the mutations lead to a gain-of-function phenotype, characterized by increased intracellular calcium levels and increased chemotaxis upon CXCL12 binding [3, 15, 16].

R334X (1013C→G) is the most common mutation. Primary human CD34⁺ cells, transfected with the WHIM-mutant R334X CXCR4, exhibited enhanced chemotaxis and calcium levels in response to CXCL12, together with impaired internalization [16]. Several other mutations in the CXCR4 receptor have been identified so far in WHIM patients, all of them have responsible for the deletion of a portion of the C-terminus. These mutations include E343X, S339fs342X, and G336X [3, 6, 9]. In addition to truncating mutations, a missense mutation was identified in a family with WHIM syndrome. This mutation, E343K (1027G- > A), was found to be responsible for changes in the charge of the CXCR4 C-terminus, leading to impaired negative regulation of the receptor and gain of function [17]. A frameshift mutation causing the replacement of the last 24 amino acids of the C-terminus of CXCR4 with 12 missense amino acids has also been reported. The frameshift occurred at codon 329 of the receptor (CXCR4 L329 fs) [18]. A novel sequence variant c.966_967delAG of CXCR4 has been recently identified in a Korean child with hypogammaglobulinemia, myelokathexis, and recurrent infections, which confirmed a diagnosis of WHIM syndrome [19]. In some cases, WHIM symptoms were reported in the absence of mutations in CXCR4 [15] thus complicating the clinical picture. For example, reduced mRNA level of GRK3, which is a regulator of CXCR4 attenuation, was found to be associated with enhanced activity of CXCR4 and WHIM syndrome in one patient [20].

14.3 WHIM-Related Defects in Innate Immunity: A Problem of Neutrophil Retention in the Bone Marrow

Neutropenia is one of the most common symptoms of the WHIM syndrome; retention of neutrophils with an apoptotic cellular phenotype has been demonstrated in the bone marrow of several WHIM patients [2, 21, 22]. As hinted above, the molecular basis of myelokathexis in WHIM has been extensively studied. The generation of animal models enabled the demonstration of a direct connection between the presence of a WHIM-mutant form of CXCR4 with the retention of neutrophils in the bone marrow. For example, NOD/SCID mice were used as recipients of xenotransplanted human $CD34^+$ hematopoietic stem cells transduced with the WHIM-mutant R334X CXCR4; neutrophils that developed from the transduced $CD34^+$ hematopoietic stem cells showed increased retention within the bone marrow and higher propensity to apoptosis. The latter was not interpreted as a direct effect of the CXCR4 mutation, but rather a consequence of the overaccumulation of neutrophils in the bone marrow [23]. A zebra fish model of WHIM syndrome provided further in vivo evidence that neutrophil retention in the hematopoietic compartment is CXCL12-dependent [24]. A WHIM knock-in mouse model, bearing the $Cxcr4^{+/1013}$ mutant gene, was generated and developed features of the disease such as neutropenia and lymphopenia [25]. The correction of neutropenia via use of the CXCR4 antagonist, AMD3100, offered further support for a link between WHIM mutations in CXCR4 and neutrophil retention in the bone marrow [17, 26].

14.4 WHIM-Related Defects in Adaptive Immunity: Defective Lymphocyte Trafficking and Function

Many features of the WHIM syndrome, such as lymphopenia, hypogammaglobulinemia, and impaired antibody class-switching, have not been fully elucidated yet. These symptoms are mostly related to a defective adaptive immunity. A WHIM patient immunized with tetanus-toxoid vaccine displayed an inability to maintain the production of specific anti-tetanus-toxoid antibodies for longer than 1 year. A severe reduction in both switched and unswitched circulating memory B cells was also reported, indicative of a defects in the ability of B cells to receive costimulation from T helper cells [3]. Further, the response to immunization to bacteriophage ΦX174 was studied in one subject by Mc Guire and colleagues [27]. The antibody response was robust after the first immunization, but—even though total immunoglobulin levels were normal—there was delayed and reduced isotype switching after the boost. The patient also displayed oligoclonality in their B cells, examined by spectratyping analysis. These observations are compatible with a defective affinity maturation of B cells, a process physiologically occurring during T cell-B cell interactions within germinal centers. Another WHIM patient immunophenotyped in the same studies also displayed circulating B cell pool with reduced isotype-switched memory B cells [27].

Indeed, defects in the initiation of adaptive immune responses were hinted at by one of the earliest studies on the disease: in a study published four decades ago, two patients suffering of chronic neutropenia and hypogammaglobulinemia showed disrupted germinal center formation in inguinal lymph node biopsies following diphtheria toxin immunization [28]. These findings were recapitulated in the absence of immunization conditions in a WHIM knock-in mouse model [25]. Despite neutropenia and lymphopenia, this mouse model displayed normal bone marrow architecture. The thymus was found to be deficient in T cells, lymph nodes showed reduced lymphatic vascularization, and the spleen contained reduced numbers of naïve B and T cells compared to wild-type controls. Primary follicles were reduced in the spleen and absent in lymph nodes [25]. The disorganized structure of secondary lymphoid organs found in the WHIM knock-in mouse model, even at the steady state, suggested that the functional defect of WHIM-mutant T and B cells could be partially explained by their mislocalization or by the aberrant spatial orchestration of their interactions.

14.5 WHIM-Mutant CXCR4 as a Regulator of T Cell Activation

We have demonstrated that the chemokine receptors CCR5 and CXCR4 are not only involved in the chemotaxis of T lymphocytes but can also modulate their activation. CXCR4 acts as a costimulatory molecule during T cell activation by becoming recruited at the immunological synapse, the specialized junction formed between T cells and antigen presenting cells (APC). At the IS, CXCR4 mediates costimulatory signals after being triggered by chemokine ligands produced by the APC with which the T cell is interacting [5]. Thus, we supposed that mutations in CXCR4 could have consequences not only on T cell migration but also on their activation and therefore on their ability to respond to pathogens. Given the recurring nature of the infections in WHIM, any T cell functional defect would help explain the lack of memory responses to pathogens. To this end, we investigated the effect of WHIM mutations on T cell activation, at the time of formation of the immunological synapse (IS). We demonstrated that WHIM-mutant CXCR4, much like wild-type CXCR4, is appropriately recruited to the IS when the T cell antigen receptor (TCR) is activated by its cognate antigen. Yet, surprisingly, we found that the presence of exogenous CXCL12 during T cell activation was able to prevent WHIM-mutant but not wild-type CXCR4 recruitment to the IS. In other words, in the wild type, chemokine produced by the APC can lead to costimulation of the T cell, while chemokines arriving from the extracellular space have no effect. However, with the hyperfunctional WHIM-mutant CXCR4, chemokines that arrive from the extracellular space "distract" the receptor away from the IS, as if the migratory function of the mutant receptor is dominant over the costimulatory function. A predicted consequence of reduced costimulation would be shorter and weaker T-APC interactions, and thus unstable T-APC IS formation. This was shown ex vivo using human patient samples, as well as in a lymph node slice culture 2-photon video microscopy system. In order to obtain unactivated WHIM-mutant or wild-type T cells that could be activated on demand, we prepared mice expressing WHIM-mutant or wild-type CXCR4 on OVA-antigen-specific T cells. To achieve this, we took advantage of the retrogenic technology, where the myeloid and lymphoid compartment of mice is generated by reconstitution with donor immune cell populations that have been modified via retroviral transduction (Holst et al., 2006). Our 2-photon imaging results revealed that the hyperfunctional nature of the WHIM-mutant CXCR4 receptor affect the IS formation, leading to unstable T-APC interactions. These effects were reversible by treating with AMD3100, the CXCR4 antagonist. As a downstream consequence, impaired WHIM T cell activation and impaired T cell-dependent B cell functions (antibody class-switching) were observed after antigen-specific immunization [29].

14.6 WHIM-Mutant CXCR4 as a Regulator of B Cell Activation

The molecular basis underlying the defective B cell responses in WHIM has been studied in the WHIM knock-in mouse model following antigenic challenge. Immunization with a thymus-dependent antigen revealed that the hyperfunctional WHIM-mutant CXCR4 promoted B cell activation and differentiation. In fact, despite the reduced number of B cells and germinal centers in the spleen of knock-in mice, germinal centers formed correctly after immunization, and B cells differentiated into plasma cells. However, antigen-specific plasma cells did not accumulate in the bone marrow – where they normally reside – but rather in the spleen. In parallel, an inability to maintain antigen-specific antibody titers over time was observed. Therefore, although the knock-in mice were able to mount an antigen-specific immune response, they were not able to maintain this response over time, matching findings in earlier human patient studies [30].

We observed that the reduced B cell frequency in the spleen of WHIM knock-in mice was associated with an increased propensity of these cells to undergo apoptosis. Yet surprisingly, the frequency of plasma cells, which are the end-products of B cell activation, was higher in these mice even in the absence of any immunization. We found that the increased plasma cell differentiation was a consequence of a spontaneous activation of WHIM-mutant B cells. In similarity to the previously described costimulatory effect of CXCR4 on wild-type T cells, we found that CXCL12 was able to costimulate WHIM-mutant B cells, possibly contributing to their spontaneous activation. Yet, unlike with WHIM-mutant T cells, where WHIM-mutant CXCR4 led to a disruption from stable IS formation and reduced strength of activation, WHIM-mutant B cell activation was boosted by presence of the chemokine. This is most likely due to the fact that B cells, unlike T cells, do not require formation of an IS in order to receive antigenic stimulation; thus there is no complex IS structure to disrupt, and (soluble) CXCL12 adds a boosting costimulatory signal, enhancing any B cell activation that may have arisen from cross-reactions with self-antigens.

Yet, when WHIM-mutant B cells were activated, the CXCL12-mediated costimulation boosted the activation but did not provide the pro-survival signals required for optimal B cell function. As a result, more apoptosis was observed in WHIM-mutant B cells. Compatible observations were made on WHIM patient B cells [31]. Productive B and T cell activation depends on the fine-tuning between signals delivered by the antigen receptor and the costimulatory molecules. In the absence of optimal costimulation, the antigen-activated cell undergoes activation induced cell death (AICD) [32]. Thus, these findings suggest an additional reason for the B cell lymphopenia in the WHIM syndrome.

We thus speculated that CXCL12 costimulation in WHIM-mutant B cells could lead to aberrant activation, which in turn could promote apoptosis. This hypothesis was supported by increased Caspase 3/Caspase 7 levels, as well as the reduced mRNA levels of the anti-apoptotic molecule Bcl-X in WHIM B cells upon activation. Given that AICD is dependent on the antigenic stimulation load [33], we attempted to reduce the antigenic load during immunization in WHIM knock-in mice; the result was better B cell survival and higher number of class-switched plasma cells in the bone marrow. While these conclusions cannot be readily translated to human patients without further work, they do suggest that the optimal immunization conditions may be different in WHIM-mutant subjects. Given the importance of vaccination for infection prevention in WHIM patients, this could be of relevance for the design of more effective vaccination strategies [31].

14.7 Association of the WHIM Syndrome with Other Diseases

14.7.1 Tetralogy of Fallot

Tetralogy of Fallot (TOF) is a genetically inherited cardiac disease featuring pulmonary outflow tract obstruction, ventricular septal defect, overriding aortic root, and right ventricular hypertrophy. Some of these features develop at the embryo stage, while hypertrophy occurs as a consequence of pulmonary blood flow obstruction. While a number of mutations have been previously identified, a report identified three non-related WHIM syndrome patients with TOF. This raises the possibility that WHIM-mutant CXCR4 may play a role, along with other factors, in TOF development. WHIM-mutant CXCR4 is associated with increased risk of cardiac defect development during embryogenesis, while CXCR7, an alternative receptor of CXCL12, is known to have a role in cardiac development [34].

14.7.2 Waldenstrom Macroglobulinemia

Waldenstrom macroglobulinemia (WM), a low-grade lymphoma with aberrant immunoglobulin secretion, is associated with somatic mutations identified in MyD88 (L265P-MyD88) in the malignant cells of 90–95% of patients [35]. MyD88 triggering activates downstream signals through BTK and IRAK (interleukin-1 receptor-associated kinase), resulting in NF (nuclear factor)-κB activation, thus affecting cell growth and survival. In 27–35% of WM patients, CXCR4 WHIM-like mutations are also present in the WM cells [36]; likewise, a case of WHIM syndrome has been recently reported featuring a CXCR4 frameshift mutation that matches a mutation found in WM patients [18]. WHIM-associated CXCR4 mutations may cause resistance to the standard therapy for WM, which is based on the use of ibrutinib, a small-molecule antineoplastic agent that inactivates BTK and induces apoptosis. CXCR4 inhibition by AMD3100 partially restored the ability of WM cells to respond to ibrutinib treatment in vitro, suggesting that CXCR4 may have a clinically important relevance in WM disease [35].

14.8 Therapeutic Regimes for the WHIM Syndrome

Given the ability of AMD3100 to inhibit CXCR4 signaling, it has been suggested as a therapy for myelokathexis in WHIM syndrome [37]. The pharmacokinetic features of a single injection of AMD3100, as a treatment of WHIM syndrome, was evaluated in a phase I safety study by McDermott and colleagues [26] who reported increased white blood cell count and the absence of side effects in treated WHIM syndrome patients. In a second study, AMD3100 was administered to a group of WHIM patients at increasing doses every 2–4 days, leading to an increase in peripheral blood leukocyte count in a dose-dependent manner, with a decline within 24 h [37]. Again, no side effects were reported [38]. A phase I clinical trial of a long-term treatment (6 months) of WHIM syndrome patients with AMD3100 was further conducted by McDermott and colleagues [39]. Results provided evidence for the safety of the treatment and efficacy in improving panleukopenia, even at the lowest dose tested (0.02 mg/kg, 8% of the FDA-approved dose for stem cell mobilization (0.24 mg/kg per day)). This study also offered the first evidence for the usage of AMD3100 in the treatment of chronic diseases which require a down-modulation of CXCR4 signaling.

Current recommendations for WHIM syndrome include vaccinations and antibiotics to prevent infections, as well as usage of G-CSF as an immune cell-mobilizing agent to combat myelokathexis. Additionally, intravenous immunoglobulin (IVIG) injections tare used to treat hypogammaglobulinemia. Unfortunately, G-CSF and IVIG are not resolving and are very expensive. A patient under treatment with IVIG but still manifesting recurrent infections found a beneficial effect after being transplanted with umbilical cord blood [38]. For the treatment of HPV infection, a prophylactic HPV vaccine was administered to a 12-year-old girl with WHIM syndrome [11], who was then able to produce HPV-specific antibodies and a cellular immune response. Two other patients received vaccination at 3 and 5 years of age and did not develop warts afterward [40]. The HPV vaccine, Cervarix, has not been tested yet on WHIM patients [41].

An interesting case of chromothripsis, which is the disruption and random reassembly of a chromosome, occurred in a 59-year-old woman affected by WHIM syndrome. The phenomenon resulted in the loss of the affected CXCR4^{R334X} allele and consequent spontaneous resolution of WHIM symptoms. This observation suggests that a partial inactivation of CXCR4 in the hematopoietic stem cells may be considered as a therapeutic strategy for the treatment of WHIM syndrome [42].

In a report of 60 cases of WHIM syndrome, five deaths were reported: two due to lymphoma, one due to advanced HPV-related genital disease, one due to bacterial meningitis, and one fetus aborted for cardiac anomaly [40]. The risk of developing malignancy or bacterial infections are indeed the most life-threatening features of the WHIM syndrome. An early recognition of the disease may thus lead to administration of preventive therapies that, combined with specific antagonists of CXCR4, could potentially improve the life span of WHIM patients [38].

14.9 Concluding Remarks

The reports described in this chapter are an elegant example of how the systematic deciphering of the physiopathological mechanisms affected by a monogenic disease can lead to substantial insight into disease pathogenesis. It is now clear that the WHIM mutations in CXCR4 affect both innate and adaptive immunity, as well as immune cell localization, activation, and function. The combined result of these effects is the multifaceted syndrome observed in WHIM patients. It is interesting to note how point mutations in a single chemokine receptor can have a very wide range of effects in the orchestration of innate and adaptive responses, testament of the key role of these molecules in the defense of our body from pathogens. Yet this same central role opens a key opportunity for therapy: as described above, treatment with a CXCR4 inhibitor was able to reverse many of the experimentally observed phenotypes. Indeed, the results in the clinic are accordingly positive; one can only wish that future experimentation will bring even further improvements in the therapeutic solutions available to WHIM syndrome patients.

References

1. O'Regan S, Newman AJ, Graham RC. "Myelokathexis". Neutropenia with marrow hyperplasia. Am J Dis Child. 1977;131:655–8.
2. Wetzler M, Talpaz M, Kleinerman ES, et al. A new familial immunodeficiency disorder characterized by severe neutropenia, a defective marrow release mechanism, and hypogammaglobulinemia. Am J Med. 1990;89:663–72.
3. Gulino AV, Moratto D, Sozzani S, et al. Altered leukocyte response to CXCL12 in patients with warts hypogammaglobulinemia, infections, myelokathexis (WHIM) syndrome. Blood. 2004;104:444–52. https://doi.org/10.1182/blood-2003-10-3532.
4. Sallusto F, Lenig D, Forster R, et al. Two subsets of memory T lymphocytes with distinct homing potentials and effector functions. Nature. 1999;401:708–12. https://doi.org/10.1038/44385.
5. Molon B, Gri G, Bettella M, et al. T cell costimulation by chemokine receptors. Nat Immunol. 2005;6:465–71. https://doi.org/10.1038/ni1191.
6. Hernandez PA, Gorlin RJ, Lukens JN, et al. Mutations in the chemokine receptor gene CXCR4 are associated with WHIM syndrome, a combined immunodeficiency disease. Nat Genet. 2003;34:70–4. https://doi.org/10.1038/ng1149.
7. Eash KJ, Greenbaum AM, Gopalan PK, Link DC. CXCR2 and CXCR4 antagonistically regulate neutrophil trafficking from murine bone marrow. J Clin Invest. 2010;120:2423–31. https://doi.org/10.1172/JCI41649.
8. Ma Q, Jones D, Springer TA. The chemokine receptor CXCR4 is required for the retention of B lineage and granulocytic precursors within the bone marrow microenvironment. Immunity. 1999;10:463–71.
9. Kawai T, Malech HL. WHIM syndrome: congenital immune deficiency disease. Curr Opin Hematol. 2009;16:20–6. https://doi.org/10.1097/MOH.0b013e32831ac557.
10. Chow KYC, Brotin É, Ben Khalifa Y, et al. A pivotal role for CXCL12 signaling in HPV-mediated transformation of keratinocytes: clues to understanding HPV-pathogenesis in WHIM syndrome. Cell Host Microbe. 2010;8:523–33. https://doi.org/10.1016/j.chom.2010.11.006.
11. Handisurya A, Schellenbacher C, Reininger B, et al. A quadrivalent HPV vaccine induces humoral and cellular immune responses in WHIM immunodeficiency syndrome. Vaccine. 2010;28:4837–41. https://doi.org/10.1016/j.vaccine.2010.04.057.
12. Dotta L, Tassone L, Badolato R. Clinical and genetic features of Warts, Hypogammaglobulinemia, Infections and Myelokathexis (WHIM) syndrome. Curr Mol Med. 2011;11:317–25.
13. Lagane B, Chow KYC, Balabanian K, et al. CXCR4 dimerization and beta-arrestin-mediated signaling account for the enhanced chemotaxis to CXCL12 in WHIM syndrome. Blood. 2008;112:34–44. https://doi.org/10.1182/blood-2007-07-102103.
14. McCormick PJ, Segarra M, Gasperini P, et al. Impaired recruitment of GrK6 and β-arrestin2 causes delayed internalization and desensitization of a WHIM syndrome-associated CXCR4 mutant receptor. PLoS One. 2009;4:e8102. https://doi.org/10.1371/journal.pone.0008102.
15. Balabanian K, Lagane B, Pablos JL, et al. WHIM syndromes with different genetic anomalies are accounted for by impaired CXCR4 desensitization to CXCL12. Blood. 2005;105:2449–57. https://doi.org/10.1182/blood-2004-06-2289.
16. Kawai T, Choi U, Whiting-Theobald NL, et al. Enhanced function with decreased internalization of carboxy-terminus truncated CXCR4 responsible for WHIM syndrome. Exp Hematol. 2005;33:460–8. https://doi.org/10.1016/j.exphem.2005.01.001.
17. Liu Q, Chen H, Ojode T, et al. WHIM syndrome caused by a single amino acid substitution in the carboxy-tail of chemokine receptor CXCR4. Blood. 2012;120:181–9. https://doi.org/10.1182/blood-2011-12-395608.
18. Liu Q, Pan C, Lopez L, et al. WHIM Syndrome Caused by Waldenstrom's Macroglobulinemia-Associated Mutation CXCR4 (L329fs). J Clin Immunol. 2016;36:397–405. https://doi.org/10.1007/s10875-016-0276-3.
19. Shin DW, Park SN, Kim SM, et al. WHIM syndrome with a novel CXCR4 variant in a Korean Child. Ann Lab Med. 2017;37:446–9.

20. Balabanian K, Levoye A, Klemm L, et al. Leukocyte analysis from WHIM syndrome patients reveals a pivotal role for GRK3 in CXCR4 signaling. J Clin Invest. 2008;118:1074–84. https://doi.org/10.1172/JCI33187.
21. Aprikyan AA, Liles WC, Park JR, et al. Myelokathexis, a congenital disorder of severe neutropenia characterized by accelerated apoptosis and defective expression of bcl-x in neutrophil precursors. Blood. 2000;95:320–7.
22. Taniuchi S, Yamamoto A, Fujiwara T, et al. Dizygotic twin sisters with myelokathexis: mechanism of its neutropenia. Am J Hematol. 1999;62:106–11.
23. Kawai T, Choi U, Cardwell L, et al. WHIM syndrome myelokathexis reproduced in the NOD/SCID mouse xenotransplant model engrafted with healthy human stem cells transduced with C-terminus—truncated CXCR4. Blood. 2007;109:78–84. https://doi.org/10.1182/blood-2006-05-025296.
24. Walters KB, Green JM, Surfus JC, et al. Live imaging of neutrophil motility in a zebrafish model of WHIM syndrome. Blood. 2010;116:2803–11. https://doi.org/10.1182/blood-2010-03-276972.
25. Balabanian K, Brotin E, Biajoux V, et al. Proper desensitization of CXCR4 is required for lymphocyte development and peripheral compartmentalization in mice. Blood. 2012;119:5722–30. https://doi.org/10.1182/blood-2012-01-403378.
26. McDermott DH, Liu Q, Ulrick J, et al. The CXCR4 antagonist plerixafor corrects panleukopenia in patients with WHIM syndrome. Blood. 2011;118:4957–62. https://doi.org/10.1182/blood-2011-07-368084.
27. Mc Guire PJ, Cunningham-Rundles C, Ochs H, Diaz GA. Oligoclonality, impaired class switch and B-cell memory responses in WHIM syndrome. Clin Immunol. 2010;135:412–21. https://doi.org/10.1016/j.clim.2010.02.006.
28. Mentzer WCJ, Johnston RBJ, Baehner RL, Nathan DG. An unusual form of chronic neutropenia in a father and daughter with hypogammaglobulinaemia. Br J Haematol. 1977;36:313–22.
29. Kallikourdis M, Trovato AE, Anselmi F, et al. The CXCR4 mutations in WHIM syndrome impair the stability of the T-cell immunologic synapse. Blood. 2013;122:666–73. https://doi.org/10.1182/blood-2012-10-461830.
30. Biajoux V, Natt J, Freitas C, et al. Efficient plasma cell differentiation and trafficking require Cxcr4 desensitization. Cell Rep. 2016;17:193–205. https://doi.org/10.1016/j.celrep.2016.08.068.
31. Roselli G, Martini E, Lougaris V, et al. CXCL12 mediates aberrant costimulation of B lymphocytes in warts, hypogammaglobulinemia, infections, myelokathexis immunodeficiency. Front Immunol. 2017;8:1–12. https://doi.org/10.3389/fimmu.2017.01068.
32. Sharpe AH. Mechanisms of costimulation. Immunol Rev. 2009;229:5–11. https://doi.org/10.1111/j.1600-065X.2009.00784.x.
33. Kehry MR. CD40-mediated signaling in B cells. Balancing cell survival, growth, and death. J Immunol. 1996;156:2345–8.
34. Badolato R, Dotta L, Tassone L, et al. Tetralogy of fallot is an uncommon manifestation of warts, hypogammaglobulinemia, infections, and myelokathexis syndrome. J Pediatr. 2012;161:763–5. https://doi.org/10.1016/j.jpeds.2012.05.058.
35. Cao Y, Hunter ZR, Liu X, et al. The WHIM-like CXCR4(S338X) somatic mutation activates AKT and ERK, and promotes resistance to ibrutinib and other agents used in the treatment of Waldenstrom's Macroglobulinemia. Leukemia. 2015;29:169–76. https://doi.org/10.1038/leu.2014.187.
36. Hunter ZR, Xu L, Yang G, et al. The genomic landscape of Waldenstrom macroglobulinemia is characterized by highly recurring MYD88 and WHIM-like CXCR4 mutations, and small somatic deletions associated with B-cell lymphomagenesis. Blood. 2014;123:1637–46. https://doi.org/10.1182/blood-2013-09-525808.
37. Dale DC, Bolyard AA, Kelley ML, et al. The CXCR4 antagonist plerixafor is a potential therapy for myelokathexis, WHIM syndrome. Blood. 2011;118:4963–6. https://doi.org/10.1182/blood-2011-06-360586.

38. Al Ustwani O, Kurzrock R, Wetzler M. Genetics on a WHIM. Br J Haematol. 2014;164:15–23. https://doi.org/10.1111/bjh.12574.
39. McDermott DH, Liu Q, Velez D, et al. A phase 1 clinical trial of long-term, low-dose treatment of WHIM syndrome with the CXCR4 antagonist plerixafor. Blood. 2014;123:2308–16. https://doi.org/10.1182/blood-2013-09-527226.
40. Beaussant Cohen S, Fenneteau O, Plouvier E, et al. Description and outcome of a cohort of 8 patients with WHIM syndrome from the French Severe Chronic Neutropenia Registry. Orphanet J Rare Dis. 2012;7:71. https://doi.org/10.1186/1750-1172-7-71.
41. Rezaei N, Hedayat M, Aghamohammadi A, Nichols KE. Primary immunodeficiency diseases associated with increased susceptibility to viral infections and malignancies. J Allergy Clin Immunol. 2011;127:1323–9. https://doi.org/10.1016/j.jaci.2011.02.047.
42. McDermott DH, Gao J-L, Murphy PM. Chromothriptic cure of WHIM syndrome: implications for bone marrow transplantation. Rare Dis (Austin, Tex). 2015;3:e1073430. https://doi.org/10.1080/21675511.2015.1073430.

Class-Switch Recombination Defects

15

Mirjam van der Burg, Andrew R. Gennery, and Qiang Pan-Hammarström

15.1 Introduction: Basic Immunology Section Including CSR Mechanism

Class-switch recombination (CSR), also known as isotype switching, is the biological mechanism that changes the isotype of an antibody (immunoglobulin) from one type to the other (i.e., from IgM to IgG, IgA or IgE). During this process, the constant region of the Ig molecule is replaced, while leaving the variable region, which is generated via V(D)J recombination intact. This implies that the antigen specificity of the Ig molecule does not change; however, the effector function and tissue distribution of the Ig molecule change as a result of CSR.

15.1.1 Germinal Center Reaction

CSR takes place in activated B-cells in the germinal centers of the lymph nodes and tonsils [1, 2]. The immune response starts with transport of antigens to the

M. van der Burg (✉)
Department of Pediatrics, Laboratory for Immunology, Leiden University Medical Center, Leiden, The Netherlands
e-mail: m.van_der_burg@lumc.nl

A. R. Gennery
Department of Pediatrics, Institute of Cellular Medicine Paediatric Immunology, Great North Children's Hospital, Newcastle Upon Tyne, UK
e-mail: andrew.gennery@newcastle.ac.uk

Q. Pan-Hammarström
Department of Laboratory Medicine, Karolinska University Hospital Huddinge, Stockholm, Sweden
e-mail: Qiang.Pan-Hammarstrom@ki.se

M. M. D'Elios, M. Rizzi (eds.), *Humoral Primary Immunodeficiencies*,
Rare Diseases of the Immune System, https://doi.org/10.1007/978-3-319-91785-6_15

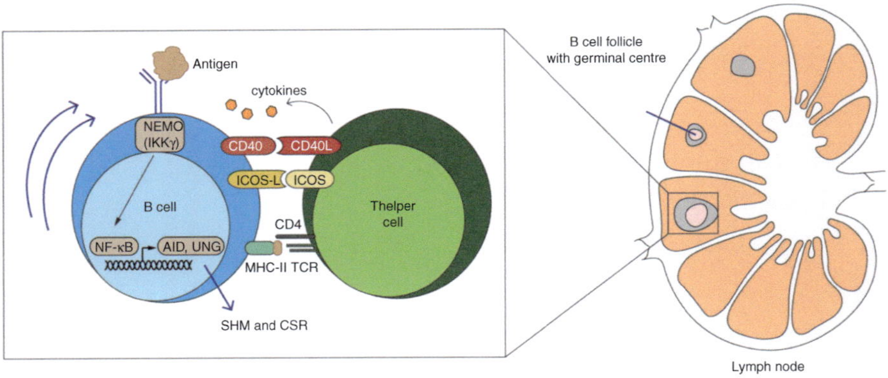

Fig. 15.1 Lymph node with B-cell follicle with germinal center and cognate B-T interaction outlined

spleen and lymph nodes by dendritic cells. After antigen uptake, dendritic cells become activated and express antigen in the context of MHC class II. Together with naïve T-cells, they migrate (in response to CCL19 and CCL21) to the T-cell zone of the lymph nodes. Antigen-specific CD4+ T-cells recognize with their T-cell receptor (TCR) the MHCII-peptide complex (immunological synapse 1) and get activated. This interaction is supported by co-stimulatory molecules and adhesion molecules with its ligands. Activated T-cells express CD40L, produce several cytokines, differentiate into CD4+ effector T-cells (Tfh cells), and migrate to the border of the T-cell zone and the B-cell follicle (see Fig. 15.1 for cognate B-T interaction). B-cells that have recognized antigen followed by uptake and presentation and MHCII-peptide complex also migrate to this border, where they can encounter the activated T-follicular helper (Tfh) cells. The recognition is based on the interaction between the TCR on the Tfh cell and the MHC-II-peptide complex on the B-cell and the co-stimulation via CD40L expressed on the T-cell and CD40 expressed on the B-cell (synapse 2). Both interactions (signals) are required to fully activate the B-cell under influence of cytokines produced by the activated Tfh cells. Subsequently B-cells can proliferate and differentiate in the germinal center. B-cells start proliferating forming a dark zone of centroblasts in the germinal center. During this phase the cells express AID, which is induced upon NFκFB signaling. AID induces somatic hypermutations (SHM) in the variable regions of the Ig molecules thereby changing the affinity of the B-cell receptor. The proliferative phase is followed by differentiation into nonproliferating centrocytes in the light zone of the germinal center. The light zone consists of a large network of follicular dendritic cells (FDCs) that bind long-term antigen-antibody complexes on its cell surface via their Fc receptors, which allow presentation of unprocessed antigen to B-cells. B-cells with BCRs with the highest affinity can best uptake antigen from the FDCs and will express the most MHCII-peptide complex that will lead to the best co-stimulation by the Tfh cells, which are also present in the light zone. Via this mechanism B-cells with the highest affinity have the best survival

(survival of the fittest). Other cells die via apoptosis. Positive selected B-cells undergo class-switch recombination (CSR) and become either memory B-cell and leave the germinal center, recirculate into the dark zone to start another found of proliferation and mutation, or become plasma cell.

15.1.2 SHM and CSR at the Molecular Level

15.1.2.1 Somatic Hypermutation (SHM)

During the germinal center reaction, SHM are induced prior to induction of CSR [3]. The first step in SHM is deamination of dC into dU by AID (i.e., activation-induced cytidine deaminase) in the rearranged V(D)J exons creating U:G mismatches (Fig. 15.2). If replication occurs without repair of these mismatches, transitions occur at C:G pairs. However, these mismatches can also be repaired via base excision repair (BER) or mismatch repair (MMR). During BER, the dU can be recognized and removed by uracil-N-glycosylase (UNG), which creates an abasic site that is recognized by BER proteins. Apyrimidinic endonuclease

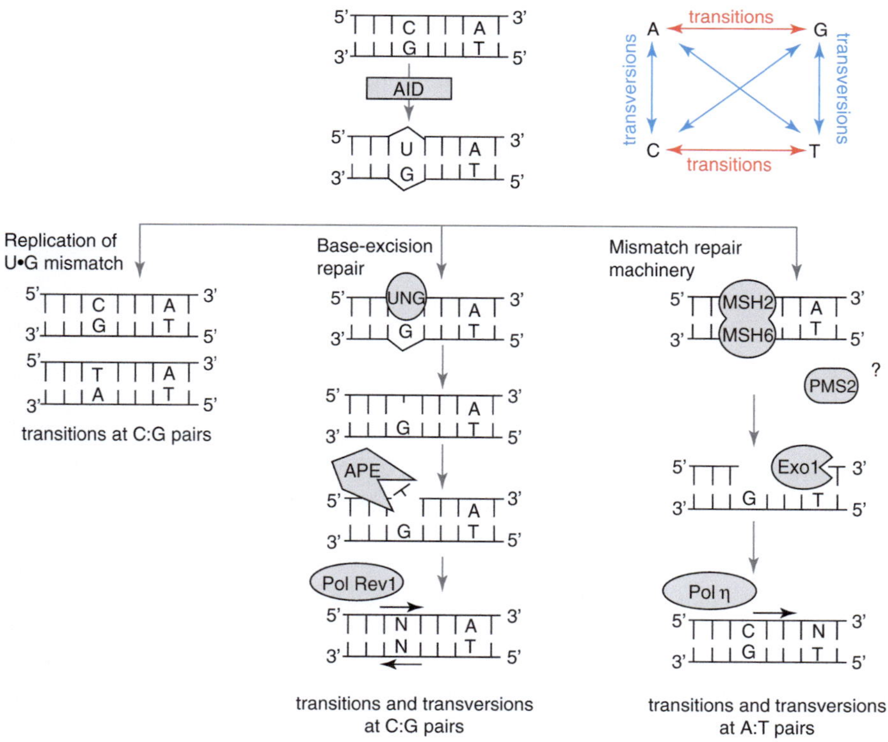

Fig. 15.2 Somatic hypermutations are induced by deamination of dC to dU by AID. The resulting U:G mismatch can be normally replicated resulting in transitions at C:G pairs or repaired via BER or MMR involving error-prone polymerases resulting in transitions and transversions at C:G pair (BER) or A:T pairs (MMR) [3]. Transitions and transversions are indicated in the top right corner

(APE) nicks the phosphate backbone creating a single-strand (ss)DNA gap, which is filled by error-prone polymerases (Pol rev1) resulting in transitions and transversions at C:G pairs. Alternatively, the U:G mismatch is recognized by the MSH2/MSH6 complex, which recruits other MMR proteins, including exonuclease 1 (Exo1), which removes surrounding nucleotides leaving a ssDNA gap. The error-prone polymerase η (Polη) fills this gap and inserts random nucleotides at A:T pairs. Therefore, repair of U:G mismatches via MMR results primarily in transitions and transversions at A:T pairs.

15.1.2.2 Class-Switch Recombination (CSR)

The constant region of the IGH locus consists of several constant regions encoding the different isotypes (Cμ, Cδ, Cγ3, Cγ1, Cα1, Cγ2, Cγ4, Cε, and Cα2), which determine the effector functions of the corresponding antibodies (Fig. 15.3a). Every constant region is preceded by a switch (S) region. S regions are composed of tandem repeats of G-rich sequences (20–80 bp) with a total length of approximately 1–12 kb, which are unique for a giving S region [4]. Only Cδ is not preceded by a switch region, because it formed upon alternative splicing of IGM-IGD transcripts. CSR is initiated by the AID (i.e., activation-induced cytidine deaminase), which deaminates dC to become dU in the top and bottom strands of the S regions, which are transcriptionally active via germline transcription (e.g., Sμ and Sα; see Fig. 15.3b) [5]. Via UNG and APE activity, these AID-initiated ssDNA breaks, which are located in close proximity, are then converted into DNA double-strand breaks (Fig. 15.3c), which can either be repaired by the non-homologous end-joining (NHEJ) pathway or via alternative end joining (aEJ) forming a Sμ-Sα hybrid joint [5]. Via this mechanism the constant region can be replaced with a different isotype leading to a different effector function while leaving the antigen recognition part (i.e., the V(D)J exon) unaffected.

15.2 CSR Deficiencies

Class-switch recombination deficiencies are a heterogeneous group of primary immunodeficiencies characterized by normal or increased levels of serum IgM in combination with reduced or absence of serum IgG, IgA, or IgE. The former name of CSR deficiency was hyper-IgM syndrome. The estimated frequency of CSR defects is around 1:500,000 newborns. There are different underlying genetic causes of CSR deficiencies, and they can be divided into groups with genetic defects hampering the cognate T-B interaction (CD40L, CD40, and NEMO), a group with intrinsic B-cell defects (AID and UNG), and finally a group with DNA repair defects involving the non-homologous end-joining (NHEJ) pathway or the mismatch repair (MMR) pathway [5–7]. The different CSR deficiencies have their specific immunological and clinical characteristics, which also require different treatment strategies. In the next sections, we describe characteristics of the involved genes and the different clinical and pathological findings together with laboratory findings followed by a section about treatment and prognosis.

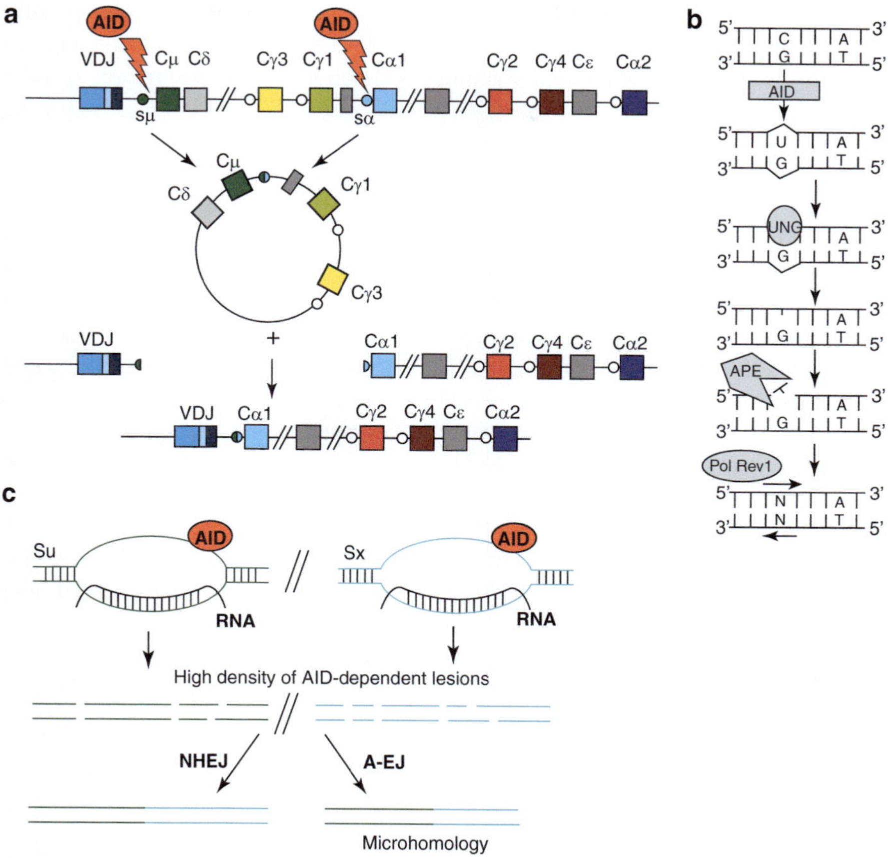

Fig. 15.3 (**a**) Schematic representation of the IGH locus with the different constant regions preceded by Switch regions (S). S regions which are transcriptionally active (germline transcription) are targeted by AID, which induces lesion that result in DNA double-strand breaks. Switch regions are joined forming a switch junction. The intervening part is excised as excision circle. Here switching from IgM to IgA1 is visualized. (**b**) AID deaminates dC into dG which results via UNG and APE activity into a ssDNA gap. (**c**) The high density of AID-dependent lesions in a S region results in the generation of a DNA double-strand break. Two ends of a switch regions (here Sμ and Sα) are repaired via NHEJ or aEJ

15.2.1 Defects in T-B Interaction

15.2.1.1 CD40L Deficiency (OMIM 308230) and CD40 Deficiency (OMIM 606843)

Genes

The X-linked gene CD40LG (*Xq26.3*) codes for CD40 ligand, which is a type II transmembrane belonging to the TNF protein family. It is expressed on activated CD4+ T-helper cells (especially the follicular T-helper cells in the germinal centers) as trimer and interacts with constitutively expressed CD40 on B-cells and other immune cells. CD40 (20q13.12) is a member of the TNF-receptor superfamily which is constitutively expressed as trimer on B-cells, on dendritic cells, and on monocytes. CD40L-CD40 interaction induces B-cell intracellular signaling, via the NFκB signaling pathway and expression of AID and UNG, the two B-cell-specific proteins that play a key role in CSR and SHM.

Clinical Presentation

X-linked CD40L deficiency is the most common CSR deficiency, whereas autosomal recessive CD40 deficiency is much more rare. Most patients present in early childhood with recurrent upper and lower respiratory tract infections. They have a high susceptibility for *Pneumocystis jirovecii* pneumonia, which is often the first clinical finding [6]. This infection is a sign of impaired cell-mediated immunity due to abnormal T-cell-monocyte interaction. Respiratory infections with CMV, respiratory syncytial virus, *Cryptococcus*, and mycobacteria have also been reported. Protracted diarrhea is another frequently occurring problem, which may require parenteral nutrition. *Giardia lamblia* or *Cryptosporidium* infections are often associated with diarrhea and the latter also with later-onset sclerosing cholangitis, which is a severe and often fatal complication. About 50% of the patients develop neutropenia, which causes oral ulcers. CD40L and CD40 deficiencies are associated with an increased risk of malignancies such as lymphomas, hepato-carcinomas, cholangiocarcinomas, and gastrointestinal and pancreatic tumors. Finally, other less frequent complications are hepatosplenomegaly, lymphadenopathy, and autoimmune manifestations such as hemolytic anemia, thrombocytopenia, and immune-complex (IgM)-mediated nephritis [8].

Laboratory Results

CD40L and CD40 deficiencies have elevated or normal levels of serum IgM with a markedly reduced level of IgG and IgA. A low level of IgM does not exclude the diagnosis of CD40L or CD40 deficiency. Sometimes normal or elevated IgA levels might be observed, which results from the T-cell-independent pathway. In CD40L deficiencies CD40L is not expressed on activated T-cells, which can be demonstrated upon in vitro stimulation with PMA and Ca-ionophore. CD40 expression is absent on B-cells of CD40 deficient patients. The number of B-cells is normal; however, due to impairment of the T-cell-dependent response, switched memory B-cells are absent. However, natural effector/marginal zone B-cells (IgM + IgD + CD27+) are present as well as CD27-IgA+ B-cells, which both arise from the T-cell-independent pathway [9]. The proliferative response to mitogens such as phytohemagglutinin (PHA) is normal, whereas the response to specific antigens is often reduced and there is a low production of TH1 cytokines. The absolute number of CD4+ and CD8+ T-cells is normal.

Treatment and Prognosis

The number of patients with CD40 deficiency is extremely small, and outcome and treatment options are the same as those of patients with CD40L deficiency—they will be therefore considered together. The majority of reported cohorts from developed countries are historic, and caution should be taken when inferring current outcomes from these historic cohorts, as diagnosis and management has significantly changed. Published data from 79 patients in the US registry in the early 2000s showed an overall mortality in the cohort of 10%, although the majority of patients were <10 years of age and none were >30 years of age. Deaths were from a number of causes including pneumonia, encephalitis, and malignancy, with the median age of death being 14 years (range 9 months–25 years) [10]. Similar causes of death were reported in an historic UK cohort [11]. A more recent report from a Latin American cohort of 35 patients confirms that pneumonia was the most common complication, but encephalitis was also reported, and three of the four deaths (10% of the cohort) were due to central nervous system infections despite immunoglobulin replacement [12]. In a small much younger Indian cohort (seven patients, median age 2.6 years, range 1.6–8 years), pneumonia remains the most common infection, and no encephalitis was reported, although the patients were young [13]. The most recent multicenter international study of patients with CD40L deficiency reported on 176 patients [14]. The median age was 11 years (range, 0.1–60.7 years). Median survival was 25 years, with no statistical difference between those treated conventionally and those receiving hematopoietic stem cell transplantation, although the Karnofsky/Lansky age performance scores were significantly better in the transplanted group. In this cohort, malignancy and hepatic disease were the most common causes of mortality in the non-transplant group, and there was an annual mortality of 2.2%. A multicenter international survey of 93 patients transplanted for CD40L deficiency between 1993 and 2014, from 23 different centers, in 15 countries documented an overall survival of 77.4% [15]. Results were better in transplants performed after the year 2000 (83% overall survival) and in children transplanted when <10 years of age (88.7% overall survival). The median follow-up was 4.3 years (range 0.4–17.1 years). Survival was 96.1% in patients transplanted with no pre-existing chronic lung disease and/or liver disease. While many patients were able to discontinue prophylactic medication, there were patients who required continued immunoglobulin substitution because of poor donor chimerism, and 13% rejected the first transplant, predominantly those who had received reduced intensity conditioning. For patients with severe liver disease, hepatic transplant can be performed before hematopoietic stem cell transplantation [16]. The most concerning feature about these data is the occurrence of potentially fatal complications despite adequate prophylaxis, particularly central nervous system infection and cryptosporidial infection leading to sclerosing cholangitis and hepatocellular carcinoma. Given that most successful transplants occurred in patients <10 years of age, without pre-existing respiratory or hepatic disease, and that the Karnofsky/Lansky age performance scores are better, there is a strong argument to offer stem cell transplant early to these patients, particularly as these will most readily tolerate myeloablative conditioning which is more likely to correct the defect. However, this has to be balanced with the potential long-term toxicities of chemotherapy, particularly on fertility.

Within the field of primary immunodeficiencies, gene therapy in the form of gene addition to defective hematopoietic stem cells using viral vectors is emerging as a potential corrective therapy for some types of severe combined immunodeficiency.

Correction of CD40L deficiency by gene addition in murine models has led to thymic lymphoproliferative disorders, probably because gene expression needs to be tightly controlled [17]. An alternative approach could be to use gene-editing to remove the faulty *CD40LG* gene from peripheral T-cells and replace it with a functional gene, thus restoring function in T-helper cells and enabling T-cell interaction with B-cells and antigen-presenting cells. This method has been shown to be effective in murine models [18], but clinical trials have yet to be developed.

15.2.1.2 NEMO Deficiency (OMIM 300248)

Gene

The IKBKG gene (Xq28) encodes the protein NEMO (NFκB essential modulator), which is the founding member of an evolutionarily conserved family of NEMO-like kinases that function in numerous cell signaling pathways. NEMO/IKKγ is one of the three catalytic subunits of the IKK complex (together with IKKα and IKKβ) [19]. NFκB is a transcription factor sequestered in the cytoplasm of resting cells through binding to inhibitor of NFκB (IκB) proteins. Upon cell stimulation, IκB are phosphorylated by IKK leading to degradation and release of NFκB, which can translocate to the nucleus where it can bind DNA and regulate gene transcription of genes such as AID and UNG.

Clinical Presentation

Hypomorphic mutations in the X-linked NEMO gene result in ectodermal dysplasia, anhidrotic with immunodeficiency (EDA-ID), which is characterized by sparse hair, cone-shaped teeth and hypohidrosis with lack of sweating and a tendency to develop hyperpyrexia [20]. More severe mutations also result in osteopetrosis and lymphedema, but loss-of-function mutations are lethal [21]. Female carriers have signs of incontinentia pigmenti syndrome, characterized by skin abnormalities including blistering rash at birth and in early infancy followed by development of wart-like skin growths [19]. There are signs of hyperpigmentation occurring in a swirled pattern, which fade with time. In adulthood incontinentia pigmenti usually shows lines of hypopigmentation on their arms and legs. Other signs are alopecia and dental and eye abnormalities. NEMO-deficient patients are susceptible to infections with pyogenic bacteria (*S. pneumoniae*, *H. influenzae*, and *S. aureus*) and to infections with mycobacteria (*M. avium* or *M. kansasii*), which causes meningitis, sepsis, arthritis, and osteomyelitis [21, 22]. Opportunistic infections with *Pneumocystis jirovecii* and chronic mucocutaneous candidiasis (CMC) have also been reported in a minority of patients. The overall clinical presentation is heterogeneous and ranges in severity. This might be caused by the nature of the mutation and the level of residual NEMO activity.

Laboratory Findings

NEMO deficiency is immunologically characterized by hypogammaglobulinemia in combination with poor antibody response to polysaccharide antigens. Serum IgM or IgA can be increased. NK cell function is reduced, and the T-cell responses to mitogens and recall antigens in vitro are variable. T- and B-cell counts in the peripheral blood are normal, although the number of memory B-cells can be reduced. Persistent lymphocytosis in combination with a normal distribution of T, B, and NK cells is also a common finding. In vitro NFκB function can be evaluated by stimulation of peripheral blood mononuclear cells with TLR or IL1R ligands and measurement of IL6 (reduced in NEMO deficiency). Another functional test suitable for evaluation of NEMO variants is measurement of degradation of IκB in patient's fibroblast upon stimulation with IL1β or TNFα [23].

Treatment and Prognosis

While the immunological defects in patients with CD40 or CD40L deficiency can be simply explained by interruption of ligand to receptor binding and signaling in hematopoietically derived cells, and thus restoration of function by replacement of defective hematopoietic stem cells, the solution is not so straightforward for patients with NEMO deficiency. NF-kB and NEMO are widely expressed in many tissues and are involved in many signal transduction pathways, including at least three non-hematopoietic pathways. Therefore, while replacement of defective hematopoietic stem cells may resolve some immunological features, other manifestations, such as lymphedema or ectodermal dysplasia, may remain.

B-cell and antibody deficiencies are the most commonly reported immunological abnormalities reported in a cohort of 72 individuals with NEMO deficiency (median age 4.6 years, range 0–48 years), of which 50% of patients who were alive were receiving immunoglobulin replacement therapy [21]. Twenty-seven patients had died (median age 2.75 years, range 0–48 years), and only 15 were >10 years of age. Serious viral infection occurred in 21% of patients and opportunistic infections occurred in 10%. While most patients do not warrant consideration for hematopoietic stem cell transplantation, one fairly large transplant cohort of 29 patients has been described [24]. Median age at transplantation was 3.4 years, range 0.33–18.8 years. The majority of patients experienced opportunistic infection with mycobacterial or fungal species, and many required nutritional support pre-transplantation. The overall survival was 74% at 108 months after transplantation with a median follow-up of 57 months and an engraftment rate of 93%. Age at transplantation did not influence the survival rate, which was better with matched siblings than unrelated donors. However, patients receiving stem cells from carrier female relatives appeared to have only partial correction of the immunodeficiency. Patients with mycobacterial infection had a worse outcome than those without. Some patients with colitis pre-transplant did not have resolution of symptoms, and two others developed colitis post-transplant, a phenomenon previously reported [25]. These observations suggest that the pathogenesis of NEMO deficiency-related colitis may involve a non-hematopoietic pathway and that transplantation may not correct IBD, possibly reflecting the importance of the NF-κB pathway in intestinal epithelial cells for controlling epithelial gut integrity.

15.2.2 Intrinsic B-Cell Defects

15.2.2.1 AID Deficiency (OMIM 605258)

Gene

Activating-induced cytidine deaminase (AICDA; 12p13.31) is the gene encoding AID, which is exclusively expressed in germinal center B-cells. AID is a DNA-specific cytidine deaminase, which is involved in the induction of CSR and SHM by deamination of cytidine to uracil during transcription of Ig-variable (V) and Ig-switch (S) regions (see Sect. 15.1.2). Mutations located in the C-terminal part of AID result in severe CSR deficiency while SHM is not affected.

Clinical Presentation

AID deficiency is characterized by recurrent bacterial infections of the respiratory tract, mostly due to encapsulated bacteria, which can lead to bronchiectasis [26]. Also, gastrointestinal bacterial infections are a prominent feature, which are sometimes related to persistent *Giardia lamblia* infections. Opportunistic infections and neutropenia, which are characteristic for CD40 and CD40L deficiency, are not observed because in AID deficiency, the T-cell responses are unaffected. Lymphoid hyperplasia is a striking feature affecting mainly cervical lymph nodes and tonsils, which may even require resection. In addition, arthritis and autoimmune features (hemolytic anemia, thrombocytopenia, and autoimmune hepatitis) are frequently found [8].

Laboratory Findings

AID-deficient patients have normal to elevated serum IgM levels and reduced or absent serum IgG and IgA levels. IgM isohemagglutinins and anti-polysaccharide IgM are normally present [6, 26]. The total number of T-cells and B-cells is within the normal range; however, switched memory B-cells are absent. B-cells are able to proliferate in vitro; however, upon stimulation with anti-CD40 and cytokines, they do not undergo CSR, which is characteristic for an intrinsic B-cell defect. The level of SHM is strongly impaired. The lymphoid hyperplasia can be characterized by follicular hyperplasia with giant germinal centers and small mantle zone interfollicular area.

15.2.2.2 UNG Deficiency (OMIM 608106)

Gene

Uracil-DNA glycosylase (UNG; 12q24.11) is expressed in germinal center B-cells in parallel with AID and removes uracil from DNA molecules via cleaving the N-glycosylic bond that has been generated by AID activity. This subsequently induces the error-prone base excision repair (BER) pathway of the SHM process, which generally results in transitions and transversions at C:G pairs. Mutations in the UNG gene result in increased accumulation of genomic uracil [27]. UNG-deficient patients have profound impairment in CSR at a DNA precleavage step and with a partial disturbance of the SHM pattern [28].

Clinical Presentation and Laboratory Findings
Only a few patients with UNG deficiency have been described [28]. They described patients have susceptibility to bacterial infections of the respiratory tract, cervical and mediastinal lymph node hyperplasia, increased serum IgM concentrations, and profoundly decreased serum IgG and IgA concentrations. At the time of diagnosis, antibody titers to pneumococcal and tetanus antigens were reduced. The T-cell counts and functions are normal, including the expression of CD40L on activated T-cells. B-cells also proliferate normally; however, they do not undergo class-switch recombination. The CSR defect occurs between the switch region transcription and induction of DNA double-strand breaks. The frequency of SHM in UNG is unaffected. However, the pattern of SHM is biased toward transitions at G/C pairs (i.e., G > A; C > T), whereas the ratio of transitions and transversions at A/T pairs is normal [28].

Treatment and Prognosis AID and UNG Deficiencies
There are few patients described with deficiency of AID or particularly of UNG, and treatment and prognosis will be considered jointly. Infections in these patients are characteristic of those associated with antibody deficiency, in contrast to patients with CD40, CD40L, or NEMO deficiency who also experience opportunistic infections [12, 26, 28]. Patients with deficient of AID have also been described as having gastrointestinal infections due to giardia. However, in contrast to patients with agammaglobulinemia, these patients appear not to experience enteroviral infections of the central nervous system. Treatment with immunoglobulin replacement should resolve the symptoms. AID-deficient patients may experience extreme lymphoid hyperplasia, for which surgery may provide symptomatic relief. Autoimmunity is also described [29] which may be severe and life-threatening and require treatment with anti-CD20 antibody with or without other immunosuppression.

15.2.3 DNA Repair Defects

15.2.3.1 Ataxia Telangiectasia (OMIM 208900)

Gene
Ataxia telangiectasia mutated (ATM;11q22.3) is a member of the phosphatidylinositol3 kinase family, which includes DNA-PKcs and ATR, which all function in DNA break responses. It exists as an inactive dimer/tetramer that is activated and recruited to sites of double-strand breaks. ATM accumulates at repair foci and regulates binding and activation of double-strand break (DSB) repair proteins and subsequent repair of the DSBs. ATM also initiates a cell-cycle checkpoint until repair is complete [30, 31]. It responses to DNA damage through phosphorylation of essential substrates involved in DSB repair and cell-cycle control. During CSR, ATM organizes the repair complex and might contribute to the correct juxtaposition of DSBs during the long-range interaction required for accurate switch

recombination [32]. However, defective switch to distal constant regions in patients with AT could also (in part) be explained by an impaired ability of B-cells to undergo multiple successful GC responses [33].

Clinical Presentation

AT is characterized by cerebellar ataxia, oculocutaneous telangiectasias, radiosensitivity, chromosomal instability, a propensity for development of (mainly hematologic) malignancies, growth retardation, and endocrine abnormalities. The prevalence of cancer in AT patients is 10–30% [34]. AT patients also have signs of immunodeficiency, predominantly antibody deficiency. However the extent and severity is highly variable. Classical AT refers to patients with an early-onset disease (childhood) in contrast to variant AT, which presents at adulthood. A subset of patients with classical AT has a severe early-onset hypogammaglobulinemia reminiscent of a CSR deficiency [35, 36]. Some patients experience lung infections, chronic lung disease, and recurrent infections, which are associated with immune deficiency. The majority of infections in childhood are caused by *Staphylococcus aureus*, *Haemophilus influenza*, and *Streptococcus pneumoniae*, whereas in older patients *Pseudomonas aeruginosa* is more frequent [37].

Laboratory Findings

The laboratory findings related to CSR deficiency in AT patients are characterized by a frequent reduction in serum IgA and IgG subclass levels. Most patients have disturbed naïve B-cell and T-cell homeostasis, as evidenced by low cell numbers, increased proliferation, a large proportion $CD21^{low}CD38^{low}$ anergic B-cells, and decreased antigen receptor repertoire diversity [33]. AT patients presenting with an early-onset hypogammaglobulinemia have impaired formation of T-cell-dependent memory B-cells. Sμ-Sa junctions in patients with AT showed increased microhomology, whereas the Sμ-Sγ junctions from these patients have severely reduced mutations or insertions, indicating that the predominantly used error-prone NHEJ pathway in CSR is impaired in patients with AT [38] and the proportion of CSR to the distal IGHG2, IGHG4, and IGHA2 constant regions is reduced [33]. However, the frequency of SHM in switched transcripts is not reduced in AT.

Treatment and Prognosis

Ataxia telangiectasia is a chronic, progressive disease, with no curative treatment available and with which patients face a high risk of infection, malignancy, and neurodegeneration. Median survival is into the mid-twenties, with most deaths due to chronic lung disease or malignancy [39]. A multidisciplinary team is best placed to consider the multidimensional aspects to supportive care and management of these patients. The newborn screening test for severe combined immunodeficiency detects T-cell receptor recombination excision circles (TRECs) from infant dried blood spots. Infants with T-cell lymphocytopenia and ataxia telangiectasia have been identified with the SCID newborn screening test in combination with exome sequencing [40]. Early diagnosis enables early family education, genetic counseling, and early, proactive supportive care.

Bacterial infections predominantly affect the sino-pulmonary tract and can be complicated by neuromuscular incoordination leading to aspiration. There is an increased risk of autoimmune or chronic inflammatory disease, including idiopathic thrombocytopenia, arthritis, and vitiligo, and likely related to the immunodeficiency rather than a direct effect of ATM protein dysfunction. There is a relationship between propensity to infection, or to development of lymphoid tumors and breast cancer, and severity of the mutation, with null mutations associated with a greater risk [41, 42]. For patients with antibody deficiency and evidence of recurrent infection, immunoglobulin substitution should be initiated, with or without antibiotic prophylaxis. There should be careful periodic assessment of oro-pharyngeal coordination, to assess swallowing and avoid malnutrition and aspiration. Use of thickened feeds may help, and placement of a gastrostomy may be required in cases of significant neuromuscular dysfunction. Malignancy is particularly challenging in these patients, as tumors are often aggressive, but patients are poorly tolerant of highly cytotoxic chemotherapy and of radiotherapy. Investigation of symptoms can be demanding, as exposure to irradiation should be minimized, alternative imaging modalities are used where possible, and areas not relevant to the diagnosis must be protected from exposure to radiation. The role of hematopoietic stem cell transplantation is controversial, and most results indicate a poor outcome [43]. However, many of these patients are treated for malignancy, and preemptive hematopoietic stem cell transplantation may prevent the development of lympho-reticular malignancy and the need for aggressive conditioning—however, such approaches should only be considered as part of an approved clinical study, with the recognition that successful treatment is unlikely to halt the neurological deterioration. Potential future therapies include the use of antisense morpholino oligonucleotides, to correct aberrant splicing and allow translation of normal ATM protein [44], or the use of aminoglycosides or small molecules for chemical-induced read through of premature stop codons in ATM to produce some functional protein [45]. However, these treatments are some way off clinical use.

Ataxia telangiectasia carriers have one mutated copy of ATM and are healthy. However, they appear to have a reduced lifespan due to breast cancer and gastrointestinal tract carcinoma and of ischemic heart disease [46]. Female carriers have a 2.3-fold increased risk for the development of breast cancer as compared to the general population [47], with the cumulative risk of breast cancer of approximately 6% by age 50 years and approximately 30% by age 80 years [48]. Currently, only standard breast cancer surveillance (monthly breast self-exams and routine mammography at the usual schedule for age) is recommended unless there is family history of breast cancer.

15.2.3.2 Nijmegen Breakage Syndrome (NBS) (OMIM 251260)

Gene

The NBN (Nibrin) gene encoding the NBS1 protein is located at chromosome location 8q21.3. It is a member of the MRE11/RAD50/NBS1 (MRN) complex, which acts as a marker of DNA breaks as it has been shown to accumulate in large nuclear foci within minutes after DSB formation [49]. It is activated in response to DSBs and keeps the two DNA ends in close proximity [50]. A second function of the MRN complex is ATM activation [51]. MRN recruits ATM to DNA breaks, which results in dissociation of the ATM dimer enabling ATM activity [52]. Furthermore, NBS1 is involved in maintenance of chromosomal integrity, telomere stability, and cell-cycle checkpoint control [53].

Clinical Presentation

Nijmegen breakage syndrome (NBS) is a rare autosomal recessive inherited condition, characterized by microcephaly, dysmorphic "birdlike" face, chromosomal instability, immunodeficiency, and predisposition to malignancy [54]. Recurrent infections are part of the clinical presentation and are mainly found in the upper respiratory tract and lungs but also in the urinary tract. Some patients develop bronchiectasis and chronic lung disease. Opportunistic infections are not part of phenotype. Autoimmune complications were found in a minority of patients and include skin changes, ITP, and AIHA [54].

Laboratory Findings

The immunodeficiency in NBS patients is considerably variable and can affect both humoral and cellular immunity. Reduced serum IgG and/or IgA levels are frequently observed. Sometimes, a normal level of IgG masks an IgG subclass deficiency. IgM concentrations are normal in the majority of cases and sometimes even elevated [54]. NBS patients can have reduced B- and T-cell numbers. In the B-cell compartment, especially the numbers of naïve and memory, B-cells are reduced, whereas the number of natural effector B lymphocytes is increased [55]. The reduction in the number of naïve B-cells can be explained by a loss of juxtaposition of RAG-induced breaks during V(D)J recombination in bone marrow [56]. Regarding the T-cell compartment, the numbers of $\alpha\beta$ + T-cells are reduced, but a number of γT+ cells are normal. In addition, T-cells from NBS patients show signs of a senescent phenotype [57]. Analysis of the CSR pathway in NBS patients showed that the NBS1 protein localizes to chromosomal sites of class switching [58] and that the switch junctions show an enhanced presence of microhomology [58, 59].

Treatment and Prognosis

Patients with Nijmegen breakage syndrome are at increased risk of immunodeficiency and malignancy. Overall survival probabilities at 5, 10, 20, and 30 years of age were 95, 85, 50, and 35% in one large cohort study [54]. Recurrent infections tend to be bacterial, affecting the sino-pulmonary tract, and should be treated with appropriate antibiotics—opportunistic infections are generally not a problem. Patients with hypogammaglobulinemia can be treated with immunoglobulin replacement. Autoimmunity can be severe and should be treated with appropriate immunosuppression—anti-CD20 antibody may be required for life-threatening cytopenias.

Malignancy is a leading cause of death [54, 60]. Patients do not tolerate standard chemotherapy protocols well, and regimens need to be adapted—however, the malignancies are often aggressive [61]. As for patients with ataxia telangiectasia, radiological examination for investigation of malignancy should be judicious and appropriately directed. Hematopoietic stem cell transplantation may have more of a role in the management of these patients [43, 60, 62], with survival of around 75% when reduced intensity conditioning is used. However, whether this approach should be routinely or preemptively offered is yet to be determined.

While heterozygote carriers are unaffected, they do have an increased risk of malignancy, particularly for breast and prostate carcinoma and melanoma [63–65], although there is no consensus on screening for these individuals.

15.2.3.3 DNA Ligase 4 (OMIM 606593) and Cernunnos (OMIM 611291)

Gene

LIG4 located on 13q33.3 encodes the Ligase 4, which is involved the final ligation step of the non-homologous end-joining pathway. The protein forms a complex with XRCC4. NHEJ1 gene (non-homologous end-joining factor 1) also called Cernunnos or XLF (XRCC4-like factor) is located on 2q35. The XLF protein can form a stable complex with XRCC4 where it can bridge DNA ends with its filamentous structure [66]. It binds to DNA and stimulates the XRCC4/ligase IV activity [67]. XRCC4 and Cernunnos are both part of the classical NHEJ pathway, which is primary mechanism for CSR [5]. XRCC4-deficient patients have impaired CSR, however, no clinical signs of immunodeficiency [68–70].

Clinical Presentation

LIG4 deficiency can present with a spectrum of clinical conditions ranging from radiosensitive leukemia [71], radiosensitive T-B-SCID [72] to the LIG4 syndrome characterized by microcephaly and growth retardation [73] and primordial dwarfism [74, 75]. Cernunnos deficiency presents similarly as the LIG4 syndrome with combined immunodeficiency and growth retardation [76]. All patients have recurrent respiratory tract infections caused by *Pneumocystis jirovecii*, CMV, and bacteria [77].

Laboratory Findings

LIG4- and Cernunnos-deficient patients have reduced numbers of peripheral B- and T-cells in combination with a normal number of NK cells. The number of B- and T-cells is dependent on the severity of the mutation. The number of switched memory B-cells is reduced in patients with LIG4 syndrome, and the Sμ-Sα junctions show dramatic shift in using long microhomologies, suggesting an impaired NHEJ during CSR [78]. The Sμ-Sγ junctions however show an increased frequency of insertions but no increase in microhomology [78]. In Cernunnos deficiency, CSR is also affected, and the junctions show similarities with the junctions of LIG4 syndrome patients [79].

Treatment and Prognosis

There are few patients described with deficiency of Cernunnos, and the phenotype is similar to that of patients with DNA ligase 4 syndrome; therefore, treatment and prognosis will be considered jointly. For patients presenting with a severe combined immunodeficiency phenotype, hematopoietic stem cell transplantation should be performed, with best results obtained when reduced intensity conditioning regimens are employed, without radiotherapy [43]. Long-term follow-up of these patients will be required to monitor for late-occurring complications given the systemic nature of the defect, which is uncorrected by transplantation. For patients with less severe immunodeficiencies, treatment with immunoglobulin replacement is recommended, with antibiotic prophylaxis as appropriate. Unfortunately, despite this, there is a high risk of malignancy [80]. The role of preemptive hematopoietic stem cell transplantation is yet to be determined.

15.2.3.4 *PMS2, MHL1, MSH2,* and *MHS6* and Deficiency (OMIM 276300)

Genes

PMS2 (postmeiotic segregation increased, S cerevisiae 2) also called mismatch repair gene PMSL2 is located on 7p22.1 and is a protein required for mismatch repair. MLH1 (MutL homolog 1) is located on 3p22.2. PMS2 and MHL1 can heterodimerize to form MutL alpha, part of the DNA mismatch repair (MMR) system. The exact role of PMS2-MHL1 in CSR remains unclear; however, it has been shown to play a role in inducing DNA double-strand breaks. The other MMR component is MutS homolog consisting of MSH2–6. MutS homology 2 gene (MSH2) is located on 2p21 and forms a complex with MSH6 (2p16.3), which binds AID-induced mismatches in the absence of UNG.

Clinical Presentation

Autosomal recessive mutations in PMS2, MHL1, MSH2, and MHS6 are found in patients with constitutional mismatch repair deficiency syndromes (CMMRD). CMMRD is a rare pediatric autosomal recessive childhood cancer predisposition syndrome with four main tumor types: hematologic malignancies, brain/central nervous system tumors, colorectal tumors and multiple intestinal polyps, and other malignancies including embryonic tumors and rhabdomyosarcoma. Heterozygous germline mutations in *MLH1*, *MSH2*, *MSH6*, and *PMS2* cause Lynch syndrome (LS), an autosomal dominant cancer syndrome associated with hereditary nonpolyposis colorectal cancer (HNPCC), endometrium carcinoma, and other malignancies, occurring on average in the fourth and fifth decades of life.

Many CMMRD patients show signs reminiscent of neurofibromatosis type I, particularly multiple cafe-au-lait macules. It remains unclear whether IgA and/or IgG deficiency is a common feature of CMMRD, because severe bacterial infections do not occur at high frequencies. However, in PMS2 deficiency, defective PMS2 has been shown to be associated with impaired CSR [81]. In these patients CSR was found partially defective in vivo resulting in reduced serum Ig and reduced numbers of memory B-cells. The SHM frequency was also found to be reduced. The CSR defect is characterized by defective occurrence of double-strand DNA breaks (DSBs) in switch regions and abnormal formation of switch junctions. No detailed immunological laboratory information is available for CMMRD patients.

Treatment and Prognosis

While recurrent bacterial infection may lead to the institution of immunoglobulin replacement therapy, the major issue for these patients is development of malignancy in early childhood, predominantly hematological malignancies, brain tumors, or early-onset gastrointestinal tumors [82]. T-cell lymphomas are usually the first tumors to present, but patients are likely to develop additional tumors. Treatment should be directed at specific tumors, but the prognosis is poor, with few patients reaching adulthood.

References

1. Shlomchik MJ, Weisel F. Germinal center selection and the development of memory B and plasma cells. Immunol Rev. 2012;247(1):52–63.
2. Victora GD, Nussenzweig MC. Germinal centers. Annu Rev Immunol. 2012;30:429–57.
3. Hwang JK, Alt FW, Yeap LS. Related mechanisms of antibody somatic hypermutation and class switch recombination. Microbiol Spectr. 2015;3(1):MDNA3-0037-2014.
4. Dunnick W, Hertz GZ, Scappino L, Gritzmacher C. DNA sequences at immunoglobulin switch region recombination sites. Nucleic Acids Res. 1993;21(3):365–72.
5. Stavnezer J, Bjorkman A, Du L, Cagigi A, Pan-Hammarstrom Q. Mapping of switch recombination junctions, a tool for studying DNA repair pathways during immunoglobulin class switching. Adv Immunol. 2010;108:45–109.
6. Qamar N, Fuleihan RL. The hyper IgM syndromes. Clin Rev Allergy Immunol. 2014;46(2):120–30.
7. Min IM, Selsing E. Antibody class switch recombination: roles for switch sequences and mismatch repair proteins. Adv Immunol. 2005;87:297–328.
8. Jesus AA, Duarte AJ, Oliveira JB. Autoimmunity in hyper-IgM syndrome. J Clin Immunol. 2008;28(Suppl 1):S62–6.
9. Berkowska MA, Driessen GJ, Bikos V, Grosserichter-Wagener C, Stamatopoulos K, Cerutti A, et al. Human memory B cells originate from three distinct germinal center-dependent and -independent maturation pathways. Blood. 2011;118(8):2150–8.
10. Winkelstein JA, Marino MC, Ochs H, Fuleihan R, Scholl PR, Geha R, et al. The X-linked hyper-IgM syndrome: clinical and immunologic features of 79 patients. Medicine (Baltimore). 2003;82(6):373–84.
11. Banatvala N, Davies J, Kanariou M, Strobel S, Levinsky R, Morgan G. Hypogammaglobulinaemia associated with normal or increased IgM (the hyper IgM syndrome): a case series review. Arch Dis Child. 1994;71(2):150–2.
12. Cabral-Marques O, Klaver S, Schimke LF, Ascendino EH, Khan TA, Pereira PV, et al. First report of the Hyper-IgM syndrome Registry of the Latin American Society for Immunodeficiencies: novel mutations, unique infections, and outcomes. J Clin Immunol. 2014;34(2):146–56.
13. Madkaikar M, Gupta M, Chavan S, Italia K, Desai M, Merchant R, et al. X-linked hyper IgM syndrome: clinical, immunological and molecular features in patients from India. Blood Cells Mol Dis. 2014;53(3):99–104.
14. de la Morena MT. Clinical phenotypes of hyper-IgM syndromes. J Allergy Clin Immunol Pract. 2016;4(6):1023–36.

15. Ferrua F, Courteille V, Janda A, Slatter M, Albert MH, Al-Mousa H. Haematopoietic stem cell transplantation for CD40 ligand deficiency: results from an EBMT Inborn Errors Working Party (IEWP) study. Bone Marrow Transplant. 2015;50(Suppl 1):S45–S6.
16. Hadzic N, Pagliuca A, Rela M, Portmann B, Jones A, Veys P, et al. Correction of the hyper-IgM syndrome after liver and bone marrow transplantation. N Engl J Med. 2000;342(5):320–4.
17. Brown MP, Topham DJ, Sangster MY, Zhao J, Flynn KJ, Surman SL, et al. Thymic lymphoproliferative disease after successful correction of CD40 ligand deficiency by gene transfer in mice. Nat Med. 1998;4(11):1253–60.
18. Hubbard N, Hagin D, Sommer K, Song Y, Khan I, Clough C, et al. Targeted gene editing restores regulated CD40L function in X-linked hyper-IgM syndrome. Blood. 2016;127(21):2513–22.
19. Courtois G, Israel A. NF-kappa B defects in humans: the NEMO/incontinentia pigmenti connection. Sci STKE. 2000;2000(58):pe1.
20. Doffinger R, Smahi A, Bessia C, Geissmann F, Feinberg J, Durandy A, et al. X-linked anhidrotic ectodermal dysplasia with immunodeficiency is caused by impaired NF-kappaB signaling. Nat Genet. 2001;27(3):277–85.
21. Hanson EP, Monaco-Shawver L, Solt LA, Madge LA, Banerjee PP, May MJ, et al. Hypomorphic nuclear factor-kappaB essential modulator mutation database and reconstitution system identifies phenotypic and immunologic diversity. J Allergy Clin Immunol. 2008;122(6):1169–77. e16
22. Picard C, Casanova JL, Puel A. Infectious diseases in patients with IRAK-4, MyD88, NEMO, or IkappaBalpha deficiency. Clin Microbiol Rev. 2011;24(3):490–7.
23. Frans G, van der Werff Ten Bosch J, Moens L, Gijsbers R, Changi-Ashtiani M, Rokni-Zadeh H, et al. Functional evaluation of an IKBKG variant suspected to cause immunodeficiency without ectodermal dysplasia. J Clin Immunol. 2017;37(8):801–10.
24. Miot C, Imai K, Imai C, Mancini AJ, Kucuk ZY, Kawai T, et al. Hematopoietic stem cell transplantation in 29 patients hemizygous for hypomorphic IKBKG/NEMO mutations. Blood. 2017;130(12):1456–67.
25. Pai SY, Levy O, Jabara HH, Glickman JN, Stoler-Barak L, Sachs J, et al. Allogeneic transplantation successfully corrects immune defects, but not susceptibility to colitis, in a patient with nuclear factor-kappaB essential modulator deficiency. J Allergy Clin Immunol. 2008;122(6):1113–8. e1
26. Revy P, Muto T, Levy Y, Geissmann F, Plebani A, Sanal O, et al. Activation-induced cytidine deaminase (AID) deficiency causes the autosomal recessive form of the Hyper-IgM syndrome (HIGM2). Cell. 2000;102(5):565–75.
27. Kavli B, Andersen S, Otterlei M, Liabakk NB, Imai K, Fischer A, et al. B cells from hyper-IgM patients carrying UNG mutations lack ability to remove uracil from ssDNA and have elevated genomic uracil. J Exp Med. 2005;201(12):2011–21.
28. Imai K, Slupphaug G, Lee WI, Revy P, Nonoyama S, Catalan N, et al. Human uracil-DNA glycosylase deficiency associated with profoundly impaired immunoglobulin class-switch recombination. Nat Immunol. 2003;4(10):1023–8.
29. Hase K, Takahashi D, Ebisawa M, Kawano S, Itoh K, Ohno H. Activation-induced cytidine deaminase deficiency causes organ-specific autoimmune disease. PLoS One. 2008;3(8):e3033.
30. Bakkenist CJ, Kastan MB. DNA damage activates ATM through intermolecular autophosphorylation and dimer dissociation. Nature. 2003;421(6922):499–506.
31. Downs JA, Nussenzweig MC, Nussenzweig A. Chromatin dynamics and the preservation of genetic information. Nature. 2007;447(7147):951–8.
32. Guikema JE, Schrader CE, Brodsky MH, Linehan EK, Richards A, El Falaky N, et al. p53 represses class switch recombination to IgG2a through its antioxidant function. J Immunol. 2010;184(11):6177–87.
33. Driessen GJ, Ijspeert H, Weemaes CM, Haraldsson A, Trip M, Warris A, et al. Antibody deficiency in patients with ataxia telangiectasia is caused by disturbed B- and T-cell homeostasis and reduced immune repertoire diversity. J Allergy Clin Immunol. 2013;131(5):1367–75. e9
34. Swift M, Morrell D, Massey RB, Chase CL. Incidence of cancer in 161 families affected by ataxia-telangiectasia. N Engl J Med. 1991;325(26):1831–6.

35. Noordzij JG, Wulffraat NM, Haraldsson A, Meyts I, van't Veer LJ, Hogervorst FB, et al. Ataxia-telangiectasia patients presenting with hyper-IgM syndrome. Arch Dis Child. 2009;94(6):448–9.
36. Mohammadinejad P, Abolhassani H, Aghamohammadi A, Pourhamdi S, Ghosh S, Sadeghi B, et al. Class switch recombination process in ataxia telangiectasia patients with elevated serum levels of IgM. J Immunoassay Immunochem. 2015;36(1):16–26.
37. Schroeder SA, Zielen S. Infections of the respiratory system in patients with ataxia-telangiectasia. Pediatr Pulmonol. 2014;49(4):389–99.
38. Pan Q, Petit-Frere C, Lahdesmaki A, Gregorek H, Chrzanowska KH, Hammarstrom L. Alternative end joining during switch recombination in patients with ataxia-telangiectasia. Eur J Immunol. 2002;32(5):1300–8.
39. Crawford TO, Skolasky RL, Fernandez R, Rosquist KJ, Lederman HM. Survival probability in ataxia telangiectasia. Arch Dis Child. 2006;91(7):610–1.
40. Mallott J, Kwan A, Church J, Gonzalez-Espinosa D, Lorey F, Tang LF, et al. Newborn screening for SCID identifies patients with ataxia telangiectasia. J Clin Immunol. 2013;33(3):540–9.
41. Staples ER, McDermott EM, Reiman A, Byrd PJ, Ritchie S, Taylor AM, et al. Immunodeficiency in ataxia telangiectasia is correlated strongly with the presence of two null mutations in the ataxia telangiectasia mutated gene. Clin Exp Immunol. 2008;153(2):214–20.
42. Reiman A, Srinivasan V, Barone G, Last JI, Wootton LL, Davies EG, et al. Lymphoid tumours and breast cancer in ataxia telangiectasia; substantial protective effect of residual ATM kinase activity against childhood tumours. Br J Cancer. 2011;105(4):586–91.
43. Slack J, Albert MH, Balashov D, Belohradsky BH, Bertaina A, Bleesing J, et al. Outcome of hematopoietic cell transplantation for DNA double-strand break repair disorders. J Allergy Clin Immunol. 2018;141(1):322–8. e10
44. Du L, Pollard JM, Gatti RA. Correction of prototypic ATM splicing mutations and aberrant ATM function with antisense morpholino oligonucleotides. Proc Natl Acad Sci U S A. 2007;104(14):6007–12.
45. Du L, Jung ME, Damoiseaux R, Completo G, Fike F, Ku JM, et al. A new series of small molecular weight compounds induce read through of all three types of nonsense mutations in the ATM gene. Mol Ther. 2013;21(9):1653–60.
46. van Os NJ, Roeleveld N, Weemaes CM, Jongmans MC, Janssens GO, Taylor AM, et al. Health risks for ataxia-telangiectasia mutated heterozygotes: a systematic review, meta-analysis and evidence-based guideline. Clin Genet. 2016;90(2):105–17.
47. Renwick A, Thompson D, Seal S, Kelly P, Chagtai T, Ahmed M, et al. ATM mutations that cause ataxia-telangiectasia are breast cancer susceptibility alleles. Nat Genet. 2006;38(8):873–5.
48. Marabelli M, Cheng SC, Parmigiani G. Penetrance of ATM gene mutations in breast cancer: a meta-analysis of different measures of risk. Genet Epidemiol. 2016;40(5):425–31.
49. Maser RS, Monsen KJ, Nelms BE, Petrini JH. hMre11 and hRad50 nuclear foci are induced during the normal cellular response to DNA double-strand breaks. Mol Cell Biol. 1997;17(10):6087–96.
50. Hopfner KP, Craig L, Moncalian G, Zinkel RA, Usui T, Owen BA, et al. The Rad50 zinc-hook is a structure joining Mre11 complexes in DNA recombination and repair. Nature. 2002;418(6897):562–6.
51. Zhou J, Lim CU, Li JJ, Cai L, Zhang Y. The role of NBS1 in the modulation of PIKK family proteins ATM and ATR in the cellular response to DNA damage. Cancer Lett. 2006;243(1):9–15.
52. Lee JH, Paull TT. ATM activation by DNA double-strand breaks through the Mre11-Rad50-Nbs1 complex. Science. 2005;308(5721):551–4.
53. Zhang Y, Zhou J, Lim CU. The role of NBS1 in DNA double strand break repair, telomere stability, and cell cycle checkpoint control. Cell Res. 2006;16(1):45–54.
54. Wolska-Kusnierz B, Gregorek H, Chrzanowska K, Piatosa B, Pietrucha B, Heropolitanska-Pliszka E, et al. Nijmegen breakage syndrome: clinical and immunological features, long-term outcome and treatment options—a retrospective analysis. J Clin Immunol. 2015;35(6):538–49.
55. Piatosa B, van der Burg M, Siewiera K, Pac M, van Dongen JJ, Langerak AW, et al. The defect in humoral immunity in patients with Nijmegen breakage syndrome is explained by defects in peripheral B lymphocyte maturation. Cytometry A. 2012;81(10):835–42.

56. van der Burg M, Pac M, Berkowska MA, Goryluk-Kozakiewicz B, Wakulinska A, Dembowska-Baginska B, et al. Loss of juxtaposition of RAG-induced immunoglobulin DNA ends is implicated in the precursor B-cell differentiation defect in NBS patients. Blood. 2010;115(23):4770–7.
57. Meijers RW, Dzierzanowska-Fangrat K, Zborowska M, Solarska I, Tielemans D, van Turnhout BA, et al. Circulating T cells of patients with Nijmegen breakage syndrome show signs of senescence. J Clin Immunol. 2017;37(2):133–42.
58. Kracker S, Bergmann Y, Demuth I, Frappart PO, Hildebrand G, Christine R, et al. Nibrin functions in Ig class-switch recombination. Proc Natl Acad Sci U S A. 2005;102(5):1584–9.
59. Lahdesmaki A, Taylor AM, Chrzanowska KH, Pan-Hammarstrom Q. Delineation of the role of the Mre11 complex in class switch recombination. J Biol Chem. 2004;279(16):16479–87.
60. Deripapa E, Balashov D, Rodina Y, Laberko A, Myakova N, Davydova NV, et al. Prospective Study of a Cohort of Russian Nijmegen breakage syndrome patients demonstrating predictive value of low kappa-deleting recombination excision circle (KREC) numbers and beneficial effect of hematopoietic stem cell transplantation (HSCT). Front Immunol. 2017;8:807.
61. Pastorczak A, Szczepanski T, Mlynarski W. International Berlin-Frankfurt-Munster ALLhgvwg. Clinical course and therapeutic implications for lymphoid malignancies in Nijmegen breakage syndrome. Eur J Med Genet. 2016;59(3):126–32.
62. Albert MH, Gennery AR, Greil J, Cale CM, Kalwak K, Kondratenko I, et al. Successful SCT for Nijmegen breakage syndrome. Bone Marrow Transplant. 2010;45(4):622–6.
63. Seemanova E, Jarolim P, Seeman P, Varon R, Digweed M, Swift M, et al. Cancer risk of heterozygotes with the NBN founder mutation. J Natl Cancer Inst. 2007;99(24):1875–80.
64. Cybulski C, Gorski B, Debniak T, Gliniewicz B, Mierzejewski M, Masojc B, et al. NBS1 is a prostate cancer susceptibility gene. Cancer Res. 2004;64(4):1215–9.
65. Steffen J, Varon R, Mosor M, Maneva G, Maurer M, Stumm M, et al. Increased cancer risk of heterozygotes with NBS1 germline mutations in Poland. Int J Cancer. 2004;111(1):67–71.
66. Lescale C, Abramowski V, Bedora-Faure M, Murigneux V, Vera G, Roth DB, et al. RAG2 and XLF/Cernunnos interplay reveals a novel role for the RAG complex in DNA repair. Nat Commun. 2016;7:10529.
67. Hammel M, Rey M, Yu Y, Mani RS, Classen S, Liu M, et al. XRCC4 protein interactions with XRCC4-like factor (XLF) create an extended grooved scaffold for DNA ligation and double strand break repair. J Biol Chem. 2011;286(37):32638–50.
68. Soulas-Sprauel P, Le Guyader G, Rivera-Munoz P, Abramowski V, Olivier-Martin C, Goujet-Zalc C, et al. Role for DNA repair factor XRCC4 in immunoglobulin class switch recombination. J Exp Med. 2007;204(7):1717–27.
69. Murray JE, van der Burg M, IJspeert H, Carroll P, Wu Q, Ochi T, et al. Mutations in the NHEJ component XRCC4 cause primordial dwarfism. Am J Hum Genet. 2015;96(3):412–24.
70. Guo C, Nakazawa Y, Woodbine L, Bjorkman A, Shimada M, Fawcett H, et al. XRCC4 deficiency in human subjects causes a marked neurological phenotype but no overt immunodeficiency. J Allergy Clin Immunol. 2015;136(4):1007–17.
71. Riballo E, Critchlow SE, Teo SH, Doherty AJ, Priestley A, Broughton B, et al. Identification of a defect in DNA ligase IV in a radiosensitive leukaemia patient. Curr Biol. 1999;9(13):699–702.
72. van der Burg M, van Veelen LR, Verkaik NS, Wiegant WW, Hartwig NG, Barendregt BH, et al. A new type of radiosensitive T-B-NK+ severe combined immunodeficiency caused by a LIG4 mutation. J Clin Invest. 2006;116(1):137–45.
73. O'Driscoll M, Cerosaletti KM, Girard PM, Dai Y, Stumm M, Kysela B, et al. DNA ligase IV mutations identified in patients exhibiting developmental delay and immunodeficiency. Mol Cell. 2001;8(6):1175–85.
74. IJspeert H, Warris A, van der Flier M, Reisli I, Keles S, Chishimba S, et al. Clinical spectrum of LIG4 deficiency is broadened with severe dysmaturity, primordial dwarfism, and neurological abnormalities. Hum Mutat. 2013;34(12):1611–4.
75. Murray JE, Bicknell LS, Yigit G, Duker AL, van Kogelenberg M, Haghayegh S, et al. Extreme growth failure is a common presentation of ligase IV deficiency. Hum Mutat. 2014;35(1):76–85.

76. Buck D, Malivert L, de Chasseval R, Barraud A, Fondaneche MC, Sanal O, et al. Cernunnos, a novel nonhomologous end-joining factor, is mutated in human immunodeficiency with microcephaly. Cell. 2006;124(2):287–99.
77. IJspeert H, Rozmus J, Schwarz K, Warren RL, van Zessen D, Holt RA, et al. XLF deficiency results in reduced N-nucleotide addition during V(D)J recombination. Blood. 2016;128(5):650–9.
78. Pan-Hammarstrom Q, Jones AM, Lahdesmaki A, Zhou W, Gatti RA, Hammarstrom L, et al. Impact of DNA ligase IV on nonhomologous end joining pathways during class switch recombination in human cells. J Exp Med. 2005;201(2):189–94.
79. Du L, Peng R, Bjorkman A, Filipe de Miranda N, Rosner C, Kotnis A, et al. Cernunnos influences human immunoglobulin class switch recombination and may be associated with B cell lymphomagenesis. J Exp Med. 2012;209(2):291–305.
80. Bacon CM, Wilkinson SJ, Spickett GP, Barge D, Lucraft HH, Jackson G, et al. Epstein-Barr virus-independent diffuse large B-cell lymphoma in DNA ligase 4 deficiency. J Allergy Clin Immunol. 2013;131(4):1237–9, 9 e1
81. Peron S, Metin A, Gardes P, Alyanakian MA, Sheridan E, Kratz CP, et al. Human PMS2 deficiency is associated with impaired immunoglobulin class switch recombination. J Exp Med. 2008;205(11):2465–72.
82. Wimmer K, Kratz CP. Constitutional mismatch repair-deficiency syndrome. Haematologica. 2010;95(5):699–701.

Selective IgA Deficiency

16

K. Sofia Appelberg, Hassan Abolhassani, and Lennart Hammarström

16.1 Definition

IgAD was tentatively shown by Giedion and Scheidegger in 1957 [1], but not formally described until 1963 (in patients with Ataxia Telangiectasia) [2]. Today IgAD is defined as a serum IgA level of ≤0.07 g/L with normal serum level of total IgG and IgM after the age of 4 years [3]. A common observation in IgAD patients is a defect in B-lymphocyte maturation and subsequent IgA production [4–7]. However, since the mechanism(s) involved in IgAD and the pathogenesis of the diseases is not fully known, other defects affecting IgA production, such as impairment of T helper cell function and cytokine production, could also play a role [8–10]. Insufficient production of IgA can also be caused by the use of selected drugs [11, 12] and hepatitis C infection [13]. The latter is often reversible and should, together with other acquired causes of hypogammaglobulinemia, be excluded before a definite diagnosis.

IgAD can occur in different forms (Table 16.1): permanent IgAD, with a constant serum IgA level ≤0.07 g/L [3]; partial IgAD, with a IgA level above 0.07 g/L but 2 standard deviations below the normal, age-matched level [14]; and transient IgAD, where IgA levels normalize after the age of 4 years [15]. Many individuals with IgAD are asymptomatic, but approximately one-third have been shown to display an increased susceptibility to infections, especially in the respiratory and gastrointestinal tracts [16–18]. Allergies and atopic manifestations are also more common in the IgAD population [19], as well as multiple autoimmune disorders such as systemic lupus erythematosus, thyroid disorders, and celiac disease [20, 21]. In some cases IgAD can progress into common variable immunodeficiency (CVID), a more severe form of immunodeficiency [22, 23].

K. Sofia Appelberg · H. Abolhassani · L. Hammarström (✉)
Division of Clinical Immunology, Department of Laboratory Medicine,
Karolinska Institute, Karolinska University Hospital, Stockholm, Sweden
e-mail: Lennart.Hammarstrom@ki.se

M. M. D'Elios, M. Rizzi (eds.), *Humoral Primary Immunodeficiencies*,
Rare Diseases of the Immune System, https://doi.org/10.1007/978-3-319-91785-6_16

Table 16.1 Different forms of IgA deficiency based on levels and development of IgA

Type of IgAD	Diagnostic criteria	References
Permanent IgAD	Serum IgA levels constantly below 0.07 g/L	[3]
Partial IgAD	IgA level over 0.07 g/L but 2 standard deviations below normal, age-matched means	[14]
Transient IgAD	Serum IgA levels normalize after the age of 4 years	[15]

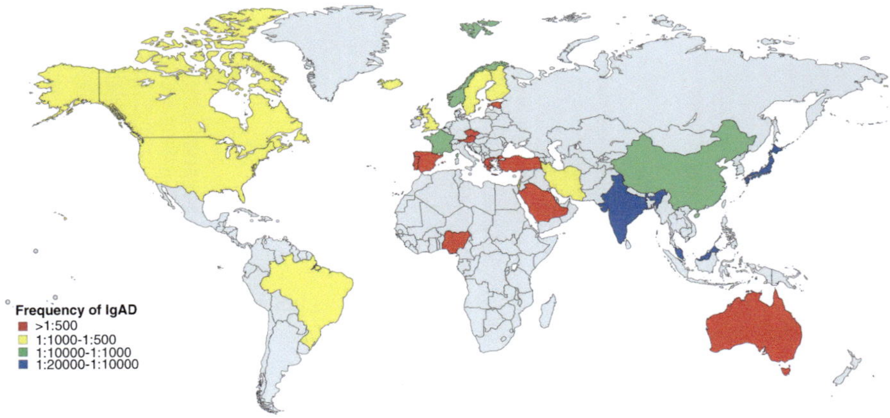

Fig. 16.1 Frequency of IgA deficiency in normal populations across the world. The map has been made based on the data extracted from repots of following countries: Austria [126, 127], the USA [128–130], France [131, 132], Spain [133], China [134, 135], Sweden [136], Japan [26], Canada [137], Nigeria [138], Australia [139], Iran [140], Saudi Arabia [25], Norway [141, 142], Finland [143], Czech [144], Turkey [30], Brazil [145, 146], Iceland [147], Estonia [148], Lithuania [149], Greece [150, 151], India [152], Israel [153], Portugal [154], Malaysia [155], and the UK [156, 157]. Figure used and updated by permission from Yazdani et al. [158]

16.2 Epidemiology

IgAD affects both males and females equally, but the frequency of the disorder varies between ethnic groups. The occurrence of IgAD in the Caucasian population is 1:600 [24], while the lowest incidence, 1:18,550, is found in East Asia and the highest, 1:142, in Saudi Arabia [25–27] (Fig. 16.1). In addition to ethnicity, family relations also affect the occurrence of IgAD. Observations of familial clustering provide evidence for genetic predisposition for IgAD, and family history of IgAD or common variable immunodeficiency is the most significant risk factor for having IgAD [28, 29].

Due to the transient form of the disease and the fact that in some individuals normal IgA levels are not reached until the age of 10 [15], the prevalence of IgAD in the pediatric population is higher than in adults [30].

16.3 Physiology of IgA and Pathogenesis of IgAD

IgA is the predominant immunoglobulin class in the body with a total production of IgA around 40–60 mg/kg per day compared to the second most produced antibody isotype, IgG, with a total production of 30 mg/kg per day [31, 32]. Most of the IgA is produced and secreted by plasma cells in the gastrointestinal tract [33, 34]. Thus, IgA is critical for mucosal immunity and maintenance of the intestinal microbial homeostasis. Binding to IgA leads to neutralization and prevention of adhesion and penetration of toxins and microbes through the mucosa [34–38]. IgA can also activate the complement system via the lectin pathway by binding of mannan-binding lectin, as well as enhance phagocytosis of IgA-antigen complex via interaction with Fcα receptors (CD89) on phagocytes [39, 40].

Due to an immature immune system, newborns show low immunoglobulin levels but are protected by maternal IgG and IgA transferred via placenta and breast milk [41–43]. Secreted IgA can be found in tears or nasal secretion from infants as early as day 10–20 after birth [44, 45]. However, serum IgA is almost undetectable at birth, and normal levels of serum IgA are reached around the age of 4. In some individuals it may take as long as 10–15 years to reach normal serum IgA levels [15]. IgA delivery by breast milk is not only important for passive immunity but also for immunomodulation and shaping of the gut microbiota [43, 46]. IgA is crucial for regulation of our bacterial flora throughout life, and there is a significant difference in the bacterial composition in fecal samples from IgAD patients compared with individuals producing normal levels of IgA.

From our understanding of the mechanisms involved in IgA production, IgAD may result from impaired IgA class switching or failure of maturation of IgA-producing B-lymphocytes. Therefore, impairment of signaling pathways involved in B cell maturation, cytokine and immunoglobulin production, and apoptosis have all been suggested to cause IgAD [10, 47, 48]. However, the true pathogenesis of IgAD is still unknown, and there might be varying underlying etiologies in different patients.

16.3.1 Genetic Basis of IgAD

The majority of IgAD cases occur sporadically, but reports show increased frequency of primary antibody deficiencies in first-degree relatives (i.e., siblings, twins, parents, and offspring) is a strong indicator for the involvement of genetic components in IgAD [28, 49]. The relative risk for siblings of IgAD patients to be affected is 50 times higher compared to siblings of healthy individuals [28], and the frequency of IgAD in monozygotic and dizygotic twins is increased as well (1:241 and 1:198, respectively, compared to 1:600 in the normal Caucasian population) [50].

Genetic linkage analysis has identified a susceptibility locus on chromosome 6, within the major histocompatibility complex (MHC) region [51, 52] (Table 16.2), and studies on multiple-affected families with IgAD (and CVID) have shown an increased MHC haplotype sharing [29]. More detailed genetic analyses have shown that the ancestral human leukocyte antigen (HLA)-A1, B8, DR3, and DQ2 (8.1) haplotype is strongly associated with disease development [53, 54]. Interestingly, while some MHC haplotypes mediate susceptibility to IgAD, others are linked to disease resistance [55].

In addition, non-MHC genes, such as interferon-induced helicase 1 (*IFIH1*) and C-type lectin domain family 16, member A (*CLEC16A*), have also been associated with IgAD [56, 57]. Recent genome-wide association studies have shown linkage to IgAD of additional genes, including *CTLA4*, *ICOS*, *PVT1*, *ATG13-AMBRA1*, and *AHI1* (Table 16.2) [56–58].

The genetic background to IgAD is complex, and there is not an apparent mode of inheritance or cause. Development of IgAD may require the presence of predisposing gene(s) in combination with as yet unknown triggering factors.

Table 16.2 Genes associated with IgA deficiency

Region	Genes/alleles	Nature of association	References
MHC-*associated genes*			
MHC class I	A1, A28, B8, B14, B44	Susceptibility	[49, 110–114]
	HLA-B*0801	Susceptibility	
	HLA-B*1402	Susceptibility	
MHC class II	DR1, DR3, DR7	Susceptibility	[52, 55, 111, 115–120]
	HLA-DQB1*02	Susceptibility	
	DRB1*0102	Susceptibility	
	DRB1*0301	Susceptibility	
	DRB1*0701	Susceptibility	
	DQB1*05	Susceptibility	
	BTNL2-HLA-DRA	Susceptibility	
	HLA-DQB1	Susceptibility	
	DRB1*1501	Protective	
MHC class III	*C2* (complement factor 2)	Susceptibility	[116, 121–123]
	C4A (complement factor 4A)	Susceptibility	
	CYP21A2	Susceptibility	
Non-MHC associated genes			
Chromosome 2q	*IFIH1*	Protective	[56, 57]
	CTLA4, ICOS	Susceptibility	[58]
Chromosome 8q	*PVT1*	Protective	[56, 57]
Chromosome 6q	*AHI1*	Susceptibility	[57]
Chromosome 11p	*ATG13-AMBRA1*	Susceptibility	[57]
Chromosome 16p	*CLEC16A*	Protective	[56, 57]
Chromosome 17q	*TNFRSF13B*	Susceptibility	[124, 125]

16.3.2 Cytokine Stimulation, IgA Production, and IgAD

The primary site of IgA production is the gut mucosal tissue where switching to IgA is the result of cytokines, including Transforming growth factor beta (TGF-β), B cell-activating factor (BAFF), and a proliferation-inducing ligand (APRIL), locally produced by epithelial cells, dendritic cells, regulatory T cells, and RORγt-positive innate lymphoid cells located in the mucosa associated lymph nodes and in the lamina propria [59–61]. Furthermore, cytokines, such as interleukin (IL)-4, IL-6, IL-7, IL-10, and, most recent, IL-21, have been found to affect IgA production [8–10, 62]. These results indicate a role for different cytokines in IgA production and potential defects in their signaling pathways in the pathogenesis of IgAD. In line with this notion, we recently described cytokine-induced IgA production in both IgAD patients and healthy controls where stimulation of peripheral blood mononuclear cells (PBMCs) with CD40 ligand (CD40L) and IL-21 induces enhanced IgA production. IgA levels in IgAD patients are on average 10% of the levels seen in healthy controls [10]. The importance of IL-21 in IgA production, and especially intestinal IgA production, has also been demonstrated in a mouse model. Mice lacking IL-21 show impaired IgA production, while IL-21 stimulation of intestinal mouse cells increased B cell differentiation and IgA class switching by inducing TGF-β and promoted B cells migration by increasing $\alpha_4\beta_7$ expression [63].

While interactions between T- and B-lymphocytes via CD40L and CD40 are necessary for T cell-dependent antibody production and class-switch recombination, BAFF and APRIL, two molecules belonging to the tumor necrosis factor (TNF)-family [64], play a role in CD40L- and T cell-independent immunoglobulin production [65–67]. BAFF and APRIL are primarily produced by innate immune cells [68], T cells and activated B cells [69, 70]. They share receptors binding to B cell maturation antigen (BCMA or TNFRSF17) and transmembrane activator and calcium modulator and cyclophilin ligand interactor (TACI or TNFRSF13B) [71]. In addition, BAFF can bind to the BAFF receptor (BAFFR, BR3, or TNFRSF13C) [71]. These three different receptors are mainly expressed on B cells [72, 73].

The importance of APRIL and BAFF in IgA class switching has been demonstrated in several studies. In APRIL-deficient mice, B and T cell development is normal, but the IgA response is significantly impaired [60, 74]. The receptors responsible for IgA isotype switching are TACI and BAFFR with TACI being the most important [67]. Stimulation of human peripheral B cells with APRIL or BAFF in combination with different cytokines (e.g., IL-10 or TGFβ) and/or Toll-like receptor (TLR) ligands (e.g., flagellin) results in increased IgA class switching and IgA secretion compared with APRIL or BAFF stimulation alone [65, 67, 75, 76]. APRIL and BAFF are thus suggested to provide an important link between the innate and adaptive immune responses due to their role in T cell-independent IgA production. Intestinal epithelial cells and dendritic cells in the intestinal mucosa stimulated by TLR ligands or interferons increase their production of APRIL and BAFF, which subsequently leads to an increased IgA production [65, 75].

16.4 Clinical Features

IgAD is generally considered to be a mild disorder. This is due to the fact that most patients are clinically asymptomatic and discovered when they volunteer as blood donors or seek medical attention for other diseases [77]. Why so many IgAD patients are asymptomatic is not fully understood. Even though individuals with IgAD produce IgM, IgD, IgG, and IgE, these antibody classes do not fully replace IgA functionally in the respiratory [19, 78] and gastrointestinal [79] tracts, so the theory of a compensatory mechanism is not completely convincing. In addition, some IgAD patients present symptoms, which vary from minor infections to more severe complications such as autoimmune disorders or progression to common variable immunodeficiency [21, 22]. The absence or presence of symptoms, as well as the differences in the severity of the symptoms, results in a very heterogeneous phenotype in IgAD.

Several studies have also demonstrated different types of allergy associated with IgAD, including allergic conjunctivitis, rhinitis, urticaria, eczema, food allergy, and asthma [18, 19, 77, 80]. In addition, the risk for chronic complications and permanent sequels (e.g., nodular lymphoid hyperplasia, bronchiectasis, and impaired lung function) increases with age in IgAD patients [81–83]. Predisposition to allergic disorders in IgAD individuals may be due to impaired clearance of dietary/environmental antigens at mucosal sites, causing an increased permeability of macromolecules and proteins into the circulation, thereby facilitating antibody production [84, 85].

The prevalence of autoimmunity in IgAD patients is markedly increased and ranges from 7 to 36% in the symptomatic IgAD population compared with 3–5% in the general population [21, 77]. Systemic lupus erythematosus, type 1 diabetes, thyroid disorders, and rheumatoid arthritis are example of autoimmune disorders associated with IgAD [21, 86–88].

Anti-IgA antibodies of the IgG class have been observed in 24–32% of IgAD patients [89]. The mechanism behind the production of anti-IgA antibodies is unknown since it occurs without known exposure to immunoglobulin or other blood products including IgA. One hypothesis is that the anti-IgA is produced against a protein/epitope expressed on intestinal bacteria that structurally mimic IgA. The concern of anti-IgA antibodies in blood transfusions and the potential involvement in anaphylactoid transfusion reactions is debated. While some conclude that anti-IgA cause anaphylactoid reactions and IgAD patients should therefore only receive blood/blood products from IgAD donors [90, 91], others suggest that it is not proven that anti-IgA antibodies are the cause of anaphylactoid reactions [92, 93].

Severe forms and allergy clinical phenotypes tend to occur during childhood, while mild infections and autoimmunity are usually diagnosed during middle age. Of note, it is possible that during the course of disease, asymptomatic IgAD develops into symptomatic phenotypes and patients with an initial minor infection phenotype may progress to show allergy, autoimmunity, and/or other severe phenotypes.

16.5 Diagnosis and Laboratory Features

Since the hallmark for IgAD is low or undetectable serum IgA with normal levels of IgM and IgG, immunoglobulin measurements are the standard for diagnosis of the disease. With the possibility of both progression and reversal of the disease, regular evaluation of IgA, IgM, and IgG levels could be suggested for IgAD patients to monitor the disease, especially in individuals with recurrent infections, allergic manifestation, or autoimmunity. It should be noted though that abnormalities in IgG production, with both increased and decreased levels, have been observed in IgAD patients [16, 94]. IgAD is occasionally combined with the lack of IgG2, and in these individuals the prevalence of infections is enhanced [95]. In addition, patients with IgA and IgG2 deficiency are also more likely to produce anti-IgA antibodies [96].

Elevated cytokine plasma levels (e.g., IFNγ, TNFα, IL-2, and IL-10) in IgAD patients with autoimmunity have been reported [97]. Furthermore, a significant decrease in regulatory T cells (T_{reg}) compared to healthy controls has been observed in IgAD patients and particularly those with chronic inflammation [98]. Reduction in the proportion of switched memory B cells ($CD19^{+}CD27^{+}IgD^{-}$) and lower levels of IgG have been associated with IgAD in combination with autoimmunity and increased frequency of pneumonia [99].

16.6 Management and Treatment

Management of IgAD is determined by the clinical symptoms of the patient, and there is no specific curative treatment. For asymptomatic patients, generally, no therapeutic intervention is needed, except possibly considering IgA-free blood components at blood transfusion to prevent potential anaphylactic reactions due to anti-IgA antibodies. Asymptomatic children as well as adults may be monitored for changes in their IgA levels and informed about the risks of developing allergies/autoimmunity [19]. Minor bacterial infections in IgAD patients should be treated with antibiotics just as in healthy individuals, and in IgAD patients with atopic symptoms, common treatments for allergy could be applied.

In cases of IgAD and autoimmune disorders, IgA antibody-based assays for diagnosis of the autoimmune disease can obviously not be used, since it will give a false-negative result. However, IgG-based tests or pathological investigation (gastrointestinal biopsies) provides alternative approaches [100, 101].

In the cases where it is needed, the primary treatment for IgAD is prophylactic use of antibiotics and/or immunoglobulin therapy [102–104]. In case of progression to common variable immunodeficiency or addition of IgG subclass deficiency, immunoglobulin replacement could be used as treatment, preferably using an immunoglobulin brand with a low IgA concentration. Immunoglobulin therapy has shown to decrease the incidence of infections in IgAD patients, and with subcutaneous administration, no severe reactions due to anti-IgA antibodies have been observed [103, 104].

The induction of IgA production after CD40L stimulation in combination with different cytokines [10, 105, 106] has opened up a novel avenue for the development of a potential treatment where administration of CD40L and specific cytokines could become a new therapy for IgAD.

16.7 Summary

Individuals with IgA deficiency have an increased risk of death the first 10–15 years after diagnosis compared to the general population [107]. Additionally, they also feel an enhanced fear of contracting infections compared with healthy individuals, which significantly correlate with a poorer physical health [108, 109]. There is also a difference between asymptomatic and symptomatic IgAD patients when it comes to health-related quality of life (HRQL). Based on both physical and mental components, the HRQL is significantly reduced in the symptomatic IgAD population, even if the phenotype is mild (e.g., infections and/or allergies). Based on these studies, IgAD significantly affects the patients HRQL in a negative way. Therefore, it is important to continue the research investigating the pathogenesis of IgAD and the underlying genetic defect(s) or environmental risk factor(s). By increasing our understanding and knowledge regarding the disease clinical prognosis, management and treatment strategies can be improved.

References

1. Giedion A, Scheidegger JJ. Congenital immunological paresis in the absence of specific beta 2-globulin & normal quantities of gamma-globulin. Helv Paediatr Acta. 1957;12(3):241–59.
2. Gutmann L, Lemli L. Ataxia-telangiectasia associated with hypogammaglobulinemia. Arch Neurol. 1963;8:318–27.
3. Primary Immunodeficiency Diseases. Report of an IUIS Scientific Committee. International Union of Immunological Societies. Clin Exp Immunol. 1999;118(Suppl 1):1–28.
4. Wang Z, Yunis D, Irigoyen M, Kitchens B, Bottaro A, Alt FW, et al. Discordance between IgA switching at the DNA level and IgA expression at the mRNA level in IgA-deficient patients. Clin Immunol. 1999;91(3):263–70. https://doi.org/10.1006/clim.1999.4702.
5. Suzuki H, Kaneko H, Fukao T, Jin R, Kawamoto N, Asano T, et al. Various expression patterns of alpha1 and alpha2 genes in IgA deficiency. Allergol Int. 2009;58(1):111–7.
6. Conley ME, Cooper MD. Immature IgA B cells in IgA-deficient patients. N Engl J Med. 1981;305(9):495–7.
7. Lawton AR, Royal SA, Self KS, Cooper MD. IgA determinants on B-lymphocytes in patients with deficiency of circulating IgA. J Lab Clin Med. 1972;80(1):26–33.
8. Ramsay AJ, Husband AJ, Ramshaw IA, Bao S, Matthaei KI, Koehler G, et al. The role of interleukin-6 in mucosal IgA antibody responses in vivo. Science. 1994;264(5158):561–3.
9. Okahashi N, Yamamoto M, Vancott JL, Chatfield SN, Roberts M, Bluethmann H, et al. Oral immunization of interleukin-4 (IL-4) knockout mice with a recombinant Salmonella strain or cholera toxin reveals that CD4+ Th2 cells producing IL-6 and IL-10 are associated with mucosal immunoglobulin A responses. Infect Immun. 1996;64(5):1516–25.
10. Borte S, Pan-Hammarstrom Q, Liu C, Sack U, Borte M, Wagner U, et al. Interleukin-21 restores immunoglobulin production ex vivo in patients with common variable immunodeficiency and selective IgA deficiency. Blood. 2009;114(19):4089–98.

11. Farr M, Struthers GR, Scott DG, Bacon PA. Fenclofenac-induced selective IgA deficiency in rheumatoid arthritis. Br J Rheumatol. 1985;24(4):367–9.
12. Matsuoka H, Okada J, Takahashi T, Matsuoka M, Sato C, Torii S. Immunological study of IgA deficiency during anticonvulsant therapy in epileptic patients. Clin Exp Immunol. 1983;53(2):423–8.
13. Ilan Y, Shouval D, Ashur Y, Manns M, Naparstek Y. IgA deficiency associated with chronic hepatitis C virus infection. A cause or an effect? Arch Intern Med. 1993;153(13):1588–92.
14. Latiff AH, Kerr MA. The clinical significance of immunoglobulin A deficiency. Ann Clin Biochem. 2007;44(Pt 2):131–9. https://doi.org/10.1258/000456307780117993.
15. Lim CK, Dahle C, Elvin K, Andersson BA, Ronnelid J, Melen E, et al. Reversal of immunoglobulin A deficiency in children. J Clin Immunol. 2015;35(1):87–91.
16. Ammann AJ, Hong R. Selective IgA deficiency: presentation of 30 cases and a review of the literature. Medicine (Baltimore). 1971;50(3):223–36.
17. Edwards E, Razvi S, Cunningham-Rundles C. IgA deficiency: clinical correlates and responses to pneumococcal vaccine. Clin Immunol. 2004;111(1):93–7.
18. Janzi M, Kull I, Sjoberg R, Wan J, Melen E, Bayat N, et al. Selective IgA deficiency in early life: association to infections and allergic diseases during childhood. Clin Immunol. 2009;133(1):78–85.
19. Jorgensen GH, Gardulf A, Sigurdsson MI, Sigurdardottir ST, Thorsteinsdottir I, Gudmundsson S, et al. Clinical symptoms in adults with selective IgA deficiency: a case-control study. J Clin Immunol. 2013;33(4):742–7.
20. Jesus AA, Liphaus BL, Silva CA, Bando SY, Andrade LE, Coutinho A, et al. Complement and antibody primary immunodeficiency in juvenile systemic lupus erythematosus patients. Lupus. 2011;20(12):1275–84.
21. Wang N, Shen N, Vyse TJ, Anand V, Gunnarson I, Sturfelt G, et al. Selective IgA deficiency in autoimmune diseases. Mol Med. 2011;17(11–12):1383–96.
22. Aghamohammadi A, Mohammadi J, Parvaneh N, Rezaei N, Moin M, Espanol T, et al. Progression of selective IgA deficiency to common variable immunodeficiency. Int Arch Allergy Immunol. 2008;147(2):87–92.
23. Hammarstrom L, Vorechovsky I, Webster D. Selective IgA deficiency (SIgAD) and common variable immunodeficiency (CVID). Clin Exp Immunol. 2000;120(2):225–31.
24. Primary Immunodeficiency Diseases. Report of a WHO scientific group. Clin Exp Immunol. 1997;109(Suppl 1):1–28.
25. al-Attas RA, Rahi AH. Primary antibody deficiency in Arabs: first report from eastern Saudi Arabia. J Clin Immunol. 1998;18(5):368–71.
26. Kanoh T, Mizumoto T, Yasuda N, Koya M, Ohno Y, Uchino H, et al. Selective IgA deficiency in Japanese blood donors: frequency and statistical analysis. Vox Sang. 1986;50(2):81–6.
27. Schaffer FM, Monteiro RC, Volanakis JE, Cooper MD. IgA deficiency. Immunodefic Rev. 1991;3(1):15–44.
28. Vorechovsky I, Zetterquist H, Paganelli R, Koskinen S, Webster AD, Bjorkander J, et al. Family and linkage study of selective IgA deficiency and common variable immunodeficiency. Clin Immunol Immunopathol. 1995;77(2):185–92.
29. Vorechovsky I, Webster AD, Plebani A, Hammarstrom L. Genetic linkage of IgA deficiency to the major histocompatibility complex: evidence for allele segregation distortion, parent-of-origin penetrance differences, and the role of anti-IgA antibodies in disease predisposition. Am J Hum Genet. 1999;64(4):1096–109.
30. Basturk B, Sari S, Aral A, Dalgic B. Prevalence of selective immunoglobulin A deficiency in healthy Turkish school children. Turk J Pediatr. 2011;53(4):364–8.
31. Conley ME, Delacroix DL. Intravascular and mucosal immunoglobulin A: two separate but related systems of immune defense? Ann Intern Med. 1987;106(6):892–9.
32. Fagarasan S, Honjo T. Intestinal IgA synthesis: regulation of front-line body defences. Nat Rev Immunol. 2003;3(1):63–72.
33. Brandtzaeg P, Johansen FE. Mucosal B cells: phenotypic characteristics, transcriptional regulation, and homing properties. Immunol Rev. 2005;206:32–63.

34. Gommerman JL, Rojas OL, Fritz JH. Re-thinking the functions of IgA(+) plasma cells. Gut Microbes. 2014;5(5):652–62.
35. Mantis NJ, Rol N, Corthesy B. Secretory IgA's complex roles in immunity and mucosal homeostasis in the gut. Mucosal Immunol. 2011;4(6):603–11.
36. Helander A, Miller CL, Myers KS, Neutra MR, Nibert ML. Protective immunoglobulin A and G antibodies bind to overlapping intersubunit epitopes in the head domain of type 1 reovirus adhesin sigma1. J Virol. 2004;78(19):10695–705.
37. Apter FM, Lencer WI, Finkelstein RA, Mekalanos JJ, Neutra MR. Monoclonal immunoglobulin A antibodies directed against cholera toxin prevent the toxin-induced chloride secretory response and block toxin binding to intestinal epithelial cells in vitro. Infect Immun. 1993;61(12):5271–8.
38. Mathias A, Pais B, Favre L, Benyacoub J, Corthesy B. Role of secretory IgA in the mucosal sensing of commensal bacteria. Gut Microbes. 2014;5(6):688–95.
39. Roos A, Bouwman LH, van Gijlswijk-Janssen DJ, Faber-Krol MC, Stahl GL, Daha MR. Human IgA activates the complement system via the mannan-binding lectin pathway. J Immunol. 2001;167(5):2861–8.
40. Monteiro RC, Van De Winkel JG. IgA Fc receptors. Annu Rev Immunol. 2003;21:177–204.
41. Simister NE. Placental transport of immunoglobulin G. Vaccine. 2003;21(24):3365–9.
42. Hurley WL, Theil PK. Perspectives on immunoglobulins in colostrum and milk. Nutrients. 2011;3(4):442–74.
43. Munblit D, Sheth S, Abrol P, Treneva M, Peroni DG, Chow LY, et al. Exposures influencing total IgA level in colostrum. J Dev Orig Health Dis. 2016;7(1):61–7.
44. McKay E, Thom H. Observations on neonatal tears. J Pediatr. 1969;75(6):1245–56.
45. Cohen AB, Goldberg S, London RL. Immunoglobulins in nasal secretions of infants. Clin Exp Immunol. 1970;6(5):753–60.
46. Sutherland DB, Fagarasan S. IgA synthesis: a form of functional immune adaptation extending beyond gut. Curr Opin Immunol. 2012;24(3):261–8.
47. Husain Z, Holodick N, Day C, Szymanski I, Alper CA. Increased apoptosis of CD20+ IgA + B cells is the basis for IgA deficiency: the molecular mechanism for correction in vitro by IL-10 and CD40L. J Clin Immunol. 2006;26(2):113–25.
48. Yazdani R, Fatholahi M, Ganjalikhani-Hakemi M, Abolhassani H, Azizi G, Hamid KM, et al. Role of apoptosis in common variable immunodeficiency and selective immunoglobulin A deficiency. Mol Immunol. 2016;71:1–9.
49. Oen K, Petty RE, Schroeder ML. Immunoglobulin A deficiency: genetic studies. Tissue Antigens. 1982;19(3):174–82.
50. Frankowiack M, Kovanen RM, Repasky GA, Lim CK, Song C, Pedersen NL, et al. The higher frequency of IgA deficiency among Swedish twins is not explained by HLA haplotypes. Genes Immun. 2015;16(3):199–205.
51. Schroeder HW Jr. Genetics of IgA deficiency and common variable immunodeficiency. Clin Rev Allergy Immunol. 2000;19(2):127–40.
52. Schroeder HW Jr, Zhu ZB, March RE, Campbell RD, Berney SM, Nedospasov SA, et al. Susceptibility locus for IgA deficiency and common variable immunodeficiency in the HLA-DR3, -B8, −A1 haplotypes. Mol Med. 1998;4(2):72–86.
53. Kralovicova J, Hammarstrom L, Plebani A, Webster AD, Vorechovsky I. Fine-scale mapping at IGAD1 and genome-wide genetic linkage analysis implicate HLA-DQ/DR as a major susceptibility locus in selective IgA deficiency and common variable immunodeficiency. J Immunol. 2003;170(5):2765–75.
54. Mohammadi J, Ramanujam R, Jarefors S, Rezaei N, Aghamohammadi A, Gregersen PK, et al. IgA deficiency and the MHC: assessment of relative risk and microheterogeneity within the HLA A1 B8, DR3 (8.1) haplotype. J Clin Immunol. 2010;30(1):138–43.
55. Olerup O, Smith CI, Hammarstrom L. Different amino acids at position 57 of the HLA-DQ beta chain associated with susceptibility and resistance to IgA deficiency. Nature. 1990;347(6290):289–90.

56. Ferreira RC, Pan-Hammarstrom Q, Graham RR, Gateva V, Fontan G, Lee AT, et al. Association of IFIH1 and other autoimmunity risk alleles with selective IgA deficiency. Nat Genet. 2010;42(9):777–80.
57. Bronson PG, Chang D, Bhangale T, Seldin MF, Ortmann W, Ferreira RC, et al. Common variants at PVT1, ATG13-AMBRA1, AHI1 and CLEC16A are associated with selective IgA deficiency. Nat Genet. 2016;48(11):1425–9.
58. Haimila K, Einarsdottir E, de Kauwe A, Koskinen LL, Pan-Hammarstrom Q, Kaartinen T, et al. The shared CTLA4-ICOS risk locus in celiac disease, IgA deficiency and common variable immunodeficiency. Genes Immun. 2009;10(2):151–61.
59. Reboldi A, Cyster JG. Peyer's patches: organizing B-cell responses at the intestinal frontier. Immunol Rev. 2016;271(1):230–45.
60. Castigli E, Scott S, Dedeoglu F, Bryce P, Jabara H, Bhan AK, et al. Impaired IgA class switching in APRIL-deficient mice. Proc Natl Acad Sci U S A. 2004;101(11):3903–8.
61. Reboldi A, Arnon TI, Rodda LB, Atakilit A, Sheppard D, Cyster JG. IgA production requires B cell interaction with subepithelial dendritic cells in Peyer's patches. Science. 2016;352(6287):aaf4822.
62. Cunningham-Rundles C. Physiology of IgA and IgA deficiency. J Clin Immunol. 2001;21(5):303–9.
63. Cao AT, Yao S, Gong B, Nurieva RI, Elson CO, Cong Y. Interleukin (IL)-21 promotes intestinal IgA response to microbiota. Mucosal Immunol. 2015;8(5):1072–82.
64. Mackay F, Schneider P. Cracking the BAFF code. Nat Rev Immunol. 2009;9(7):491–502.
65. Litinskiy MB, Nardelli B, Hilbert DM, He B, Schaffer A, Casali P, et al. DCs induce CD40-independent immunoglobulin class switching through BLyS and APRIL. Nat Immunol. 2002;3(9):822–9.
66. Bergqvist P, Gardby E, Stensson A, Bemark M, Lycke NY. Gut IgA class switch recombination in the absence of CD40 does not occur in the Lamina Propria and is independent of germinal centers. J Immunol. 2006;177(11):7772–83.
67. Castigli E, Wilson SA, Scott S, Dedeoglu F, Xu S, Lam KP, et al. TACI and BAFF-R mediate isotype switching in B cells. J Exp Med. 2005;201(1):35–9.
68. Cerutti A, Rescigno M. The biology of intestinal immunoglobulin A responses. Immunity. 2008;28(6):740–50.
69. Mackay F, Leung H. The role of the BAFF/APRIL system on T cell function. Semin Immunol. 2006;18(5):284–9.
70. Chu VT, Enghard P, Riemekasten G, Berek C. In vitro and in vivo activation induces BAFF and APRIL expression in B cells. J Immunol. 2007;179(9):5947–57.
71. Bossen C, Schneider P. BAFF, APRIL and their receptors: structure, function and signaling. Semin Immunol. 2006;18(5):263–75.
72. Ng LG, Sutherland AP, Newton R, Qian F, Cachero TG, Scott ML, et al. B cell-activating factor belonging to the TNF family (BAFF)-R is the principal BAFF receptor facilitating BAFF costimulation of circulating T and B cells. J Immunol. 2004;173(2):807–17.
73. Darce JR, Arendt BK, Wu X, Jelinek DF. Regulated expression of BAFF-binding receptors during human B cell differentiation. J Immunol. 2007;179(11):7276–86.
74. Hardenberg G, van Bostelen L, Hahne M, Medema JP. Thymus-independent class switch recombination is affected by APRIL. Immunol Cell Biol. 2008;86(6):530–4.
75. He B, Xu W, Santini PA, Polydorides AD, Chiu A, Estrella J, et al. Intestinal bacteria trigger T cell-independent immunoglobulin A(2) class switching by inducing epithelial-cell secretion of the cytokine APRIL. Immunity. 2007;26(6):812–26.
76. Xu W, He B, Chiu A, Chadburn A, Shan M, Buldys M, et al. Epithelial cells trigger frontline immunoglobulin class switching through a pathway regulated by the inhibitor SLPI. Nat Immunol. 2007;8(3):294–303.
77. Aghamohammadi A, Cheraghi T, Gharagozlou M, Movahedi M, Rezaei N, Yeganeh M, et al. IgA deficiency: correlation between clinical and immunological phenotypes. J Clin Immunol. 2009;29(1):130–6.

78. Brandtzaeg P, Karlsson G, Hansson G, Petruson B, Bjorkander J, Hanson LA. The clinical condition of IgA-deficient patients is related to the proportion of IgD- and IgM-producing cells in their nasal mucosa. Clin Exp Immunol. 1987;67(3):626–36.
79. Richman LK, Brown WR. Immunochemical characterization of IgM in human intestinal fluids. J Immunol. 1977;119(4):1515–9.
80. Sloper KS, Brook CG, Kingston D, Pearson JR, Shiner M. Eczema and atopy in early childhood: low IgA plasma cell counts in the jejunal mucosa. Arch Dis Child. 1981;56(12):939–42.
81. Bjorkander J, Bake B, Oxelius VA, Hanson LA. Impaired lung function in patients with IgA deficiency and low levels of IgG2 or IgG3. N Engl J Med. 1985;313(12):720–4.
82. Stead A, Douglas JG, Broadfoot CJ, Kaminski ER, Herriot R. Humoral immunity and bronchiectasis. Clin Exp Immunol. 2002;130(2):325–30.
83. Vendrell M, de Gracia J, Rodrigo MJ, Cruz MJ, Alvarez A, Garcia M, et al. Antibody production deficiency with normal IgG levels in bronchiectasis of unknown etiology. Chest. 2005;127(1):197–204.
84. McNabb PC, Tomasi TB. Host defense mechanisms at mucosal surfaces. Annu Rev Microbiol. 1981;35:477–96.
85. Allardyce RA, Bienenstock J. The mucosal immune system in health and disease, with an emphasis on parasitic infection. Bull World Health Organ. 1984;62(1):7–25.
86. Mantovani AP, Monclaro MP, Skare TL. Prevalence of IgA deficiency in adult systemic lupus erythematosus and the study of the association with its clinical and autoantibody profiles. Rev Bras Reumatol. 2010;50(3):273–82.
87. Cerutti F, Urbino A, Sacchetti C, Palomba E, Zoppo M, Tovo PA. Selective IgA deficiency in juvenile-onset insulin-dependent diabetes mellitus. Pediatr Med Chir. 1988;10(2):197–201.
88. Chow MA, Lebwohl B, Reilly NR, Green PH. Immunoglobulin A deficiency in celiac disease. J Clin Gastroenterol. 2012;46(10):850–4.
89. Rachid R, Bonilla FA. The role of anti-IgA antibodies in causing adverse reactions to gamma globulin infusion in immunodeficient patients: a comprehensive review of the literature. J Allergy Clin Immunol. 2012;129(3):628–34.
90. Vyas GN, Perkins HA, Fudenberg HH. Anaphylactoid transfusion reactions associated with anti-IgA. Lancet. 1968;2(7563):312–5.
91. Laschinger C, Shepherd FA, Naylor DH. Anti-IgA-mediated transfusion reactions in Canada. Can Med Assoc J. 1984;130(2):141–4.
92. Sandler SG, Eder AF, Goldman M, Winters JL. The entity of immunoglobulin A-related anaphylactic transfusion reactions is not evidence based. Transfusion. 2015;55(1):199–204.
93. Sandler SG, Mallory D, Malamut D, Eckrich R. IgA anaphylactic transfusion reactions. Transfus Med Rev. 1995;9(1):1–8.
94. Hammarstrom L, Persson MA, Smith CI. Immunoglobulin subclass distribution of human anti-carbohydrate antibodies: aberrant pattern in IgA-deficient donors. Immunology. 1985;54(4):821–6.
95. Aittoniemi J, Koskinen S, Laippala P, Laine S, Miettinen A. The significance of IgG subclasses and mannan-binding lectin (MBL) for susceptibility to infection in apparently healthy adults with IgA deficiency. Clin Exp Immunol. 1999;116(3):505–8.
96. Ferreira A, Garcia Rodriguez MC, Lopez-Trascasa M, Pascual Salcedo D, Fontan G. Anti-IgA antibodies in selective IgA deficiency and in primary immunodeficient patients treated with gamma-globulin. Clin Immunol Immunopathol. 1988;47(2):199–207.
97. Kowalczyk D, Mytar B, Zembala M. Cytokine production in transient hypogammaglobulinemia and isolated IgA deficiency. J Allergy Clin Immunol. 1997;100(4):556–62.
98. Soheili H, Abolhassani H, Arandi N, Khazaei HA, Shahinpour S, Hirbod-Mobarakeh A, et al. Evaluation of natural regulatory T cells in subjects with selective IgA deficiency: from senior idea to novel opportunities. Int Arch Allergy Immunol. 2013;160(2):208–14.
99. Aghamohammadi A, Abolhassani H, Biglari M, Abolmaali S, Moazzami K, Tabatabaeiyan M, et al. Analysis of switched memory B cells in patients with IgA deficiency. Int Arch Allergy Immunol. 2011;156(4):462–8.

100. Cataldo F, Marino V, Ventura A, Bottaro G, Corazza GR. Prevalence and clinical features of selective immunoglobulin A deficiency in coeliac disease: an Italian multicentre study. Italian Society of Paediatric Gastroenterology and Hepatology (SIGEP) and "Club del Tenue" Working Groups on Coeliac Disease. Gut. 1998;42(3):362–5.
101. Villalta D, Alessio MG, Tampoia M, Tonutti E, Brusca I, Bagnasco M, et al. Diagnostic accuracy of IgA anti-tissue transglutaminase antibody assays in celiac disease patients with selective IgA deficiency. Ann N Y Acad Sci. 2007;1109:212–20.
102. Albin S, Cunningham-Rundles C. An update on the use of immunoglobulin for the treatment of immunodeficiency disorders. Immunotherapy. 2014;6(10):1113–26.
103. Garcia JM, Espanol T, Gurbindo MD, Casas CC. Update on the treatment of primary immunodeficiencies. Allergol Immunopathol (Madr). 2007;35(5):184–92.
104. Gustafson R, Gardulf A, Granert C, Hansen S, Hammarstrom L. Prophylactic therapy for selective IgA deficiency. Lancet. 1997;350(9081):865.
105. Marconi M, Plebani A, Avanzini MA, Maccario R, Pistorio A, Duse M, et al. IL-10 and IL-4 co-operate to normalize in vitro IgA production in IgA-deficient (IgAD) patients. Clin Exp Immunol. 1998;112(3):528–32.
106. Briere F, Bridon JM, Chevet D, Souillet G, Bienvenu F, Guret C, et al. Interleukin 10 induces B lymphocytes from IgA-deficient patients to secrete IgA. J Clin Invest. 1994;94(1):97–104.
107. Ludvigsson JF, Neovius M, Hammarstrom L. IgA deficiency and mortality: a population-based cohort study. J Clin Immunol. 2013;33(8):1317–24.
108. Jorgensen GH, Gardulf A, Sigurdsson MI, Arnlaugsson S, Hammarstrom L, Ludviksson BR. Health-related quality of life (HRQL) in immunodeficient adults with selective IgA deficiency compared with age- and gender-matched controls and identification of risk factors for poor HRQL. Qual Life Res. 2014;23(2):645–58.
109. Routes J, Costa-Carvalho BT, Grimbacher B, Paris K, Ochs HD, Filipovich A, et al. Health-related quality of life and health resource utilization in patients with primary immunodeficiency disease prior to and following 12 months of immunoglobulin G treatment. J Clin Immunol. 2016;36(5):450–61.
110. Cobain TJ, French MA, Christiansen FT, Dawkins RL. Association of IgA deficiency with HLA A28 and B14. Tissue Antigens. 1983;22(2):151–4.
111. Ferreira RC, Pan-Hammarstrom Q, Graham RR, Fontan G, Lee AT, Ortmann W, et al. High-density SNP mapping of the HLA region identifies multiple independent susceptibility loci associated with selective IgA deficiency. PLoS Genet. 2012;8(1):e1002476.
112. Ambrus M, Hernadi E, Bajtai G. Prevalence of HLA-A1 and HLA-B8 antigens in selective IgA deficiency. Clin Immunol Immunopathol. 1977;7(3):311–4.
113. Cuccia-Belvedere M, Monafo V, Martinetti M, Plebani A, De Paoli F, Burgio GR. Recurrent extended HLA haplotypes in children with selective IgA deficiency. Tissue Antigens. 1989;34(2):127–32.
114. Mohammadi J, Pourpak Z, Jarefors S, Saghafi S, Zendehdel K, Pourfathollah AA, et al. Human leukocyte antigens (HLA) associated with selective IgA deficiency in Iran and Sweden. Iran J Allergy Asthma Immunol. 2008;7(4):209–14.
115. Hammarstrom L, Smith CI. HLA-A, B, C and DR antigens in immunoglobulin A deficiency. Tissue Antigens. 1983;21(1):75–9.
116. Schaffer FM, Palermos J, Zhu ZB, Barger BO, Cooper MD, Volanakis JE. Individuals with IgA deficiency and common variable immunodeficiency share polymorphisms of major histocompatibility complex class III genes. Proc Natl Acad Sci U S A. 1989;86(20):8015–9.
117. French MA, Dawkins RL. Central MHC genes, IgA deficiency and autoimmune disease. Immunol Today. 1990;11(8):271–4.
118. Fiore M, Pera C, Delfino L, Scotese I, Ferrara GB, Pignata C. DNA typing of DQ and DR alleles in IgA-deficient subjects. Eur J Immunogenet. 1995;22(5):403–11.
119. Reil A, Bein G, Machulla HK, Sternberg B, Seyfarth M. High-resolution DNA typing in immunoglobulin A deficiency confirms a positive association with DRB1*0301, DQB1*02 haplotypes. Tissue Antigens. 1997;50(5):501–6.

120. De La Concha EG, Fernandez-Arquero M, Martinez A, Vidal F, Vigil P, Conejero L, et al. HLA class II homozygosity confers susceptibility to common variable immunodeficiency (CVID). Clin Exp Immunol. 1999;116(3):516–20.
121. Wilton AN, Cobain TJ, Dawkins RL. Family studies of IgA deficiency. Immunogenetics. 1985;21(4):333–42.
122. Volanakis JE, Zhu ZB, Schaffer FM, Macon KJ, Palermos J, Barger BO, et al. Major histocompatibility complex class III genes and susceptibility to immunoglobulin A deficiency and common variable immunodeficiency. J Clin Invest. 1992;89(6):1914–22.
123. Cucca F, Zhu ZB, Khanna A, Cossu F, Congia M, Badiali M, et al. Evaluation of IgA deficiency in Sardinians indicates a susceptibility gene is encoded within the HLA class III region. Clin Exp Immunol. 1998;111(1):76–80.
124. Castigli E, Wilson SA, Garibyan L, Rachid R, Bonilla F, Schneider L, et al. TACI is mutant in common variable immunodeficiency and IgA deficiency. Nat Genet. 2005;37(8):829–34.
125. Pan-Hammarstrom Q, Salzer U, Du L, Bjorkander J, Cunningham-Rundles C, Nelson DL, et al. Reexamining the role of TACI coding variants in common variable immunodeficiency and selective IgA deficiency. Nat Genet. 2007;39(4):429–30.
126. Winter PM, Manndorff P. The frequency of IgA-deficiency in the Austrian population. A protocol for large-scale screening by ELISA and a study on 3056 blood donors. Infusionstherapie. 1988;15(5):221–4.
127. Weber-Mzell D, Kotanko P, Hauer AC, Goriup U, Haas J, Lanner N, et al. Gender, age and seasonal effects on IgA deficiency: a study of 7293 Caucasians. Eur J Clin Investig. 2004;34(3):224–8.
128. Clark JA, Callicoat PA, Brenner NA, Bradley CA, Smith DM Jr. Selective IgA deficiency in blood donors. Am J Clin Pathol. 1983;80(2):210–3.
129. Vyas GN, Perkins HA, Yang YM, Basantani GK. Healthy blood donors with selective absence of immunoglobulin A: prevention of anaphylactic transfusion reactions caused by antibodies to IgA. J Lab Clin Med. 1975;85(5):838–42.
130. Cassidy JT, Burt A, Petty R, Sullivan D. Selective IgA deficiency in connective tissue diseases. N Engl J Med. 1969;280(5):275.
131. Frommel D, Moullec J, Lambin P, Fine JM. Selective serum IgA deficiency. Frequency among 15,200 French blood donors. Vox Sang. 1973;25(6):513–8.
132. Ropars C, Muller A, Paint N, Beige D, Avenard G. Large scale detection of IgA deficient blood donors. J Immunol Methods. 1982;54(2):183–9.
133. Pereira LF, Sapina AM, Arroyo J, Vinuelas J, Bardaji RM, Prieto L. Prevalence of selective IgA deficiency in Spain: more than we thought. Blood. 1997;90(2):893.
134. Feng L. Epidemiological study of selective IgA deficiency among 6 nationalities in China. Zhonghua Yi Xue Za Zhi. 1992;72(2):88–90, 128.
135. Feng ML, Zhao YL, Shen T, Huang H, Yin B, Liu RZ, Qian KC, Liu DZ. Prevalence of immunoglobulin A deficiency in Chinese blood donors and evaluation of anaphylactic transfusion reaction risk. Transfus Med. 2011;21(5):338–43.
136. Bachmann R. Studies on the serum gamma-A-globulin level. 3. The frequency of A-gamma-A-globulinemia. Scand J Clin Lab Invest. 1965;17(4):316–20.
137. Palmer DS, O'Toole J, Montreuil T, Scalia V, Yi QL, Goldman M, et al. Screening of Canadian Blood Services donors for severe immunoglobulin A deficiency. Transfusion. 2010;50(7):1524–31.
138. Ezeoke A. Selective IgA deficiency (SIgAD) in Eastern Nigeria. Afr J Med Med Sci. 1988;17(1):17–21.
139. Wells JV, McNally MP, King MA. Selective IgA deficiency in Australian blood donors. Aust NZ J Med. 1980;10(4):410–3.
140. Shiva S, Zahra P, Asghar A, Akbar PA, Azam S, Maryam F, et al. Selective immunoglobulin A deficiency in Iranian blood donors: prevalence, laboratory and clinical findings. Iran J Allergy Asthma Immunol. 2008;7(3):157–62.
141. Kornstad L, Nordhagen R. Immunodeficiency and autoimmunity I Selective IgA deficiency in thyroid autoimmunity. Int Arch Allergy Appl Immunol. 1974;47(6):942–5.

142. Natvig JB, Harboe M, Fausa O, Tveit A. Family studies in individuals with selective absence of gamma-A-globulin. Clin Exp Immunol. 1971;8(2):229–36.
143. Koistinen J. Selective IgA deficiency in blood donors. Vox Sang. 1975;29(3):192–202.
144. Litzman J, Sevcikova I, Stikarovska D, Pikulova Z, Pazdirkova A, Lokaj J. IgA deficiency in Czech healthy individuals and selected patient groups. Int Arch Allergy Immunol. 2000;123(2):177–80.
145. Carneiro-Sampaio MM, Carbonare SB, Rozentraub RB, de Araujo MN, Riberiro MA, Porto MH. Frequency of selective IgA deficiency among Brazilian blood donors and healthy pregnant women. Allergol Immunopathol (Madr). 1989;17(4):213–6.
146. Gandolfi L, Pratesi R, Cordoba JC, Tauil PL, Gasparin M, Catassi C. Prevalence of celiac disease among blood donors in Brazil. Am J Gastroenterol. 2000;95(3):689–92.
147. Ulfarsson J, Gudmundsson S, Birgisdottir B, Kjeld JM, Jensson O. Selective serum IgA deficiency in Icelanders. Frequency, family studies and Ig levels. Acta Med Scand. 1982;211(6):481–7.
148. Velbri S, Pärlist M, Leito K. Primaarne immuunpuudulikkus. Eestis Eesti Arst. 2005;84:310–4.
149. Urbonas V, Sadauskaite J, Cerkauskiene R, Kaminskas A, Maki M, Kurppa K. Population-based screening for selective Immunoglobulin A (IgA) deficiency in lithuanian children using a rapid antibody-based fingertip test. Med Sci Monit. 2016;22:4773–8.
150. Giza S, Kotanidou E, Papadopoulou-Alataki E, Antoniou MC, Maggana I, Kyrgios I, et al. Prevalence of selective immunoglobulin A deficiency in Greek children and adolescents with type 1 diabetes. World J Pediatr. 2016;12(4):470–6.
151. Foudoulaki-Paparizos LVT, Stamoulis K, Kyriakis K, Fakitsa V, Stayropoulou-Gioka E. Prevalence of IgA deficiency in Greek blood donors. Haema. 2002;5:330–2.
152. Chandran S, Khetan D, Chaudhary R, Misra R, Aggarwal A. Low prevalence of IgA deficiency in north Indian population. Indian J Med Res. 2006;123(5):653–6.
153. Sharon R, Amar A. IgA deficiency in Israeli blood donors. J Clin Pathol. 1982;35(5):582–3.
154. Duran J, Lopes C, Rangel G, Ruivo I. IgA deficiency in a Portuguese donor population. Vox Sang. 2008;95(S1):170–7.
155. Yadav M, Iyngkaran N. Low incidence of selective IgA deficiency in normal Malaysians. Med J Malaysia. 1979;24:145–8.
156. Holt PD, Tandy NP, Anstee DJ. Screening of blood donors for IgA deficiency: a study of the donor population of South-West England. J Clin Pathol. 1977;30(11):1007–10.
157. Hunt AF, Allen DL, Aries DL, Strange JJ. A protocol for sensitive large-scale screening of blood donors for IgA deficiency. Vox Sang. 1975;29:192–202.
158. Yazdani R, Azizi G, Abolhassani H, Aghamohammadi A. Selective IgA deficiency: epidemiology, pathogenesis, clinical phenotype, diagnosis, prognosis and management. Scand J Immunol. 2017;85(1):3–12.

IgG Subclass and Anti-polysaccharide Antibody Deficiency

17

Esther de Vries

17.1 Definitions

Of all primary immunodeficiencies, predominantly antibody deficiencies (PADs) [1] form the largest group. These patients—by definition—do *not* have relevant T-cell deficiency (in laboratory investigations and/or clinically). If they do, they belong to another group (e.g., late-onset combined immunodeficiency (LOCID); see Chap. 4). In the previous chapters, many PADs of varying severity, mainly monogenetic in origin, have been described. Although a lot of questions remain to be answered, these entities are well classifiable. Unfortunately, on a population-wide basis by far the largest group of PADs is much more difficult to classify. Traditionally, common variable immunodeficiency disorders (CVID; see Chap. 3) are considered a separate entity, comprising the most severe hypogammaglobulinemia patients. However, even for CVID expert opinion varies as to which patients with decreased IgG and disturbed specific antibody responses should be classified under this diagnosis, some considering combination with decreased IgM *or* decreased IgA sufficient, others only diagnosing CVID in case IgA is decreased (± decreased IgM) [2]. Less clear-cut cases are often referred to as "other hypogammaglobulinemia" or "dysgammaglobulinemia" and more recently as "unclassified primary antibody deficiency (unPAD)" [3]. Within the unPAD group, clinical severity as well as the results of immunological laboratory investigations and potential underlying pathophysiology may differ greatly.

E. de Vries
Department of Tranzo, Tilburg School of Social and Behavioral Sciences, Tilburg University, Tilburg, The Netherlands

Laboratory for Medical Microbiology and Immunology, Elisabeth Tweesteden Hospital, Tilburg, The Netherlands
e-mail: e.devries@tilburguniversity.edu; esther.devries@etz.nl

M. M. D'Elios, M. Rizzi (eds.), *Humoral Primary Immunodeficiencies*,
Rare Diseases of the Immune System, https://doi.org/10.1007/978-3-319-91785-6_17

Over time, subgroups of hypogammaglobulinemia patients have been defined in the literature in many ways, often (partially) overlapping each other. The following entities have been defined by the Registry Working Party of the European Society for Immunodeficiencies ESID [3]:

- IgA/IgGsc*def*—IgA with IgG subclass deficiency—a combination of sIgA*def* (see Chap. 16) and sIgGsc*def* features (see below)
- sIgG*def*—selective (isolated) IgG deficiency—decreased IgG with normal IgA and IgM (thymoma with IgG deficiency is a separate, well-classified entity; it is described in Chap. 18)
- sIgGsc*def*—selective (isolated) IgG subclass deficiency—≥1 of IgG_1, IgG_2, and/or IgG_3 subclass deficiency with normal total IgG, IgA, and IgM and normal specific antibody responses (isolated IgG_4 deficiency is considered clinically irrelevant [4])
- SPAD—deficiency of specific IgG/specific antibody deficiency—abnormal specific antibody responses to polysaccharide antigens with normal IgG, IgG subclasses, IgA, and IgM
- sIgM*def*—selective (isolated) IgM deficiency—IgM deficiency with normal IgG, IgG subclasses, IgA, and specific antibody responses
- unPAD—unclassified antibody deficiency—≥1 of decreased IgG, IgG1, IgG2, IgG3, IgA, IgM, or vaccination response, not fitting any of the other definitions of primary antibody deficiency (≈ combinations of decreased values and incompletely investigated cases)

All these definitions are solely based upon the results of immunological laboratory investigations. It is not clear how useful they really are. There is no consensus about the cutoff levels below which the conclusion "deficiency" can be drawn. Often words like "marked" or "at least 2SD" are used to indicate that the decrease should be large enough to be considered relevant for the clinical situation of the patient (age-matched reference values in Table 17.1; these can differ somewhat between laboratories). Also, it is important to realize that these definitions can only be used to classify a patient if all relevant laboratory investigations included in the definition have been performed. Because this is often not the case, and because there is currently insufficient evidence that these laboratory-based subgroups have clinical relevance, it might be better to combine all these patients under the umbrella definition of unclassified primary antibody deficiency (unPAD) [3].

17.2 Epidemiology

Hypogammaglobulinemia can be found at any age; however, the clinical significance may differ in different age groups. Newborns produce low levels of immunoglobulins themselves but—when born at term—have high serum IgG levels due to placental transfer of maternal IgG in the third trimester [6]. Their own production slowly increases during the first year of life, while their maternal IgG shows a steady decline.

Table 17.1 Age-matched reference values for IgG subclasses in serum (g/L)

	IgG_1	IgG_2	IgG_3	IgG_4
0–1 months	2.4–10.6	0.87–4.1	0.14–0.55	0.039–0.56
1–4 months	1.8–6.7	0.38–2.1	0.14–0.70	0.022–0.36
4–6 months	1.8–7.0	0.34–2.1	0.15–0.80	0.017–0.23
6–12 months	2.0–7.7	0.34–2.3	0.15–0.97	0.012–0.43
1–1.5 years	2.5–8.2	0.38–2.4	0.15–1.07	0.011–0.62
1.5–2 years	2.9–8.5	0.45–2.6	0.15–1.13	0.011–0.79
2–3 years	3.2–9.0	0.52–2.8	0.14–1.20	0.012–1.06
3–4 years	3.5–9.4	0.63–3.0	0.13–1.26	0.015–1.27
4–6 years	3.7–10.0	0.72–3.4	0.13–1.33	0.017–1.58
6–9 years	4.0–10.8	0.85–4.1	0.13–1.42	0.023–1.89
9–12 years	4.0–11.5	0.98–4.8	0.15–1.49	0.030–2.1
12–18 years	3.7–12.8	1.06–6.1	0.18–1.63	0.034–2.3
Adults	4.9–11.4	1.50–6.4	0.20–1.10	0.080–1.40

Source: Vademecum Diagnostisch onderzoek, Sanquin Diagnostiek, 2014, p.101 [5]

Together, this results in a physiological nadir of IgG at 4–6 months of age [7]. In some children, immunoglobulin production matures at a slower rate, resulting in so-called transient hypogammaglobulinemia of infancy (THI); this is characterized by the fact that it resolves with increasing age. There is no consensus about the cutoff age after which normalization can no longer be expected. In the past, the age of 3 was used as limit, but it seems that it might be as high as 8–10 years. Some but not all of these children in fact have an underlying persistent immunodeficiency [8].

Milder hypogammaglobulinemia patients are often missed [9], because of a lack of awareness and—even when immunologically screened—incomplete investigations. Therefore, the true prevalence is unknown. In the literature, around 5–25% and 10–25% of patients tested for recurrent respiratory infections are described to have sIgGsc*def* and SPAD, respectively [10, 11]. Truly isolated sIgM*def* is probably very rare [12]. Estimates using insurance databases in the USA showed a prevalence of all primary antibody deficiencies combined of around 1.5–3 per 10,000 [13].

In hypogammaglobulinemic children, there is a slight but significant predominance of boys [14], whereas this is the case for women in hypogammaglobulinemic adults. The reason for this is not yet known.

17.3 Pathophysiology

The five immunoglobulin isotypes (IgA, IgD, IgE, IgG, and IgM) are described in more detail in Chaps. 1, 2, and 15. IgG is the most important isotype in the blood; it is composed of four different subclasses, IgG_1, IgG_2, IgG_3, and IgG_4. IgG_1 is the largest fraction of IgG; it contains a lot of anti-protein antibodies (e.g., anti-tetanus). IgG_2 contains a lot of anti-polysaccharide antibodies (e.g., antipneumococcal capsular antigens). IgG_3 can also contain anti-protein antibodies. IgG_4 is the smallest fraction; IgG_4 deficiency is considered clinically irrelevant [4]. Immunoglobulins attach themselves to microorganisms (opsonization), facilitating uptake by phagocytes. Therefore, immunoglobulin deficiency leads to an increased frequency of infections.

It is currently unknown how the different forms of milder hypogammaglobulinemia arise. It seems likely that affected patients form a heterogeneous group, where several genetic and environmental factors together determine the clinical phenotype, severity, and outcome.

17.4 Clinical Features

Hypogammaglobulinemic patients generally present with recurrent "normal" ENT and airway infections caused by ordinary bacterial respiratory agents like pneumococci, *Haemophilus influenzae*, and *Moraxella* (*Branhamella*) *catarrhalis*. The infections can generally be cured by regular antibiotic therapy [14]. When IgA deficiency is also present, gastrointestinal infections with *Giardia lamblia* are also more frequent. However, patients can also be asymptomatic, especially if only IgG subclass or IgA deficiency is present. In general, SPAD as well as combinations of abnormal laboratory results seem to be associated with more symptoms and more sequelae [15]. Specific antibody deficiency against protein antigens is generally symptomatic and associated with serious clinical problems.

Most cases do not show a clear Mendelian inheritance pattern; however, affected patients can have affected members somewhere in the family with some form of hypogammaglobulinemia upon detailed investigation. This can be associated with increased incidence of consanguinity [16]. Therefore, it is important to investigate family members, at the least by taking a detailed family history.

Chronic fatigue with serious lack of energy is seen in many hypogammaglobulinemic patients, often leading to decreased quality of life and less participation in society [17]. The recurrent infections may lead to irreversible damage to the middle ear, causing hearing loss [18]; the sinuses, causing local obstructive problems [19]; and the lungs, causing bronchiectasis with loss of pulmonary function and a further increased tendency to develop lower respiratory tract infections [20]. This is already found in children [21] and prevalence increases with increasing age [22].

In children, hypogammaglobulinemia should be suspected when the frequency of upper respiratory infections does not subside with increasing age. Recurrent lower respiratory infections, especially when bacterial in origin, suggest immunological screening is warranted. When hypogammaglobulinemia is found in a young child, this may be THI (see 17.2). Only follow-up over time will show whether this is indeed the case. The hypogammaglobulinemia may also worsen over time and develop into overt CVID. Unfortunately, currently no absolute predictions can be made as to which children that will be. Therefore, follow-up is essential once hypogammaglobulinemia has been diagnosed in a child.

Adult hypogammaglobulinemic patients may be "hidden" among patients with a diagnosis of chronic bronchitis, difficult-to-treat asthma, COPD, unexplained bronchiectasis, chronic sinusitis, or atypical autoimmunity. Also, in adults hematological malignancy may present with hypogammaglobulinemia. It is important to always keep this in mind. In children as well as adults, hypogammaglobulinemia may develop during treatment for a hematological malignancy. Especially in adults, it is not always clear in those cases which of the two (malignancy or antibody deficiency) is the primary disease.

17.5 Diagnosis and Laboratory Features

Determination of IgG, IgA, and IgM in serum is widely available, but IgG subclasses cannot be determined in every country. It is important to draw a sample outside of active infections and before administering immunoglobulin substitution therapy (this will interfere with the determination of IgG produced by the patient). It is important to realize that the lower limit of detection in the laboratory test used may overlap the normal age-matched reference values for IgA, IgG_3, and IgG_4 in young children. More sensitive techniques are more expensive, and these are not uniformly available.

Determination of vaccination responses is more difficult; techniques to determine specific antibody titers are generally only present in specialized immunological laboratories. It requires comparison between two samples, one taken before and one 3–4 weeks after vaccination with a tetanus booster (protein antigen) and *un*conjugated pneumococcal vaccine (polysaccharide antigen). This should be performed and interpreted by an immunologist, and preferably not before 3–4 years of age, because of the physiological immaturity of the immune system. Interpretation of the results is not straightforward and depends on the age and vaccination history of the patient. Moreover, there are no validated age-matched reference values available.

Diagnosing hypogammaglobulinemia as a laboratory phenomenon can thus be performed in one or two small blood samples. However, determining when to perform these tests and, once done, how to interpret the results is quite another story. Many young children present with recurrent ENT and airway infections, especially when they visit day care on a regular basis. Also, allergy, parental smoking, bronchial hyperreactivity, and adenoidal hypertrophy may play a role in respiratory symptoms in children, and a vicious cycle of symptoms, malaise, insufficient diet resulting in iron deficiency, viral infections, and superimposed bacterial infections may arise [23]. Immunological differential diagnosis in children with recurrent ENT and airway infections includes neutropenia (mostly autoimmune, rarely congenital) and the rare case of X-linked or autosomal recessive agammaglobulinemia (see previous chapters). Other, more rare, non-immunological conditions may also be the underlying cause (e.g., cystic fibrosis, ciliary dyskinesia). In adults, smoking, asthma, allergy, and COPD are well-known causes of recurrent respiratory symptoms. However, these can occur together with antibody deficiency or may be misinterpretations of symptoms that are in fact caused by antibody deficiency. It is also important to clearly distinguish primary from secondary causes of antibody deficiency such as renal or intestinal protein loss, adverse drug events, and malignancy, especially in adults, where secondary forms are much more frequent (Table 17.2).

Table 17.2 Secondary causes of hypogammaglobulinemia

Cause	Examples	Diagnose by
Drug-induced	E.g., steroids, immunosuppressants, certain anti-epileptics	History
Infection	E.g., HIV, EBV	Serology, PCR
Malignancy	E.g., CLL, non-Hodgkin lymphoma, multiple myeloma	Appropriate lab tests, imaging
Protein loss	E.g., nephrotic syndrome, severe burns, protein-losing enteropathy	Urinary protein, history, fecal alpha-fetoprotein

Source (adapted from): Bonilla FA, et al. *International Consensus Document (ICON): Common Variable Immunodeficiency Disorders* [2]

A particularly difficult group is formed by children with syndromal abnormalities. When they have recurrent infections, this is generally interpreted as caused by abnormal swallowing with aspiration or a result of abnormal airway anatomy. Although these factors are often present in these children, many syndromes are accompanied by forms of hypogammaglobulinemia of varying severity [24]. Recognizing and treating this (with immunoglobulin substitution therapy) may greatly increase the quality of life of these children and their families.

17.6 Management and Treatment: Children

Treatment depends on the age of the child, the severity of clinical problems, the family history, and the outcome of laboratory investigations [25]. There is not enough evidence to support clinical decisions. These are generally taken based on experience and expertise, in communication with the parents. It is on the one hand important to stress the potential presence of other factors influencing the clinical picture (e.g., day care, parental smoking), and on the other hand, it is important to follow up the child. It may be THI, but it may also be CVID in development. With increasing age, THI becomes less and developing CVID becomes more likely. Bridging these years of watchful waiting can be supported by rigorous treatment of occurring infections; trials of antibiotic prophylaxis with, e.g., co-trimoxazole (there is no evidence for this, but experts use it widely); or in selected cases a trial of subcutaneous or intravenous immunoglobulin substitution therapy (see Chap. 20).

17.7 Management and Treatment: Adults

Treatment in adults depends on the severity of symptoms, the outcome of laboratory investigations, the family history, and on the presence or absence of bronchiectasis and comorbidities. Active and passive smoking should be discouraged. Also in adults, milder hypogammaglobulinemia can be a sign of developing CVID, so follow-up is important. If bronchiectasis is present, antibiotic prophylaxis, with, e.g., doxycycline or azithromycin, may be warranted. Many adults present with a CVID-like phenotype, but never develop the full-blown laboratory abnormalities required for a diagnosis of CVID. They often also have asthma or COPD, with very frequent, prolonged, and severe exacerbations. In those cases, a trial of subcutaneous or intravenous immunoglobulin substitution therapy should certainly be considered (see Chap. 21). These are complex decisions that should be taken by an experienced immunologist.

Summary and Take-Home Messages
1. *Which types of "milder" primary hypogammaglobulinemia*[a] *are encountered in the clinic (for definitions see main text)?* – IgA ± IgG subclass deficiency (see also Chap. 16) – Selective IgG deficiency (≥1 of serum IgG subclasses may be below age-matched reference values) – Selective IgG subclass deficiency (decreased IgG4 is considered clinically irrelevant) – Selective IgM deficiency – Selective anti-polysaccharide antibody deficiency – Unclassified primary antibody deficiency: any combination of the above that does not fulfil the definition of common variable immunodeficiency disorders (see Chap. 3) and that is not explained by a known genetic cause (see previous chapters) – (Unclassified) syndromic immunodeficiency: any of the above alone or in combination, with concomitant syndromic features ± a known genetic cause
2. *What is the immunological background?* • Immunoglobulins are needed for protection against extracellular, encapsulated bacteria such as pneumococci.
3. *What is the typical clinical presentation, and which complications can be expected?* – Patients with "milder" hypogammaglobulinemia generally present with recurrent ENT and/or airway infections caused by "common" bacterial pathogens like pneumococci, *Haemophilus influenzae*, and *Moraxella (Branhamella) catarrhalis.* – Infections can generally be cured by regular antibiotics but continue to recur. – Chronic fatigue and lack of energy are often present, with considerable personal and societal impact. – Affected individuals can be asymptomatic (especially isolated, selective forms). – *Giardia lamblia* intestinal infections are more frequent and more difficult to eradicate (especially in IgA deficient patients). – Both allergy and autoimmunity can accompany the hypogammaglobulinemia, leading to additional problems and loss of quality of life. – Recurring lower respiratory tract infections can lead to bronchiectasis, which can be severe, leading to substantial morbidity and decreased life span.
4. *What is the appropriate diagnostic work-up?* – Determine serum levels of IgG, IgA, and IgM (any age; take maternal IgG into account when interpreting results in young infants). – Determine serum levels of IgG subclasses (not before 3–4 years of age). – Determine anti-polysaccharide antibody titers in serum directed against pneumococcal serotypes before and 3–4 weeks after vaccination with unconjugated (polysaccharide) pneumococcal vaccine (not before 3–4 years of age; use serotypes not present in conjugate vaccines to reach conclusions regarding anti-polysaccharide antibody formation). – Always use age-matched reference values that are valid for your laboratory.

5. *What is the appropriate treatment and follow-up?*
   - Prompt, adequate diagnosis and treatment of infections.
   - Consider antibiotic prophylaxis (there is currently no conclusive evidence on efficacy, choice of antibiotic, or dose, but experts widely use it).
   - If clinical problems continue, consider referral to an experienced immunologist; such patients need repeated immunological evaluations (do not repeat pneumococcal polysaccharide vaccination within 5 years), yearly lung function tests including TLCO[b], and a baseline HRCT[c] scan of the thorax which is repeated every 2–10 years depending on results and severity of symptoms.
   - In selected cases, subcutaneous or intravenous immunoglobulin substitution can be warranted; refer to an experienced immunologist for this.

[a]In all cases classified as "milder" primary hypogammaglobulinemia laboratory and/or clinical signs of T-cell deficiency (T-lymphocytopenia, T-cell functional defect, opportunistic infections) as well as secondary causes (e.g., protein loss, medication) should be absent

[b]*TLCO* transfer factor of the lung for carbon monoxide (measurement of diffusion capacity of the lung)

[c]*HRCT* high-resolution computed tomography (can show bronchiectasis and interstitial lung disease)

References

1. Bousfiha A, Jeddane L, Al-Herz W, Ailal F, Casanova JL, Chatila T, Conley ME, Cunningham-Rundles C, Etzioni A, Franco JL, Gaspar HB, Holland SM, Klein C, Nonoyama S, Ochs HD, Oksenhendler E, Picard C, Puck JM, Sullivan KE, Tang ML. The 2015 IUIS Phenotypic Classification for Primary Immunodeficiencies. J Clin Immunol. 2015;35:727–38.
2. Bonilla FA, Barlan I, Chapel H, Costa-Carvalho BT, Cunningham-Rundles C, de la Morena MT, Espinosa-Rosales FJ, Hammarström L, Nonoyama S, Quinti I, Routes JM, Tang ML, Warnatz K. International Consensus Document (ICON): Common Variable Immunodeficiency Disorders. J Allergy Clin Immunol Pract. 2016;4:38–59.
3. https://esid.org/Working-Parties/Registry/Diagnosis-criteria. Accessed October 2017.
4. Ochs HD, Stiehm ER, Winkelstein JA, et al. Antibody deficiencies. In: Ochs HD, Stiehm ER, Winkelstein JA, editors. Immunologic disorders in infants and children. 5th ed. Philadelphia: Elsevier; 2004.
5. https://www.sanquin.nl/repository/documenten/nl/product-dienst/diagnostiek/algemeen/vademecum-2014.pdf. Accessed October 2017.
6. Palmeira P, Quinello C, Silveira-Lessa AL, Zago CA, Carneiro-Sampaio M. IgG placental transfer in healthy and pathological pregnancies. Clin Dev Immunol. 2012;2012:985646.
7. Johansson SG, Berg T. Immunoglobulin levels in healthy children. Acta Paediatr Scand. 1967;56:572.
8. Keles S, Artac H, Kara R, Gokturk B, Ozen A, Reisli I. Transient hypogammaglobulinemia and unclassified hypogammaglobulinemia: 'similarities and differences'. Pediatr Allergy Immunol. 2010;21:843–51.
9. de Vries E. Clinical Working Party of the European Society for Immunodeficiencies (ESID) (2006) Patient-centred screening for primary immunodeficiency: a multi-stage diagnostic protocol designed for non-immunologists. Clin Exp Immunol. 145:204–14.
10. Stiehm ER. The four most common pediatric immunodeficiencies. J Immunotoxicol. 2008;5:227–34.
11. Perez E, Bonilla FA, Orange JS, Ballow M. Specific antibody deficiency: controversies in diagnosis and management. Front Immunol. 2017;8:586.
12. Janssen LM, Macken T, Creemers MC, Pruijt JF, Eijk JJ, de Vries E. Truly selective primary IgM deficiency is probably very rare. Clin Exp Immunol. 2017;6 https://doi.org/10.1111/cei.13065.

13. Kobrynski L, Powell RW, Bowen S. Prevalence and morbidity of primary. immunodeficiency diseases, United States 2001-2007. J Clin Immunol. 2014;34:954–61.
14. Schatorjé EJ, Gathmann B, van Hout RW, de Vries E, PedPAD consortium. The PedPAD study: boys predominate in the hypogammaglobulinaemia registry of the ESID online database. Clin Exp Immunol. 2014;176:387–93.
15. Cheng YK, Decker PA, O'Byrne MM, Weiler CR. Clinical and laboratory characteristics of 75 patients with specific polysaccharide antibody deficiency syndrome. Ann Allergy Asthma Immunol. 2006;97:306–11.
16. Aghamohammadi A, Sedighipour L, Saeed SE, Kouhkan A, Heydarzadeh M, Pourpak Z. Alterations in humoral immunity in relatives of patients with common variable immunodeficiency. J Investig Allergol Clin Immunol. 2008;18:266–71.
17. Barton JC, Bertoli LF, Barton JC, Acton RT. Fibromyalgia in 300 adult index patients with primary immunodeficiency. Clin Exp Rheumatol. 2017;105(Suppl):68–73.
18. Tavakol M, Kouhi A, Abolhassani H, Ghajar A, Afarideh M, Shahinpour S, Aghamohammadi A. Otological findings in pediatric patients with hypogammaglobulinemia. Iran. J Allergy Asthma Immunol. 2014;13:166–73.
19. Chiarella SE, Grammer LC. Immune deficiency in chronic rhinosinusitis: screening and treatment. Expert Rev Clin Immunol. 2017;13:117–23.
20. Ruffner MA, Aksamit TR, Thomashow B, Choate R, DiMango A, Turino GM, O'Donnell AE, Johnson MM, Olivier KN, Fennelly K, Daley CL, Winthrop KL, Metersky ML, Salathe MA, Knowles MR, Daniels MLA, Noone PG, Tino G, Griffith DE, Sullivan KE. Frequency of untreated hypogammaglobulinemia in bronchiectasis. Ann Allergy Asthma Immunol. 2017;119:83–5.
21. Schatorjé EJ, de Jong E, van Hout RW, García Vivas Y, de Vries E. The challenge of Immunoglobulin-G subclass deficiency and specific polysaccharide antibody deficiency—a Dutch Pediatric Cohort Study. J Clin Immunol. 2016;36:141–8.
22. Maarschalk-Ellerbroek LJ, Hoepelman AI, van Montfrans JM, Ellerbroek PM. The spectrum of disease manifestations in patients with common variable immunodeficiency disorders and partial antibody deficiency in a university hospital. J Clin Immunol. 2012;32:907–21.
23. De Vries E, Driessen G. Educational paper: primary immunodeficiencies in children: a diagnostic challenge. Eur J Pediatr. 2011;170:169–77.
24. Schatorjé E, van der Flier M, Seppänen M, Browning M, Morsheimer M, Henriet S, Neves JF, Vinh DC, Alsina L, Grumach A, Soler-Palacin P, Boyce T, Celmeli F, Goudouris E, Hayman G, Herriot R, Förster-Waldl E, Seidel M, Simons A, de vries E. Primary immunodeficiency associated with chromosomal aberration—an ESID survey. Orphanet J Rare Dis. 2016;11:110.
25. Driessen G, van der Burg M. Educational paper: primary antibody deficiencies. Eur J Pediatr. 2011;170:693–702.

Good's Syndrome (GS): Thymoma with Immunodeficiency

18

Hans-Hartmut Peter

18.1 Incidence, Etiology, and Pathogenesis

Good's syndrome (GS) is a very rare disease affecting adults between 40 and 90 years of age. The most salient clinical characteristic of GS is the association of thymoma, immunodeficiency, and various forms of autoimmunity [1]. How these three phenotypic features tie together in etiology and pathogenesis remains even 64 years after the first description of GS largely unclear [2]. Two systematic reviews covering 152 [2] and 47 GS cases [3], respectively, came to similar observations regarding the histopathological types of thymoma. Based on the new WHO thymoma classification [4, 5], benign A and AB thymomas (formerly spindle cell thymoma, epithelial and lymphoepithelial thymomas) make up for >80% of GS associated thymomas, while lymphocyte-rich B1 and B2 thymomas amount to 10–12% and malignant thymomas to 4–10%. In the Kelesidis cohort [2], diagnosis of thymoma preceded the emergence of infections and hypogammaglobulinemia in 42% of the cases, occurred simultaneously in 38%, and followed the emergence of symptoms in 20%. The respective figures in the Chinese cohort [3] were 26, 20, and 54%.

Consecutive large thymoma series from France and Thailand, showing a preponderance of B2 and AB thymomas, outlined a strong association with autoimmune diseases (55%), notably myasthenia gravis (39%), and observed GS only rarely [6, 7]. In the Thai thymoma study [7], the prevalence of autoimmune diseases, immunodeficiency states, and secondary neoplasms was 34.5, 10.3, and 10.3%, respectively. Thymoma patients showed significantly lower percentages of CD4+ T cells and interferon-γ production but elevated regulatory T cells compared to healthy controls [7].

H.-H. Peter
Center for Chronic Immunodeficiency, University Medical Center Freiburg, Freiburg, Germany
e-mail: hans-hartmut.peter@uniklinik-freiburg.de

M. M. D'Elios, M. Rizzi (eds.), *Humoral Primary Immunodeficiencies*,
Rare Diseases of the Immune System, https://doi.org/10.1007/978-3-319-91785-6_18

A causal relationship between thymoma, severe B cell deficiency (87%), and hypogammaglobulinemia (100%) in GS patients has been attributed to pre-B-cell suppression by thymoma patients' lymphocytes [8]. Another case report observed a block in early B-cell differentiation [9], but this finding has not been confirmed in a larger series nor elucidated at the molecular level. An interferon-like cytokine Limitin being produced by bone marrow stroma cell lines has been shown to preferentially suppress early B-cell growth and differentiation [10] rendering it an interesting candidate to link thymus stroma cell hyperplasia to inhibition of early B-cell growth.

Low CD4+ T cells counts (73%), low NK cells (57%), and elevated CD8+ T cells are common findings in GS [2] and are confirmed in part by the Thai thymoma study [7], in which GS was rare. The different prevalence of thymoma histologies in both studies may provide some explanation: whereas in cohorts of GS thymomas of type AB and A prevail [2, 3], the lymphocyte-rich B2 type is more common in the French and Thai thymoma studies [6, 7], which both associate strongly with autoimmune diseases but barely with immunodeficiency or GS.

Another interesting case report correlates a thymoma-associated T-cell immunodeficiency to an increase of naïve T cells with a reduced ζ-chain (CD247) expression in the TCR complex of both γδ- and αβ-T cells [11]. The patient presented with cutaneous anergy, expansion of γδ-T cells (30%), a polyclonal hypergammaglobulinemia, hepatosplenomegaly, lymphadenopathy, and opportunistic infections (leishmaniosis), thus a distinctly different phenotype from GS. The thymoma histology was B2 with a malignant phenotype requiring cytoreductive chemotherapy. In vitro stimulation of naïve CD4+ T cells exhibited a substantially reduced IL2 and IFN-γ production. The author did not observe mutations in the ζ-chain. Although they found similar reduced ζ-chain expression in three additional thymoma biopsies, their findings do not provide a pathophysiological model for GS but underline the broad spectrum of possible thymoma-associated immunodysregulation.

18.2 Clinical Presentation of GS

18.2.1 Infections

The clinical picture is dominated by severe, recurrent upper, and lower respiratory tract infections with encapsulated bacteria (e.g., *S. pneumoniae*, *H. influenzae*, *K. pneumoniae*) typical for hypogammaglobulinemia [2, 3, 12, 13]. In this respect, GS resembles X-linked agammaglobulinemia (XLA) or common variable immune deficiency (CVID). However, frequent opportunistic infections, such as CMV, *Candida*, *Mycobacteria tuberculosis*, *Pneumocystis jirovecii*, toxoplasma, cryptococcus, disseminated nocardiosis, and JC virus a.o., distinguish GS from XLA and CVID indicating an impaired cellular immunity [12–21]. Table 18.1 lists pathogens that have been associated with infections in GS patients.

Table 18.1 Pathogens observed in infections of GS patients (ref. 12–21)

Bacteria	Fungi	Viruses	Protozoa
Streptococcus pneumoniae	*Candida albicans*	Cytomegalovirus (CMV)	*Giardia lamblia*
Haemophilus influenzae	*Pneumocystis jirovecii*	Herpes simplex (HSV)	*Leishmania*
Staphylococcus aureus	*Toxoplasma gondii*	Varicella zoster (VZV)	
Klebsiella pneumoniae	*Cryptococcus*	Human herpesvirus type 8	
Moraxella catarrhalis	*Aspergillus fumigatus*	JC virus	
Salmonella spp.			
Campylobacter jejuni			
Helicobacter pylori			
Mycobacteria spp.			
Nocardia spp.			

Chronic diarrhea is another prominent feature occurring in up to 50% of GS patients [2, 22, 23]. Pathogens isolated from these patients comprise enterobacteria, *Campylobacter jejuni*, *Salmonella* species, *Giardia lamblia*, and CMV. But in the majority of GS patients with diarrhea, no pathogens can be isolated, and the local and histological pictures resemble secretory diarrhea or inflammatory bowel disease as has been described in CVID patients. Idiopathic diarrhea may improve with immunoglobulin substitution and in some cases fully resolved following thymectomy [22, 24].

18.2.2 Autoimmune Disease

As has been mentioned above [6, 7], autoimmune diseases are frequently associated with thymomas notably the lymphocyte-rich forms. Not surprisingly, the GS subset (thymoma with hypogammaglobulinemia) presents also with a considerable degree of autoimmunity [2]. Interestingly, while myasthenia gravis (MG) prevails in thymoma without hypogammaglobulinemia [6, 7], pure red cell aplasia (PRCA) with and without myelodysplastic syndrome [2, 25–28] and other forms of autoimmune anemias (aplastic, macrocytic, autoimmune hemolytic) [2, 14, 28] are the dominant autoimmune diseases in GS; together they account for anemic states in over 50% of GS patients. In the largest GS cohort [2, 14], PRCA leads the ranking list with 34.8% followed by MG with 15.7% and oral and vulvovaginal lichen planus [2, 30, 31] at 13.5% (Table 18.2). Viewing the total spectrum of autoimmune disease in GS, it is obvious that bone marrow-associated autoimmune manifestations are prevailing (Table 18.2).

Table 18.2 Autoimmune manifestations observed in 89 patients with Good's syndrome (Adapted according to ref. 2, 14)

Autoimmune manifestation associated with hematopoietic system	Other autoimmune diseases
Pure red cell aplasia (34.8%)	
	Myasthenia gravis (15.7%)
	Oral and vulvovaginal lichen planus (13.5%)
Aplastic anemia (7.9%)	
Macrocytic anemia (5.6%)	
Autoimmune hemolytic anemia (3.4%)	
Monoclonal gammopathy (3.4%)	
	Diabetes mellitus (2.2%)
	Polyarthropathy (2.2%)
Myelodysplastic syndrome (2.2%)	
Paroxysmal nocturnal hemoglobinuria (1.1%)	
Agranulocytosis (1.1%)	
Thrombocytopenia (1.1%)	
Idiopathic myelofibrosis (1.1%)	
	Dermatomyositis (1.1%)
	Primary sclerosing cholangitis (1.1%)
	Sweet's syndrome (1.1%)
	Ulcerative colitis (1.1%)
61.7% Total	**38.0% Total**

18.3 Laboratory Features of GS

18.3.1 Hematology

Over 50% of GS patients present with various forms of anemia, predominantly PRCA [25–28]. A similar percentage of GS patients present with low white blood cell counts [3, 32]. Thrombocytopenia has been observed in up to 20% [2, 3, 13]. Multilineage pancytopenia seen in GS patients may be driven by bone marrow-infiltrating autoreactive T cells [33]. Pernicious, macrocytic anemia can be associated with atrophic pangastritis and autoantibodies to parietal cells producing intrinsic factor [29]. Regular substitution with vitamin B12 is mandatory in these cases. Benign monoclonal gammopathy has been observed in a minority of GS patients [34].

18.3.2 Immunology

The immunological hallmark in GS patients is hypogammaglobulinemia of all isotypes associated with low B-cell counts and reduced CD4+ T cells and NK cells. Table 18.3 summarizes cumulative findings of 45 patients from the recently published Chinese GS cohort [3] and 75 GS patients collected by Kelleher and Misbah [13].

Table 18.3 Immunological findings in two cohorts of GS patients [3, 13]

	Dong et al. [3]		Kelleher [13]	
	n	Percent	*n*	Percent
Hypogammaglobulinemia	45/45	100	75/75	100
Low IgG, IgA, IgM	39/45	87	75/75	100
Low/absent B cells	42/42	100	33/38	87
Low CD4+ T cells	37/39	95	9/20	45
Reversed CD4/CD8 ratio	41/42	97	22/30	73
Low NK cell counts	12/13	92	n.d.	
Reduced PHA stimulation	n.d.		8/20	40
Absent skin DTH[a]	n.d.		12/14	86

[a]Delayed-type hypersensitivity

18.4 Diagnosis and Differential Diagnosis of GS

Adult-onset acquired immunodeficiency with frequent opportunistic infections requires first of all the definite exclusion of HIV infection and idiopathic or acquired low CD4 syndromes [35]. However, as hypogammaglobulinemia is untypical in these conditions, the most obvious differential diagnosis of GS is CVID or XLA which can be distinguished by lower rates of opportunistic infections. The diagnosis of thymoma together with hypogammaglobulinemia usually sparks the diagnosis of GS particularly when thymoma precedes or occurs simultaneously with symptoms of immunodeficiency, which is the case in 46–80% of GS patients [2, 3]. Delayed diagnosis of thymoma may obscure the diagnosis of GS for quite some time. Patients may be treated for years for various autoimmune diseases, anemia, or hypogammaglobulinemia before hitting the diagnostic clue with a chest X-ray revealing an enlarged anterior mediastinum [2, 36].

18.5 Therapy

Treatment of respiratory tract and gastrointestinal infections require anti-infective therapy. As most GS patients are not only hypogammaglobulinemic but lack also specific antipathogen antibodies, they usually improve with the institution of iv or sc IgG replacement therapy. Whenever possible, thymectomy is certainly indicated to establish the histological diagnosis of thymoma [37]. Moreover thoracic surgeons who incidentally remove a thymoma should always test for serum immunoglobulin levels and B-cell counts and consult a clinical immunologist to check for autoimmune diseases. Thymectomy often has a beneficial effect on autoimmune manifestations such as MG and PRCA or on chronic diarrhea [22, 24]. It may, however, not cure myelodysplastic syndromes. Immunosuppressive drugs such as cyclosporine A or even antithymocyte globulin (ATG) in combination with colony-stimulating factor (G-CSF) may be tried to fight CD8+ T cells infiltrating the bone marrow and impeding hematopoiesis. In a spectacular case, complete hematopoietic recovery of an aplastic syndrome occurred under Eltrombopag, a thrombopoietin receptor agonist [33]. Another inspiring case report concerns a 90-year-old man with a large thoracic mass, PRCA, MG, and a history of recurrent HSV infections. Histology of a punch biopsy revealed a lymphocyte-rich B1 thymoma. Serum Ig levels and B cells were low confirming GS [38]. As the patient was no candidate for surgical thymoma resection, he was by way of trial put on rituximab and surprisingly greatly improved his PRCA by stabilizing the erythropoiesis. The MG improved under pyridostigmine.

As underlined by many case reports, autoimmune manifestations and hematopoietic disturbances are amenable to various, often successful, therapeutic attempts including immunosuppressants, cytokines (e.g., G-CSF), thrombopoietin receptor agonist, and rituximab. However hypogammaglobulinemia is usually not reverted by thymectomy necessitating long-term IgG replacement therapy. The few cases in which flow cytometric analysis of blood lymphocyte subsets was performed before and after thymectomy did not reveal any significant changes of the low B-cell, CD4 cell, and NK cell counts [39] indicating that the severe thymoma-induced immunodysregulation is of long-term, persisting nature.

18.6 Prognosis

Given the broad spectrum of complications and opportunistic infections, it is very difficult to predict the prognosis of GS patients. If they just suffer from hypogammaglobulinemia and infections, they may fare as well as CVID and XLA patients. A 20-year single-center survey of 240 patients with CVID, 44 with XLA, and 7 with GS [40] suggested that the prognosis of GS is worse than that of CVID and XLA. Thus, after 5 and 10 years, 70% and 33% of GS patients, respectively, survived, compared with 99% and 95% of CVID and/or XLA patients [13, 40]. While thymoma itself does not contribute to excess mortality, the main causes of death are infections, autoimmune diseases, and hematological complications [13, 40].

References

1. Good RA. Agammaglobulinaemia—a provocative experiment of nature. Bull Univ Minn. 1954;26:1–19.
2. Kelesidis T, Yang O. Good's syndrome remains a mystery after 55 years: a systematic review of the scientific evidence. Clin Immunol. 2010;135(3):347–63. https://doi.org/10.1016/j.clim.2010.01.006. Review
3. Dong JP, Gao W, Teng GG, Tian Y, Wang HH. Characteristics of Good's Syndrome in China: a systematic review. Chin Med J. 2017;130:1604–9.
4. Masaoka A, Monden Y, Nakahara K, Tanioka T. Follow-up study of thymomas with special reference to their clinical stages. Cancer. 1981;48:2485–92.
5. den Bakker MA, Roden AC, Marx A, Marino M. Histologic classification of thymoma: a practical guide for routine cases. J Thorac Oncol. 2014;9(9 Suppl 2):S125–30. https://doi.org/10.1097/JTO.0000000000000297. Review
6. Bernard C, Frih H, Pasquet F, Kerever S, Jamilloux Y, Tronc F, Guibert B, Isaac S, Devouassoux M, Chalabreysse L, Broussolle C, Petiot P, Girard N, Sève P. Thymoma associated with autoimmune

diseases: 85 cases and literature review. Autoimmun Rev. 2016;15(1):82–92. https://doi.org/10.1016/j.autrev.2015.09.005. Review

7. Thongprayoon C, Tantrachoti P, Phatharacharukul P, Buranapraditkun S, Klaewsongkram J. Associated immunological disorders and cellular immune dysfunction in thymoma: a study of 87 cases from Thailand. Arch Immunol Ther Exp. 2013;61(1):85–93. https://doi.org/10.1007/s00005-012-0207-9. Epub 2012 Dec 11
8. Hayward AR, Paolucci P, Webster ADB, et al. Pre-B cell suppression by thymoma patients' lymphocytes. Clin Exp Immunol. 1982;48:437–42.
9. Yamazaki K, Watanabe N, Hasegawa A, Yamaguchi E, Miyamoto K, Sakiyama Y, Kawakami Y. Good's syndrome with a block in the early stage of B cell differentiation and complicated by Campylobacter fetus sepsis. Intern Med. 1994;33(8):496–500. Review
10. Oritani K, Medina KL, Tomiyama Y, Ishikawa J, Okajima Y, Ogawa M, Yokota T, Aoyama K, Takahashi I, Kincade PW, Matsuzawa Y. Limitin: an interferon-like cytokine that preferentially influences B-lymphocyte precursors. Nat Med. 2000;6(6):659–66.
11. Christopoulos P, Dopfer EP, Malkovsky M, Esser PR, Schaefer HE, Marx A, Kock S, Rupp N, Lorenz MR, Schwarz K, Harder J, Martin SF, Werner M, Bogdan C, IWW S, Fisch P. A novel thymoma-associated immunodeficiency with increased naive T cells and reduced CD247 expression. J Immunol. 2015;194(7):3045–53. https://doi.org/10.4049/jimmunol.1402805.
12. Sun X, Shi J, Wang M, Xu K, Xiao Y. Good's syndrome patients hospitalized for infections: a single-center retrospective study. Medicine (Baltimore). 2015;94(47):e2090. https://doi.org/10.1097/MD.0000000000002090.
13. Kelleher P, Misbah SA. What is Good's syndrome? Immunological abnormalities in patients with thymoma. J Clin Pathol. 2003;56(1):12–6.
14. Joven MH, Palalay MP, Sonido CY. Case report and literature review on Good's syndrome, a form of acquired immunodeficiency associated with thymomas. Hawaii J Med Public Health. 2013;72(2):56–62.
15. Ide S, Koga T, Rikimaru T, Katsuki Y, Oizumi K. Good's syndrome presenting with cytomegalovirus pneumonia. Intern Med. 2000;39(12):1094–6.
16. Wargo JJ, Kim AH, Hart A, Berg A. It took a village: Good's syndrome. Am J Med. 2015;128(7):699–701. https://doi.org/10.1016/j.amjmed.2015.03.002.
17. Tachdjian R, Keller JJ, Pfeffer M. A bad case of Good's syndrome. Infect Dis Ther. 2014;3(2):333–7. https://doi.org/10.1007/s40121-014-0045-7.
18. Ueno S, Sekimoto-Tsuboi S, Ishiguro Y, Koinuma T, Eguchi H, Machida Y, HattoriN MH. Good's syndrome with opportunistic infection of the central nervous system: a case report. BMC Neurol. 2015;15:150. https://doi.org/10.1186/s12883-015-0406-1.
19. Sveinsson O, Matell H, Herrman L. Progressive multifocal leukoencephalopathy in a patient with Good's syndrome. BMJ Case Rep. 2013;2013:pii: bcr2013009763. https://doi.org/10.1136/bcr-2013-009763.
20. Sasson SC, Davies S, Chan R, Davies L, Garsia R. Cerebral toxoplasmosis in a patient with myasthenia gravis and thymoma with immunodeficiency/Good's syndrome: a case report. BMC Infect Dis. 2016;16(1):457. https://doi.org/10.1186/s12879-016-1801-y.
21. Akinosoglou K, Melachrinou M, Siagris D, Koletsis E, Marangos M, Gogos CA, Solomou EE. Good's syndrome and pure white cell aplasia complicated by cryptococcus infection: a case report and review of the literature. J Clin Immunol. 2014;34(3):283–8. https://doi.org/10.1007/s10875-014-0014-7.
22. Disselhorst MJ, Dickhoff C, Alhan C. Good's syndrome: an uncommon cause of therapy-resistant diarrhoea. Neth J Med. 2016;74(7):309–12.
23. Rawat A, Dhir V, Gupta A, Suri D, Burad DK, Nada R, Singh S. Good's syndrome presenting with recurrent giardiasis. J Clin Immunol. 2014;34(7):751–2. https://doi.org/10.1007/s10875-014-0080-x.
24. Verne GN, Amann ST, Cosgrove C, Cerda JJ. Chronic diarrhea associated with thymoma and hypogammaglobulinemia (Good's syndrome). South Med J. 1997;90(4):444–6.
25. Murray WD, Webb JN. Thymoma associated with hypogammaglobulinaemia and pure red cell aplasia. Am J Med. 1966;41:974–80.

26. Taniguchi T, Usami N, Kawaguchi K, Yokoi K. Good syndrome accompanied by pure red cell aplasia. Interact Cardiovasc Thorac Surg. 2009;9(4):750–2. https://doi.org/10.1510/icvts.2009.210393.
27. Kuribayashi K, Fujimi A, Kobune M, Takimoto R, Kikuchi S, Iyama S, Kato J, Niitsu Y, Watanabe N. Pure red cell aplasia associated with Good's syndrome accompanied by decreased stem cell factor production in the bone marrow. Intern Med. 2010;49(5):377–82.
28. Nitta H, Harada Y, Okikawa Y, Fujii M, Arihiro K, Kimura A, Harada H. Good's syndrome-associated pure red cell aplasia with myelodysplastic syndrome. Intern Med. 2011;50(18):2011–4.
29. Hashizume T. Good's syndrome and pernicious anemia. Intern Med. 2002;41(11):1062–4.
30. Kaku Y, Shimamoto N, Matsunaga H, Makiura M, Fujisawa A, Morita K. Oral erosive lichen planus and alopecia areata with Good's syndrome (thymoma with hypogammaglobulinemia). Eur J Dermatol. 2011;21(1):124–5. https://doi.org/10.1684/ejd.2010.1183.
31. Hanafusa T, Umegaki N, Yamaguchi Y, Katayama I. Good's syndrome (hypogammaglobulinemia with thymoma) presenting intractable opportunistic infections and hyperkeratotic lichen planus. J Dermatol. 2010;37(2):171–4. https://doi.org/10.1111/j.1346-8138.2009.00781.x.
32. Ohuchi M, Inoue S, Hanaoka J, Igarashi T, Tezuka N, Ozaki Y, et al. Good syndrome coexisting with leukopenia. Ann Thorac Surg. 2007;84:2095–7. https://doi.org/10.1016/j.athoracsur.2007.06.070.
33. Kristiansen HA, Spetalen S, Fløisand Y, Heldal D. Eltrombopag in Good's Syndrome. Case Rep Hematol. 2014;2014:172139. https://doi.org/10.1155/2014/172139.
34. Soppi E, Eskola J, Veromaa T, et al. Thymoma with immunodeficiency (Good's syndrome) associated with myasthenia gravis and benign IgG gammopathy. Arch Intern Med. 1985;145:1704–7.
35. Zonios D, Sheikh V, Sereti I. Idiopathic CD4 lymphocytopenia: a case of missing, wandering or ineffective T cells. Arthritis Res Ther. 2012;14(4):222. https://doi.org/10.1186/ar4027.
36. Glück J, Rymarczyk B, Paluch U, Rogala B, Brzoza Z. A case of Good's syndrome diagnosed after more than 20 years since onset of myasthenia in a patient with psoriasis. Neurol Sci. 2016;37(7):1179–80. https://doi.org/10.1007/s10072-016-2526-9.
37. Habib AM, Thornton H, Sewell WC, Loubani M. Good's syndrome: Is thymectomy the solution? Case report and literature review. Asian Cardiovasc Thorac Ann. 2016;24(7):712–4. https://doi.org/10.1177/0218492316655641.
38. Antar AI, Otrock ZK, Kharfan-Dabaja MA, Mahfouz RA, Alameddine RS, El-Majzoub NM, Salem ZM. Thymoma with concomitant pure red cell aplasia, Good's syndrome and myasthenia gravis responding to rituximab. Indian J Hematol Blood Transfus. 2016;32(Suppl 1):219–22. https://doi.org/10.1007/s12288-014-0478-x.
39. Ternavasio-de la Vega HG, Velasco-Tirado V, Pozo-Rosado L, Soler-Fernández MC, Pérez-Andres M, Orfao A, Sánchez-Sánchez R, González-Villaron L. Persistence of immunological alterations after thymectomy in Good's syndrome: a clue to its pathogenesis. Cytometry B Clin Cytom. 2011;80(5):339–42. https://doi.org/10.1002/cyto.b.20595.
40. Hermaszewski RA, Webster AD. Primary hypogammaglobulinaemia: a survey of clinical manifestations and complications. Q J Med. 1993;86(1):31–**42**.

Differential Diagnosis in Hypogammaglobulinemia

19

Isabella Quinti, Cinzia Milito, Rossella Carello, and Federica Pulvirenti

19.1 Hypogammaglobulinemias

Hypogammaglobulinemias are characterized by low or deficient levels of any of the immunoglobulins (IgG, IgA, IgM, IgE, and IgG subclasses). This condition represents a diagnostic challenge for clinicians, due to its association with many pathological entities with different manifestations and outcomes. At the initial evaluation, several factors should be considered to correctly recognize the possible cause of hypogammaglobulinemia, including age of onset, sex, number and type immunoglobulin class involved, vaccine responses, clinical manifestations, comorbidities, and medications. Clinician must have a high level of suspicion for antibody deficiency for all patients when a serum hypogammaglobulinemia is evident. In the registry of European Society for Immunodeficiencies (ESID), the vast majority of cases of antibody disorders involve a hypogammaglobulinemia, including common variable immunodeficiency disorder (CVID), the most reported one. As described in Chap. 3, CVID is characterized by marked decrease of IgG and IgA serum levels, recurrent respiratory infections and/or autoimmune features, and impaired vaccine response in association with pathological B subset immunophenotype. Some patients with a low IgG level and impaired vaccine responses may not fulfill criteria for CVID because IgA or IgM level is not low. This form of hypogammaglobulinemia with antibody deficiency should be classified as "unspecified IgG deficiency" or "unspecified hypogammaglobulinemia" (see Chap. 17). Alternatively, IgG and IgA levels may be low, but vaccine responses may appear normal. In all these cases, patients should be assessed repeatedly over time because immunoglobulin levels and antibody function may wane to the point that the above criteria are

I. Quinti (✉) · C. Milito · R. Carello · F. Pulvirenti
Department of Molecular Medicine, Sapienza University of Rome, Rome, Italy
e-mail: isabella.quinti@uniroma1.it

M. M. D'Elios, M. Rizzi (eds.), *Humoral Primary Immunodeficiencies*,
Rare Diseases of the Immune System, https://doi.org/10.1007/978-3-319-91785-6_19

met and a diagnosis of CVID can be conferred [1]. The age of onset of a serum hypogammaglobulinemia should also be taken into account since a physiological condition of hypogammaglobulinemia is observed in infants below 2 years of age. Thus, before 2 years of age, children with low level of serum immunoglobulins may be cautiously defined as having hypogammaglobulinemia and be monitored over the time such as most of the patients with hypogammaglobulinemias of infancy can normalize IgG values within 2–4 years of age (transient hypogammaglobulinemia of infancy) (see Chap. 17). Moreover, serum immunoglobulin levels vary with age, so age-specific cutoffs should be used when performing laboratory testing (see Chap. 17 for normal values). A basic laboratory work-up that includes testing complete blood count with differential, and measurement of serum immunoglobulin and complement levels for human immunodeficiency virus (HIV) antibody, can identify children who need further testing and referral to a subspecialist for a suspected immunodeficiency disease [2, 3].

In addition to primary antibody defect, hypogammaglobulinemia can be due to a broad spectrum of conditions, which can be divided into immunoglobulin production diseases such as lymphoid malignancies, infections, and medications and immunoglobulin loss diseases such as enteropathies or renal amyloidosis. Due to this complexity, at initial evaluation of all patients with low serum immunoglobulin level, defined causes of hypogammaglobulinemias must be investigated, according to a list of differential diagnosis (Table 19.1), to differentiate primary from secondary forms of hypogammaglobulinemia and prescribe treatment when possible.

19.2 Primary Hypogammaglobulinemias

Primary hypogammaglobulinemias are defined as an impaired production of antibodies caused by defects in B-cell number and maturation, reduced survival and activation of B cells, and faulty interaction between B and T cells. This condition is an immunological feature common to many primary immunodeficiencies [4, 5]. Differential diagnosis of primary hypogammaglobulinemia is quite broad. The laboratory work-up that should be performed during initial evaluation of suspected primary hypogammaglobulinemia should include measurement of serum immunoglobulin levels and vaccine responses to a T-dependent and a T-independent antigen. To improve diagnostic specificity, flow cytometry analysis of peripheral circulating lymphocytes is essential, in order to define T-, B-, and natural killer-cell populations and exclude combined immunodeficiency. Measurement of B-cell subsets may also be helpful for differentiating CVID from other disorders. Primary immunodeficiencies with autosomal recessive inheritance should be considered in patients with early-onset hypogammaglobulinemia mimicking CVID, particularly in a consanguineous family. Thus, the differential diagnosis for panhypogammaglobulinemia can vary depending on age of onset and includes XLA, transient hypogammaglobulinemia of infancy, autosomal recessive B-cell deficiency, X-linked lymphoproliferative syndrome, and combined T- and B-cell immunodeficiency with hypogammaglobulinemia and CVID. As general rule, lack of B lymphocytes excludes transient hypogammaglobulinemia of infancy (Chap. 17) and other causes of primary hypogammaglobulinemias, such as X-linked

Table 19.1 List of differential diagnosis in hypogammaglobulinemia

Primary immunodeficiencies
X-linked agammaglobulinemia
CVID and CVID-like disorders
Severe combined immunodeficiency
Hyper-IgM
Selective IgA deficiency
Isolated IgG subclass deficiency
ADA deficiency
Wiskott-Aldrich syndrome
Congenital agammaglobulinemias
Others (LOCID, ICOS deficiency, CD19 deficiency, CD20 deficiency, CD21 deficiency, TACI deficiency, LRBA deficiency, BAFF receptor deficiency, TWEAK defects, NFKB2 deficiency, WHIM syndrome, thymoma with immunodeficiency, PRKC delta, and PI3K delta-associated diseases)
Chromosomal abnormalities
18q syndrome
Trisomy 8
Trisomy 21
Monosomy 22
Secondary hypogammaglobulinemias
B-cell malignancies
Chronic lymphocytic leukemia
Multiple myeloma
Others
Viral infections
Congenital AIDS
EBV
CMV
Drug induced
Steroids
Anti-CD20 therapy and B-cell targeting therapies
Bone marrow transplantation HSCT
Immunosuppressive regimes in solid organ transplantation
Immunosuppressive regimes in autoimmune disease
Antiepileptic drugs
Others
Hypogammaglobulinemia due to reduced Ig half-life
Autoimmune diseases
Protein-losing syndromes
Enteropathy
Lymphangiectasis
Nephropathy
Severe burns

hyper-IgM (Chap. 15) and X-linked lymphoproliferative disease. Absence of T cells directs the work-up toward defects associated with severe combined immunodeficiency. The isolated congenital deficiency of B cells supports the diagnosis of XLA in a male subject, but the clinical phenotype can be mimicked by rare mutations in genes encoding the μ heavy chain, Igα, Igβ, λ5, B-cell linker (BLNK), leucine-rich repeat-containing 8 (LRRC8), or the p85α subunit of phosphoinositide 3-kinase (PI3K).

Details of diagnostic criteria for primary immunodeficiencies with a humoral defect are illustrated in other chapters of this volume. A comprehensive search for mutations in known primary immunodeficiency genes may be warranted in hypogammaglobulinemic patients with unusual clinical features. According to the clinical spectrum of clinical manifestations, the age of the patient, and the molecular and immunological phenotypes, many of these primary immunodeficiencies should be excluded in this differential diagnostic work-up.

19.3 Chromosomal Abnormalities

Several chromosomal abnormalities (chromosome 18q-syndrome, monosomy 22, trisomy 8, and trisomy 21) are currently identified as causes of hypogammaglobulinemia and can manifest with recurrent infections and mimic CVID. On the other hand, patients with genetic abnormalities and recurrent infections should be evaluated for hypogammaglobulinemia, in order to early identify humoral deficiency, allow the treatment, and prevent complications and sequelae [6].

19.3.1 18q Syndrome

The incidence of 18q deletion syndrome is reported as 1 in 10,000 live births. The characteristic features of the syndrome are short stature, hearing loss, hypotonia, mental retardation, and endocrine disorders, accompanied by autoimmunity. However, the pathogenesis of the hypogammaglobulinemia is unclear since no immunoglobulin genes are encoded on the 18th chromosome. IgA deficiency is seen approximately in 24% of patients. Moreover, IgA deficiency has been also reported in other 18th chromosomal abnormalities (ring chromosome 18 and 18q deletion syndrome) as well as from 18q deletion syndrome [7]. The immunological deficit was limited to an inability to synthesize chains of the IgA molecule in normal amounts and justify the occurrence of repeated infections of the respiratory tract [7, 8]. Additionally, in other patients, moderate IgM hypogammaglobulinemia has been reported, due to deletion of the long arm of chromosome 18.

19.3.2 Trisomy 8

Trisomy 8 is currently identified as a cause of hypogammaglobulinemia and can be characterized by recurrent infections, mimicking CVID. Few cases of hypogammaglobulinemia associated with trisomy 8 mosaicism were also described. Immunoglobulin levels should be routinely tested in patients with trisomy 8 presenting with recurrent sinopulmonary infections, diarrhea, malnutrition, and pernicious anemia. To date, no data are available about the link of genes on the chromosome 8 and CVID [9].

19.3.3 Trisomy 21

Down syndrome is associated with characteristic manifestations of primary immunodeficiencies, such as susceptibility to infection, autoimmunity, and a high malignancy risk. However, Down syndrome is not considered a primary immunodeficiency but rather a syndromic deficiency, due to the relevance of the characteristic neurological delay. Down syndrome individuals may have a high frequency of infections, usually of the upper respiratory tract, characterized by increased severity and prolonged course of disease, which are partially attributed to defects of the immune system. The abnormalities of the immune system associated with Down syndrome include mild to moderate T- and B-cell lymphopenia, with marked decrease of naive lymphocytes, impaired mitogen-induced T-cell proliferation, impaired specific antibody responses to immunizations, and defects of neutrophil chemotaxis associated with infections predominantly of the respiratory tract. Recently, a severe reduction of switched memory B cells in Down syndrome was demonstrated [10].

19.4 Secondary Hypogammaglobulinemias

The process of generating a different diagnosis in a patient with hypogammaglobulinemia should include a vigorous search for secondary treatable causes. Differential diagnosis could be difficult because of similar clinical aspects in primary and secondary forms of hypogammaglobulinemias. Secondary immune deficiencies (SID) develop in the course of different diseases and/or as consequence of immune suppressive or immune modulatory treatment. Deficiencies may involve innate immunity, adaptive T- and B-cell immunity. Thus, SID patients represent a heterogeneous population, including subjects with HIV infection, haematological malignancies, malignant solid tumors, hematopoietic stem cell transplant (HSCT) and solid organ transplant recipients, patients on immune suppressive or immune modulatory treatment for systemic autoimmune and inflammatory diseases, and other minor conditions [11]. Given the broad differential diagnosis of hypogammaglobulinemia and that primary hypogammaglobulinemia is often a diagnosis of exclusion, an extensive diagnostic work-up should be performed in order to identify a SID (Table 19.2).

Classical conditions of SID due to malignant B-cell lymphoproliferation or conditioning regimes with alkylating agents in transplant recipients are being outnumbered by SID conditions caused by an ever-increasing number of therapeutic monoclonal antibodies, fusion proteins, and engineered T cells with potential to directly or indirectly target the B-cell lineage and plasma cells. With the advent of many new potent therapeutic options and their combination with classical drugs, the spectrum of hypogammaglobulinemic states caused by innovative treatment strategies has greatly broadened.

Table 19.2 Diagnostic work-up for the exclusion of secondary immunodeficiencies in patients with hypogammaglobulinemias

Physical exam	Splenomegaly
	Hepatomegaly
	Lymphadenopathy
	Sings of malnutrition
Symptoms	Refractory diarrhea
	Chronic cough, sputum, or rhinitis
	Dyspnea
	Refractory fever
Medical history	Number of infections
	Similar manifestations in relatives
	Age of onset
	Diagnosis of chronic diseases, including malignancies
	Hospital admissions for infections
	Medications
Laboratory evaluation	Complete blood count (WBC, RBC, PLT count, Hb)
	Blood smear
	Biochemistry (LDH, bilirubin)
	Complete urine analysis
	Stool chemical and physical analysis
	Immunoelectrophoresis-serum and urine test
	Dosage of serum free light chains
	Beta2 microglobulin serum levels
	Peripheral Lymphocytes subsets: CD3+, CD3+/CD4+, CD3+/CD8+, CD3+/CD4-CD8-; CD19+, CD20+, CD20kappa+, CD20lamda+, CD8+/CD57+/CD16+
	Peripheral B-cell subsets: naïve, MZ, and switched memory B cells
Imaging	Chest CT scan: evaluation of nodules, bronchiectasis, consolidation, interstitial lung disease, lymph nodes enlargement, mediastinal mass
	Abdominal complete ultrasound (or abdominal CT scan): evaluation of the spleen, liver diameter and lesions, lymph node number and diameter
Endoscopy	Upper gastrointestinal endoscopy with tissue biopsies: to evaluate stomach and duodenum
	Lower gastrointestinal endoscopy with tissue biopsies: to evaluate ileum and colon
	Search for *Helicobacter pylori*, *Chlamydia*, *Campylobacter*, *Borrelia*, and CMV by PCR on biopsy specimens
Microbiology	Search for CVM, EBV, HIV, HCV, HHV8, and HHV6 by PCR on peripheral blood samples
	Search for *Campylobacter* and *Protozoa* on stool samples
Histology	Bone marrow
	Lymph nodes
	Stomach, duodenum, ileum, colon

19.4.1 Hypogammaglobulinemia and Malignancies

Immunocompetent patients with cancer can develop immune suppression after chemotherapy and to post-transplant immunosuppressive therapy. In particular, the finding of a hypogammaglobulinemia is recurrent for patients affected by B-cell chronic lymphocytic leukemia (CLL), lymphoproliferative disorders, or plasma cell dyscrasias, conditions that must be carefully ruled out at initial evaluation of every patient with low immunoglobulin serum levels. Patients suffering from B-cell malignancies are prone to acquired hypogammaglobulinemia with specific antibody failure and suffer from severe, recurrent, or opportunistic infections, all hallmarks of antibody failure. Clinical manifestations can range from recurrent and prolonged respiratory or gastrointestinal infections by agents with low pathogenicity to severe life-threatening infections. These manifestations are an important cause of morbidity, mortality, hospital admissions, and intensive care treatments in this group of patients.

Due to the recurrence of lymphoproliferative disorders in patients with primary immunodeficiency such as CVID, it could be difficult to differentiate a hypogammaglobulinemia secondary to lymphoma from lymphomas complicating a newly diagnosed primary antibody defect. Past medical history positive for recurrent infections or hypogammabulinemia, presence of bronchiectasis or other clinical features associated to primary antibody deficiency (ie autoimmune diseases) are more consistent with malignancy following a primary immunodeficiency. An observation period after the first finding of hypogammaglobulinemia could also be useful for differential diangosis. The diagnosis of lymphoma could be puzzling in patients with CVID and other primary antibody deficiency. The histology can be indistinguishable from a primary tumor, including absence of EBV antigens on immune histology. This may be an important distinction from those lymphoid tumors associated with another condition confused with CVID, namely, X-linked lymphoproliferative disease, in which EBV-driven tumors are seen. Moreover, it should be noted that the histology of lymphoid tissues and bone marrow from hypogammaglobulinemic patients without a suspected malignancy varies from microscopically normal to grossly abnormal. In addition, the validity of clonality as a marker of lymphoma in antibody deficiency is not resolved, as monoclonal proliferations have been reported in patients without progression. The histological specimens should be analyzed by morphological identification, immunostaining, Epstein–Barr virus by in situ hybridization to detect EBV-encoded short RNA species (EBER 1 and EBER 2), TCR and IgH clonality.

19.4.1.1 Hypogammaglobulinemia in Chronic Lymphocytic Leukemia

Hypogammaglobulinemia is the most recognized inherent immune defect in patients with CLL during their disease course. It occurs in 20–70% of unselected patients with CLL, and it is a continuous process developing spontaneously during the untreated course of the disease. The incidence increases in patients with advanced disease stage and in those with a long disease duration and following immunosuppressive therapy. Moreover, infections are the major cause of morbidity and mortality, contributing to 25–50% of deaths. Selected patients with CLL, hypogammaglobulinemia and infections could benefit from Ig replacement treatment [12, 13].

19.4.1.2 Hypogammaglobulinemia in Multiple Myeloma

Prevalence of multiple myeloma (MM) is 4–5/10,000 with a predominance of male sex. Multiple myeloma is associated with a susceptibility to bacterial infections, specifically for encapsulated organisms such as *S. pneumoniae*. There has been an evolution in the spectrum of infections noted, and this has been related to the move away from alkylator-based therapies to newer medications such as the purine analogues and monoclonal antibodies that have their own unique impact on immune functions.

Hypogammaglobulinemia of the non-monoclonal immunoglobulin heavy chain classes has been also reported in monoclonal gammopathy of undetermined significance (MGUS) [14]. In adults with antibody deficiency, a bone marrow examination might be required to rule out all hematologic malignancies, including multiple myeloma and in particular light chain myeloma. The absence of defining organ pathology in MGUS raises the possibility that its diagnosis in patients presenting with hypogammaglobulinemia—including those diagnosed with CVID—could be missed unless a serum protein electrophoresis and serum immunofixation are performed. The dosage of serum free light chains was proven useful in the differential diagnosis and prognosis of primary and secondary hypogammaglobulinemia [15].

19.4.2 Hypogammaglobulinemia After Bone Marrow Transplantation

Allogeneic hematopoietic stem cell transplantation (HSCT) is an established treatment option for many malignant and nonmalignant disorders. In the past two decades, peripheral blood stem cells replaced bone marrow as stem cell source due to faster engraftment and practicability. As transplant indications and conditioning regimens continue to change, whether the choice of the stem cell source has an impact on transplant outcomes remains to be determined. HSCT in combination with rituximab maintenance therapy might induce persisting hypogammaglobulinemia in a considerable number of patients. Hypogammaglobulinemia in particular appears to be a contributing factor in recurring cytomegalovirus infection in organ transplant patients, leading to severe gastrointestinal disease [16].

19.4.3 Congenital AIDS and Other Viral Infections (EBV, CMV)

HIV disease is the most frequent secondary immunodeficiency. It is characterized by profound lymphopenia and high susceptibility to opportunistic infections. Infection with the human immunodeficiency virus is characteristically associated with hypergammaglobulinemia in both adult and pediatric cases. HIV virus induces T-cell lymphopenia by several mechanism: HIV-induced apoptosis, viral cytopathic effect, and apoptosis secondary to immune activation. The immunological profile of HIV infection is peculiar. In fact, patients show a condition of hypergammaglobulinemia in both adult and pediatric cases and a T-cell defect with a difficult to mount specific antibody responses to various T-cell-dependent antigens. When infection occurs early in development (by transplacental exposure to the virus or from blood transfusion in small premature infants), hypogammaglobulinemia can lead to the absence of antibody responses on which diagnosis is usually based. Due to the deficient antibody production, children might experience severe recurrent bacterial infections, including bacteremia and pneumonia. Moreover, also HIV adult patients can show profoundly impaired humoral immunity with hypogammaglobulinemia and a high susceptibility to bacterial infections [17].

Congenital and persistent cytomegalovirus (CMV) infection can induce in newborn neutropenia and other immunologic abnormalities such as decreased serum IgG and IgA, depressed T- and B-lymphocyte functions, and decreased natural killer activity [18]. Hypogammaglobulinemia is also reported in adult patients with disseminate CMV infection. Hypogammaglobulinemia occurring during cytomegalovirus infection is transient but deep [19].

Hypogammaglobulinemia is not usually observed during Epstein-Barr virus (EBV) infections. Male which developed persistent hypogammaglobulinemia following severe acute infectious mononucleosis have to be evaluated for XLP if other immunological abnormalities are observed [20].

19.4.4 Protein-Losing Syndromes (Enteropathy, Lymphangiectasis, Nephropathy, Severe Burns)

Excessive serum protein loss from the gastrointestinal tract, from renal tract, and from the skin might cause hypogammaglobulinemia. Protein-losing enteropathy should be considered in individuals with hypogammaglobulinemia, edema, and hypoalbuminemia and in absence of liver or renal diseases. Radiolabeled albumin and fecal clearance of alpha 1-antitrypsin have been used for the diagnosis of protein malabsorption and intestinal losses. Moreover, hypogammaglobulinemia might be the underlying cause of an undiagnosed celiac disease, due the lacking of the diagnostic serology. In these patients small bowel biopsies have been considered the gold standard for the diagnosis [21].

19.4.5 Hypogammaglobulinemia Secondary to Short Immunoglobulin Half-Life

Genetic defects in MOGS, the gene encoding mannosyl-oligosaccharide glucosidase (the first enzyme in the processing pathway of N-linked oligosaccharide), cause the rare congenital disorder of glycosylation type IIb (CDG-IIb), also known as MOGS-CDG. MOGS is expressed in the endoplasmic reticulum and is involved in the trimming of N-glycans. This condition has been described in two siblings with CDG-IIb who presented with multiple neurologic complications and a paradoxical immunologic phenotype characterized by severe hypogammaglobulinemia. A shortened immunoglobulin half-life was determined to be the mechanism underlying the hypogammaglobulinemia [22].

19.4.6 Drug-Induced Hypogammaglobulinemias

19.4.6.1 Glucocorticosteroids

Glucocorticoid therapy represents the first-line therapy in many disorders, especially for the treatment of acute exacerbations of the diseases. Its use however has been limited by several side effects including infection susceptibility due to secondary immunodeficiency. Besides compromising T-cell function, glucocorticoid therapy has also been reported as a cause of secondary hypogammaglobulinemia. While an initial drop is common among all patients under glucocorticoid therapy, the occurrence of manifest hypogammaglobulinemia additionally depends on pretreatment IgG serum levels. It has been demonstrated that if serum IgG had dropped below 5.0 g/L, patients did not recover from hypogammaglobulinemia. Regarding glucocorticoid use, daily doses of more than 20 mg for 14 days in individuals (or doses >2 mg/kg in children weighing <10 kg) or lower doses over longer periods (months to years) may lead to hypogammaglobulinemia. Although hypogammaglobulinemia with systemic steroid use is well documented, impaired vaccine response is more theoretical [23].

19.4.6.2 Cyclophosphamide and Mycophenolate

Mycophenolate and cyclophosphamide therapies are associated with severe hypogammaglobulinemia. The lack of immunoglobulins might be explained by the high proportion of proteinuric patients, as hypogammaglobulinemia is a common finding in patients with nephrotic syndrome. Patients with proteinuria should be monitored closely with regard to Ig levels and infections. Especially a combination with other immunosuppressive agents, such as atacicept or ocrelizumab, has been described to be associated with a higher risk for development of severe immunoglobulin deficiency and infections [24]. Prolonged hypogammaglobulinemia requiring antibody replacement therapy occurred in 21% of ANCA vasculitis patients treated with cyclophosphamide followed by rituximab. It could be assumed that hypogammaglobulinemia is also caused by the drugs used to treat SLE. Nevertheless, discontinuation of therapy does not reverse hypogammaglobulinemia.

19.4.6.3 Fenclofenac

During treatment with fenclofenac in patients affected by rheumatoid arthritis, selective IgA deficiency might develop. The hypogammaglobulinemia is temporary, and after withdrawal of drug serum, IgA level returned to normal [25].

19.4.6.4 Sulfasalazine

Sulfasalazine can induce hypogammaglobulinemia together with thrombocytopenia. After stopping the therapy, the serum immunoglobulin levels returned to normal level within 3 months [26].

19.4.6.5 Gold Salts

In patients affected by rheumatoid arthritis receiving gold salts, selective IgA deficiency and panhypogammaglobulinemia have been recorded. In some patients treated with gold therapy, the immunodeficiency persisted and even required replacement therapy [27].

19.4.6.6 Penicillamine

Serum IgA deficiency was described after the onset of D-penicillamine therapy. Special immunological examinations revealed a deficiency of the secretory component of IgA, while cellular functions of T and B lymphocytes were normal. Regular control of serum immunoglobulin levels is mandatory during D-penicillamine treatment [28].

19.4.6.7 Carbamazepine

In patients on long-term carbamazepine therapy, the physician should monitor Ig serum levels and the lymphocyte subpopulation. Carbamazepine has been implicated in a variety of immunodeficiency disorders such as agranulocytosis or neutropenia, immunosuppressant effects on T cells, absence of B cells, alteration of class switch process, impairment of the synthesis of immunoglobulins in B cells, monoclonal gammopathy of undetermined significance, and reduced serum IgA and IgM with normal numbers of T or B lymphocytes [29].

19.4.6.8 Phenytoin

Panhypogammaglobulinemia mimicking CVID and low levels of mature CD19 + B cells may be associated with phenytoin treatment. Patients on phenytoin treatment who reported symptoms indicating immunodeficiency lymphocyte subpopulations and immunoglobulin levels need to be monitored. Hypogammaglobulinemia is always reversible after stopping therapy [30].

19.4.6.9 Valproic Acid

Antibody failure due to valproic acid has been recently reported. This histone deacetylase inhibitor can inhibit early B-cell differentiation and activation leading to hypogammaglobulinemia [31].

19.4.6.10 Hypogammaglobulinemia After B-Cell Targeting Therapies (Directly or Indirectly Targeting B-Cell and Plasma Cells)

Patients receiving B-cell-directed therapies, particularly when in combination with cytotoxic drugs, are prone to develop SID, which may involve transient or long-lasting impairment of humoral and cellular immunity. The leading clinical symptoms are severe, recurrent, or opportunistic infections. Well known is therapeutic

B-cell depletion by rituximab, a monoclonal antibody against the protein CD20. CD20 is expressed on pre-B and mature B-lymphocytes but not on pro-B cells or plasma cells. Although not affecting plasma cells directly, the use of anti-CD20 in the setting of non-hematological conditions (e.g., autoimmune cytopenias, rheumatoid arthritis, desensitization prior to solid organ transplantation) has extended the spectrum of SID following anti-CD20 therapy. Indeed, prolonged anti-CD20 therapy, particularly when in association with preceding chemotherapy, considerably increases the risk of hypogammaglobulinemia [32–34].

In the last years, the number of patients with SID is rapidly increasing because of the rapid development of highly effective new drugs. Therapeutic B-cell targeting has become more and more popular to overcome various autoantibody-mediated clinical conditions. Agents are therapeutic monoclonal antibodies with specificities for CD20, CD22, IL6-receptor, BAFF have been recently released, and other are under ongoing phase I/II studies. This, together with a widening of clinical indication in B-cell malignancies, warrants a heightened vigilance with respect to recurrent severe infections. A list of therapeutic monoclonal antibodies potentially capable of inducing a secondary hypogammaglobulinemia is reported in Table 19.3.

Table 19.3 Therapeutic monoclonals potentially capable of inducing a secondary hypogammaglobulinemias

Target	Molecule	Mechanism	Indication	Ref.
CD20	Rituximab	Depletion of B-cells expressing the CD20 antigen	B-NHL and RA	[32–34]
	Ibritumomab tiuxetan	Targeting CD20+ cells by binding to CD22+ follicular B cells and destroying through 90 Yttrium (ß-radiation-emitting isotope)	Refractory, relapsing B-NHL as consolidation therapy after remission induction in previously untreated patients with follicular lymphoma; adult patients with rituximab relapsed or refractory CD20+ follicular B-cell NHL	[35]
	Obinutuzumab	Depletion of CD20 B cells	Refractory CLL; follicular lymphoma	[36]
	Ofatumumab	Depletion of CD20 B cells	Previously untreated CLL	[37]
	Ocrelizumab	Depletion of CD20 B cells	MS (phase II) RA and SLE (phase III)	[38]
BAFF	Belimumab	Neutralizing soluble BAFF	Non-renal forms in SLE	[39]
	Tabalumab	Neutralizes membrane-bound and soluble BAFF		[40]
	Blisibimod	Blocking soluble and membrane expressed biologically active BAFF	(Ongoing studies for patients affected by SLE, RA, SS, and myositis)	[41]
CD3/ CD19	Blinatumomab	Targeting and promotion of the links between cytotoxic T cell and malignant CD19+ B cells	Philadelphia chromosome negative relapsed or refractory B-precursor ALL	[42]

Table 19.3 (continued)

Target	Molecule	Mechanism	Indication	Ref.
CD22	Epratuzumab	Targets CD22 by inhibiting the production of the pro-inflammatory cytokines IL-6 and TNF-α by B cells, but not the regulatory cytokine IL-10	SLE (phase III), in refractory aggressive B-NHL (phase II)	[43]
	Inotuzumab	Binds to the endocytotic receptor CD22, expressed by majority of B cells	Acute B-ALL	[44]
	Moxetumomab pasudotox	Targeting CD22 conjugated to toxin composed of the VH and VL portions of an anti-CD22 antibody connected by a disulfide bond and fused to a truncated form of Pseudomonas exotoxin	Hairy cell leukemia and B-lymphoblastic leukemia/ lymphoma B-ALL (phase III clinical trials)	[45]
CD19	CD19-targeted chimeric antigen receptor transduced T cells	Killing CD19 expressing ALL cells	Refractory ALL, after HSCT	[46]
CD25	Daclizumab, Basiliximab	Binding CD25 on T cells	Acute GvH reaction in allograft recipients, allograft rejection, MS, and in T-cell leukemia	[47]
CD52	Alemtuzumab	Binding CD52 and promoting the cytotoxicity of CD52 bearing cells	CLL, MS, CTCL, T-cell lymphoma	[48]
IL6R	Tocilizumab	Binding-soluble and membrane-bound IL-6R, blocking the IL-6/IL-6R interactions, critical for B-cell differentiation, plasma blast growth, and plasma cell IgG production	RA, systemic juvenile idiopathic arthritis	[49]
FcRn		Inhibition of the capability of neonatal Fc receptor in salvaging IgG from lysosomal degradation	(Phase I studies)	[50]
TACI	Atacicept	Binding TACI and neutralizing soluble April and BAFF, impairing B-cell differentiation	Ongoing studies in SLE, RA and MS already showing a severe hypogammaglobulinemia in treated patients	[51]

19.4.6.11 Hypogammaglobulinemia After Immunosuppressive Regimes in Solid Organ Transplantation

Hypogammaglobulinemia has been proposed to be a risk factor for infection after solid organ transplantation. In heart transplant recipients, infection is a leading cause of morbidity and mortality. In orthotropic liver transplant recipients, hypogammaglobulinemia was observed in 26% of the individuals, and it was strongly associated with mortality. Moreover, severe hypogammaglobulinemia during the first year post-transplantation significantly increased the risk of CMV and fungal and respiratory infections, and it may be associated with higher 1-year all-cause mortality.

19.5 Conclusion

Hypogammaglobulinemia is a diagnostic challenge for clinicians. After confirmation, it is essential to differentiate primary from secondary forms. Because primary hypogammaglobulinemia is an exclusion diagnosis, an extensive work-up should be performed in order to identify a cause of SID and prescribe a specific treatment when possible. In particular, B-cell malignancies (mainly chronic lymphocytic leukemia) and plasma cell dyscrasias should be excluded in patients with low immunoglobulin serum levels. For patients with hypogammaglobulinemia and lymphomas, it is necessary to discriminate an antibody primary failure or a lymphoid malignancy complicating primary antibody defect from SID. A period of observation after the first finding of a hypogammaglobulinemia, especially in patients who not fulfilled the criteria for a primary antibody defect as CVID and in children, could be useful to better define the diagnosis. SID patients are often less well defined than primary antibody defect as the diagnosis relies only on serum Ig levels rather than on proven antibody failure, but their clinical relevance is recognized. Patients with SID are unduly susceptible to different types of pathogens depending on the overall immunological defects. As for primary antibody defect, numerous studies in patients with SID have shown beneficial effects of immunoglobulin replacement therapy, resulting in fewer infectious episodes, reduced use of antibiotics, shorter hospital stay but no difference in overall mortality [52].

Abbreviations: *ALL* acute lymphoblastic leukemia, *CLL* chronic lymphocytic leukemia, *CTCL* cutaneous T-cell lymphoma, *GvH* graft versus host disease, *HSCT* hematopoietic stem cell transplantation, *MS*, multiple sclerosis, *NHL* non-Hodgkin's lymphoma, *RA* rheumatoid arthritis, *SS* systemic sclerosis, *SLE* systemic lupus erythematosus

References

1. Bonilla FA, Barlan I, Chapel H, Costa-Carvalho BT, Cunningham-Rundles C, de la Morena MT, Espinosa-Rosales FJ, Hammarström L, Nonoyama S, Quinti I, Routes JM, Tang MLK, Warnatz K. International Consensus Document (ICON): common variable immunodefi-

ciency disorders. J Allergy Clin Immunol Pract. 2016;4:38–59. https://doi.org/10.1016/j.jaip.2015.07.025.
2. Dorsey MJ, Orange JS. Impaired specific antibody response and increased B-cell population in transient hypogammaglobulinemia of infancy. Ann Allergy Asthma Immunol. 2006;97:590–5.
3. Moschese V, Cavaliere FM, Graziani S, Bilotta C, Milito C, Chini L, Quinti I. Decreased IgM, IgA, and IgG response to pneumococcal vaccine in children with transient hypogammaglobulinemia of infancy. J Allergy Clin Immunol. 2016;137:617–9. https://doi.org/10.1016/j.jaci.2015.06.014.
4. Conley ME, Notarangelo LD, Etzioni A. Diagnostic criteria for primary immunodeficiencies representing PAGID (Pan-American Group for Immunodeficiency) and ESID (European Society for Immunodeficiencies). Clin Immunol. 1999;93:190–7.
5. Al-Herz W, Bousfiha A, Casanova JL, Chapel H, Conley ME, Cunningham-Rundles C, et al. Primary immunodeficiency diseases: an update on the classification from the International Union of Immunological Societies Expert Committee for Primary Immunodeficiency. Front Immunol. 2011;2:54.
6. Calvo Campoverde K, Gean E, Piquer Gibert M, Martinez Valdez L, Deyà-Martínez A, Rojas Volquez M, Esteve-Sole A, Juan M, Plaza AM, Alsina L. Humoral deficiency in three paediatric patients with genetic diseases. Allergol Immunopathol (Madr). 2016;44:257–62. https://doi.org/10.1016/j.aller.2015.07.007.
7. Finley SC, Cooper MD, Finley WH, Uchida IA, Noto TA, Roddam RF. Immunological profile in a chromosome 18 deletion syndrome with IgA deficiency. J Med Genet. 1969;6:388–93.
8. Cody JD, Sebold C, Heard P, Carter E, Soileau B, Hasi-Zogaj M, Hill A, Rupert D, Perry B, O'Donnell L, Gelfond J, Lancaster J, Fox PT, Hale DE. Consequences of chromsome18q deletions. J Med Genet C Semin Med Genet. 2015;169:265–80. https://doi.org/10.1002/ajmg.c.31446.
9. Yu HR, Yang MY, Yeh WT, Yang KD. Common variable immunodeficiency with mosaic trisomy 8: report of one case. Acta Paediatr Taiwan. 2000;41:331–5.
10. Valentini D, Marcellini V, Bianchi S, Villani A, Facchini M, Donatelli I, Castrucci MR, Marasco E, Farroni C, Carsetti R. Generation of switched memory B cells in response to vaccination in Down syndrome children and their siblings. Vaccine. 2015;33:6689–96. https://doi.org/10.1016/j.vaccine.2015.10.083.
11. Kerr J, Quinti I, Eibl M, Chapel H, Späth PJ, Sewell WA, Salama A, van Schaik IN, Kuijpers TW, Peter HH. Is dosing of therapeutic immunoglobulins optimal? A review of a three-decade long debate in europe. Front Immunol. 2014;12(5):629. https://doi.org/10.3389/fimmu.2014.00629.
12. Forconi F, Moss P. Perturbation of the normal immune system in patients with CLL. Blood. 2015;126:573–81. https://doi.org/10.1182/blood-2015-03-567388.
13. Visentin A, Compagno N, Cinetto F, Imbergamo S, Zambello R, Piazza F. Clinical profile associated with infections in patients with chronic lymphocytic leukemia. Protective role of immunoglobulin replacement therapy. Haematologica. 2015;100:e515–8. https://doi.org/10.3324/haematol.2015.
14. Zemble RM, Takach PA, Levinson AI. The relationship between hypogammaglobulinemia, monoclonal gammopathy of undetermined significance and humoral immunodeficiency: a case series. J Clin Immunol. 2011;31:737–43. https://doi.org/10.1007/s10875-011-9548-0.
15. Compagno N, Cinetto F, Boscaro E, Semenzato G, Agostini C. Serum free light chains in the differential diagnosis and prognosis of primary and secondary hypogammaglobulinemia. J Allergy Clin Immunol. 2015;135:1075–7.
16. Holtick U, Albrecht M, Chemnitz JM, Theurich S, Skoetz N, Scheid C, von Bergwelt-Baildon M. Bone marrow versus peripheral blood allogeneic haematopoietic stem cell transplantation for haematological malignancies in adults. Cochrane Database Syst Rev. 2014;4:CD010189. https://doi.org/10.1002/14651858.CD010189.
17. Pastori D, Esposito A, Mezzaroma I. Immunomodulatory effects of intravenous immunoglobulins (IVIGs) in HIV-1 disease: a systematic review. Int Rev Immunol. 2011;30:44–66. https://doi.org/10.3109/08830185.2010.529975.

18. Pahwa S, Kirkpatrick D, Ching C, Lopez C, Pahwa R, Smithwick E, O'Reilly R, August C, Pasquariello P, Good RA. Persistent cytomegalovirus infection: association with profound immunodeficiency and treatment with interferon. Clin Immunol Immunopathol. 1983;28:77–89.
19. Greenberger PA, Walker CL, Fitzsimons TE, Roberts M. Hypogammaglobulinemia associated with cytomegalovirus pneumonia. J Infect Dis. 1991;163:631–3.
20. Hügle B, Suchowerskyj P, Hellebrand H, Adler B, Borte M, Sack U, Overberg-Schmidt US, Strnad N, Otto J, Meindl A, Schuster V. Persistent hypogammaglobulinemia following mononucleosis in boys is highly suggestive of X-linked lymphoproliferative disease—report of three cases. J Clin Immunol. 2004;24:515–22.
21. Ameratunga R, Barker RW, Steele RH, Deo M, Woon ST, Yeong ML, Koopmans W. Profound reversible hypogammaglobulinemia caused by celiac disease in the absence of protein losing enteropathy. J Clin Immunol. 2015;35:589–94. https://doi.org/10.1007/s10875-015-0189-6.
22. Sadat MA, Moir S, Chun TW, Lusso P, Kaplan G, Wolfe L, Memoli MJ, He M, Vega H, Kim LJ, Huang Y, Hussein N, Nievas E, Mitchell R, Garofalo M, Louie A, Ireland DC, Grunes C, Cimbro R, Patel V, Holzapfel G, Salahuddin D, Bristol T, Adams D, Marciano BE, Hegde M, Li Y, Calvo KR, Stoddard J, Justement JS, Jacques J, Long Priel DA, Murray D, Sun P, Kuhns DB, Boerkoel CF, Chiorini JA, Di Pasquale G, Verthelyi D, Rosenzweig SD. Glycosylation, hypogammaglobulinemia, and resistance to viral infections. N Engl J. 2014;370:1615–25. https://doi.org/10.1056/NEJMoa1302846.
23. Wirsum C, Glaser C, Gutenberger S, Keller B, Unger S, Voll RE, Vach W, Ness T, Warnatz K. Secondary antibody deficiency in glucocorticoid therapy clearly differs from primary antibody deficiency. J Clin Immunol. 2016;36:406–12. https://doi.org/10.1007/s10875-016-0264-7.
24. Fassbinder T, Saunders U, Mickholz E, Jung E, Becker H, Schlüter B, Jacobi AM. Differential effects of cyclophosphamide and mycophenolate mofetil on cellular and serological parameters in patients with systemic lupus erythematosus. Arthritis Res Ther. 2015;17:92. https://doi.org/10.1186/s13075-015-0603-8.
25. Farr M, Struthers GR, Scott DG, Bacon PA. Fenclofenac-induced selective IgA deficiency in rheumatoid arthritis. Br J Rheumatol. 1985;24:367–9.
26. Farr M, Tunn E, Bacon PA, Smith DH. Hypogammaglobulinaemia and thrombocytopenia associated with sulphasalazine therapy in rheumatoid arthritis. Ann Rheum Dis. 1985;44:723–4.
27. Snowden N, Dietch DM, Teh LS, Hilton RC, Haeney MR. Antibody deficiency associated with gold treatment: natural history and management in 22 patients. Ann Rheum Dis. 1996;55:616–21.
28. Williams A, Scott DL, Greenwood A, Huskisson EC. The clinical value of measuring immunoglobulins when assessing penicillamine therapy in rheumatoid arthritis. Clin Rheumatol. 1988;7:347–53.
29. Pereira LF, Sanchez JF. Reversible panhypogammaglobulinemia associated with phenytoin treatment. Scand J Infect Dis. 2002;34:785–7.
30. Hoshino C, Hoshi T. Carbamazepine-induced agammagloblinaemia clinically mimicking diffuse panbronchiolitis. BMJ Case Rep. 2011; https://doi.org/10.1136/bcr.11.2010.3535.
31. Eom TH, Lee HS, Jang PS, Kim YH. Valproate-induced panhypogammaglobulinemia. Neurol Sci. 2013;34:1003–4. https://doi.org/10.1007/s10072-012-1153-3.
32. De Angelis F, Tosti ME, Capria S, Russo E, D'Elia GM, Annechini G, Stefanizzi C, Foà R, Pulsoni A. Risk of secondary hypogammaglobulinaemia after Rituximab and Fludarabine in indolent non-Hodgkin lymphomas: A retrospective cohort study. Leuk Res. 2015;39:1382–8. https://doi.org/10.1016/j.leukres.2015.10.013.
33. Diwakar L, Gorrie S, Richter A, Chapman O, Dhillon P, Al-Ghanmi F, et al. Does rituximab aggravate pre-existing hypogammaglobulinaemia? J Clin Pathol. 2010;63:275–7. https://doi.org/10.1136/jcp.2009.068940.
34. Edwards JC, Szczepanski L, Szechinski J, Filipowicz-Sosnowska A, Emery P, Close DR, Stevens RM, Shaw T. Efficacy of B-cell-targeted therapy with rituximab in patients with rheumatoid arthritis. N Engl J Med. 2004;350:2572–81.

35. Witzig TE, Flinn IW, Gordon LI, Emmanouilides C, Czuczman MS, Saleh MN, Cripe L, Wiseman G, Olejnik T, Multani PS, White CA. Treatment with ibritumomab tiuxetan radioimmunotherapy in patients with rituximab-refractory follicular non-Hodgkin's lymphoma. J Clin Oncol. 2002;20:3262–9.
36. Evans SS, Clemmons AB. Obinutuzumab: a novel anti-CD20 monoclonal antibody for chronic lymphocytic leukemia. J Adv Pract Oncol. 2015;6:370–4.
37. Österborg A, Wierda WG, Mayer J, Hess G, Hillmen P, Schetelig J, Schuh A, Smolej L, Beck C, Dreyfus B, Hellman A, Kozlowski P, Pfreundschuh M, Rizzi R, Spacek M, Phillips JL, Gupta IV, Williams V, Jewell RC, Nebot N, Lisby S, Dyer MJ. Ofatumumab retreatment and maintenance in fludarabine-refractory chronic lymphocytic leukaemia patients. Br J Haematol. 2015;170:40–9. https://doi.org/10.1111/bjh.13380.
38. Kappos L, Li D, Calabresi PA, O'Connor P, Bar-Or A, Barkhof F, Yin M, Leppert D, Glanzman R, Tinbergen J, Hauser SL. Ocrelizumab in relapsing-remitting multiple sclerosis: a phase 2, randomised, placebo-controlled, multicentre trial. Lancet. 2011;378:1779–87. https://doi.org/10.1016/S0140-6736(11)61649-8.
39. Lutalo PM, D'Cruz DP. Update on belimumab for the management of systemic lupus erythematosus. Expert Opin Biol Ther. 2014;14:1701–8. https://doi.org/10.1517/14712598.2014.959924.
40. Genovese MC, Silverman GJ, Emery P, Gupta RC, Gill A, Veenhuizen M, Xie L, Komocsar WJ, Berclaz PY, Lee C. Efficacy and safety of Tabalumab, an anti-B-cell-activating factor monoclonal antibody, in a heterogeneous rheumatoid arthritis population: results from a randomized, placebo-controlled, Phase 3 Trial (FLEX-O). J Clin Rheumatol. 2015;21:231–8. https://doi.org/10.1097/RHU.0000000000000276.
41. Furie RA, Leon G, Thomas M, Petri MA, Chu AD, Hislop C, Martin RS, Scheinberg MA, PEARL-SC Study. A phase 2, randomised, placebo-controlled clinical trial of blisibimod, an inhibitor of B cell activating factor, in patients with moderate-to-severe systemic lupus erythematosus, the PEARL-SC study. Ann Rheum Dis. 2013;74:1667–75. https://doi.org/10.1136/annrheumdis-2013-205144.
42. Topp MS, Kufer P, Gökbuget N, Goebeler M, Klinger M, Neumann S, Horst HA, Raff T, Viardot A, Schmid M, Stelljes M, Schaich M, Degenhard E, Köhne-Volland R, Brüggemann M, Ottmann O, Pfeifer H, Burmeister T, Nagorsen D, Schmidt M, Lutterbuese R, Reinhardt C, Baeuerle PA, Kneba M, Einsele H, Riethmüller G, Hoelzer D, Zugmaier G, Bargou RC. Targeted therapy with the T-cell-engaging antibody blinatumomab of chemotherapy-refractory minimal residual disease in B-lineage acute lymphoblastic leukemia patients results in high response rate and prolonged leukemia-free survival. J Clin Oncol. 2011;29:2493–8. https://doi.org/10.1200/JCO.2010.32.7270.
43. Micallef IN, Maurer MJ, Wiseman GA, Nikcevich DA, Kurtin PJ, Cannon MW, Perez DG, Soori GS, Link BK, Habermann TM, Witzig TE. Epratuzumab with rituximab, cyclophosphamide, doxorubicin, vincristine, and prednisone chemotherapy in patients with previously untreated diffuse large B-cell lymphoma. Blood. 2011;118:4053–61. https://doi.org/10.1182/blood-2011-02-336990.
44. Kantarjian H, Thomas D, Jorgensen J, Kebriaei P, Jabbour E, Rytting M, York S, Ravandi F, Garris R, Kwari M, Faderl S, Cortes J, Champlin R, O'Brien S. Results of inotuzumab ozogamicin, a CD22 monoclonal antibody, in refractory and relapsed acute lymphocytic leukemia. Cancer. 2013;119:2728–36. https://doi.org/10.1002/cncr.28136.
45. Sullivan-Chang L, O'Donnell RT, Tuscano JM. Targeting CD22 in B-cell malignancies: current status and clinical outlook. Bio Drugs. 2013;27:293–304. https://doi.org/10.1007/s40259-013-0016-7. Review.
46. Maude SL, Teachey DT, Porter DL, Grupp SA. CD19-targeted chimeric antigen receptor T-cell therapy for acute lymphoblastic leukemia. Blood. 2015;125:4017–23. https://doi.org/10.1182/blood-2014-12-580068.
47. Kappos L, Wiendl H, Selmaj K, Arnold DL, Havrdova E, Boyko A, Kaufman M, Rose J, Greenberg S, Sweetser M, Riester K, O'Neill G, Elkins J. Daclizumab HYP versus interferon beta-1a in relapsing multiple sclerosis. N Engl J Med. 2015;373:1418–28. https://doi.org/10.1056/NEJMoa1501481.

48. Obermann M, Ruck T, Pfeuffer S, Baum J, Wiendl H, Meuth SG. Simultaneous early-onset immune thrombocytopenia and autoimmune thyroid disease following alemtuzumab treatment in relapsing-remitting multiple sclerosis. Mult Scler. 2016;22:1235–41. https://doi.org/10.1177/1352458516638558.
49. Furst DE, Keystone EC, Braun J, Breedveld FC, Burmester GR, De Benedetti F, Dörner T, Emery P, Fleischmann R, Gibofsky A, Kalden JR, Kavanaugh A, Kirkham B, Mease P, Sieper J, Singer NG, Smolen JS, Van Riel PL, Weisman MH, Winthrop K. Updated consensus statement on biological agents for the treatment of rheumatic diseases. Ann Rheum Dis. 2011;2:i2–45. https://doi.org/10.1136/annrheumdis-2011-201036.
50. Nixon AE, Chen J, Sexton DJ, Muruganandam A, Bitonti AJ, Dumont J, Viswanathan M, Martik D, Wassaf D, Mezo A, Wood CR, Biedenkapp JC, TenHoor C. Fully human monoclonal antibody inhibitors of the neonatal fc receptor reduce circulating IgG in non-human primates. Front Immunol. 2015;6:176. https://doi.org/10.3389/fimmu.2015.00176.
51. Hartung HP, Kieseier BC. Atacicept: targeting B cells in multiple sclerosis. Ther Adv Neurol Disord. 2010;3:205–16. https://doi.org/10.1177/1756285610371146.
52. Kerr J, Quinti I, Eibl M, Chapel H, Späth PJ, Sewell WA, Salama A, van Schaik IN, Kuijpers TW, Peter HH. Is dosing of therapeutic immunoglobulins optimal? A review of a three-decade long debate in europe Front Immunol. 2014 Dec 12;5:629. https://doi.org/10.3389/fimmu.2014.00629. eCollection 2044.

Management of Humoral Primary Immunodeficiencies in Pediatrics

20

Chiara Azzari and Clementina Canessa

20.1 Introduction

The clinical spectrum of humoral primary immunodeficiencies (PID) is extremely broad; there are many therapeutic strategies targeted on different aspects. Besides recurrent infections occurring in the respiratory tract, gastrointestinal tract, skin, and soft tissues [1–3], inflammatory complications are frequent and include autoimmunity, chronic lung disease, bronchiectasis, gastrointestinal disease with or without malabsorption, systemic or localized granulomatous disease, liver disease, splenomegaly, and lymphadenopathy [4, 5]. Finally, patients affected by severe humoral defects are at higher risk of developing malignancies compared with normal population, especially in case of hematological neoplasia and solid tumors of the gastrointestinal tract. Over the last few years, advances have been made in the management of humoral PID, improving patients' outcomes; these include immunoglobulin (Ig) replacement, antibiotics for treatment and prevention of infections, respiratory rehabilitation programs, and appropriate therapy for noninfectious complications [6]. Ig replacement is the mainstay of treatment [5]; it has been shown that long-term Ig replacement therapy reduces the rate of infections and their long-term complications [7–10]. However, despite the reduction of bacterial infections using Ig replacement, patients remain more susceptible to complications because of an associated T-cell defect or dysregulated immune response that deserves particular attention. Management is different depending on the defect: common variable immunodeficiency disorders (CVID) and agammaglobulinemia require Ig replacement therapy, whereas selective IgA deficiency and isolated IgG subclass deficiency usually do not. Irrespective of the specific disease, children with humoral

C. Azzari · C. Canessa (✉)
Paediatric Immunology Department, Meyer Children's Hospital, Florence, Italy
e-mail: chiara.azzari@unifi.it; clementina.canessa@meyer.it

M. M. D'Elios, M. Rizzi (eds.), *Humoral Primary Immunodeficiencies*,
Rare Diseases of the Immune System, https://doi.org/10.1007/978-3-319-91785-6_20

immunodeficiency deserve a multidisciplinary approach since they could show different clinical manifestations over the lifetime. Moreover, the correct relationship between a physician and a child's family is fundamental for a correct and long-lasting follow-up. Parents need to be understood and supported by healthcare professionals. Finally, psychological support could be necessary, especially for adolescent patients. In fact, primary immunodeficiencies are lifelong conditions and that could be difficult to accept, even by younger patients. The life of the whole family can be dominated by the disease, and psychological, social, and economic aspects are involved. For all these reasons, psychological assistance should be offered. A critical point in the care of the patients is the management of the transition of 18-year-old patients from pediatric care to adult care. In fact, in many contexts all over the world, the approach of adult immunologists to the disease and to patients and their families can be very different from that of pediatricians. Pediatricians tend to give complete care to PID patients, curing their medical needs and taking on the role of coordinator, whereas in hospitals for adult patients, coordination of the whole management is often left up to the patients. Sometimes, patients feel this gap and struggle with leaving the pediatric center. For these reasons, transition should be planned carefully starting from adolescence, in order to ease patients slowly into adult. During this period of time, autonomy and awareness of their medical condition have to be progressively encouraged.

20.2 Management of Minor Antibody Defects

20.2.1 Management of Selective IgA Deficiency

Patients need a regular clinical and hematological follow-up: clinical visits and blood tests should be performed every 10–12 months until the age of 10 years; visits and blood examinations can be performed every 12–18 months in older children, depending on clinical conditions and associated manifestations. In particular, patients have to be checked for airway infections that are usually more frequent in the first years of life. Signs or symptoms of autoimmune diseases should be searched in selective IgA deficiency (sIgAD) as the patients have an increased risk for autoimmunity [11]. Antibiotic prophylaxis is usually not needed in the pediatric age range, and every single episode of infection should be treated depending on the severity of the manifestation. Periodic blood examination for autoimmunity is controversial since it cannot prevent autoimmunity itself and is not performed with the same periodicity in different countries. The Italian IPINET suggests blood testing for autoimmunity every 3 years [12]. The aim is to recognize early the onset of autoimmune diseases and to prevent clinical complications. Periodic blood examinations should include blood count, liver and kidney function, thyroid function, and specific autoimmunity of the thyroid, pancreas, and gut, with thyroglobulin antibodies, microsomal antibodies, anti-transglutaminase antibodies, and glycated hemoglobin assessment, respectively. Since selective IgA deficiency can, in a small percentage of patients, progress to common variable immunodeficiency disorder

[13], serum immunoglobulin levels and blood lymphocyte subpopulations need to be routinely checked. An allergic evaluation should be performed in all those cases presenting allergy symptoms, since prevalence of allergic disorders increases in selective IgA deficiency in children [14] and adults [15]. When concomitant IgG2 subclass deficiency or impaired antibody responses to bacterial or vaccine antigens are present, immunoglobulin replacement therapy may be necessary, especially in case of lung damage or recurrent infections. The usual therapeutic doses are indicated, using a product low in IgA, because of the higher risk of having anti-IgA antibodies. Diseases associated with sIgAD (such as allergic, intestinal, autoimmune, or tumoral diseases) need to be treated conventionally using standard therapies, and their outcome is not dissimilar to those of non-sIgAD patients [16]. Prognosis of associated diseases does not change in the presence of concomitant sIgAD. Interestingly, sIgAD asthmatic patients appear to be more resistant to standard therapies [16]. Because of the higher risk of infections, especially respiratory tract infections, prevention through vaccines is crucial (see Chap. 22). sIgAD patients can receive all vaccines (inactivated or live) included in the vaccination schedule and appropriate for their age with the exception of the yellow fever (YF) vaccine and the oral poliovirus vaccine (OPV) [17]. The OPV should be replaced by the inactivated polio vaccine (IPV). The reason why the YF vaccine is normally contraindicated is because sIgAD is a heterogeneous condition, and while most patients have no clinically significant immune deficit, others may have low levels of T cells and decreased T-cell function. Vaccines against capsulated bacteria are strongly recommended [17].

20.2.2 Management of Isolated IgG Subclass Deficiency

Asymptomatic subjects with one or more subclass deficiencies and normal antibody responses require no treatment [18]. Since a small proportion of these patients may evolve into CVID, they should be monitored periodically, and clinical visits and blood checks of subclass levels and immunoglobulins should be performed [18]. Individuals with respiratory infections and an IgG subclass deficiency but with normal specific antibody production are not candidates for replacement therapy. If severe recurrent respiratory infections are associated to a documented specific antibody deficiency, Ig therapy is indicated, especially if patients have deficient antibody responses to both protein and polysaccharide antigens. Failure of prolonged antibiotic therapy, severe symptoms, and persistent radiographic abnormalities also suggest the use of Ig replacement therapy. In those cases, therapy can be given with the same dosage and intervals as for patients with other primary antibody deficiencies [18]. In case of isolated IgG2 deficiency, physicians should make sure that their patients are vaccinated against capsulated bacteria (*Streptococcus pneumoniae*, *Neisseria meningitidis*, *Haemophilus influenzae*) with all available conjugate vaccines, because of the higher susceptibility to these pathogens due to IgG2 defect. IgG1 deficiency often manifests itself as hypogammaglobulinemia: patients need to be treated as hypogammaglobulinemic/agammaglobulinemic subjects, Ig replacement therapy has to be started as soon as possible, and all the other therapeutic strategies for hypogammaglobulinemic patients have to be undertaken. As previously described for sIgAD, patients with isolated subclass deficiency can receive all vaccines (inactivated or live) included in the vaccination schedule and appropriate for their age with the exception of the YF vaccine and the oral poliovirus (OPV) [17].

20.3 Management of Major Antibody Defects

20.3.1 Immunoglobulin Therapy

Lifelong Ig replacement therapy is the gold standard for management of primary antibody deficiency. Ig replacement therapy was first used by Bruton in a child with agammaglobulinemia in 1952 [19]. Today Ig replacement therapy can be administered intravenously (IVIG) or subcutaneously (SCIG), the latter with different preparations and administration procedures. SCIG preparations were first introduced in the 1980s in the USA and in Europe. The slow infusion technique and the low concentration of the preparations available at that time made SCIG impractical and less attractive to patients and healthcare professionals. Therefore, IVIG, which allowed infusions of higher doses and monthly intervals between infusions, remained the preferred route of administration for years. In the last two decades, subcutaneous administration of IgG (SCIG) has gained considerable acceptance among patients and doctors and is increasingly used worldwide [20–22] so that in many countries, both in pediatrics and in adult patients, the proportion of patients treated with SCIG has exceeded that of patients treated with IVIG. Different options are now available: besides the intravenous route (IVIG), Ig can be given by a standard subcutaneous (SCIG) route, by a manual rapid subcutaneous push, or by a facilitated subcutaneous route using recombinant human hyaluronidase. All routes have advantages and disadvantages, but it is very important that patients are treated with the route best suited to them and even shift from one route to another, according to changing situations and needs. Available Ig products differ in concentration of IgG and other plasma proteins, as well as in sodium or sugar content, osmolarity, and IgA content. The selection of an Ig product must be individualized, based on the clinical condition of the patient and Ig product-related factors. It is usually considered best practice not to change products and brands. Actually, different commercial products are not identical, and patients who tolerate one product may not necessarily tolerate another. However, it is extremely important to consider quality of life of patients and their need to reduce the number of infusions in some periods during the year (e.g., during travel, vacation, scout camps). In these cases, if the clinical situation allows it, transient shift from SCIG to IVIG can be planned in order to obtain a month interval free from infusions. All immunoglobulin replacement therapies now available, independent of the route of administration, have the limitation that they replace only IgG, while they are unable to correct defects in secretory antibodies. Both intravenous (concentration of IVIG 3–12%) and subcutaneous (concentration of SCIG 10–20%) routes provide sufficient amounts of IgG [23, 24]. The purpose of Ig replacement therapy is to prevent infections. The amounts of administered Ig and individualized dosage can vary, depending on the baseline level of IgG and on the presence of chronic lung or gastrointestinal (GI) damage [25]. Furthermore, the optimum trough level of IgG is not universal, and clinical response may be a better indicator for dose adjustments [26–28].

20.3.2 Intravenous Immunoglobulin

Based on the goal of preventing infections, universal IVIG routine protocols for replacement therapy recommend starting at 400–600 mg/kg every 3–4 weeks. As for SCIG, the same total dosage is used, but it should be divided into three or four doses to obtain the weekly dose. Therefore SCIG is usually started at 100–200 mg/kg followed by 160 mg/kg every week [29–32]. It is important to note that doses should be rounded to the nearest whole bottle size not to waste immunoglobulin which, as with any other blood product, is extremely precious because the supply is limited and the demand is constantly rising.

It has been largely demonstrated that patients who maintained IgG trough levels at or near the lower limit of normal (>500 mg/dL) had significantly fewer hospitalizations and infections [18, 33, 34]. Unfortunately, IgG trough levels at or near 500 mg/dL may not be sufficient to prevent chronic lung disease and chronic sinusitis in antibody-deficient patients [18, 35]. Infusion rates can be adjusted to approximately 5–7.2 mL/kg/h for 10% liquid IVIG formulation [36] which means that a 25 kg child can complete his/her infusion in less than 1 h.

Differently from SCIG, infusion volume is not a problem for IVIG, with the exception of patients with renal or cardiac disease. In these cases, SCIG can be a useful and effective alternative. IVIG administration has been demonstrated to be very safe, and adverse events (AEs) are extremely rare (Table 20.1). Side effects may occur up to 72 h after the infusion [37, 38]. The majority of IVIG side effects are mild, transient, and self-limited and do not require discontinuation of therapy [23]. The most common AEs (headache, myalgia, nausea, fever, chills) usually arise during the infusion or immediately after. These adverse events can be alleviated by reducing the infusion rate or by using acetaminophen.

20.3.3 Subcutaneous Therapy

With recent technical advances in IgG formulation, pure and highly concentrated SCIG preparations have been developed: they have relatively low viscosity (around 14–15 millipascal second (mPAs)) and can therefore be infused relatively rapidly [20–22]. IgG enters the vascular compartment from the extravascular compartment (subcutaneous space) via the lymphatics at a defined rate, which integrates IgG catabolism and total IgG distribution, so that IgG is progressively released into the circulation. SCIG therapies differ from IVIG in many aspects: as previously described, while IVIG is infused every 3–4 weeks, SCIG is typically administered

Table 20.1 Adverse events of intravenous immunoglobulins

Systemic and organic classification (SOC) MedDRA	Adverse reaction	Frequency
Infections and infestations	Aseptic meningitis	Not common
Emolymphopoietic system disorders	Anemia, hemolysis, leucopenia	Common
	Anisocytosis (microcytosis) Thrombocytosis	Not common
Immunologic disorders	Hypersensitivity	Common
	Anaphylactic shock	Not known
Nervous system disorders	Headache Dizziness Drowsiness, tremors	Very common Common Not common
Cardiac effects	Tachycardia	Not common
Vascular effects	Hypertension, flushing, hypotension	Common
	Thromboembolic events, vasculitis Acute pulmonary damage due to transfusion	Not common Not known
Respiratory, thoracic, and mediastinal effects	Dyspnea	Common
Gastrointestinal effects	Nausea Vomit, diarrhea, abdominal pain	Very common Common
Hepatobiliary disorders	Hyperbilirubinemia	Common
Cutaneous and subcutaneous reactions	Rush, itch, urticaria, maculopapular rush, erythema, exfoliation	Common
Musculoskeletal and connective tissue disorders	Myalgia (spasms, stiffness, pain)	Common
Renal and urinary disorders	Proteinuria, increase of creatinine value	Not common
	Acute renal failure	Not known
Reactions related to administration site	Pain (back, limbs, neck, facial pain, arthralgia), fever, shivers, influenza-like illness	Very common
	Fatigue, muscular weakness	Common
	Pain at injection site	Not common
Diagnostic exams	Hemoglobin decrease, positive direct Coombs test, alanine aminotransferase and aspartate aminotransferase increase, lactate dehydrogenase increase	Common

Modified from https://farmaci.agenziafarmaco.gov.it/aifa/servlet/PdfDownloadServlet?pdfFileName=footer_002278_025266_FI.pdf&retry=0&sys=m0b1l3. Document available by AIFA starting from November 28, 2017

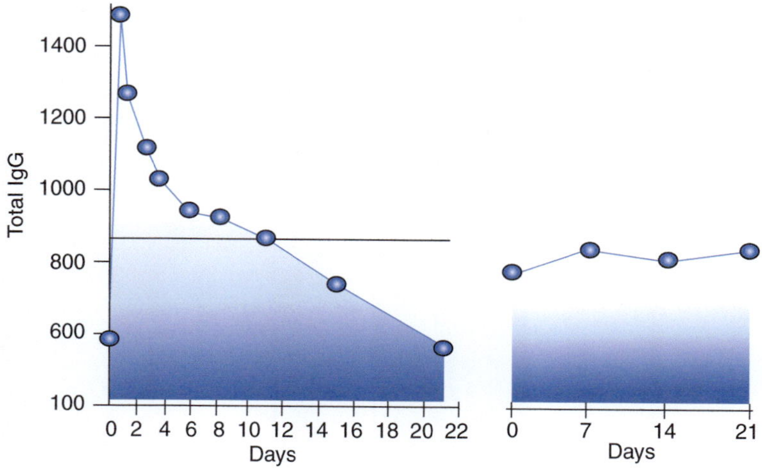

Fig. 20.1 Kinetics of serum levels of IgG in the two different routes of administration

once a week, with the total IVIG monthly dosage divided into smaller portions. Therefore SCIG is usually started at 100–200 mg/Kg[29–32]. As for IVIG, dosage and interval between infusions must be personalized looking at serum IgG levels obtained, infection prevented, and the presence of complications. SCIG results in more stable serum IgG levels, avoiding the peaks and troughs associated with IVIG [22, 39] (Fig. 20.1). SCIG is associated with fewer systemic AEs than IVIG and requires no venous access [20, 22, 39]. Finally, SCIG is easy to use and is easier to self-administer, providing patients with flexibility and an improved quality of life [40] (Fig. 20.2). Patients treated with SCIG do not need to go to the hospital or to infusion centers. Therefore they require less assistance from healthcare professionals, reducing the costs associated with Ig replacement therapy, and can take greater control over their own therapy. The recommended rate for SCIG 20% is usually 15 mL/h/site for the first infusion and 25 mL/h/site for subsequent infusions; however, an infusion rate of 35 mL/h does not increase the frequency of adverse events [41], and rapid rates (up to 70 mL/h) have been used and tolerated well [41]. These rates are usually not required in the pediatric age range but can be considered for adolescents or in special conditions. The volume infused should be carefully calculated, since it is limited to what can be tolerated comfortably by the patient. However, increasing the number of sites used simultaneously per infusion allows larger volumes to be administered. In adults, up to 80 mL per site have been infused [36]. It is unlikely that such doses are necessary in the pediatric age range, but they could be considered in adolescents needing immune-modulating doses, which are 2.5–5 times higher than replacement doses. However, increasing both infusion volumes and infusion rates may increase AEs. Therefore, to increase volume, number of sites should be increased. Up to four sites can be used simultaneously both in adults and

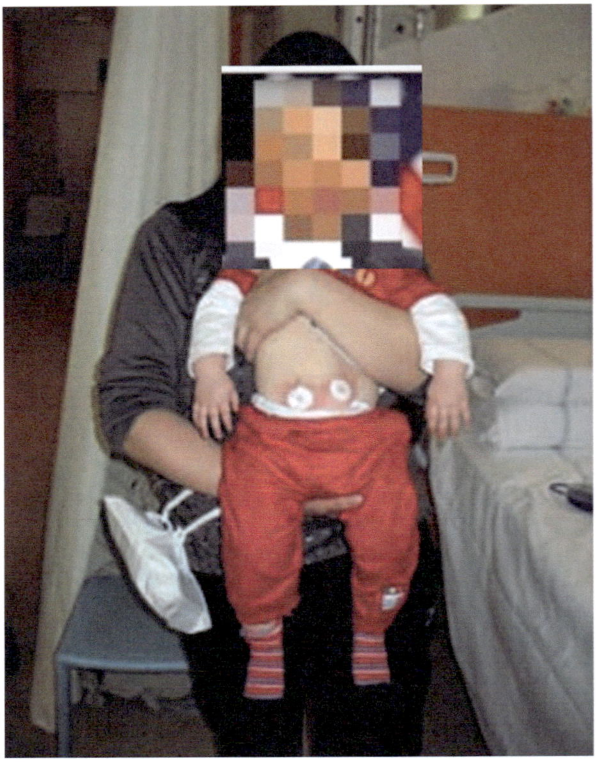

Fig. 20.2 Modified from Canessa C et al. SCIG therapy in patients with primary antibody defect: theoretical basis and center experience, Pediatric Immunology and Allergology Magazine 2010 (3):19–26 with the permission of authors

in children, and up to eight sites have been used for single infusions in adults. Bifurcated or more highly branched tubing sets can be used to increase the number of sites and help limit the total time required for each SCIG infusion. The flexibility of using different intervals, volume per site, number of sites, and infusion duration allows the best infusion regimens as well as the most comfortable ones to be found for each patient.

Generally, AEs of SCIG are of mild or moderate intensity. The most common events are local injection site reactions. Systemic AEs – such as headache, fatigue, and nausea – are relatively rare. SCIG self-administration requires older children or their parents to be trained. Training sessions are usually conducted at hospital, and the number of training sessions is variable, depending on the self-sufficiency and levels of conscientiousness of patients and families. Nursing teams teach patients and parents how to perform SCIG infusions. During the training sessions, the selection of proper subcutaneous needle gauges and lengths, the selection and rotation of infusion sites, the management of local adverse reactions, and the use of pumps and other infusion equipment are reviewed. Patients learn how to use aseptic procedures and the proper disposal of infusion materials. Generally, parents/older children can self-infuse SCIG doses independently after three to four training sessions. Recent evidence has demonstrated that the interval between two SCIG infusions can be increased to 10–15 days while respecting the monthly amount, resulting in the same clinical and hematological effects [42]. When SCIG is used in patients never treated before, it is necessary to consider that weekly SCIG will raise the serum IgG levels gradually. If a rapid increase is necessary, a daily SCIG infusion with 100 mg/kg for 3–5 days can be used and will allow serum levels of IgG of >500 mg/dL to be reached in 3–5 days.

20.3.4 Hyaluronidase-Facilitated Subcutaneous Immunoglobulins

Recently, a new strategy of delivery of SCIG has been developed to overcome many of the limitations of conventional SCIG. In fact, the flow and distribution of SCIG to the vasculature are impeded by the glycosaminoglycan hyaluronan in the extracellular matrix, which limits the infusion rate and volume per site, necessitating frequent infusions and multiple infusion sites [43]. In the new strategy, the subcutaneous infusion of IgG is preceded by an infusion of hyaluronidase, an enzyme that catalyzes the depolymerization of hyaluronan, resulting in enhanced drug delivery by increasing dispersion and absorption of IgG from the subcutaneous tissues. Consequently, larger volumes can be infused in each infusion site. Hyaluronan is depolymerized by hyaluronidase so that injectable biologics can spread more easily in the tissues and their dispersion and absorption are facilitated. Using hyaluronidase before SCIG infusion, patients can take the same IgG dose they would have taken with an IVIG and avoid the intravenous access required for intravenous infusions and the repeated SCIG infusion needed for conventional SCIG therapy. Treatment effectiveness is comparable to IVIG and conventional SCIG treatment and is well tolerated [43].

20.3.5 Subcutaneous Rapid Push (Subcutaneous Immunoglobulin Therapy Given by Subcutaneous Rapid Push)

An alternative to conventional SCIG infusion is the manual push technique, based on frequent (one to seven) infusions per week. This technique consists of the frequent manual infusion of small portions of the weekly dose using a syringe and a 23- to 25-gauge butterfly needle. A recent retrospective analysis in patients treated with SCIG showed that, if the same weekly dose is used, manual push and conventional SCIG are equivalent in terms of serum IgG levels, tolerability, and safety [44, 45]. As no pump or tubing is required with the frequent push technique, the cost of the procedure is reduced, and time for equipment preparation and maintenance are considerably reduced, making this approach attractive to patients [36]. Given the increased number of shots (1–7/week), the rapid push technique is preferred by adolescents and adults who prefer simplicity and reduced infusion time, but not by children 2–10 years of age [46].

20.3.6 Management of Comorbidities and Complications

As mentioned before, CVID and different forms of agammaglobulinemia can be variably associated to different manifestations, such as infections, pulmonary diseases, lymphoproliferative and granulomatous lesions, autoimmunity, gastrointestinal disorders, and other malignancies. The association is more or less strong, depending on the underlying humoral defect. Each of these aspects deserves a specific management (Table 20.2).

20.3.7 Management of Infectious Complications

Children and parents need to be informed about hygienic rules, such as avoiding crowded places and contact with sick people and washing hands to reduce risk of infection. Children and their families have to be educated about alarming signs of infection and the need for prompt clinical examination. Children and parents need

Table 20.2 Guidelines for management of common variable immunodeficiency and agammaglobulinemia

Primary immunodeficiency	Every 3 months	Every year	Depending on clinical advice
XLA – autosomal recessive agammaglobulinemia	– Clinic evaluation – Blood count, IgG, IgA, IgM, transaminases, azotemia, serum creatinine, plasmatic glucose, total protein Protein, urine analysis	HIV, HCV, HBV detection by PCR Abdomen ultrasound Fecal occult blood test Pulmonary function tests	Pulmonary CT scan (suggested every 5 years after 10 years old) Paranasal and nasal CT scan Periodic sputum collection Periodic evaluation by respiratory physiotherapist Digestive endoscopy
Common variable immunodeficiency	– Clinic evaluation – blood count, IgG, IgA, IgM, transaminases, azotemia, serum creatinine, plasmatic glucose, total protein Protein, urine analysis	HIV, HCV, HBV detection by PCR Lymphocytic subpopulations count Abdomen ultrasound Fecal occult blood test Pulmonary function tests	Pulmonary CT scan (suggested very 5 years after 10 years old) Paranasal and nasal CT scan Periodic sputum collection Periodic evaluation by respiratory physiotherapist Digestive endoscopy

PCR polymerase chain reaction, *CT* computed tomography

to be reminded of all these recommendations periodically. The other main point of prevention along with replacement therapy is respiratory rehabilitation. This is particularly important when chronic upper airway infections are present. In fact, 36–78% of patients with CVID have chronic sinusitis [47]. It was shown that immunoglobulin therapy increases the total survival rate and lowers the number of life-threatening infections, but does not influence the degree of clinical chronic sinusitis [48]. Because of these reasons, nasal cleaning using different techniques is crucial to prevent these manifestations.

After immunoglobulin replacement therapy and respiratory rehabilitation, the second line in pharmacological prevention of infection in humoral PID patients is antibiotic prophylaxis, especially in patients with bronchiectasis, frequent infections (generally more than three per year) or disruptive infections (hospital admission, prolonged periods away from school, and secondary complications such as empyema) [49]. Microbiology results, serial sputum testing, and antibiotic sensitivity of cultured organisms determine the choice of antimicrobial prophylaxis [50]. However, the benefit of prophylaxis is under discussion. In fact, some authors suggest that the use of prophylactic antibiotics should be avoided because of an increased risk of infection with fungi or other resistant organisms [51]. In pediatric patients, the use of antibiotic prophylaxis is limited. Finally, vaccines represent another essential tool of prevention of infections. It is fundamental to know which vaccines can be administered in each single case, in order not to miss an opportunity to protect the patient. Inactivated vaccines can always be administered, since they can be less effective but never dangerous for patients with humoral primary immunodeficiency. Different from what has been previously described for patients with sIgAD or isolated subclass deficiency, patients with major antibody deficiency should not receive live attenuated vaccines.

20.3.7.1 Follow-Up

Besides sensitizing patients, raising the awareness of medical and social caregivers concerning appropriate approaches to recurrent infection is critical. Family pediatricians and general practitioners must be informed about a patient's clinical condition as soon as possible after diagnosis. Medical examinations for early detection of infections will warrant immediate treatment. Periodic physicals should be carried out every 3–6 months. Sputum monitoring and analysis must be performed for all cases with productive cough. HBV, HCV, and HIV viral genome must be checked annually in all patients receiving Ig products. Periodical evaluation by respiratory physiotherapists is suggested, in order to manage new clinical events, to refresh rehabilitation techniques to the patient and to verify his compliance to therapy.

20.3.7.2 Treatment

Early treatment of infections at the first signs and symptoms should be considered an integral part of the treatment of humoral PID to prevent secondary structural damage. Biological samples (blood, cerebral spinal fluid (CSF), sputum, swab, stool) must be collected when appropriate before oral or intravenous antibiotic therapy, if possible. Besides culture, molecular methods by PCR (polymerase chain reaction) must always be used for detection of bacterial or viral genome, since they have greater sensitivity and specificity [52, 53]. Moreover, quantitative PCR allows a conclusive diagnosis to be obtained in less than 2 h. In the meanwhile, empiric therapy must be initiated. A prolonged course of treatment should be considered in cases with relapse of infections. Because of the nature of the disease, resistant common organisms, unusual organisms, and opportunistic infections (*Pseudomonas* spp., *Mycobacterium tuberculosis*) should be reviewed when treatment fails. Specifically, in case of persistent rhinitis, otitis, or sinusitis, common pathogens usually involved in these infections have to be considered: *H. influenzae*, *S. pneumoniae*, and *M. catarrhalis*. Otitis usually needs to be treated for 10 days whereas sinusitis for 3 weeks. Parenteral antibiotics are recommended for complicated infections, such as cellulitis and mastoiditis. In case of chronic sinusitis or other ORL complications, a specialistic evaluation could be necessary: local antibiotic therapy via aerosol could be prescribed, or prolonged oral antibiotics could be required. Endoscopic sinus surgery may be required in selected cases [54].

20.3.8 Management of Pulmonary Complications

Pulmonary complications are very frequent in patients affected by antibody deficiencies. They are the most frequent manifestation of CVID and significantly increase morbidity and mortality of these patients [55, 56]. In agammaglobulinemic patients, they represent the consequence of infections, whereas in CVID patients they can also be due to chronic inflammation. Recurrent pulmonary infections with pyogenic bacteria can determine permanent pulmonary damages such as atelectasis, bronchiectasis, reticular fibrosis, air trapping, ground-glass attenuation, and/or bronchial wall thickening [56, 57]. Even though these complications are more common in adults, they can already be present at the time of diagnosis in pediatric patients [56]. Together with Ig replacement therapy and treatment of upper and lower respiratory tract infections, respiratory rehabilitation is the best way to control lung disease progression, especially when bronchiectasis is already present. Postural drainage, inspiratory muscle training, and pulmonary rehabilitation programs are all effective strategies. Positive expiratory pressure (PEP) mask physiotherapy improves ventilation and reduces volume of trapped gas [58, 59].

20.3.8.1 Follow-Up

Pulmonary function tests, such as spirometry or the interruption technique (RINT) for preschool children, should be done at baseline and every year in pediatric patients. High-resolution computed tomography is the gold standard test for monitoring lung damage. It should be performed at baseline and every 4–5 years. Its use in pediatric patients can be limited by warning about radiation exposure and the need of anesthesia for taking the procedure. Other methods – such as multiple-breath washout test – are now studied in PID patients in order to check lung function without using radiation. Plain chest X-ray radiography is of limited value; it should be considered if the patient is febrile or has pleuritic pain and signs of consolidation, effusion, or collapse. Moreover, because of the probability of radiosensitivity in some CVID cases, lower intervals with other X-ray procedures should be avoided as screening leads to excessive radiation exposure over time [56, 57, 60–62]. However a pulmonary, nasal, and paranasal CT scan is recommended at least at 10 years of age and then every 5 years. The final choice to prescribe this test takes into account the global status of the patient and his clinical evolution. As mentioned above, periodic evaluation by a respiratory physiotherapist should be included in the follow-up program.

20.3.8.2 Treatment

Different therapeutic approaches are available, depending on type and grade of pulmonary involvement. Firstly, specific respiratory rehabilitation programs should be immediately started if not already underway. In fact, it is essential not only for prevention of pulmonary complications but also for their treatment. Reaching higher IgG trough levels (700–800 mg/dL) [63] can be useful. Patients with bronchiectasis may require IVIG higher than 600 mg/kg/month to achieve the same serum IgG level compared with patients without bronchiectasis [64, 65]. Other possible treatments of lung complications are azithromycin that has anti-inflammatory effects [66–68], inhaled corticosteroid fluticasone or nebulized gentamicin for reduction of sputum production [69, 70], oral quinolone and aerosolized colimycin or tobramycin for aggressive eradication of colonized *Pseudomonas* spp. [71, 72], NSAIDs [73], and mucolytics [74]. Obstructive airway diseases can be managed with inhaled corticosteroids [75]. Clinical response, lung function, and sputum sampling should be performed for respiratory health monitoring after starting the treatment. In CVID patients with pulmonary diseases, new therapeutic approaches focus on IL-2 therapy [76–79], short- and long-acting inhaled B_2-agonists in bronchiectasis [80, 81], and leukotriene receptor antagonists [73].

20.3.9 Management of Polyclonal Lymphocyte Infiltrative Complications

Polyclonal lymphocyte infiltrative complications are typical of CVID patients. Approximately 10–25% of all CVID patients encounter various lymphoproliferative and granulomatous diseases. Although mean age at onset of these complications is 20–40 years, they can be seen in pediatric patients as well [82]. Unfortunately, Ig replacement therapy has no effect on these manifestations, since they are due to an immune dysregulation mechanism [83].

20.3.9.1 Follow-Up

Signs of interstitial lung disease including dyspnea and reduced exercise tolerance should be considered in regular visits. Pulmonary function tests can show restrictive ventilatory patterns; high-resolution computed tomography can reveal parenchymal nodules or ground-glass opacities. Biopsy via open lung or transbronchial surgery may be required for large and persistent lymph nodes [82].

20.3.9.2 Treatment

It is not clear which therapeutic option could be the most appropriate for CVID-related lymphoproliferative diseases. High doses of systemic corticosteroids (10 mg/day or 20 mg every other day or twice daily inhaled beclomethasone) are the first choice for interstitial lung disease with restrictive ventilatory defects due to lymphoproliferative disease, such as pulmonary granulomas and lymphoid interstitial pneumonitis (LIP); but long-term treatment is limited because of the risk of infections [84, 85]. For long-term therapy, hydroxychloroquine is prescribed with dosages of 200–400 mg a day (range: 3.5–6.5 mg/kg) [86–89]. Steroid-sparing immunosuppressive agents have also been recommended in special situations when inflammation is predominantly pulmonary, including cyclosporine A (3–5 mg/kg) [83], methotrexate [89], azathioprine, mycophenolate mofetil, and 6-mercaptopurine [84]. Monoclonal antibodies as TNF-α inhibitors, such as etanercept [90] and infliximab [91–94], can be used in the case of generalized granulomatous lesions combined with autoimmunity, but no systematic clinical trials have investigated their efficacy and safety. Opportunistic infections like *Pneumocystis jirovecii* pneumonia may result when patients are under treatment for lymphoproliferative diseases [95]; for this reason prophylaxis with trimethoprim sulfamethoxazole is suggested. Treatment recommendations for hepatomegaly and lymphadenopathy are also lacking. Splenectomy should be avoided because its efficacy in the treatment of cytopenia is controversial and this surgery strongly predisposes patients to severe infections [1, 96].

20.3.10 Management of Autoimmune Complications

Autoimmune-associated disorders are other typical complications of CVID and are reported in 20–25% of patients. Agammaglobulinemic patients are less prone to autoimmunity: only rare cases of alopecia and glomerulonephritis have been described [18]. No preventive modalities are presently available for autoimmune manifestations. However, it has been shown that IVIG treatment can decrease the incidence of autoimmune diseases and especially autoimmune thrombocytopenia or autoimmune hemolytic anemia [97].

20.3.10.1 Follow-Up

General medical vigilance and hematologic laboratory monitoring with intervals of 3–6 months are ways to monitor hematologic autoimmunity. Besides routine blood testing, thyroid function and glycated hemoglobin should be checked annually in patients with CVID. Autoantibody assessment has little significance in these patients.

20.3.10.2 Treatment

Common treatment protocols for autoimmunity can be used in patients with CVID. In case of hematologic autoimmunity, management is based on intravenous corticosteroids (1 g of methylprednisolone in mild disease) or anti-CD20 monoclonal antibodies (rituximab) in severe disorders [98–100]. Persistent autoimmunity can be handled with high Ig immunomodulatory effects (1 g/kg/week) for a short time. TNF-α inhibitors might be used in overlapped phenotypes of autoimmunity (e.g., infliximab for Crohn's disease and etanercept for rheumatoid arthritis) and polyclonal lymphocytic infiltration [101].

20.3.11 Management of GI Complications and Enteropathy

At present no approach seems to be effective in preventing GI complications in patients with CVID or agammaglobulinemia. However, early recognition of viral hepatitis, hepatic autoimmunity, and granulomatous disease helps to avoid progression of CVID cases to regenerative hyperplasia leading to portal hypertension, cholestasis, and hepatic dysfunction. It remains to be proven whether fast treatment of intestinal infections improves outcomes for CVID patients [102].

20.3.11.1 Follow-Up

The caring physician should monitor over the course of periodic checkup the occurrence of new patient complaints (such as chronic diarrhea) and clinical symptoms (especially weight loss), as these may constitute alarm sign [102]. Yearly ultrasonography and fecal occult blood testing on three samples are suggested to screen for GI manifestations. Search for infectious agents in fecal samples, including parasites and opportunistic germs, should be performed in symptomatic cases (diarrhea, weight loss). *Giardia lamblia*, *Campylobacter*, *Shigella*, *Salmonella*, *E. coli enteropatogeni*, and *Cryptosporidium* must be specifically searched for since patients are more susceptible to these pathogens. If an inflammatory disease is suspected, fecal calprotectin assessment can be useful. In persistently symptomatic patients, endoscopies are indicated [103]. Almost half of CVID patients have chronic diarrhea that can evolve into moderate malabsorption. In these cases, body weight, height, and body mass index (BMI) should be periodically checked, in order to monitor the nutritional state. Besides specific therapy of enteropathy, a nutritional program should be planned with the dietitian [54].

20.3.11.2 Treatment

The management of severe inflammatory enteropathy that can occur in CVID is based on low-dose immunomodulatory drugs (azathioprine or 6-mercaptopurine) and TNF-α blockers (infliximab or etanercept) [104, 105]. Management in mild inflammatory bowel disease is the same as for immunocompetent patients. The use of long-term high-dose corticosteroids is controversial because of the increased susceptibility to intestinal CMV infection [106, 107].

20.3.12 Management of Malignancy

Decreasing unnecessary exposure of CVID patients to irradiation can reduce risk of iatrogenic cancer due to chromosomal radiosensitivity [108].

20.3.12.1 Follow-Up

Routine clinical and hematological checks with complete blood counts and differential white blood cell counts are essential for early recognition of lymphoid malignancies that are more frequent in CVID patients. In pediatric patients, yearly abdomen ultrasonography and fecal occult blood testing on three samples are indicated for screening of GI malignancies. Specific screening by endoscopy for finding mucosal changes should be performed in symptomatic cases. Histopathological investigation of enlarged nodes via excision of the whole lymph node is an important mean to screen of lymphoid malignancy [109].

20.3.12.2 Treatment

Neoplasia treatment can be done with routine chemotherapy protocols for cancerous patients [105]. Because of the relation of presentation of malignancy and impaired T-cell immunity in CVID, allogeneic stem cell transplantation is now considered in these selected CVID cases. However, it should be noticed that these potentially curative approaches are experimental and should only be proposed for therapy-refractory, life-threatening complications (late-onset combined immunodeficiency subgroup) including a careful process for donor selection [110]. The best response of allogeneic stem cell transplantation is seen in patients with non-Hodgkin lymphoma (NHL), resolving all CVID-related consequences. Graft-versus-host disease should be monitored in these patients [111].

20.3.13 Management of Arthritis

Up to 20% of XLA patients develop arthritis. Occasionally this is caused by pyogenic bacteria typical of septic arthritis and needs to be treated as in nonimmune-deficient subjects. More often arthritis is non-septic but has an inflammatory origin, as in juvenile idiopathic arthritis. In this case, besides anti-inflammatory and immunosuppressive therapy, motorial rehabilitation has a crucial role for recovery. In CVID patients, arthritis can have an inflammatory origin as well, and it needs the same therapeutic strategies undertaken in patients without PID [18, 103].

References

1. Cunningham-Rundles C, Bodian C. Common variable immunodeficiency: clinical and immunological features of 248 patients. Clin. Immunol. 1999;92:34–48.
2. Hermaszewski RA, Webster AD. Primary hypogammaglobulinaemia: a survey of clinical manifestations and complications. Q J Med. 1993;86:31–42.
3. Quinti I, Soresina A, Spadaro G, Italian Primary Immunodeficiency Network, et al. Long-term follow-up and outcome of a large cohort of patients with common variable immunodeficiency. J Clin Immunol. 2007;27(3):308–16.
4. Resnick ES, Moshier EL, Godbold JH, Cunningham-Rundles C. Morbidity and mortality in common variable immune deficiency over 4 decades. Blood. 2012;119:1650–7.

5. Bonilla FA, Bernstein IL, Khan DA, et al American Academy of Allergy, Asthma and Immunology; American College of Allergy, Asthma and Immunology; Joint Council of Allergy, Asthma and Immunology. Practice parameter for the diagnosis and management of primary immunodeficiency. Ann Allergy Asthma Immunol. 2005;94(5 Suppl. 1):S1–S63.
6. Abolhassani H, Aghamohammadi A, Abolhassani F, Eftekhar H, Heidarnia M, Rezaei N. Health policy for common variable immunodeficiency: burden of the disease. J Investig Allergol Clin Immunol. 2011;21(6):454–8.
7. Busse PJ, Razvi S. Cunningham-Rundles C Efficacy of intravenous immunoglobulin in the prevention of pneumonia in patients with common variable immunodeficiency. J Allergy Clin Immunol. 2002;109(6):1001–4.
8. Björkander J, Wadsworth C, Hanson LA. 1040 prophylactic infusions with an unmodified intravenous immunoglobulin product causing few side-effects in patients with antibody deficiency syndromes. Infection. 1985;13:102–10.
9. de Gracia J, Vendrell M, Alvarez A, et al. Immunoglobulin therapy to control lung damage in patients with common variable immunodeficiency. Int Immunopharmacol. 2004;4(6):745–53.
10. Pourpak Z, Aghamohammadi A, Sedighipour L, et al. Effect of regular intravenous immunoglobulin therapy on prevention of pneumonia in patients with common variable immunodeficiency. J Microbiol Immunol Infect. 2006;39:114–20.
11. Ludvigsson JF, Neovius M, Hammarström L. Association between IgA deficiency & other autoimmune conditions: a population-based matched cohort study. J Clin Immunol. 2014;34:444–51.
12. Selective IgA deficiency Diagnostic and therapeutic recommendations Working group Associazione Italiana di Ematologia ed Oncologia pediatrica (AIEOP)-Italian primary immunodeficiencies network (IPINET) 16th December 2010.
13. Aghamohammadi A, Mohammadi J, Parvaneh N, Rezaei N, Moin M, Espanol T, Hammarstrom L. Progression of selective IgA deficiency to common variable immunodeficiency. Int Arch Allergy Immunol. 2008;147:87–92.
14. Erkoçoğlu M, Metin A, Kaya A, Özcan C, Akan A, Civelek E, Çapanoğlu M, Giniş T, Kocabaş CN. Allergic and autoimmune disorders in families with selective IgA deficiency. Turk J Med Sci. 2017;47:592–8.
15. Jorgensen GH, Gardulf A, Sigurdsson MI, Sigurdardottir ST, Thorsteinsdottir I, Gudmundsson S, Hammarström L, Ludviksson BR. Clinical symptoms in adults with selective IgA deficiency: a case-control study. J Clin Immunol. 2013;33:742–7.
16. Yazdani R, Azizi G, Abolhassani H, Aghamohammadi A. Selective IgA deficiency: epidemiology, pathogenesis, clinical phenotype, diagnosis, prognosis and management. Scand J Immunol. 2017;85:3–12.
17. CDC. Vaccination of persons with primary and secondary immune deficiencies. https://www.cdc.gov/vaccines/pubs/pinkbook/downloads/appendices/a/immuno-table.pdf. Accessed 16 March 2018.
18. Sthiem ER, Ochs HD, Winkelstein JA. Immunologic disorders in infants and children. 5th ed. Philadelphia: Elsevier Saunders.
19. Bruton OC. Agammaglobulinemia. Pediatrics. 1952;9:722–8.
20. Gardulf A. Immunoglobulin treatment for primary antibody deficiencies: advantages of the subcutaneous route. Bio Drugs. 2007;21:105–16.
21. Moore ML, Quinn JM. Subcutaneous immunoglobulin replacement therapy for primary antibody deficiency: advancements into the 21st century. Ann Allergy Asthma Immunol. 2008;101:114–21.
22. Ochs HD, Gupta S, Kiessling P, Nicolay U, Berger M. Safety and efficacy of self-administered subcutaneous immunoglobulin in patients with primary immunodeficiency diseases. J Clin Immunol. 2006;26:265–73.
23. Rezaei N, Abolhassani H, Aghamohammadi A, Ochs HD. Indications and safety of intravenous and subcutaneous immunoglobulin therapy. Expert Rev Clin Immunol. 2011;7:301–16.
24. Weiler CR. Immunoglobulin therapy: history, indications, and routes of administration. Int J Dermatol. 2004;43:163–6.

25. Koleba T, Ensom MH. Pharmacokinetics of intravenous immunoglobulin: a systematic review. Pharmacotherapy. 2006;26:813–27.
26. Yong PL, Boyle J, Ballow M, et al. Use of intravenous immunoglobulin and adjunctive therapies in the treatment of primary immunodeficiencies: a working group report of and study by the Primary Immunodeficiency Committee of the American Academy of Allergy Asthma and Immunology. Clin Immunol. 2010;135:255–63.
27. Orange JS, Hossny EM, Weiler CR, Primary Immunodeficiency Committee of the American Academy of Allergy, Asthma and Immunology, et al. Use of intravenous immunoglobulin in human disease: a review of evidence by members of the Primary Immunodeficiency Committee of the American Academy of Allergy, Asthma and Immunology. J Allergy Clin Immunol. 2006;117(Suppl. 4):S525–53.
28. Eijkhout HW, van Der Meer JW, Kallenberg CG, Inter-University Working Party for the Study of Immune Deficiencies, et al. The effect of two different dosages of intravenous immunoglobulin on the incidence of recurrent infections in patients with primary hypogammaglobulinemia. A randomized, double-blind, multicenter crossover trial. Ann Intern Med. 2001;135:165–74.
29. Moore ML, Quinn JM. Subcutaneous immunoglobulin replacement therapy for primary antibody deficiency: advancements into the 21st century. Ann Allergy Asthma Immunol. 2008;101:114–21. quiz 122
30. Chapel HM, Spickett GP, Ericson D, Engl W, Eibl MM, Bjorkander J. The comparison of the efficacy and safety of intravenous versus subcutaneous immunoglobulin replacement therapy. J Clin Immunol. 2000;20:94–100.
31. Abolhassani H, Sadaghiani MS, Aghamohammadi A, Ochs HD, Rezaei N. Home-based subcutaneous immunoglobulin versus hospital-based intravenous immunoglobulin in treatment of primary antibody deficiencies: systematic review and meta analysis. J Clin Immunol. 2012;32:1180–92.
32. Berger M, Flebogamma 5% DIF Investigators. A multicenter, prospective, open label, historically controlled clinical trial to evaluate efficacy and safety in primary immunodeficiency diseases (PID) patients of Flebogamma 5% DIF, the next generation of Flebogamma. J Clin Immunol. 2007;27:628–33.
33. Bonagura VR, Marchlewski R, Cox A, Rosenthal DW. Biologic IgG level in primary immunodeficiency disease: the IgG level that protects against recurrent infection. J Allergy Clin Immunol. 2008;122:210–2.
34. Ballow M. Optimizing immunoglobulin treatment for patients with primary immunodeficiency disease to prevent pneumonia and infection incidence: review of the current data. Ann Allergy Asthma Immunol. 2013;111(6 Suppl):S2–5.
35. Orange JS, Grossman WJ, Navickis RJ, Wilkes MM. Impact of trough IgG on pneumonia incidence in primary immunodeficiency: A meta-analysis of clinical studies. Clin Immunol. 2010;137:21–30.
36. Jolles S, Orange JS, Gardulf A, Stein MR, Shapiro R, Borte M, Berger M. Current treatment options with immunoglobulin G for the individualization of care in patients with primary immunodeficiency disease. Clin Exp Immunol. 2015;179(2):146–60.
37. Dashti-Khavidaki S, Aghamohammadi A, Farshadi F, et al. Adverse reactions of prophylactic intravenous immunoglobulin; a 13-year experience with 3004 infusions in Iranian patients with primary immunodeficiency diseases. J Investig Allergol Clin Immunol. 2009;19:139–45.
38. Aghamohammadi A, Farhoudi A, Nikzad M, et al. Adverse reactions of prophylactic intravenous immunoglobulin infusions in Iranian patients with primary immunodeficiency. Ann Allergy Asthma Immunol. 2004;92:60–4.
39. Gardulf A, Nicolay U, Asensio O, et al. Rapid subcutaneous IgG replacement therapy is effective and safe in children and adults with primary immunodeficiencies—a prospective, multinational study. J Clin Immunol. 2006;26:177–85.
40. Gardulf A, Nicolay U. Replacement IgG therapy and self-therapy at home improve the health-related quality of life in patients with primary antibody deficiencies. Curr Opin Allergy Clin Immunol. 2006;6:434–42.

41. Hansen S, Gustafson R, Smith CI, Gardulf A. Express subcutaneous IgG infusions: decreased time of delivery with maintained safety. Clin Immunol. 2002;104:237–41.
42. Gustafson R, Gardulf A, et al. Rapid subcutaneous immunoglobulin administration every second week results in high and stable serum immunoglobulin G levels in patients with primary antibody deficiencies. Clin Exp Immunol. 2008;152:274–9.
43. Wasserman RL. Recombinant human hyaluronidase-facilitated subcutaneous immunoglobulin infusion in primary immunodeficiency diseases. Immunotherapy. 2017;9:1035–50.
44. Shapiro R. Subcutaneous immunoglobulin therapy by rapid push is preferred to infusion by pump: a retrospective analysis. J Clin Immunol. 2010;30:301–7.
45. Shapiro RS. Subcutaneous immunoglobulin therapy given by subcutaneous rapid push vs infusion pump: a retrospective analysis. Ann Allergy Asthma Immunol. 2013;111:51–5.
46. Shapiro RS. Subcutaneous immunoglobulin: rapid push vs. infusion pump in pediatrics. Pediatr Allergy Immunol. 2013;24:49–53.
47. Urschel S, Kayikci L, Wintergerst U, Notheis G, Jansson A, Belohradsky BH. Common variable immunodeficiency disorders in children: delayed diagnosis despite typical clinical presentation. J Pediatr. 2009;154:888–94.
48. Quinti I, Soresina A, Spadaro G, Martino S, Donnanno S, Agostini C, Claudio P, Franco D, Maria Pesce A, Borghese F, Guerra A, Rondelli R, Plebani A, Network IPI. Long-term follow-up and outcome of a large cohort of patients with common variable immunodeficiency. J Clin Immunol. 2007;27:308–16.
49. Lindberg K, Gustafson R, Samuelson A, Rynnel-Dagöö B. Impact of IgG replacement therapy and antibiotic treatment on the colonization of non-encapsulated *Haemophilus influenzae* in the nasopharynx in patients with hypogammaglobulinaemia. Scand J Infect Dis. 2001;33:904–8.
50. Sewell WA, Buckland M, Jolles SR. Therapeutic strategies in common variable immunodeficiency. Drugs. 2003;63:1359–71.
51. López-Boado YS, Rubin BK. Macrolides as immunomodulatory medications for the therapy of chronic lung diseases. Curr Opin Pharmacol. 2008;8:286–91.
52. Resti M, Micheli A, Moriondo M, Becciolini L, Cortimiglia M, Canessa C, Indolfi G, Bartolini E, de Martino M, Azzari C. Comparison of the effect of antibiotic treatment on the possibility of diagnosing invasive pneumococcal disease by culture or molecular methods: a prospective, observational study of children and adolescents with proven pneumococcal infection. Clin Ther. 2009;31:1266–73.
53. Azzari C, Moriondo M, Indolfi G, Massai C, Becciolini L, de Martino M, Resti M. Molecular detection methods and serotyping performed directly on clinical samples improve diagnostic sensitivity and reveal increased incidence of invasive disease by Streptococcus pneumoniae in Italian children. J Med Microbiol. 2008;57:1205–12.
54. Common Variable Immunodeficiency Diagnostic and therapeutic recommendations Working group Associazione Italiana di Ematologia ed Oncologia pediatrica (AIEOP)-Italian primary immunodeficiencies network (IPINET) december 2001.
55. Aghamohammadi A, Abolhassani H, Moazzami K, Parvaneh N, Rezaei N. Correlation between common variable immunodeficiency clinical phenotypes and parental consanguinity in children and adults. J Investig Allergol Clin Immunol. 2010;20(5):372–9.
56. Hampson FA, Chandra A, Screaton NJ, et al. Respiratory disease in common variable immunodeficiency and other primary immunodeficiency disorders. Clin Radiol. 2012;67:587–95.
57. Park MA, Li JT, Hagan JB, Maddox DE, Abraham RS. Common variable immunodeficiency: a new look at an old disease. Lancet. 2008;372:489–502.
58. Garrod R, Lasserson T. Role of physiotherapy in the management of chronic lung diseases: an overview of systematic reviews. Respir Med. 2007;101:2429–36.
59. Bradley J, Moran F, Greenstone M. Physical training for bronchiectasis. Cochrane Database Syst Rev. 2002;3:CD002166.
60. Aghamohammadi A, Moin M, Kouhi A, et al. Chromosomal radiosensitivity in patients with common variable immunodeficiency. Immunobiology. 2008;213:447–54.
61. Palanduz S, Palanduz A, Yalcin I, et al. In vitro chromosomal radiosensitivity in common variable immune deficiency. Clin Immunol Immunopathol. 1998;86:180–2.

62. Vorechovský I, Scott D, Haeney MR, Webster DA. Chromosomal radiosensitivity in common variable immune deficiency. Mutat Res. 1993;290:255–64.
63. Fried AJ, Bonilla FA. Pathogenesis, diagnosis, and management of primary antibody deficiencies and infections. Clin Microbiol Rev. 2009;22:396–414.
64. Touw CM, van de Ven AA, de Jong PA, et al. Detection of pulmonary complications in common variable immunodeficiency. Pediatr Allergy Immunol. 2010;21:793–805.
65. Busse PJ, Farzan S, Cunningham-Rundles C. Pulmonary complications of common variable immunodeficiency. Ann Allergy Asthma Immunol. 2007;98:1–8. quiz 8
66. Yalçin E, Kiper N, Ozçelik U, et al. Effects of claritromycin on inflammatory parameters and clinical conditions in children with bronchiectasis. J Clin Pharm Ther. 2006;31:49–55.
67. Koh YY, Lee MH, Sun YH, Sung KW, Chae JH. Effect of roxithromycin on airway responsiveness in children with bronchiectasis: a double-blind, placebo-controlled study. Eur Respir J. 1997;10(5):994–9.
68. Cymbala AA, Edmonds LC, Bauer MA, et al. The disease-modifying effects of twice-weekly oral azithromycin in patients with bronchiectasis. Treat Respir Med. 2005;4:117–22.
69. Lin HC, Cheng HF, Wang CH, Liu CY, Yu CT, Kuo HP. Inhaled gentamicin reduces airway neutrophil activity and mucus secretion in bronchiectasis. Am J Respir Crit Care Med. 1997;155:2024–9.
70. Tsang KW, Tan KC, Ho PL, et al. Inhaled fluticasone in bronchiectasis: a 12 month study. Thorax. 2005;60:239–43.
71. Jensen T, Pedersen SS, Garne S, Heilmann C, Høiby N, Koch C. Colistin inhalation therapy in cystic fibrosis patients with chronic Pseudomonas aeruginosa lung infection. J Antimicrob Chemother. 1987;19:831–8.
72. Chuchalin A, Csiszér E, Gyurkovics K, et al. A formulation of aerosolized tobramycin (Bramitob) in the treatment of patients with cystic fibrosis and Pseudomonas aeruginosa infection: a double-blind, placebo-controlled, multicenter study. Paediatr Drugs. 2007;9.(Suppl. 1:21–31.
73. Corless JA, Warburton CJ. Surgery vs non-surgical treatment for bronchiectasis. Cochrane Database Syst Rev. 2000;4:CD002180.
74. O'Donnell AE, Barker AF, Ilowite JS, Fick RB. Treatment of idiopathic bronchiectasis with aerosolized recombinant human DNase I. rhDNase Study Group. Chest. 1998;113:1329–34.
75. Quartier P, Debré M, De Blic J, et al. Early and prolonged intravenous immunoglobulin replacement therapy in childhood agammaglobulinemia: a retrospective survey of 31 patients. J Pediatr. 1999;134:589–96.
76. Foruny JR, Bárcena R, Moreno A, et al. Benefit of pegylated interferon-alpha-2a/ribavirin in a patient with common variable immunodeficiency and hepatitis C virus cirrhosis after liver transplantation and splenic embolization. Transplantation. 2006;82:289–90.
77. Cunningham-Rundles C, Bodian C, Ochs HD, Martin S, Reiter-Wong M, Zhuo Z. Long-term low-dose IL-2 enhances immune function in common variable immunodeficiency. Clin Immunol. 2001;100:181–90.
78. Rump JA, Jahreis A, Schlesier M, Stecher S, Peter HH. A double-blind, placebo-controlled, crossover therapy study with natural human IL-2 (nhuIL-2) in combination with regular intravenous gammaglobulin (IVIG) infusions in 10 patients with common variable immunodeficiency (CVID). Clin Exp Immunol. 1997;110:167–73.
79. Ten RM, Anderson PM, Zein NN, Temesgen Z, Clawson ML, Weiss W. Interleukin-2 liposomes for primary immune deficiency using the aerosol route. Int Immunopharmacol. 2002;2:333–44.
80. Franco F, Sheikh A, Greenstone M. Short acting beta-2 agonists for bronchiectasis. Cochrane Database Syst Rev. 2003;3:CD003572.
81. Sheikh A, Nolan D, Greenstone M. Long-acting beta-2-agonists for bronchiectasis. Cochrane Database Syst Rev. 2001;4:CD002155.
82. Abolhassani H, Sagvand BT, Shokuhfar T, Mirminachi B, Rezaei N, Aghamohammadi A. A review on guidelines for management and treatment of common variable immunodeficiency. Expert Rev Clin Immunol. 2013;9(6):561–75.

83. Davies CW, Juniper MC, Gray W, Gleeson FV, Chapel HM, Davies RJ. Lymphoid interstitial pneumonitis associated with common variable hypogammaglobulinaemia treated with cyclosporin A. Thorax. 2000;55:88–90.
84. Paramothayan S, Lasserson T. Treatments for pulmonary sarcoidosis. Respir Med. 2008;102:1–9.
85. Boursiquot JN, Gérard L, Malphettes M, et al; DEFI Study Group. Granulomatous disease in CVID: retrospective analysis of clinical characteristics and treatment efficacy in a cohort of 59 patients. J Clin Immunol. 2013;33:84–95.
86. Fazzi P. Pharmacotherapeutic management of pulmonary sarcoidosis. Am J Respir Med. 2003;2:311–20.
87. Kyburz D, Brentano F, Gay S. Mode of action of hydroxychloroquine in RA—evidence of an inhibitory effect on toll-like receptor signaling. Nat Clin Pract Rheumatol. 2006;2:458–9.
88. Knight AK, Cunningham-Rundles C. Inflammatory and autoimmune complications of common variable immune deficiency. Autoimmun Rev. 2006;5:156–9.
89. Paramothayan S, Lasserson TJ, Walters EH. Immunosuppressive and cytotoxic therapy for pulmonary sarcoidosis. Cochrane Database Syst Rev. 2006;3:CD003536.
90. Smith KJ, Skelton H. Common variable immunodeficiency treated with a recombinant human IgG, tumour necrosis factor-alpha receptor fusion protein. Br J Dermatol. 2001;144:597–600.
91. Fernández-Ruiz M, Guerra-Vales JM, Francisco-Javier CF, et al. Fever of unknown origin in a patient with common variable immunodeficiency associated with multisystemic granulomatous disease. Intern Med. 2007;46:1197–202.
92. Hatab AZ, Ballas ZK. Caseating granulomatous disease in common variable immunodeficiency treated with infliximab. J Allergy Clin Immunol. 2005;116:1161–2.
93. Baughman RP, Drent M, Kavuru M, et al; Sarcoidosis Investigators. Infliximab therapy in patients with chronic sarcoidosis and pulmonary involvement. Am J Respir Crit Care Med. 2006;174:795–802.
94. Thatayatikom A, Thatayatikom S, White AJ. Infliximab treatment for severe granulomatous disease in common variable immunodeficiency: a case report and review of the literature. Ann Allergy Asthma Immunol. 2005;95:293–300.
95. Martínez García MA, de Rojas MD, Nauffal Manzur MD, et al. Respiratory disorders in common variable immunodeficiency. Respir Med. 2001;95:191–5.
96. Sève P, Bourdillon L, Sarrot-Reynauld F, DEF-I Study Group, et al. Autoimmune hemolytic anemia and common variable immunodeficiency: a case-control study of 18 patients. Medicine (Baltimore). 2008;87:177–84.
97. Michel M, Chanet V, Galicier L, et al. Autoimmune thrombocytopenic purpura and common variable immunodeficiency: analysis of 21 cases and review of the literature. Medicine (Baltimore). 2004;83:254–63.
98. Chapel H, Cunningham-Rundles C. Update in understanding common variable immunodeficiency disorders (CVIDs) and the management of patients with these conditions. Br J Haematol. 2009;145:709–27.
99. Cunningham-Rundles C. Autoimmune manifestations in common variable immunodeficiency. J Clin Immunol. 2008;28.(Suppl. 1:S42–5.
100. Wakim M, Shah A, Arndt PA, et al. Successful anti-CD20 monoclonal antibody treatment of severe autoimmune hemolytic anemia due to warm reactive IgM autoantibody in a child with common variable immunodeficiency. Am J Hematol. 2004;76:152–5.
101. Nos P, Bastida G, Beltran B, Aguas M, Ponce J. Crohn's disease in common variable immunodeficiency: treatment with antitumor necrosis factor alpha. Am J Gastroenterol. 2006;101:2165–6.
102. Cunningham-Rundles C. How I treat common variable immune deficiency. Blood. 2010;116:7–15.
103. Shillitoe B, Gennery A. X-Linked Agammaglobulinaemia: Outcomes in the modern era. Clin Immunol. 2017;183:54–62.
104. Chua I, Standish R, Lear S, et al. Anti-tumour necrosis factor-alpha therapy for severe enteropathy in patients with common variable immunodeficiency (CVID). Clin Exp Immunol. 2007;150:306–11.

105. Agarwal S, Cunningham-Rundles C. Autoimmunity in common variable immunodeficiency. Curr Allergy Asthma Rep. 2009;9:347–52.
106. Daniels JA, Lederman HM, Maitra A, Montgomery EA. Gastrointestinal tract pathology in patients with common variable immunodeficiency (CVID): a clinicopathologic study and review. Am J Surg Pathol. 2007;31:1800–12.
107. Raeiszadeh M, Kopycinski J, Paston SJ, et al. The T cell response to persistent herpes virus infections in common variable immunodeficiency. Clin Exp Immunol. 2006;146:234–42.
108. Abolhassani H, Aghamohammadi A, Imanzadeh A, Mohammadinejad P, Sadeghi B, Rezaei N. Malignancy phenotype in common variable immunodeficiency. J Investig Allergol Clin Immunol. 2012;22:133–4.
109. Gompels MM, Hodges E, Lock RJ, et al. Associated Study Group. Lymphoproliferative disease in antibody deficiency: a multi-centre study. Clin Exp Immunol. 2003;134:314–20.
110. Ochtrop ML, Goldacker S, May AM, et al. T and B lymphocyte abnormalities in bone marrow biopsies of common variable immunodeficiency. Blood. 2011;118:309–18.
111. Rizzi M, Neumann C, Fielding AK, et al. Outcome of allogeneic stem cell transplantation in adults with common variable immunodeficiency. J Allergy Clin Immunol. 2011;128:1371–4.

Management of Humoral Primary Immunodeficiencies in Adults

21

Gianfranco Vitiello, Giacomo Emmi, and Boaz Palterer

21.1 Immunoglobulin Replacement Therapy

21.1.1 Introduction and History

The history of immunoglobulin replacement dates back in 1890, when Emil Adolf von Behring and Shibasaburo Kitasato demonstrated that protection against diphtheria or tetanus could be transferred to provide protection in animal model [1]. Around the same time, Paul Ehrlich coined the term "antibody" [2]. It was not until the World War II that immunoglobulin G became available for clinical use. Indeed, Edwin Joseph Cohn developed a technique for blood fractionation [3]. Hence, in 1952 Ogden Carr Bruton for the first time was able to use a subcutaneous gammaglobulin preparation from Cohn fraction II to prevent life-threatening infections in agammaglobulinemic patients [4]. Attempts to inject these preparations intravenously resulted in severe anaphylactoid reactions due to spontaneous complement activation from immunoglobulin aggregates [5]. For these reasons, intramuscular preparations were used at the cost of serious adverse reactions such as pain and nerve injury [6] with a poor increase of the immunoglobulin levels [7]. In the 1970s the first chemically modified intravenous immunoglobulin preparations became available and, 10 years later, enzymatic and chemical modifications helped to suppress the complement activation by reducing the ability of immunoglobulins to form aggregates [8]. Albeit subcutaneous route of administration was the first to be explored, it was then abandoned in favor of intramuscular one. Only in mid-1980s, the concept of home therapy with subcutaneous immunoglobulin infusion started to gain popularity, especially in Scandinavian countries [9].

G. Vitiello · G. Emmi (✉) · B. Palterer
Department of Experimental and Clinical Medicine, University of Florence, Florence, Italy
e-mail: giacomo.emmi@unifi.it

M. M. D'Elios, M. Rizzi (eds.), *Humoral Primary Immunodeficiencies*,
Rare Diseases of the Immune System, https://doi.org/10.1007/978-3-319-91785-6_21

21.1.2 From Donor to Recipient

Intravenous and subcutaneous immunoglobulins (IVIg and SCIg, respectively) are therapeutic preparation of normal immunoglobulins G (IgGs) usually obtained from a large pool of healthy blood or plasma donors.

Regular donors are thoroughly screened by clinical history in search for known risk factors for infectious agents according to the National Regulatory Authorities. The obtained plasma is carefully stored at constant temperature (– 20 °C) as to avoid complement or coagulation activation. Donations are screened for human immunodeficiency virus (HIV), hepatitis C virus (HCV), hepatitis B virus (HBV), hepatitis A virus (HAV), and parvovirus B19. If needed, according to the epidemiological situation of the country of origin of the donor, other screening measures could be implemented. Donations with high-titer anti-A, anti-B, and anti-D isoagglutinin are discarded. Various purification processes, usually cryoprecipitation plus chromatographic absorption, will eliminate contaminants that can be responsible for adverse events such as prekallikrein activator and activated coagulation factors. In this regard, chromatographic procedures are pivotal to the removal of IgA. To eliminate possible viral contamination several methods, possibly in combination, are employed, such as low pH treatments, pasteurization, solvent detergent, caprylic acid treatment and nanofiltration. For these reasons, the products are not identical to each other and can vary in concentration, osmolality and IgA, sugar, and amino acid content.

A thorough review about production methods and quality controls of IVIg can be found at these two references [8, 10].

21.1.3 Intravenous Immunoglobulins

IVIg are used to treat a large number of diseases. However, their approved indication can be divided in three major categories (Table 21.1).

HIV human immunodeficiency virus, *CLL* chronic lymphocytic leukemia, *ITP* idiopathic thrombocytopenic purpura, *CIDP* chronic inflammatory demyelinating polyneuropathy

IVIg are administered through a peripheral venous catheter. The placement of permanent central venous access should be discouraged as it has been associated with thrombotic and infectious complications [11]. On the contrary, difficult peripheral venous access should encourage the switch from intravenous to subcutaneous

Table 21.1 Indications of intravenous immunoglobulins

Protection	Immunomodulation	Prevention
Primary immunodeficiencies Secondary immunodeficiencies HIV CLL	ITP Guillain-Barré Syndrome CIDP Kawasaki disease	Bone marrow transplantation Infections Graft-versus-host disease

immunoglobulins therapy [12]. An infusion rate of 0.5–1 mg/kg/min is recommended at the beginning, increasing gradually up to 3–4 mg/kg/min. Rates above 5 mg/kg/min are associated with more side effects but may be well-tolerated by some patients [13]. For these reasons, infusions usually take 2–6 h.

The recommended starting dose is comprised between 400 and 600 mg/kg every 4 weeks in order to achieve trough IgG levels of 600–800 mg/dL [13]. Three to 4 months after the first infusion, a patient-centered follow-up should be implemented. Routine monitoring ought to be calibrated on age, clinical conditions, and trough IgG levels (see after), and it must include total blood cell count and liver and renal function [11]. A rapid increase in immunoglobulin level at the beginning of treatment may be observed, followed by a rapid decrease in IgG3 levels (half-life 7 days), whereas IgG1, IgG2, and IgG4 levels dawn between the third and the fourth week after infusion (half-life 21 days). In general, for each 100 mg/kg of intravenous immunoglobulin, IgG levels increase by 250 mg/dL [13].

21.1.4 Subcutaneous Immunoglobulins

Subcutaneous administration of immunoglobulin replacement therapy has gained in popularity during the last 20 years. Infusions are usually delivered using infusion pumps and administration may take 30–90 min, but it is possible to deliver therapy using 10 mL syringes and multiple site of injections. The latter is preferable in children, as the injected dose is small. Conversely, adults usually prefer to make use of a pump. Suitable infusion sites are the lower abdomen, thighs, and back of the arms. Leanest patients may use the upper outer quadrant of the buttocks. Site rotation is not always necessary but recommended, in order to find the preferred site of infusion. Needles are 4–14 mm long and 24–27 gauges in diameter. Patients should be trained to self-administer the infusion therapy in the proper way. This training is usually given by specialized nurses, who tailor patients education based on schooling and the preferred learning style. A complete review on the role of infusion nursing is available at this reference [14].

In general, it is recommended to start the replacement therapy intravenously, and then, if necessary or preferred (see after), it is possible to switch to the subcutaneous route. The first SCIg infusion may be given 1–2 weeks after the last intravenous administration. A period of 5–12 weeks is necessary to reach a new steady state and, therefore, to eventually perform dose adjustment [13]. When a switch is necessary, the following correction factors have been proposed to achieve bioequivalence:

$$\frac{\text{weight}(\text{kg}) \times \text{IVIg dosage}\left(\text{g} \times \text{kg}^{-1} \times \text{month}^{-1}\right) \times 1.37(\text{for } 10\%\,\text{products}) \text{ or} \times 1.53(\text{for } 20\%\,\text{products})}{4(\text{passage from monthly to weekly interval})}$$

Other experts, especially in Europe, use a 1:1 correction factor. It is thought that the correction factor may lose its usefulness in patients receiving higher intravenous doses [15].

21.1.5 Facilitated Subcutaneous Immunoglobulins

The flow of SCIg is limited by extracellular matrix, therefore reducing the amount of IgG that can be delivered if compared to intravenous infusions by 37% to 53% [16]. In some patients, higher doses of SCIg are necessary to reach the trough levels, and, in some cases, more than one infusion site is necessary to overcome the development of local adverse reactions, namely, a painful lump that can last for days. For these reasons, the addition of recombinant human hyaluronidase (rHuPH20) has helped to increase the permeability of subcutaneous tissues and therefore the administration of higher volumes at a single site. This approach increases the flexibility in the frequency of infusions, which now ranges from daily to monthly dosing [17].

21.1.6 When to Start Immunoglobulins Replacement [18]

It is recommended to start immunoglobulin replacement therapy in every patient that fulfills CVID diagnostic criteria (Chap. 3). Indeed, even if patients with pneumonia did not have lower IgG trough levels than patients without infection episodes, when clustered according to IgG levels, only the group with IgG lower than 400 mg/dL had an increased risk of pneumonia [19]. In addition to this, an increased risk of pneumonia was found in patients that did not reach an IgG level of 400 mg/dL when treated with intravenous immunoglobulins [19]. However, three main exceptions exist: the patient with reduced, but not absent, immunoglobulin G in the range of 400–600 mg/dL; the patient with selective antibody deficiencies; and the patients that, despite low immunoglobulin levels, do not develop recurrent and/or severe infections. In these cases, the benefits of starting replacement therapy are controversial [20]. It is important to follow these patients every 6–12 months to assess the number and the severity of bacterial infections and the development of the classical complications of CVID, such as lymphoproliferation, enteropathy, or granulomatous-lymphocytic interstitial lung disease. To date it is unclear whether or not immunoglobulins treatment can control the multi-organ involvement related to the disease [18]. What is clear is that determination of vaccine responses are pivotal to decide the therapeutic approach [18]. When vaccine responses are appropriate, a trial of prophylactic antibiotics before considering replacement immunoglobulins therapy has been suggested. Once infections become severe and frequent and antibiotic prophylaxis results ineffective, a trial of intermittent replacement therapy could be attempted, revaluating the patients 3–5 months after discontinuation [17]. Multiple cessations are not useful if the patients require restarting immunoglobulin therapy more than twice [17]. In patients with selective IgA deficiency, replacement therapy should be started only when antibiotic prophylactic therapy is not sufficient to prevent frequent and/or severe infections [17]. In this case, SCIg- or IgA-depleted intravenous immunoglobulin must be administered [21].

21.1.7 Intravenous or Subcutaneous Replacement? [14, 15, 22–24]

Intravenous and subcutaneous immunoglobulins show similar efficacy in protection. However, there are many factors that can influence the preferred route of administration, both patient-centered and health-centered. Regarding patient-centered features, compliance is a major issue. In this regard, intravenous administration requires less frequent infusions as higher doses can be easily administered with a single infusion. Moreover, hospital-based administration may help to monitor the patient closely and more frequently. On the contrary, patients that travel frequently (i.e., for work) or that live away from hospital may prefer subcutaneous administration. Another pivotal factor is the patients' ability to learn and perform the procedure. Therefore, individualized educational programs are essential in ensuring success.

In relation to health-centered features, intravenous administration should be selected when a rapid increase of immunoglobulin levels is necessary in a short time as higher doses can be easily administered. Thereafter, according to patient preference, education programs may be started in order to switch to the subcutaneous route. Subcutaneous administration should be selected when consistent and steady IgG levels are necessary, mostly when intravenous route becomes responsible for wear-off effects (see after). Moreover, this route is desirable when difficulties in venous access are present. On the contrary, intravenous immunoglobulins are preferred when one or more comorbidities related to the primary immunodeficiency are present (i.e., granulomatous-lymphocytic interstitial lung disease, cytopenias, autoimmune features) as higher doses can be used with benefit in these kinds of patients. It is important to remember that relative contraindications of subcutaneous administration are severe thrombocytopenia, bleeding disorders, anticoagulation therapy, widespread eczema, and limited subcutaneous tissue [15]. Regarding adverse reactions, intravenous route is responsible for more systemic effects (i.e., fever, headache, flushing, chills, tachycardia, hypo-/hypertension). These reactions are fewer with subcutaneous immunoglobulins, and this route of administration should be preferred in these patients. On the contrary, in patients with unacceptable local reactions (i.e., infusion site pain, swelling, erythema), facilitated subcutaneous immunoglobulins may help reduce these adverse effects. Likewise, intravenous route is an appropriate solution.

21.1.8 Trough Levels

The main goal of immunoglobulins replacement therapy is the minimization of infective complications in immunocompromised subjects. A trough level is the lowest concentration of a drug before the next dose is administered. In the case of IVIg, the optimal trough level has remained uncertain. From early studies, a level of 500 mg/dL emerged as the minimum target level of immunoglobulin replacement [25]. However, subsequent clinical evidence has suggested higher levels, in general >800 mg/dL [26]. These recommendations have been strengthened by a recent meta-analysis that found a fivefold higher risk of pneumonia in patients with 500 mg/dL trough levels when compared with those with 1000 mg/dL [25]. Since the level of immunoglobulins that is able to prevent infections varies from patient to patient (with a wide range from 500 to 1700 mg/dL), the new concept of individual trough has been developed [27]. The target is not directed to reach a particular IgG level, yet to improve the clinical outcome of the single patient, according to their clinical phenotype and the presence of complications [28]. For example, it is known that lower IgG and IgA at diagnosis and very low IgA level during follow-up reflect a severe impaired switching process and represented a major risk for lung complications [19].

21.1.9 Adverse Reactions and Side Effects

21.1.9.1 Immediate Reactions and Anaphylaxis

Immediate IVIg infusion reactions may range from mild to severe life-threatening (Fig. 21.1). Headaches, nausea, flushing, mild fever and chills, and joint, muscle, and abdominal pain are common, together with hypertension, hypotension, tachycardia, and chest pain. Fatigue, weakness and dizziness might be present the days

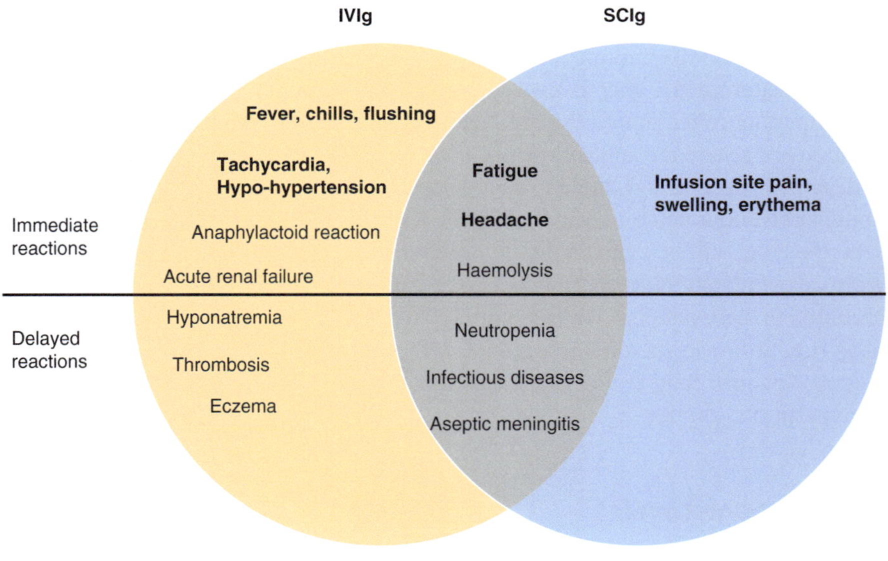

Fig. 21.1 Immediate and delayed reactions to IVIg and SCIg. *IVIg* intravenous immunoglobulins, *SCIg* subcutaneous immunoglobulins

after the administration and tend to decrease with the subsequent administrations. Anaphylactic and anaphylactoid reactions are uncommon and rarely life-threatening. Usually, the reactions can be prevented by slowing the infusion rate. Mild symptoms can be managed with antihistamines and acetaminophen. Patients can also be pretreated with nonsteroidal anti-inflammatory drug and/or antihistamines in order to prevent infusion reactions. In high-risk patients (first-time infusion, previous reaction, obstructive lung disease, etc.), corticosteroids can be added into the pre-treatment protocol.

True anaphylaxis is rarely caused by IVIg and must be treated as needed as standard allergic reactions. These reactions are classically attributed to anti-IgA antibodies, of either the IgG or IgE isotype. Patients with CVID and/or IgA deficiency might get sensitized by contaminant IgA in IVIg or other blood products [29]. The reaction mechanism of IgG anti-IgA is not clear, and it is possibly mediated by immune complex deposition. However, the significance and clinical value of anti-IgA antibodies is debated as they are found in healthy subjects as well. Moreover, they do not predict always a reaction in IgA deficient patients. In fact, numerous factors should be taken into consideration: antibody concentration and detection method sensibility (passive hemagglutination, ELISA, RIA), antibody isotype (IgG vs. IgE) and class or subclass specificity (IgA1 vs. IgA2), and the administration route (IVIg vs. SCIg) [30]. Severe reactions requiring the use of epinephrine are exceedingly rare. Patients with anaphylactic or anaphylactoid reactions can be switched to slow subcutaneous administration, as this route is usually well-tolerated [31].

21.1.9.2 Headaches and Aseptic Meningitis

Headache is one of the most common complaints after IVIg infusion, starting either during the infusion or several hours later. It usually resolves spontaneously in less than 24 h and responds to analgesics. However, sometimes it might last longer and be associated with prolonged malaise, myalgia, photophobia, neck stiffness, nausea, and vomiting. In these severe cases, cerebrospinal fluid may reveal aseptic meningitis, characterized by pleocytosis, elevated proteins, and negative research for viral PCRs and bacterial cultures. A positive history for migraine is a risk factor for aseptic meningitis, independently of preparation or infusion rate [32]. These reactions are more frequent when an immunomodulatory high-dose IVIg (1–2 g/kg) is administered, even though they have been also reported in patients with low-dose replacement therapy [33]. The mechanism of action is unclear. IVIg-mediated osmotic shifts in the meninges and a direct inflammatory reaction have been proposed. Atypical anti-neutrophil antibodies contained in IVIg preparations have been claimed to activate TNF-α primed neutrophils [34].

21.1.9.3 Thrombotic Complications

Thrombosis has been widely reported, especially with high-dose IVIg, whereas it seems to be less likely in patients receiving low dose or SCIg [35]. The majority (80%) of reported thrombotic events is arterial (stroke and myocardial infarction) and occurs early after IVIg administration. Arterial thrombotic events are associated with older age and atherosclerotic vascular disease. Venous thrombosis (deep vein thrombosis and pulmonary embolism) occurs less frequently (20%), usually later than 24 hours after IVIg administration, and is associated with factors contributing to venous stasis (i.e., obesity or immobility) [36]. Thrombotic events in the cerebral sinus and jugular vein have been reported as well [37, 38]. The mechanisms implicated in thrombotic events are platelet activation and increased adhesiveness, hyperviscosity, autoantibodies, or excess coagulation factors in the IVIg. A retrospective study reported thromboembolic events, even at low-dose regimens, in correlation with higher concentrations of clotting factor XI. Manufacturing and regulations have since been changed to test for procoagulant factors [39]. Prevention of thrombotic events includes identifying risk factors, adequate prehydration, slower infusion, premedication with antiplatelet drugs, or low molecular weight heparins [40]. Arterial thrombosis caused by IVIg can be treated with tissue plasminogen activator (tPA) [41].

21.1.9.4 Hemolysis and Cytopenias

Hemolytic reactions can occur after infusions due to the presence of isohemagglutinins in IVIg preparations. They usually involve anti-A and anti-B antibodies, even though minor groups like anti-D and anti-K have been implicated as well. In practice, most events are subclinical, with mild hemolysis presenting as hyperbilirubinemia and positive direct Coombs test. In a large cohort study, 1.6% of clinically relevant hemolytic events were reported, with a hemoglobin drop ranging from 0.8 to 5.2 g/dL. Characteristics of these patients included high-dose IVIg, female sex, non-group 0 blood and with an underlying inflammatory state [42]. Immunoaffinity chromatography is used in modern preparations to reduce the titer of isohemagglutinins [43].

Transient neutropenia can occur 2–4 days after IVIg administration and last up to weeks. However, there is no report about severe infections [44]. Naturally occurring anti-Siglec-9 (anti-sialic acid-binding Ig-like lectin 9) autoantibodies, contained in some IVIg preparations, have been found to mediate neutrophil death [45].

21.1.9.5 Pulmonary Complications

Dyspnea and wheezing are relatively frequent but usually mild. Respiratory failure can be seen during anaphylaxis and pulmonary embolism. A rare but life-threatening adverse reaction is transfusion-related acute lung injury (TRALI), mostly associated with platelets and plasma transfusions but reported also with IVIg. It manifests with noncardiogenic pulmonary edema within 6 h from the infusion. The pathogenesis of TRALI in the setting of IVIg appears to be related to anti-HLA antibodies [46].

21.1.9.6 Renal Failure and Electrolyte Imbalances

Renal failure was initially reported in patients undergoing high-dose IVIg treatment and attributed to immune complex deposition and glomerular necrosis.

The decrease in renal function peaks usually 1 week after infusion and might be severe and even irreversible, requiring dialysis and transplantation [47]. Most renal adverse reactions have been associated with IVIg formulations containing sucrose, a sugar that is not metabolized in the kidney and that can cause osmotic nephrosis in the proximal tubules [48]. Reports of renal injury with sucrose-free IVIg are very rare. There are seldom case reports with maltose containing IVIg, but in most cases concomitant risk factors were present. Single cases have been reported with D-sorbitol, glycine, and L-proline. The risk factors associated with renal failure are concomitant administration of potentially nephrotoxic drugs (loop diuretics, angiotensin-converting enzyme inhibitors, angiotensin receptor antagonists, cyclosporine, iodinated contrast agent, aminoglycosides, vancomycin), prior renal impairment, diabetes, hypertension, hypovolemia, obesity, and dysproteinemias (cryoglobulinemia, monoclonal gammopathies, multiple myeloma) [49]. Treatment and prevention aim to monitor renal function, maintain adequate hydration, and avoid IVIg overload with slower infusion and smaller dose per day [49].

IVIg infusion can cause hyponatremia through a dilutional effect resulting from sucrose-induced translocation of water from the intracellular compartment to the extracellular one [50]. Pseudo-hyponatremia caused by plasma hyperproteinemia is common [51]. In both cases the electrolyte defect is transient and does not require any treatment.

SCIg infusions are generally well-tolerated, even in the event of previous adverse events with IVIg. Local pain, swelling, and redness in SCIg injection site are common and can persist up to 3 days. However, those reactions are mild and well-tolerated, especially when compared to the IVIg ones [52]. Systemic reaction to SCIg are extremely rare, therefore premedication and monitoring of the therapy is rarely necessary [53].

21.1.9.7 Infective Complications

As with any blood product, immunoglobulins carry an intrinsic risk for the transmission of pathogens. The most notable infection transmitted by IVIg in the past has been hepatitis C (HCV). Since 1996, after the adoption of antiviral measures during IVIg preparation and PCR screening of samples HCV, transmissions have not been reported [54]. Notably, parvovirus B19 is not removed by standard IVIg preparations, but it is usually neutralized by the antibodies contained in the preparation, although few cases of infection have been reported [55]. No cases of HIV transmission have been reported so far, probably because the virus is lost during preparation due to its fragility. It has been speculated that also prion disease like Creutzfeldt-Jakob could be transmitted by IVIg [56]. A case series of patients with immunodeficiency and progressive neurodegeneration have been described, but no viral or prion etiologic factor have been identified [57].

21.2 Antibiotics

21.2.1 Antibiotic Prophylaxis

Prophylactic antibiotics are of common use in patients with primary humoral primary immunodeficiencies, even though there are no guidelines in this regard. A different approach is used in patients with or without bronchiectasis.

21.2.1.1 Antibiotic Prophylaxis in Patients Without Bronchiectasis

The use of antibiotics in these patients is common, especially when only a partial antibody deficiency or an isolated IgA deficiency is present. A prophylaxis with a continuous or seasonal intermittent scheme may be of benefit, particularly in patients with more than three infections per year [58].

21.2.1.2 Antibiotic Prophylaxis in Patients with Bronchiectasis

Most of the experience in this field is adopted from cystic fibrosis (CF) patients with bronchiectasis and bronchiectasis of other origin. Studies from bronchoalveolar lavage indicate that *H. influenzae*, *S. aureus*, *S. pneumoniae*, and viruses represent the more frequent colonizers of these patients' lungs [59]. In this subgroup of patients, antimicrobial prophylaxis is generally suggested when sinopulmonary infections occur despite pushing up IgG replacement therapy [60].

The most popular prophylactic antibiotics are macrolides, since they present an additional anti-inflammatory effect [61]. Azithromycin 500 mg 3 days/week is the most common approach [18]. Nontuberculosis mycobacterial (NTM) infection is common among patients with bronchiectasis. Azithromycin monotherapy is associated to mycobacterial resistance when NTMs are present. For this reason, their presence should be excluded before initiating the antimicrobic prophylaxis.

21.2.1.3 Pseudomonas Aeruginosa

Pseudomonas aeruginosa is a frequent colonizer of bronchiectasis, but true infections seldom occur. However, this colonization has been associated with the decline of lung function and poor prognosis. In CF and non-CF bronchiectasis patients, the use of azithromycin for 3 days each week has reduced exacerbations without a clear effect on lung function [58, 60].

Nebulized antibiotics may reduce the load of *P. aeruginosa* in bronchiectasis. Inhaled colistin and tobramycin may help reducing exacerbation frequency and lung function decline [62, 63]. Premedication with beta2-agonists may be needed in order to avoid bronchospasm [64].

21.2.2 Antibiotic Therapy

Most infections in patients with hypogammaglobulinemia are in the upper and lower respiratory tract, including sinusitis, otitis, bronchitis, and pneumonia. Therefore, empiric antibiotic therapy should be targeted to encapsulated bacteria as

S. pneumoniae while waiting for cultures. In patients with bronchiectasis, *P. aeruginosa* coverage should be taken into consideration. Early treatment of infections is necessary, especially in the presence of purulent sputum, in order to avoid secondary structural damage. Before initiating any antibiotic therapy, samples should be collected to obtain cultures and antibiogram, as unusual microorganisms or antibiotic resistance can occur. However, in the setting of upper respiratory tract symptoms, viruses are a common cause. Indeed, upper respiratory tract infections respond poorly to antibiotics, suggesting that antibiotic usage should be targeted better [65].

Gastrointestinal infections are the second common localization, and therapy should be first aimed at rehydration and nutrition and then targeted on the basis of biopsies and cultures. The most common cause of infectious diarrhea is *Giardia lamblia*, followed by *Campylobacter jejuni* and *Salmonella* species. Other pathogens reported are *Cytomegalovirus* and *Clostridium difficile*. Notably, despite using more antibiotics than the general population, CVID patients aren't more susceptible to *C. difficile* infection. Unusual parasites and fungi, or pathogens like *Microsporidia* or *Cryptosporidia*, should raise the suspicion of combined immunodeficiency [66].

In recent years, *Norovirus* has been recognized as an important pathogen. While in the healthy population it only causes a self-limiting acute diarrhea, in CVID patients it can lead to a severe chronic enteropathy, and clearance of the infection may be associated with the improvement of villous atrophy. Oral immunoglobulins and nitazoxanide have been used to treat *Norovirus* infections, although only ribavirin has been linked to viral clearance [67].

Atypical gram-negative rods like *Helicobacter bilis*, also known as *Flexispira rappini*, can cause bacteremia, skin ulcers, arthritis, and osteomyelitis in deeply hypogammaglobulinemic patients. Isolation of those pathogens is difficult, as it requires selective culture conditions. Therefore, a strict cooperation with microbiologist is needed [68].

Chronic enterovirus meningoencephalitis is a rare complication of deeply hypogammaglobulinemic patients, usually seen in Bruton's agammaglobulinemia or hyper-IgM syndromes. Cases have been reported also in patients with CVID, successfully treated with pleconaril [69].

21.2.3 Non-pharmacological Interventions

Bronchiectatic patients may benefit from pulmonary rehabilitation, as it improves the removal of secretions from the airways and exercise tolerance [70].

21.3 Hematopoietic Stem Cell Transplantation

Infections in CVID are usually well controlled with IVIg/SCIg. However, a subgroup of patients has severe autoimmune, autoinflammatory, lymphoproliferative, and neoplastic complications that negatively impact the prognosis. Although these manifestations are usually controlled by immunosuppressive and immunomodulatory therapies, more invasive treatments are needed when treatment-resistant and life-threating complications are present. In all these cases, allogeneic hematopoietic stem cell transplantation (HSCT) should be considered as a valid option. The most common indications for HSCT are immunologic dysregulation and lymphoma. The reported mortality is very high (52%), even though HSCT was curative in most patients that survived and half of the patients have also suspended immunoglobulin therapy [71]. The diffusion of newborn screening and next-generation sequencing will enable the early recognition of genetic forms of combined immunodeficiency and CVID associated with severe complications, like LRBA deficiency [72] or ADA2 deficiency [73], which might benefit more from early HSCT.

References

1. von Behring E, Kitasato S. The mechanism of diphtheria immunity and tetanus immunity in animals. 1890. Mol Immunol. 1991;28(1317):1319–20.
2. Lindenmann J. Origin of the terms "antibody" and "antigen". Scand J Immunol. 1984;19:281–5.
3. Cohn EJ, Strong LE, Hughes WL, Mulford DJ, Ashworth JN, Melin M, Taylor HL. Preparation and properties of serum and plasma proteins. IV. A system for the separation into fractions of the protein and lipoprotein components of biological tissues and fluids 1a,b,c,d. J Am Chem Soc. 1946;68:459–75.
4. Bruton OC. Agammaglobulinemia Pediatrics. 1952;9:722–8.
5. Barandun S, Kistler P, Jeunet F, Isliker H. Intravenous administration of human gamma-globulin. Vox Sang. 1962;7:157–74.
6. Lieberman P, Berger M. Intramuscular versus intravenous immunoglobulin replacement therapy and measurement of immunoglobulin levels during immunoglobulin replacement therapy. J Allergy Clin Immunol Pract. 2013;1:705–6.
7. Smith GN, Griffiths B, Mollison D, Mollison PL. Uptake of IgG after intramuscular and subcutaneous injection. Lancet. 1972;1:1208–12.
8. Radosevich M, Burnouf T. Intravenous immunoglobulin G: trends in production methods, quality control and quality assurance. Vox Sang. 2010;98:12–28.
9. Ashida ER, Saxon A. Home intravenous immunoglobulin therapy by self-administration. J Clin Immunol. 1986;6:306–9.
10. Afonso AFB, João CMP. The production processes and biological effects of intravenous immunoglobulin. Biomol Ther. 2016;6:1–20.
11. Bonilla FA, Khan DA, Ballas ZK, et al. Practice parameter for the diagnosis and management of primary immunodeficiency. J Allergy Clin Immunol. 2014;136:1–20e78.
12. Torgerson TR. Overview of routes of IgG administration. J Clin Immunol. 2013;33:2012–4.
13. Sriaroon P, Ballow M. Immunoglobulin Replacement Therapy for Primary Immunodeficiency. Immunol Allergy Clin N Am. 2015;35:713–30.
14. Younger MEM, Blouin W, Duff C, Epland KB, Murphy E, Sedlak D. Subcutaneous immunoglobulin replacement therapy: Ensuring success. J Infus Nurs. 2015;38:70–9.
15. Wasserman RL. Progress in gammaglobulin therapy for immunodeficiency: From subcutaneous to intravenous infusions and back again. J Clin Immunol. 2012;32:1153–64.
16. Frost GI. Recombinant human hyaluronidase (rHuPH20): an enabling platform for subcutaneous drug and fluid administration. Expert Opin Drug Deliv. 2007;4:427–40.
17. Perez EE, Orange JS, Bonilla F, et al. Update on the use of immunoglobulin in human disease: A review of evidence. J Allergy Clin Immunol. 2017;139:S1–S46.
18. Jolles S, Chapel H, Litzman J. When to initiate immunoglobulin replacement therapy (IGRT) in antibody deficiency: a practical approach. Clin Exp Immunol. 2017;188:333–41.

19. Quinti I, Soresina A, Guerra A, et al. Effectiveness of immunoglobulin replacement therapy on clinical outcome in patients with primary antibody deficiencies: Results from a multicenter prospective cohort study. J Clin Immunol. 2011;31:315–22.
20. Wolf HM, Thon V, Litzman J, Eibl MM. Detection of impaired IgG antibody formation facilitates the decision on early immunoglobulin replacement in hypogammaglobulinemic patients. Front Immunol. 2015;6:32. https://doi.org/10.3389/fimmu.2015.00032.
21. Björkander J, Hammarström L, Smith CI, Buckley RH, Cunningham-Rundles C, Hanson LA. Immunoglobulin prophylaxis in patients with antibody deficiency syndromes and anti-IgA antibodies. J Clin Immunol. 1987;7:8–15.
22. Lingman-Framme J, Fasth A. Subcutaneous immunoglobulin for primary and secondary immunodeficiencies: An evidence-based review. Drugs. 2013;73:1307–19.
23. Shabaninejad H, Asgharzadeh A, Rezaei N, Rezapoor A. A Comparative Study of Intravenous Immunoglobulin and Subcutaneous Immunoglobulin in Adult Patients with Primary Immunodeficiency Diseases: A Systematic Review and Meta-Analysis. Expert Rev Clin Immunol. 2016;12:595–602.
24. Peter JG, Chapel H. Immunoglobulin replacement therapy for primary immunodeficiencies. Immunotherapy. 2014;6:853–69.
25. Orange JS, Grossman WJ, Navickis RJ, Wilkes MM. Impact of trough IgG on pneumonia incidence in primary immunodeficiency: A meta-analysis of clinical studies. Clin Immunol. 2010;137:21–30.
26. Orange JS, Hossny EM, Weiler CR, et al. Use of intravenous immunoglobulin in human disease: a review of evidence by members of the Primary Immunodeficiency Committee of the American Academy of Allergy, Asthma and Immunology. J Allergy Clin Immunol. 2006;117:S525–53.
27. Lucas M, Lee M, Lortan J, Lopez-Granados E, Misbah S, Chapel H. Infection outcomes in patients with common variable immunodeficiency disorders: Relationship to immunoglobulin therapy over 22 years. J Allergy Clin Immunol. 2010;125:1354–1360.e4.
28. Bonagura VR. Illustrative cases on individualizing immunoglobulin therapy in primary immunodeficiency disease. Ann Allergy Asthma Immunol. 2013;111:S10–3.
29. Burks AW, Sampson HA, Buckley RH. Anaphylactic reactions after gamma globulin administration in patients with hypogammaglobulinemia. Detection of IgE antibodies to IgA. N Engl J Med. 1986;314:560–4.
30. Rachid R, Bonilla FA. The role of anti-IgA antibodies in causing adverse reactions to gamma globulin infusion in immunodeficient patients: a comprehensive review of the literature. J Allergy Clin Immunol. 2012;129:628–34.
31. Sundin U, Nava S, Hammarström L. Induction of unresponsiveness against IgA in IgA-deficient patients on subcutaneous immunoglobulin infusion therapy. Clin Exp Immunol. 1998;112:341–6.
32. Sekul EA, Cupler EJ, Dalakas MC. Aseptic meningitis associated with high-dose intravenous immunoglobulin therapy: frequency and risk factors. Ann Intern Med. 1994;121:259.
33. Kaarthigeyan K, Burli VV. Aseptic meningitis following intravenous immunoglobulin therapy of common variable immunodeficiency. J Pediatr Neurosci. 2011;6:160–1.
34. Jarius S, Eichhorn P, Albert MH, Wagenpfeil S, Wick M, Belohradsky BH, Hohlfeld R, Jenne DE, Voltz R. Intravenous immunoglobulins contain naturally occurring antibodies that mimic antineutrophil cytoplasmic antibodies and activate neutrophils in a TNFalpha-dependent and Fc-receptor-independent way. Blood. 2007;109:4376–82.
35. Caress JB, Hobson-Webb L, Passmore LV, Finkbiner AP, Cartwright MS. Case-control study of thromboembolic events associated with IV immunoglobulin. J Neurol. 2009;256:339–42.
36. Paran D, Herishanu Y, Elkayam O, Shopin L, Ben-Ami R. Venous and arterial thrombosis following administration of intravenous immunoglobulins. Blood Coagul Fibrinolysis. 2005;16:313–8.
37. Barada W, Muwakkit S, Hourani R, Bitar M, Mikati M. Cerebral sinus thrombosis in a patient with humoral immunodeficiency on intravenous immunoglobulin therapy: a case report. Neuropediatrics. 2008;39:131–3.

38. Iroh Tam P-Y, Richardson M, Grewal S. Fatal case of bilateral internal jugular vein thrombosis following IVIg infusion in an adolescent girl treated for ITP. Am J Hematol. 2008;83:323–5.
39. Funk MB, Gross N, Gross S, Hunfeld A, Lohmann A, Guenay S, Hanschmann KM, Keller-Stanislawski B. Thromboembolic events associated with immunoglobulin treatment. Vox Sang. 2013;105:54–64.
40. Huang L, Kanellis J, Mulley W. Slow and steady. Reducing thrombotic events in renal transplant recipients treated with IVIg for antibody-mediated rejection. Nephrology (Carlton). 2011;16:239–42.
41. Okuda D, Flaster M, Frey J, Sivakumar K. Arterial thrombosis induced by IVIg and its treatment with tPA. Neurology. 2003;60:1825–6.
42. Daw Z, Padmore R, Neurath D, Cober N, Tokessy M, Desjardins D, Olberg B, Tinmouth A, Giulivi A. Hemolytic transfusion reactions after administration of intravenous immune (gamma) globulin: a case series analysis. Transfusion. 2008;48:1598–601.
43. Gerber S, Gaida A, Spiegl N, Wymann S, Antunes AM, El MI, Zurbriggen B, Hubsch A, Imboden M. Reduction of isoagglutinin in intravenous immunoglobulin (IVIG) using blood Group A- and B-specific immunoaffinity chromatography: industry-scale assessment. BioDrugs. 2016;30:441–51.
44. Ben-Chetrit E, Putterman C. Transient neutropenia induced by intravenous immune globulin. N Engl J Med. 1992;326:270–1.
45. von Gunten S, Schaub A, Vogel M, Stadler BM, Miescher S, Simon H-U. Immunologic and functional evidence for anti-Siglec-9 autoantibodies in intravenous immunoglobulin preparations. Blood. 2006;108:4255–9.
46. Ibrahim J, Al Amri A, Ghatasheh G. Transfusion-related acute lung injury after immunoglobulin infusion for Kawasaki disease: a case report and literature review. Glob Pediatr Heal. 2017;4:2333794X17746545.
47. Rault R, Piraino B, Johnston JR, Oral A. Pulmonary and renal toxicity of intravenous immunoglobulin. Clin Nephrol. 1991;36:83–6.
48. Centers for Disease Control and Prevention (CDC). Renal insufficiency and failure associated with immune globulin intravenous therapy—United States 1985-1998. MMWR Morb Mortal Wkly Rep. 1999;48:518–21.
49. Dantal J. Intravenous Immunoglobulins: in-depth review of excipients and acute kidney injury risk. Am J Nephrol. 2013;38:275–84.
50. Nguyen MK, Rastogi A, Kurtz I. True hyponatremia secondary to intravenous immunoglobulin. Clin Exp Nephrol. 2006;10:124–6.
51. Lawn N, Wijdicks EFM, Burritt MF. Intravenous immune globulin and pseudohyponatremia. N Engl J Med. 1998;339:632.
52. Gardulf A. Immunoglobulin treatment for primary antibody deficiencies: advantages of the subcutaneous route. BioDrugs. 2007;21:105–16.
53. Krivan G, Jolles S, Granados EL, Paolantonacci P, Ouaja R, Cissé OA, Bernatowska E. New insights in the use of immunoglobulins for the management of immune deficiency (PID) patients. Am J Clin Exp Immunol. 2017;6:76–83.
54. Razvi S, Schneider L, Jonas MM, Cunningham-Rundles C. Outcome of intravenous immunoglobulin-transmitted hepatitis C virus infection in primary immunodeficiency. Clin Immunol. 2001;101:284–8.
55. Hayakawa F, Imada K, Towatari M, Saito H. Life-threatening human parvovirus B19 infection transmitted by intravenous immune globulin. Br J Haematol. 2002;118:1187–9.
56. Zou S, Fang CT, Schonberger LB. Transfusion transmission of human prion diseases. Transfus Med Rev. 2008;22:58–69.
57. Ziegner UHM, Kobayashi RH, Cunningham-Rundles C, et al. Progressive neurodegeneration in patients with primary immunodeficiency disease on IVIG treatment. Clin Immunol. 2002;102:19–24.
58. Tarzi MD, Grigoriadou S, Carr SB, Kuitert LM, Longhurst HJ. Clinical immunology review series: An approach to the management of pulmonary disease in primary antibody deficiency. Clin Exp Immunol. 2009;155:147–55.

59. Kainulainen L, Nikoskelainen J, Vuorinen T, Tevola K, Liippo K, Ruuskanen O. Viruses and bacteria in bronchial samples from patients with primary hypogammaglobulinemia. Am J Respir Crit Care Med. 1999;159:1199–204.
60. Kuruvilla M, de la Morena MT. Antibiotic prophylaxis in primary immune deficiency disorders. J Allergy Clin Immunol Pract. 2013;1:573–82.
61. Steel HC, Theron AJ, Cockeran R, Anderson R, Feldman C. Pathogen- and host-directed anti-inflammatory activities of macrolide antibiotics. Mediat Inflamm. 2012;2012:584262.
62. Jensen T, Pedersen SS, Garne S, Heilmann C, Høiby N, Koch C. Colistin inhalation therapy in cystic fibrosis patients with chronic Pseudomonas aeruginosa lung infection. J Antimicrob Chemother. 1987;19:831–8.
63. Moss RB. Long-term benefits of inhaled tobramycin in adolescent patients with cystic fibrosis. Chest. 2002;121:55–63.
64. Quon BS, Goss CH, Ramsey BW. Inhaled antibiotics for lower airway infections. Ann Am Thorac Soc. 2014;11:425–34.
65. Sperlich JM, Grimbacher B, Workman S, Haque T, Seneviratne SL, Burns SO, Reiser V, Vach W, Hurst JR, Lowe DM. Respiratory Infections and Antibiotic Usage in Common Variable Immunodeficiency. J Allergy Clin Immunol Pract. 2018;6:159–168.e3.
66. Uzzan M, Ko HM, Mehandru S, Cunningham-Rundles C. Gastrointestinal Disorders Associated with Common Variable Immune Deficiency (CVID) and Chronic Granulomatous Disease (CGD). Curr Gastroenterol Rep. 2016;18:17.
67. Woodward J, Gkrania-Klotsas E, Kumararatne D. Chronic norovirus infection and common variable immunodeficiency. Clin Exp Immunol. 2017;188:363–70.
68. Brachet-Castang C, Viallard JF, Fourche J, Le Flèche A, Grimont PA, Pellegrin JL, Maugein J. Bactériémie à Flexispira rappini et déficit immunitaire commun variable. Médecine Mal Infect. 2005;35:95–7.
69. Radanović I, Rkman D, Zekan P, Kutleša M, Baršić B. Chronic meningoencephalitis caused by Echo virus 6 in a patient with common variable immunodeficiency. Wien Klin Wochenschr. 2018;130:70–2.
70. Bradley J, Moran F, Greenstone M. Physical training for bronchiectasis. Cochrane Database Syst Rev. 2002;3:CD002166.
71. Wehr C, Gennery AR, Lindemans C, et al. Multicenter experience in hematopoietic stem cell transplantation for serious complications of common variable immunodeficiency. J Allergy Clin Immunol. 2015;135:988–97e6.
72. Kostel Bal S, Haskologlu S, Serwas NK, et al. Multiple presentations of LRBA deficiency: a single-center experience. J Clin Immunol. 2017;37:790–800.
73. Hsu AP, West RR, Calvo KR, Cuellar-Rodriguez J, Parta M, Kelly SJ, Ganson NJ, Hershfield MS, Holland SM, Hickstein DD. Adenosine deaminase type 2 deficiency masquerading as GATA2 deficiency: successful hematopoietic stem cell transplantation. J Allergy Clin Immunol. 2016;138:628–630.e2.

Vaccines in Humoral Primary Immunodeficiencies

22

Lorenzo Lodi and Maurizio de Martino

22.1 Introduction

Vaccines in humoral immunodeficiencies play a pivotal role both in prevention and diagnosis.

In predominantly antibody deficiencies (PADs), the increased susceptibility to infectious diseases, in addition to autoimmune and malignant complications, results in increased morbidity and mortality and has a major role in determining the prognosis. Due to the generally severe course of infections and to the poor response to conventional antimicrobial treatment, prevention is crucial in this population. Therefore, vaccination, as well as immunoglobulin replacement therapy and antibiotic and antifungal prophylaxis, represents the mainstay of individual prevention; moreover, on a population scale, vaccines contribute to protection through herd immunity [1].

However, several issues need to be considered when performing vaccinations in humoral immunodeficiencies:

1. Hazard of vaccine-induced infection
2. Likelihood of adequate immune response
3. Susceptibility to specific pathogens

The first concern is about safety and takes into account the risk of proliferation and dissemination of live viral or bacterial agents mainly depending on the degree of immune

L. Lodi
Post-Graduate School of Pediatrics, University of Florence, Florence, Italy

M. de Martino (✉)
Pediatric Clinic 1, Anna Meyer University Campus, Anna Meyer Children's University Hospital, University of Florence, Florence, Italy
e-mail: maurizio.demartino@unifi.it

M. M. D'Elios, M. Rizzi (eds.), *Humoral Primary Immunodeficiencies*,
Rare Diseases of the Immune System, https://doi.org/10.1007/978-3-319-91785-6_22

impairment. Providing specific recommendations for each type of PADs is made difficult by multiple factors as the rarity of the single conditions, the exclusion of immunocompromised individuals from prelicensure vaccines tests, the lack of high-quality data and the extreme heterogeneity of clinical expression even among patients with the same diagnosis. A tailor-made approach based on the combination of general principles and specific evaluation of the patient's immune function has to be considered the most appropriate.

The second issue, probably even more important, concerns lower immunogenicity of vaccines in immunocompromised patients and the consequent possibility of not obtaining specific protection against pathogens. Besides their primary inability to mount an adequate immune response, also the interference generated by immunoglobulin substitutive therapy or the secondary immunosuppression caused by immunomodulatory drugs can contribute to the scarce response to vaccination.

Eventually, the specific pathogen susceptibility in the different types of primary immunodeficiencies (PIDs) should be considered, guiding specific vaccine recommendation.

Mainly because of safety issues, the proportion of vaccinated immunocompromised individuals is below the one of the general population, even though these patients have increased susceptibility to vaccine-preventable infections and do not have contraindications to vaccination in several cases [2, 3].

22.2 Vaccination in Pad: Prophylactic Use

22.2.1 General Principles

The International Union of Immunological Societies (IUIS) Expert Committee for Primary Immunodeficiencies has recently catalogued and classified all known prevalent antibody deficiencies into four main groups [4]. This classification, based on serum immunoglobulin isotype reduction and B cell number, is of paramount importance during the diagnostic process. Nevertheless, with respect to a practical approach to vaccination, PADs can be broadly classified into mild and severe basing on the degree of B cell function impairment and the consequent infection susceptibility [5–7]. Mild antibody deficiencies include conditions like transient hypogammaglobulinemia of infancy (THI), selective IgA deficiency (sIGAD), IgG subclass deficiency (IGGSD), or specific antibody deficiency. On the other hand, common variable immunodeficiency disorders (CVID), X-linked agammaglobulinemia (XLA), all forms of autosomal recessive agammaglobulinemias, and E47 transcription factor deficiency necessarily have to be included, among others, in the severe group.

Viable and nonviable vaccines have different general indications and contraindications in the above mentioned categories (Table 22.1). Inactivated vaccines can be considered safe in all immunocompromised hosts. However, in patients with profound immune impairment, their benefit is unlikely, and their use is not fully justified especially when receiving immunoglobulin replacement therapy. On the other side, the main concern about live vaccine is to cause vaccine-induced infections, for which reason they should be used with greater caution in patients with PADs.

Table 22.1 Vaccination in prevalent antibody deficiencies

	Nonviable vaccines		Viable vaccines	
	General principle	Exceptions	General principle	Exceptions
	– Follow vaccination schedule of healthy individuals		– Follow vaccination schedule of healthy individuals in industrialized countries	– Avoid administration of: – LAIV (use IIV) – OPV (use IPV) – Adenovirus vaccine – Ty21a (use ViCPS) – YF
Mild PADs	– Hyporesponsiveness should not restrain administration	—	– Check T cell absolute n.° and function if doubts about associate cellular impairment (Table 22.2)	– Caution is urged with BCG – Rule out severe PID (e.g., SCID, severe PAD) before ROTA
Severe PADs	– Not recommended because ineffectiveness especially in patients receiving IVIG/SCIG	– Recommended also in patient on IVIG/SCIG: – IIV – 4vHPV or 9vHPV – AVA and rabies only in postexposure setting		Consider BCG with extreme caution only in XLA and only in settings at high risk of contagion[c]
	– Use if there is evidence of partial immune response	– Consider active vaccination in CVID group II[a] receiving IVIG/SCIG in particular with: PCV13, PPVS23, MCV4, MPSV4, MenB, Hib[b]	Avoid administration	

Abbreviations: *PADs* prevalent antibody deficiencies, *LAIV* live attenuated influenza vaccine, *IIV* inactivated influenza vaccine, *OPV* oral poliovirus vaccine, *IPV* inactivated poliovirus vaccine, *Ty21a* live oral typhoid vaccine, *ViCPS* Vi capsular polysaccharide (inactivated typhoid) vaccine, *YF* yellow fever vaccine, *BCG Bacillus* Calmette-Guérin vaccine, *THI* transient hypogammaglobulinemia of infancy, *SCID* severe combined immunodeficiency, *ROTA* rotavirus vaccine, *IVIG* intravenous immunoglobulins G, *SCIG* subcutaneous immunoglobulins G, *4v/9vHPV* quadrivalent/9-valent human papillomavirus vaccine, *AVA* anthrax vaccine, *CVID* common variable immunodeficiencies, *PCV13* pneumococcal conjugate vaccine (13-valent), *PPSV23* pneumococcal polysaccharide vaccine (23-valent), *MCV4* meningococcal conjugate vaccine (quadrivalent), *MPSV4* meningococcal polysaccharide vaccine (quadrivalent), *MenB* serogroup B meningococcal vaccine, *Hib Haemophilus influenzae* type b vaccine, *XLA* X-linked agammaglobulinemia

[a]Freiburg classification of CVID

[b]Vaccines against pathogens for which severe PAD patients are particularly susceptible and for which replacement therapy has shown variable levels of protection

[c]Evidence about safety of BCG in XLA is extremely low for the moment being [6]

22.2.2 Mild Antibody Deficiencies

In mild PADs the possibility of decreased specific immune response should not discourage vaccine utilization. For the lack of safety data in the immunocompromised host and for the significant possibility of harm with a low potential benefit, all the following vaccines should be avoided in these group: live oral polio (OPV), live attenuated influenza (LAIV), adenovirus, live typhoid (Ty21a), and yellow fever (YF) vaccines [7, 8]. In the *2015 report of the Committee on Infectious Diseases* and in the *Pink Book* (13th Edition – 2015), *Bacillus* Calmette-Guérin vaccine (BCG) is considered contraindicated too. However, for the absence of systemic infection after BCG administration in 50 XLA infants, the risk of disseminated disease in mild PADs can be considered even lower than in severe forms, but caution is urged because evidence is extremely low [5, 6, 9]. OPV should be avoided in these patients and in their household contacts due to several reported cases of paralytic polio after vaccine administration [10]. With regard to adenovirus vaccine, the Food and Drug Administration has approved its use only in military personnel, and no safety data are available in the immunocompromised population [7, 11]. LAIV and Ty21a are not listed among contraindicated vaccines in the *Red Book: 2015*, presumptively because their use can easily be substituted by safer inactivated vaccines [5, 7]. Moreover, LAIV is licensed only for healthy individuals aged 2–49 [5] years. For all the other live vaccines in mild PADs, the possibility of harm is considered small and the benefit likely so that the administration is recommended [7].

Among nonviable vaccines *Haemophilus influenzae B* and pneumococcal vaccines are specially recommended [6] due to increased susceptibility in mild PADs, and a slightly modified schedule can be followed [7] also basing on laboratory detection of specific immune response in the patient (see Sect. 22.2.7).

Accordingly, patients with mild antibody deficiency can safely follow the normal vaccination schedule with both viable and nonviable vaccines, only in industrialized countries where the contraindicated vaccines are not included for epidemiological reasons or for the existence of safer alternatives [7]. In the sporadic case of patients with mild antibody deficiency on immunoglobulin substitutive therapy, specific recommendations should be followed as described separately in this chapter (Table 22.1).

22.2.3 Specific Mild Antibody Deficiencies

sIGAD has a tremendously variable clinical phenotype: from completely asymptomatic to more severe with recurrent infections, autoimmune comorbidity, decreased T cell proliferation, and high possibility of evolving to CVID [12]. For this reason a small proportion of patients with sIGAD could theoretically be harmed by live attenuated vaccines [13]. However, in the absence of reported cases of vaccine-induced infections in this population and the rarity of such a profound immune impairment, children with SIGAD should follow the same vaccination schedule of healthy children, also considering that is impossible to define this condition before 4 years of age [1]. It is otherwise advisable that SIGAD patients which start showing manifestations of severe clinical phenotype [12, 14] undergo a complete evaluation of immune system before further administration of live vaccines. This should be done in order to promptly detect the evolution to CVID or a possibly associated T cell impairment. For T cell function assessment, with regard to live vaccine administration, it is possible to adopt cutoff levels used in children with partial combined immunodeficiencies for the separate administration of measles/mumps/rubella (MMR) and varicella (VAR) vaccines (see Table 22.2). Generally accepted cutoffs are ≥500 CD4+ T lymphocytes/μL, ≥200 CD8+ T lymphocytes/μL, and normal mitogen response [6, 15]. Basing on data extrapolated from HIV-infected patients and partial DiGeorge syndrome, the separate administration of MMR and VAR is considered safe when CD4+ T cell count is ≥500 cells/μL [16, 17]. However, even minor absolute numbers or percentages of CD4+ T cells could probably be considered safe, but more studies are needed to lower these cutoffs [7, 18] (Table 22.2). Of note, age-related levels of immunocompetence are as follows [19]:

- ≥1500 CD4+ T lymphocytes/μL for children 1–11 months
- ≥750 CD4+ T lymphocytes/μL for children 12–23 months
- ≥500 CD4+ T lymphocytes/μL for children 24 months through 5 years
- ≥200 CD4+ T lymphocytes/μL for children older than 6 years

These values are obtained from the guidelines for prophylaxis against *pneumocystis* pneumonia in children with HIV [19] and may be helpful, together with functional tests, when evaluating children younger than 1 year of age with suspected PID before the administration of live vaccines as rotavirus vaccine (ROTA).

Table 22.2 Safety cutoff levels for MMR and VAR separate administration[a]

CD4+ T lymphocytes	≥500 cells/μL[b]
CD8+ T lymphocytes	≥200 cell/μL
T cell proliferation to PHA	Normal[c]

All parameters have to be met

Abbreviations: *MMR* measles, mumps, rubella vaccine, *VAR* varicella vaccine, *MMRV* measles, mumps, rubella, varicella vaccine, *PHA* phytohemoagglutinin

[a]MMRV in immunocompetent individuals has shown to produce higher fever and higher risk of febrile seizure than separate administration of MMR and VAR [8]. No data are available for MMRV in the immunocompromised so that its administration is not recommended [7]

[b]A proliferation >50% of control is roughly considered "normal" depending on laboratories

[c]Lower cutoffs of CD4+ T cell ≥200 cell/μL or percentage >15% have shown to be safe in DiGeorge syndrome but still have to be confirmed by further studies [7, 18]

Infants with presumptive diagnosis of THI have to undergo complete immune evaluation to rule out SCID or other forms of immune impairment as severe PADs before the administration of ROTA [5, 20, 21]. Newborn screening programs for PIDs should be available in all those countries where ROTA is offered in the first year of life, and ROTA should not be administered in nursery before discharge because of the risk of spread. Infants with THI can normally follow vaccine schedule with nonviable vaccines, but if hypogammaglobulinemia persists beyond 1 year of age, complete immune assessment has to be carried out before the administration of live vaccines.

22.2.4 Severe Antibody Deficiencies

All live attenuated vaccines are contraindicated in this group of patients [5]. The hazard of vaccine-induced infections sums up with a low potential benefit in patients that are almost always receiving immunoglobulin substitutive therapy and have exogenous protective antibody titers. The likelihood to produce a protective response after vaccination is very low in patients with such a profound immune impairment. Furthermore, the neutralizing effect exerted on live vaccines by therapeutic IgG makes this possibility even lower, as shown for measles, rubella, and varicella in several studies [5, 22]. Among live vaccines the only options that may be considered are BCG [7], MMR, and VAR [5, 6]; however, there is no consensus in literature, and potential risk for the patient should be carefully evaluated in consideration of environmental hazard of contagion, immunoglobulin replacement therapy, and specific pathology (e.g., XLA vs. CVID). No safety data are currently available about varicella or rotavirus in this group of patients [6].

Nonviable vaccines are not recommended for prevention in severe PADs because, despite being safe, they are unnecessary and ineffective [7], especially for polysaccharide vaccines that should elicit a T-independent response (e.g., PPV23 and MPSV4) [5]. No data are available about efficacy of pneumococcal vaccination in severe PADs [6]. All these vaccines can be administered safely to evaluate specific immune response before the administration of substitutive IgG (see Sect. 22.4). Administration of nonviable vaccines has to be considered only in all those individuals who still have some residual antibody response and do not receive substitutive IgG. Inactivated influenza vaccine (IIV) is the first exception to this general principle and has to be administered in all patients with severe PADs because it can induce cellular immunity and because replacement immunoglobulin preparations may not contain protective titers against seasonal strains [23–25]. Human papillomavirus (HPV) vaccine constitutes the second exception and is recommended with the same schedule of healthy individuals as it can induce cellular protective immunity [26, 27]. The third and last exception is postexposure prophylaxis of anthrax and rabies. Both diseases have no widespread immunity among general population, and immunoglobulin preparation does not generally contain protective antibodies. For this reason, even if not approved for prevention under the 18 years of age, in a postexposure setting, anthrax vaccine should be administered in all individuals including children and immunocompromised patients [28]. Similarly, in pre-exposure setting rabies vaccine is offered only to high-risk categories. After exposure to infected animals, immunocompromised subjects should receive the 5-dose vaccine regimen together with specific immunoglobulins [29].

Different from mild antibody deficiencies, smallpox vaccine is contraindicated in severe PADs with reference to pre-exposure settings even if no absolute contraindication exists [7, 9].

22.2.5 Specific Severe Antibody Deficiencies

All agammaglobulinemias with extremely low numbers or absent B cells are included in the first group of the 2015 IUIS classification of PADs [4] and represent the classical example of isolated B cell deficiency. With regard to vaccination, they are classified in the severe group together with other PADs like CVID. However, their pathogenesis does not primarily involve cellular immunity, and the immune defect is severe but apparently limited to the humoral compartment. This could be a critical point in differential management of agammaglobulinemias versus other disorders of the severe group like CVID that can have a less profound reduction of serum immunoglobulins but a variably associated T cell function impairment. No killed vaccines can be effective in agammaglobulinemias, unless detection of some remnant Ig production as it can happen in XLA. For the previously mentioned reasons, IIV, HPV, rabies, and anthrax vaccines are the main exceptions to this principle. However, mainly basing on studies on T cell response in XLA [30–32], some authors [2] suggest that all vaccines with protein antigens could be helpful because even a partial immune response could contribute to the protection offered by substitutive IgG. Among these, PCV13 should be the first considered in these patients because of possibly insufficient titers in the immunoglobulin preparation [13] and patients' increased susceptibility to pneumococcal invasive diseases.

On the other hand, all live vaccines should be avoided, but Shearer et al. [6] agree that measles, varicella, and BCG could be considered if strictly necessary and with extreme caution in isolated agammaglobulinemic patients like XLA but not in CVID or CVID-like disorders. It is the opinion of the authors that MMR and VAR administrations constitute a risk that should not be taken, at least in all individuals receiving substitutive IgG. No data are available about safety of ROTA in these patients, for which reason newborn screening programs that include KRECs detection on dried blood spot [33, 34] can be of paramount importance to avoid vaccine-induced infections.

In CVID, due to the variable level of T cell function impairment, it is difficult to produce general vaccine recommendations. Different patterns of vaccine exposure, due to the late onset of the disease, can also play a role in determining the risk of vaccine-induced infections which is difficult to evaluate [6]. No cases of disseminate infection after administration of LAIV in CVID patients have ever been reported, but there is some evidence of transmission from close contacts who received the viable vaccine to patient with CVID [6]. For this reason, in CVID, all live vaccines should be avoided with no exceptions [7].

Nonviable vaccines are generally not recommended in CVID as for all the other severe PADs, especially in patients receiving immunoglobulin substitutive therapy. IIV and HPV are the only exceptions of proved efficacy. In particular IIV in CVID has been recently reviewed, and available data suggest benefits from its administration in these patients and in their household contacts [35]. Moreover, a recent study of Goldacker et al. encourages active immunization of CVID patients with anti-peptide and anti-polysaccharide vaccines in addition to IgG replacement therapy [36]. This practice is not currently considered a standard care component [1, 37], but it could be advisable in those patients with higher probability of specific immune response (CVID group II of Freiburg classification) and for those vaccines for which replacement therapy has shown variable levels of protection [38].

22.2.6 Other Humoral PIDs

Some other PIDs with a major component of humoral impairment, like class switch recombination defects (e.g., CD40 and CD40L deficiency), have been recently classified in the combined immunodeficiency (CID) group because of their pathogenesis and their associated cellular dysfunction [4]. ICOS and LRBA deficiency are part of this group too [4]. For these disorders, despite the striking impairment of humoral component, vaccine recommendation for CID should be followed. Inactivated vaccines can have some residual efficacy in mild CIDs when IgG replacement therapy is not in use, while live vaccines are generally proscribed. Milder CID can also tolerate live vaccines, but in this case a patient-specific assessment of cellular compartment is mandatory and should rely on safety cutoff levels derived from partial DiGeorge syndrome and HIV-infected patients (Table 22.2) [7].

With regard to vaccination in PADs like TWEAK defects; TACI, NFKB2, BAFF receptor, CD19, and CD21 deficiencies [4]; and all other novel humoral immunodeficiencies with recent phenotypical characterization, an approach similar to the one used in CID should be adopted in order to rule out a major immune impairment that can pose the patient at risk of vaccine-induced infection. This approach may be considered cautionary, but even if pathogenesis has been clearly elucidated and seems to affect only the humoral compartment, these defects can show tremendous variability in clinical and immune phenotype. To date, only few reports are available for each of these defects, and categorization into severe or mild group is difficult, so that a complete assessment of immune function is imperative.

PRKC delta deficiency, despite the significant impairment of B cell lineage with low memory B cells and hypo-IgG, is classified among immune dysregulation diseases and in particular among autoimmune lymphoproliferative syndromes (ALPS) because of its intrinsic defect in apoptosis and because of its clinical and laboratory phenotype [4]. For this reason vaccination in PRKC delta deficiency may arouse some concerns about possible triggering of autoimmune flares [7] derived from studies on rheumatic diseases [39]. However, the theoretic possibility of disproportionate immune response and consequent increase of disease activity should not refrain the current immunization practice because benefits of infection prevention

Table 22.3 Drug-related levels of immunosuppression [5]

Mild immunosuppression	Heavy immunosuppression
Patients receiving: • <20 mg/day of prednisone or equivalent for ≥14 days • <2 mg/kg/day of prednisone or equivalent for ≥14 days for patients weighing <10 kg • Alternate-day corticosteroid therapy • ≤0.4 mg/kg/week of methotrexate • ≤3 mg/kg/day of azathioprine • ≤1.5 mg/kg/day of 6-mercaptopurine	Patients receiving: • ≥20 mg/day of prednisone or equivalent for ≥14 days • ≥2 mg/kg/day of prednisone or equivalent for ≥14 days for patients <10 kg • TNF-α antagonists • Anti-B-lymphocyte monoclonal antibodies • Cancer chemotherapy • Within 2 months after SOT • Within 2 months after HSCT[a]

Abbreviations: *SOT* solid organ transplant, *HSCT* hematopoietic stem cell transplant, *GVHD* graft versus host disease

[a]Heavy immunosuppression is frequently longer depending on the type of transplant, donor, and stem cell source. Posttransplant complications like GVHD and their treatment is also to be considered

are much more relevant than possible damages produced by an eventual disease flare [40]. Lower immunogenicity and risk of infection by attenuate pathogens should be considered carefully with proper evaluation of protective antibody titers and the definition of the degree of immunosuppression caused by immunosuppressive drugs [7, 40] (Table 22.3 and Section on 22.2.8.2 "Specific Population: Patients on Immunosuppressive Drugs").

Warts, hypogammaglobulinemia, infections, myelokathexis (WHIM) syndrome is a disorder of intrinsic and innate immunity that shows also an important impairment of the humoral compartment with low immunoglobulin levels and reductions of B cell number. In these patients the increased susceptibility to HPV infections gives HPV vaccine special importance mostly because safety and efficacy of quadrivalent HPV (4vHPV) vaccine have been demonstrated [41]. No studies on 9-valent HPV vaccine (9vHPV) in WHIM are available. However, 9vHPV has been approved for immunocompromised persons [42] and expands the protection offered by 4vHPV, so that it likely constitutes the best option for these patients.

22.2.7 Increased Susceptibility to Specific Pathogens: Dedicated Vaccines

In addition to group-specific recommendations, some vaccines deserve specific analysis because of their importance in patients with humoral immunodeficiencies. Increased susceptibility to bacteremias and sepsis and central nervous system and gastrointestinal infections caused by several pathogens have been observed in PAD patients [1]. Encapsulated bacteria, like *Streptococcus pneumoniae* or *Haemophilus influenzae type B* (Hib), are responsible for the great majority of infections [43].

Because of this increased susceptibility, modified schedule should be considered in these patients in order to obtain a complete protection, especially in those individuals that are not receiving substitutive IgG. Therapeutic immunoglobulin preparations contain variable but generally protective antibody levels against pneumococcus and Hib, while titers against meningococcus are even more variable [7, 38]. For these reasons vaccines against these pathogens should be offered to all those patients who show at least a partial immune response, according to some authors, even if they are receiving substitutive IgG [36].

In the light of the accumulating data regarding possible PPSV23-related immune tolerance, immunization with PCV13 has to be the one of choice; moreover, PCV13 booster doses can be administered every 5 years after normal vaccination schedule [1, 7]. However, to expand protection against more serotypes, a PPV13/PPSV23 combined schedule may be used with the following timing: PPSV23 may be administered in children older than 2 years of age at least 8 weeks after the last PCV13 administration, and it can be followed by a PPV23 booster dose after at least 5 years [44]. The administration of more than two doses of PPVS23 before the age of 65 has to be avoided [45]. Children with IGGSD (in particular IgG2 deficiency), eventually associated with SAD or sIGAD, may receive two doses of pneumococcal conjugate vaccine at ages when one would normally be sufficient in order to enhance immunity [1, 46].

Patients with PADs should receive at least one dose of Hib during their life, even after the 5 years of age when the vaccine is no more recommended in the general population [7].

Different from complement component deficiencies and anatomic or functional asplenia, PADs are not listed among those conditions that increase the risk of meningococcal infection, so that these patients should follow normal schedule and, in the USA, avoid MCV4 between 2 months through 10 years of age unless traveling or residing in endemic areas or communities with meningococcal disease outbreak [47]. In all those countries, like many European ones (e.g., Italy, Spain, Portugal, France, Germany, the UK, etc.), where monovalent C conjugate meningococcal vaccine (MenC) is recommended, vaccination should be scheduled as for healthy individuals before 10 years of age [48]. Similar risk categories (asplenias and complement deficiencies) have been identified for MenB, so that humoral immunodeficiencies do not need specific scheduling and normal administration timing can be followed in the countries where the vaccine is licensed [49]. MCSV4 is not recommended in individuals younger than 55 years of age when the conjugate vaccine is available [50].

MMR and VAR are listed among risk-specific vaccines in severe antibody deficiencies, and indication is given to consider the administration [9]. This indication likely refers to agammaglobulinemias and to the possibility of inducing cellular immunity; however, there is no consensus in literature, and other authors consider the possibility of harm significant, the benefit unlikely so that administration is not recommended [7].

22.2.8 Special Populations

22.2.8.1 Vaccination in Patients with Humoral Immunodeficiency Receiving Immunoglobulin Therapy

IgG replacement therapy is the mainstay of treatment of severe PADs, but occasionally intravenous or subcutaneous immunoglobulins (IVIG or SCIG) are used also in milder defects when chemoprophylaxis is not effective in preventing recurrent infections. Moreover, exogenous IgG can be used to modulate a dysregulated immune response that can be part of the clinical picture in some humoral immunodeficiencies like CVID. With regard to infection prevention, therapeutic IgG play several roles like neutralization of toxins and opsonization of pathogens with consequent complement-mediated lysis and killing by phagocytes and NK cells. Common immunoglobulin preparations contain protective antibodies against most of the pathogens included in the primary childhood immunization schedule with variable but generally protective titers against Hib and the different pneumococcal serotypes [7]. Even more variability is encountered with anti-meningococcal antibodies [38]. No protection can be granted against seasonal strains of influenza and against all those pathogens that do not have diffuse immunity in the general population which constitutes the pool of donors.

Circulating antibodies, regardless if endogenous or exogenous, do not generally interfere with the immune response elicited by the antigens contained in nonviable vaccines so that their administration can be previous, simultaneous, or subsequent to the immunoglobulins [51]. A different anatomic site should be chosen for vaccine administration if the patient is receiving SCIG [5]. Simultaneous administration of immunoglobulins and the specific vaccine is recommended for prophylaxis after exposure to certain diseases like HBV, tetanus, and rabies [51].

For the abovementioned principle and for their capacity to evoke a cellular immune response, IIV and HPV are recommended in all patients receiving IVIG or SCIG [23–27]. Moreover, antigenic shift and drift of influenza virus do not allow the creation of herd immunity in the general population, so that common immunoglobulin preparations cannot be considered protective against seasonal strains and annual vaccination is recommended in all patients receiving substitutive IgG [1]. Conjugate polysaccharide vaccines can be considered in all those individuals who maintain at least a partial immune response, especially if the vaccine is offered in order to protect against pathogens with increased susceptibility in the disease [5, 7, 36].

Different from nonviable vaccines that are generally not affected by circulating antibodies to the antigen, live vaccines may be affected because specific antibodies can interfere with pathogen replication that is necessary to evoke the immune response [51]. In particular, response to measles, rubella, and varicella is affected, while response to YF and OPV does not seem to be altered [5, 22, 52]. Anyhow, YF and OPV are generally contraindicated in humoral immunodeficiencies so that special recommendations about timing have to be observed only when talking about MMR and VAR. A minimum of 2 weeks, broadly corresponding to the incubation period, should be waited before the administration of immunoglobulins if the vaccine was the first given product [51]. If this period has not been respected, specific immune response should be tested or the vaccine repeated [51]. Conversely, if therapeutic Ig was first administered, complete degradation should be waited to avoid interference, and this period may vary from 3 to 11 months depending on the concentration of antibody in the product [51]. A complete list of recommended intervals between the administration of immune globulin preparations and measles- or varicella-containing vaccines can be found in the *Appendix A* of the *Pink Book* (13th Edition – 2015), but the generally accepted interval after IVIG given for substitutive therapy in immunodeficiencies (300–400 mg/kg) is 8 months [9].

22.2.8.2 Vaccination in Patients with Humoral Immunodeficiency Receiving Immunosuppressive Drugs

Patients with humoral immunodeficiencies can exhibit autoimmune diseases and need immunosuppressive treatment. Although necessary, pharmacological immunomodulation can produce secondary immunodeficiency that goes beyond the humoral compartment. In these patients, in addition to the evaluation of the primary immune defect, it is essential to assess the degree of drug-related immunosuppression, especially with regard to vaccination. High- or low-level immunosuppression can be identified basing on drug type, dosage, duration of therapy, and route of administration (Table 22.3) [5].

Patients with low-level immunosuppression can safely receive viable and nonviable vaccines [5, 53]. Individuals on steroid physiological replacement therapy or receiving steroids by topical skin application, local injection, or aerosol inhalation can be incorporated in the previous category, and no concern should be raised about safety or efficacy of the vaccination [5].

Patients with heavy immunosuppression should receive nonviable vaccines at least 2 weeks before the initiation of therapy and live vaccines at least 4 weeks before, especially when a long period of treatment is planned. When high-dose immunosuppressive therapy was not planned, inactivated vaccines can safely be administered even during therapy, but their efficacy may be impaired so that administration should be repeated after cessation of treatment [7]. Live vaccines are contraindicated during high-dose immunosuppressive medication.

With regard to intervals for vaccine administration after cessation of therapy, 2 weeks should be waited when high-dose steroids have been administered for less than 14 days, even if some authors recommend immediate administration. When high-dose steroid treatments have lasted more than 14 days, vaccine administrations have to be delayed for 4 weeks after stopping therapy [5]. Immune reconstitution after termination of drugs other than corticosteroids is extremely variable and depends on several factors. Therefore, it is difficult to define recommendations about the time frame after cessation of therapy that could grant immunogenicity for inactivated vaccines and safety as well as efficacy for live vaccines [5].

22.2.8.3 Household Contacts of Patients with Humoral Immunodeficiency

OPV should be avoided in household contacts of patients with humoral immunodeficiency because of documented risk of transmission and possible vaccine-related complications in immunodeficient patients [5]. All other vaccines, including live ones like MMR, VAR, MMRV, and ROTA, should be administered following normal routine schedule with no restrictions, neither for travel vaccinations including YF and Ty21a [5].

Annual immunization with IIV is particularly recommended in household members who are 6 months of age or older, in order to prevent possible close sources of contagion. In particular, IIV is to be preferred to LAIV even if risk of transmission is mainly theoretical and explicit contraindication does not include household contacts of patients with humoral immunodeficiency [5]. LAIV, in fact, should not be administered (or contact avoided for at least 7 days if LAIV is given) only in household members of:

- Patients with SCID
- Patients who received hematopoietic stem cell transplantation (HSCT) within 2 months
- Patients receiving treatment for graft versus host disease (GVHD) [5]

In order to diminish the risk of transmission, individuals living with immunocompromised patients should schedule periodic vaccination with pertussis vaccine, while MMR and VAR should be up to date [6]. Immunocompromised patients should avoid contact with individuals developing varicella rash after VAR, and isolation of the immunodeficient person is recommended until skin lesions have cleared. If contact occurs, risk of transmission is low, and when it has occurred, the vaccine-strain varicella virus has maintained its attenuated characteristics. For this reasons, in the *Red Book: 2015*, the administration of varicella zoster immunoglobulin preparation or IVIG is not indicated even if some authors still consider it adequate [5–7].

22.2.8.4 Vaccination in Pregnancy: Women at High Risk to Deliver a Child with Humoral Immunodeficiency

Pregnant women without an up-to-date immunization history should routinely receive tetanus, diphtheria, pertussis vaccine (Tdap), and IIV. However, when there is high suspicion of being pregnant with a child at risk of humoral immunodeficiency, the mother should also be offered with PCV13, Hib, and meningococcal vaccines [6]. This practice, thanks to the placental passage of maternal antibodies, would grant to the newborn passive immunity against the abovementioned pathogens at least during the first months of life, while diagnosis is better defined and treatment can be initiated.

22.2.8.5 Vaccination for Travel in Patients with Humoral Immunodeficiency

Patients with humoral immunodeficiency planning a travel to regions with different endemics should be evaluated by a specialist in travel medicine together with a physician aware of the patient's immunocompromised state [54]. When feasible, vaccination should be started soon enough to allow serological testing and eventual booster immunizations before departure. Beside the selection of appropriate travel vaccines depending on the itinerary, travel counseling can be a good opportunity to review routine immunizations status.

Travel vaccines may include YF, typhoid vaccines, polio, Japanese encephalitis, meningococcus, cholera, rabies, and HAV. Safety and effectiveness, especially of live vaccines, must be weighted with the risk of contracting natural infection together with the availability of alternatives for passive protection. For instance, immunocompromised patients, who are not likely to respond to hepatitis A (HAV) vaccine or those who do not have enough time for immunization, should receive specific intramuscular immunoglobulin prior to travel [5]. Patients that are already receiving IVIG or SCIG do not need additional antibody protection against HAV. However, awareness should be raised in the patients receiving IVIG or SCIG that common immunoglobulin preparations do not contain protective titers against pathogens, like rabies, whose immunity is not widespread in the general population. For this reason, when risk of exposure is high and vaccination is contraindicated or likely ineffective, hyperimmune globulins can be administered preventively in order to grant passive protection.

Inducing immunity to cholera can be challenging in patients with humoral immunodeficiencies because protection is mainly based on mucosal humoral immunity [55]. In June 2016 an oral live attenuated single-dose vaccine against cholera (lyophilized CVD 103-HgR) was approved in the USA for adult travelers (aged 18 to 64 years) to risk areas [56]. Apparently, no difference in adverse events was reported among HIV-infected recipients of an older formulation of CVD 103-HgR [57]. However, safety and effectiveness have not been established among immunocompromised people, so that vaccination should be avoided in these individuals and in their household contacts [56]. Killed whole cell monovalent (O1) vaccine with recombinant B subunit of cholera toxin (WC-rBS) and killed modified whole cell bivalent (O1 and O139) without the B subunit (WC) have been proved safe in extremely large populations including HIV-positive and other immunocompromised individuals [55]. Eventually, in patients with humoral immunodeficiency, concerns should be raised regarding efficacy, as long as lower immunogenicity has been observed in HIV-infected individuals with the lowest CD4 counts [55]. Further studies are needed to evaluate additional dose regimens in these populations. Of note, heat-labile toxin (LT) of enterotoxinogenic *Escherichia coli* (ETEC) is structurally similar to cholera toxin B, and immunological cross-reaction has been demonstrated. For this reason WC-rBS, different from WCs, may provide some protection against ETEC [55]. As for general population, food and water precautions together with frequent handwashing are fundamental for cholera prevention especially in immunocompromised hosts.

Adequate counseling about prophylactic and preventive measures should be offered to patients with humoral immunodeficiencies which have a higher risk to be harmed by diseases that cannot be prevented by vaccination, like travelers' diarrhea or malaria [54].

22.2.8.6 Vaccination in Patients with Humoral Immunodeficiency Undergoing HSCT

HSCT does not constitute a primary therapeutic option in patients with antibody deficiencies [58]. Thus far, only limited experiences with XLA and CVID are available [59, 60], but new strategies to minimize ablative regimens are under study for patients with PADs [58]. Approach to vaccination in candidate and recipients of HSCT can rely on national and international guidelines [61, 62]. In particular, patients with PADs already have peculiar immune features in a pretransplant setting, so that in case of HSCT, an appropriate immunization strategy for pre- and posttransplant period should be planned by the specialist in clinical immunology together with the hematologist that will conduct the HSCT.

22.3 Vaccination in PADs: Diagnostic Use

Vaccines can be used as a diagnostic tool to evaluate the capacity of the immune system to mount an adequate response against specific antigens. This response relates to patients' possibility of defending themselves from natural infections [63]. For this reason, specific antibody production is of paramount importance for the evaluation of the humoral immune system, and it is part of the diagnostic criteria of many clinical entities like SAD or CVID. The assessment of specific response to protein and polysaccharide antigens, in fact, is considered the main functional test in the evaluation of B cell compartment, and it is generally used together with quantitative determination of serum immunoglobulin levels.

Assessing response to both protein and polysaccharide antigens is fundamental in order to identify two well-described patterns of nonresponse:

1. Failure to respond solely to polysaccharide antigens
2. Failure to respond both to polysaccharide and protein antigens [63]

Distinct clinical entities generally show one of these two phenotypes. When protein response is impaired, it is extremely unusual to find a preserved response to polysaccharide antigens. T-dependent antigens, in fact, constitute a strong stimulus in evoking a specific immune response, so that when this is impaired, we are generally facing a major immunodeficiency with a global impairment of immune function. Response to protein-polysaccharide conjugate vaccines represents a hybrid, and it is not routinely used in the primary assessment as its effects are not fully standardized [64].

At the present time, the procedure for qualitative assessment of antibody function involves in vitro assays (ELISA is considered the one of choice) used to detect specific antibody titers produced in vivo as a response to standardized antigens [63]. Vaccines used in routine immunization schedules represent the main source of these standardized antigens. However, novel vaccine antigens can be used in specific situations of interference, like immunoglobulin substitutive therapy or infusions with plasma products. In particular ΦX174 bacteriophage, rabies and Japanese encephalitis may be administered. Nonetheless, they are all protein antigens, and each of them shows specific limitations. The ΦX174 bacteriophage is available only in selected research centers [65], normal response to rabies vaccine has not been fully defined [63], and Japanese encephalitis can be an option only in selected countries like European ones where the vaccine is licensed but at the same time is not routinely administered nor endemic [66].

When evaluating specific antibody response, IgG is the only immunoglobulin isotype that has to be considered, because, differently from IgA and IgM, it is the only one representing a long-term protection [63].

When poor antibody response is detected in a *baseline* setting, it is necessary to administer an immunization booster in order to prove, with an antigenic challenge, if a pattern of nonresponse is actually present [63]. Pre- and postvaccination titers have to be determined in the same laboratory with the same method 4–8 weeks after vaccine administration. Earlier testing would not allow completion of seroconversion, while later testing would not permit to perceive the difference between poor response and rapid loss of immunologic memory.

The response to protein antigens is generally tested through the quantitative determination of antibody titers against tetanus and diphtheria toxoids. It is considered protective a level of:

- 0.01–0.1 IU/mL for diphtheria
- >0.1 IU/mL for tetanus [67]

In children, antibody titers should be determined only after a complete immunization series, which includes three doses of anti-tetanus and anti-diphtheria vaccine. In adults, immunization history is fundamental, because after several years from the last booster dose, antibody titers may have naturally decreased, especially diphtheria's one [68]. In those cases, administration of a booster dose will restore protection and will allow to document a normal humoral response to protein antigens.

The assessment of polysaccharide antigen response is more complex than that to proteins, and it is generally carried out through the determination of antibody titers against multiple pneumococcal serotypes [63, 69].

Antibody response to polysaccharide antigens is not a component of routine immune investigation in children younger than 2 years. In fact, it has historically been determined that children younger than this age have a minor and variable capacity to respond to T-independent antigens because of age-dependent immunologic maturation [70]. Moreover, pure polysaccharide vaccines may endanger the patient inducing tolerance and impairing the efficacy of conjugate vaccine administered subsequently [71]. In these age groups, polysaccharide response can be tested indirectly with quantitative determination of isohemagglutinin titers: anti-A and anti-B. These antibodies are naturally produced against gut flora polysaccharides, and only their complete absence in patients older than 6 months of age can be suggestive of an antibody production defect. Moreover, normal titers, composed of IgG and IgM, do not exclude immunodeficiency and are naturally absent in individuals with AB blood group [72].

In individuals older than 2 years of age, responsiveness to polysaccharide antigens is generally tested through the determination of antibody titers against 23 pneumococcal serotypes. A single-serotype IgG concentration is considered protective when ≥1.3 μg/mL [63, 73], but it has scarce significance if considered singularly. In fact, different pneumococcal serotypes have completely different immunogenicities so that a high isolated response to one serotype cannot be considered as indicative of normal polysaccharide response.

If the patient has already received PCV13, when evaluating polysaccharide response, only those serotypes that are not included in the conjugated vaccine have to be considered. In particular, when studying a child with a history of recurrent infections, normal serological response to pneumococcus requires:

- ≥50% of protective titers (≥1.3 μg/mL) against serotypes not included in the conjugate vaccine if previously administered, in patients 2 to 5 years of age
- ≥70% of protective titers (≥1.3 μg/mL) against serotypes not included in the conjugate vaccine if previously administered, in patients older than 6 years of age [63]

This means that if PCV13 has normally been administered in the first year of life, the response have to be evaluated basing on the 11 serotypes (2, 8, 9 N, 10A, 11A, 12F, 15B, 17F, 20, 22, and 33F) included in PPV23 and not in PCV13.

For instance, a child under 6 years of age with recurrent infections but normal polysaccharide response will have protective titers against 6 or more serotypes out of these 11. If the same child were older than 6 years of age, a normal response would be identified by the presence of protective titers against 8 or more of the 11 serotypes not included in PCV13.

When children with recurrent infections have lower proportions of protective titers, they can be considered deficient, and PPV23 may be administered (at least at 8 weeks from PCV13 and after 2 years of age) in order to expand protection and to test specific antibody response against pure polysaccharide. Repeated booster doses of PPV23 are not recommended because they can induce tolerance and efficacy is absent especially in non-responder [73–75].

Deficient responsiveness to PPV23 can be classified as follows, basing mainly on the percentage of protective titers (≥1.3 μg/mL) documented against the different serotypes:

- Severe phenotype has ≤2 protective titers, and protective titers present are low (<2.0 μg/mL).
- Moderate phenotype has ≥3 protective titers, but proportion is <70% in over 6 and < 50% in under 6.

- Mild phenotype.
- Rapid memory loss [63].

When evaluating relative increase in a postvaccination setting, proportion of neo-protective titers is fundamental, but it should be determined through the accurate analysis of single-serotype pre- and postimmunization titers. In fact, the higher the single titer was in a pre-vaccination setting, the lower the increase will be after PPV23 administration [76, 77]. Limited data are available about how much an already protective titer should increase after a booster dose. However, a twofold increase is considered adequate if preimmunization titers were lower than 4.4 to 10.3 μg/mL depending on the pneumococcal serotype [76]. Accordingly, mild phenotype is identified as the incapacity to generate a twofold increase in patients that had lower pre-vaccination titers compared with the one mentioned above or a general failure to generate protective titers against multiple serotypes.

Rapid memory loss can be identified when, despite a good vaccine-response, the patient continues to suffer from recurrent infections. In this case retesting of antibody titers is repeated within 6 months from the last immunization, and titers have already decreased below the protective levels. Isolated hyporesponsiveness to polysaccharide antigens with normal response to proteins is typical of mild humoral immunodeficiencies like SAD, IGGSD, and sIGAD.

22.4 Herd Immunity: A Social Issue

The importance of vaccinations in humoral immunodeficiencies as prophylactic and diagnostic tool is crucial. Moreover, their role is not confined to the single-patient care, but it obviously goes further being relevant on a population scale. The term "herd immunity" refers to the reduction of infections in the general population even among susceptible individuals because of presence and proximity of immune individuals [78]. The advent of immunizations is the reason of rare occurrence of potentially deadly childhood infections like rubella, varicella, measles, or pertussis. In industrialized countries, population have become complacent with this rarity which has generated the misbelief that these diseases are disappeared and will not return [6]. Moreover, population is everyday more sophisticated and likely to oppose to vaccine recommendations so that maintenance of high coverage is more difficult as the diseases decline in incidence. *Anti-vax* sentiment is a complex issue whose roots slip into clear disinformation, fear of conspiracy, new libertarian philosophies, religious views, and fear of severe side effects like development of autism, despite vast evidence of the contrary [6, 78]. Immunodeficient individuals are obviously the most endangered from the loss of indirect protection in the general population. It would be desirable that all healthcare providers contribute to patients and parents adequate information and that national and international programs are implemented to fight the phenomenon and correctly spread scientific evidence among the public.

References

1. Bonilla FA, Khan DA, Ballas ZK, et al. Practice parameter for the diagnosis and management of primary immunodeficiency. J Allergy Clin Immunol. 2015;136:1186–1205.e1-78.
2. Eibl MM, Wolf HM. Vaccination in patients with primary immune deficiency, secondary immune deficiency and autoimmunity with immune regulatory abnormalities. Immunotherapy. 2015;7:1273–92.
3. Pinkbook|Immunization Strategies|Epidemiology of VPDs|CDC. https://www.cdc.gov/vaccines/pubs/pinkbook/strat.html. Accessed 21 Oct 2017.
4. Picard C, Al-Herz W, Bousfiha A, et al. Primary immunodeficiency diseases: an update on the classification from the International Union of Immunological Societies Expert Committee for Primary Immunodeficiency 2015. J Clin Immunol. 2015;35:696–726.
5. American Academy of Pediatrics, Committee on Infectious Diseases; Kimberlin DW, Brady MT, Jackson MA, Long SS (2015) Red book: 2015 report of the Committee on infectious diseases.
6. Medical Advisory Committee of the Immune Deficiency Foundation, Shearer WT, Fleisher TA, et al. Recommendations for live viral and bacterial vaccines in immunodeficient patients and their close contacts. J Allergy Clin Immunol. 2014;133:961–6.
7. Sobh A, Bonilla FA. Vaccination in primary immunodeficiency disorders. J Allergy Clin Immunol Pract. 2016;4:1066–75.
8. Rubin LG, Levin MJ, Ljungman P, et al. 2013 IDSA clinical practice guideline for vaccination of the immunocompromised host. Clin Infect Dis Off Publ Infect Dis Soc Am. 2014;58:e44–100.
9. (2017) Pinkbook|Schedules and Recommendations|Epidemiology of Vaccine Preventable Diseases|CDC. https://www.cdc.gov/vaccines/pubs/pinkbook/appendix/appdx-a.html. Accessed 23 Oct 2017.
10. Guo J, Bolivar-Wagers S, Srinivas N, Holubar M, Maldonado Y. Immunodeficiency-related vaccine-derived poliovirus (iVDPV) cases: a systematic review and implications for polio eradication. Vaccine. 2015;33:1235–42.
11. Research C for BE and Approved Products—October 20, 2014 Approval Letter—Adenovirus Type 4 and Type 7 Vaccine, Live, Oral. https://www.fda.gov/BiologicsBloodVaccines/Vaccines/ApprovedProducts/ucm419764.htm. Accessed 6 Oct 2017.
12. Yazdani R, Azizi G, Abolhassani H, Aghamohammadi A. Selective IgA deficiency: epidemiology, pathogenesis, clinical phenotype, diagnosis, prognosis and management. Scand J Immunol. 2017;85:3–12.
13. Principi N, Esposito S. Vaccine use in primary immunodeficiency disorders. Vaccine. 2014;32:3725–31.
14. Aghamohammadi A, Cheraghi T, Gharagozlou M, Movahedi M, Rezaei N, Yeganeh M, Parvaneh N, Abolhassani H, Pourpak Z, Moin M. IgA deficiency: correlation between clinical and immunological phenotypes. J Clin Immunol. 2009;29:130–6.
15. Diseases AC on. Red Book. 29th ed. Elk Grove Village: American Academy of Pediatrics; 2012.
16. Moylett EH, Wasan AN, Noroski LM, Shearer WT. Live viral vaccines in patients with partial DiGeorge syndrome: clinical experience and cellular immunity. Clin Immunol Orlando Fla. 2004;112:106–12.
17. Al-Sukaiti N, Reid B, Lavi S, Al-Zaharani D, Atkinson A, Roifman CM, Grunebaum E. Safety and efficacy of measles, mumps, and rubella vaccine in patients with DiGeorge syndrome. J Allergy Clin Immunol. 2010;126:868–9.
18. Hofstetter AM, Jakob K, Klein NP, Dekker CL, Edwards KM, Halsey NA, Baxter R, Williams SE, Graham PL, LaRussa P. Live vaccine use and safety in DiGeorge syndrome. Pediatrics. 2014;133:e946–54.
19. Centers for Disease Control (CDC). Guidelines for prophylaxis against Pneumocystis Carinii pneumonia for persons infected with human immunodeficiency virus. MMWR Suppl. 1989;38:1–9.

20. Addition of Severe Combined Immunodeficiency as a Contraindication for Administration of Rotavirus Vaccine. https://www.cdc.gov/mmwr/preview/mmwrhtml/mm5922a3.htm. Accessed 19 Oct 2017.
21. Prevention of Rotavirus Gastroenteritis Among Infants and Children Recommendations of the Advisory Committee on Immunization Practices (ACIP). https://www.cdc.gov/mmwr/preview/mmwrhtml/rr5802a1.htm. Accessed 19 Oct 2017.
22. Siber GR, Werner BG, Halsey NA, Reid R, Almeido-Hill J, Garrett SC, Thompson C, Santosham M. Interference of immune globulin with measles and rubella immunization. J Pediatr. 1993;122:204–11.
23. Beck CR, BC MK, Hashim AB, Harris RC, University of Nottingham Influenza and the Immuno Compromised (UNIIC) Study Group, Nguyen-Van-Tam JS. Influenza vaccination for immunocompromised patients: systematic review and meta-analysis by etiology. J Infect Dis. 2012;206:1250–9.
24. Muller RB, Maier R, Hoschler K, Zambon M, Ludewig B, Herrmann M, Schulze-Koops H, von Kempis J. Efficient boosting of the antiviral T cell response in B cell-depleted patients with autoimmune rheumatic diseases following influenza vaccination. Clin Exp Rheumatol. 2013;31:723–30.
25. Oren S, Mandelboim M, Braun-Moscovici Y, et al. Vaccination against influenza in patients with rheumatoid arthritis: the effect of rituximab on the humoral response. Ann Rheum Dis. 2008;67:937–41.
26. Committee on Infectious Diseases. HPV vaccine recommendations. Pediatrics. 2012;129:602–5.
27. Markowitz LE, Dunne EF, Saraiya M, Chesson HW, Curtis CR, Gee J, Bocchini JA, Unger ER, Centers for Disease Control and Prevention (CDC). Human papillomavirus vaccination: recommendations of the Advisory Committee on Immunization Practices (ACIP). MMWR Recomm Rep. 2014;63:1–30.
28. Advisory Committee on Immunization Practices. Use of anthrax vaccine in the United States. MMWR Recomm Rep. 2000;49:1–20.
29. Centers for Disease Control and Prevention. Use of a reduced (4-dose) vaccine schedule for postexposure prophylaxis to prevent human rabies-recommendations of the Advisory Committee on Immunization Practice. Ann Emerg Med. 2010;56:64–7.
30. Plebani A, Fischer MB, Meini A, Duse M, Thon V, Eibl MM. T cell activity and cytokine production in X-linked agammaglobulinemia: implications for vaccination strategies. Int Arch Allergy Immunol. 1997;114:90–3.
31. Paroli M, Accapezzato D, Francavilla V, Insalaco A, Plebani A, Balsano F, Barnaba V. Long-lasting memory-resting and memory-effector CD4+ T cells in human X-linked agammaglobulinemia. Blood. 2002;99:2131–7.
32. Amedei A, Romagnani C, Benagiano M, Azzurri A, Fomia F, Torrente F, Plebani A, D'Elios MM, Del Prete G. Preferential Th1 profile of T helper cell responses in X-linked (Bruton's) agammaglobulinemia. Eur J Immunol. 2001;31:1927–34.
33. Barbaro M, Ohlsson A, Borte S, Jonsson S, Zetterström RH, King J, Winiarski J, von Döbeln U, Hammarström L. Newborn screening for severe primary immunodeficiency diseases in Sweden—a 2-year Pilot TREC and KREC screening study. J Clin Immunol. 2017;37:51–60.
34. Lodi L, Ricci S, Romano F, Ghiori F, Canessa C, Lippi F, Bianchi L, Azzari C. Newborn screening for PIDs using both TREC and KREC identifies late occurrence of B cells. Pediatr Allergy Immunol. 2017;28:498–500.
35. Mieves JF, Wittke K, Freitag H, Volk H-D, Scheibenbogen C, Hanitsch LG. Influenza vaccination in patients with common variable immunodeficiency (CVID). Curr Allergy Asthma Rep. 2017;17:78.
36. Goldacker S, Draeger R, Warnatz K, Huzly D, Salzer U, Thiel J, Eibel H, Schlesier M, Peter HH. Active vaccination in patients with common variable immunodeficiency (CVID). Clin Immunol Orlando Fla. 2007;124:294–303.

37. Bonilla FA, Barlan I, Chapel H, et al. International Consensus Document (ICON): common variable immunodeficiency disorders. J Allergy Clin Immunol Pract. 2016;4:38–59.
38. Adam E, Church JA. Antibody levels to Bordetella pertussis and Neisseria meningitidis in immunodeficient patients receiving immunoglobulin replacement therapy. J Clin Immunol. 2015;35:213–7.
39. Chen RT, Pless R, Destefano F. Epidemiology of autoimmune reactions induced by vaccination. J Autoimmun. 2001;16:309–18.
40. Groot N, Heijstek MW, Wulffraat NM. Vaccinations in paediatric rheumatology: an update on current developments. Curr Rheumatol Rep. 2015; https://doi.org/10.1007/s11926-015-0519-y.
41. Handisurya A, Schellenbacher C, Reininger B, Koszik F, Vyhnanek P, Heitger A, Kirnbauer R, Förster-Waldl E. A quadrivalent HPV vaccine induces humoral and cellular immune responses in WHIM immunodeficiency syndrome. Vaccine. 2010;28:4837–41.
42. Petrosky E, Bocchini JA, Hariri S, Chesson H, Curtis CR, Saraiya M, Unger ER, Markowitz LE, Centers for Disease Control and Prevention (CDC). Use of 9-valent human papillomavirus (HPV) vaccine: updated HPV vaccination recommendations of the advisory committee on immunization practices. MMWR Morb Mortal Wkly Rep. 2015;64:300–4.
43. Conley ME, Dobbs AK, Farmer DM, Kilic S, Paris K, Grigoriadou S, Coustan-Smith E, Howard V, Campana D. Primary B cell immunodeficiencies: comparisons and contrasts. Annu Rev Immunol. 2009;27:199–227.
44. Prevention of pneumococcal disease among infants and children—use of 13-valent pneumococcal conjugate vaccine and 23-valent pneumococcal polysaccharide vaccine. https://www.cdc.gov/mmwr/preview/mmwrhtml/rr5911a1.htm#Tab12. Accessed 18 Oct 2017.
45. Use of 13-valent pneumococcal conjugate vaccine and 23-valent pneumococcal polysaccharide vaccine among children Aged 6–18 years with immunocompromising conditions: Recommendations of the Advisory Committee on Immunization Practices (ACIP). https://www.cdc.gov/mmwr/preview/mmwrhtml/mm6225a3.htm. Accessed 18 Oct 2017.
46. Zielen S, Bühring I, Strnad N, Reichenbach J, Hofmann D. Immunogenicity and tolerance of a 7-valent pneumococcal conjugate vaccine in nonresponders to the 23-valent pneumococcal vaccine. Infect Immun. 2000;68:1435–40.
47. Use of MenACWY-CRM vaccine in children aged 2 through 23 months at increased risk for meningococcal disease: Recommendations of the Advisory Committee on Immunization Practices, 2013. https://www.cdc.gov/mmwr/preview/mmwrhtml/mm6324a2.htm. Accessed 18 Oct 2017.
48. Vaccine Schedule. http://vaccine-schedule.ecdc.europa.eu/Pages/Scheduler.aspx. Accessed 31 Oct 2017.
49. European Medicines Agency—Find medicine—Bexsero. http://www.ema.europa.eu/ema/index.jsp?curl=pages/medicines/human/medicines/002333/human_med_001614.jsp&mid=WC0b01ac058001d124. Accessed 18 Oct 2017.
50. Pinkbook|Meningococcal|Epidemiology of Vaccine Preventable Diseases|CDC. https://www.cdc.gov/vaccines/pubs/pinkbook/mening.html#vaccines. Accessed 18 Oct 2017.
51. Pinkbook|General Recommendations|Epidemiology of VPDs|CDC. https://www.cdc.gov/vaccines/pubs/pinkbook/genrec.html. Accessed 23 Oct 2017.
52. Kaplan JE, Nelson DB, Schonberger LB, Hatch MH, Monath TP, Lazuick JS, Calisher CH, Rosa FW. The effect of immune globulin on the response to trivalent oral poliovirus and yellow fever vaccinations. Bull World Health Organ. 1984;62:585–90.
53. Glück T, Müller-Ladner U. Vaccination in patients with chronic rheumatic or autoimmune diseases. Clin Infect Dis. 2008;46:1459–65.
54. 2018 Yellow Book Home|Travelers' Health|CDC. https://wwwnc.cdc.gov/travel/page/yellowbook-home. Accessed 2 Nov 2017.
55. Cholera vaccines: WHO position paper—August 2017. Releve Epidemiol Hebd. 2017;92:477–98.

56. Cholera—Chapter 3-2018 Yellow Book|Travelers' Health|CDC. https://wwwnc.cdc.gov/travel/yellowbook/2018/infectious-diseases-related-to-travel/cholera. Accessed 28 Nov 2017.
57. Perry RT, Plowe CV, Koumaré B, Bougoudogo F, Kotloff KL, Losonsky GA, Wasserman SS, Levine MM. A single dose of live oral cholera vaccine CVD 103-HgR is safe and immunogenic in HIV-infected and HIV-noninfected adults in Mali. Bull World Health Organ. 1998;76:63–71.
58. Ballow M. Primary immunodeficiency disorders: antibody deficiency. J Allergy Clin Immunol. 2002;109:581–91.
59. Howard V, Myers LA, Williams DA, Wheeler G, Turner EV, Cunningham JM, Conley ME. Stem cell transplants for patients with X-linked agammaglobulinemia. Clin Immunol Orlando Fla. 2003;107:98–102.
60. Wehr C, Gennery AR, Lindemans C, et al. Multicenter experience in hematopoietic stem cell transplantation for serious complications of common variable immunodeficiency. J Allergy Clin Immunol. 2015;135:988–97. e6
61. Tomblyn M, Chiller T, Einsele H, Gress R, Sepkowitz K, Storek J, Wingard JR, Young J-AH, Boeckh MA. Guidelines for preventing infectious complications among hematopoietic cell transplant recipients: a global perspective. Biol Blood Marrow Transplant. 2009;15:1143–238.
62. (2017) ACIP Altered Immunocompetence Guidelines for Immunizations|Recommendations |CDC. https://www.cdc.gov/vaccines/hcp/acip-recs/general-recs/immunocompetence.html. Accessed 7 Nov 2017.
63. Orange JS, Ballow M, Stiehm ER, et al. Use and interpretation of diagnostic vaccination in primary immunodeficiency: a working group report of the Basic and Clinical Immunology Interest Section of the American Academy of Allergy Asthma & Immunology. J Allergy Clin Immunol. 2012;130:S1–24.
64. Shrimpton A, Duddridge M, Ziegler-Heitbrock L. Vaccination with polysaccharide-conjugate-vaccines in adult patients with specific antibody deficiency. Vaccine. 2006;24:3574–80.
65. Smith LL, Buckley R, Lugar P. Diagnostic immunization with bacteriophage ΦX 174 in patients with common variable immunodeficiency/hypogammaglobulinemia. Front Immunol. 2014;5:410.
66. Seidel MG, Planitzer CB, Kreil TR, Förster-Waldl E. Tick-borne encephalitis virus vaccine as additional alternative neoantigen for the clinical immunologist's toolbox. J Allergy Clin Immunol. 2013;131:617.
67. Plotkin SA. Correlates of protection induced by vaccination. Clin Vaccine Immunol. 2010;17:1055–65.
68. McQuillan GM, Kruszon-Moran D, Deforest A, Chu SY, Wharton M. Serologic immunity to diphtheria and tetanus in the United States. Ann Intern Med. 2002;136:660–6.
69. Paris K, Sorensen RU. Assessment and clinical interpretation of polysaccharide antibody responses. Ann Allergy Asthma Immunol. 2007;99:462–4.
70. Leinonen M, Säkkinen A, Kalliokoski R, Luotonen J, Timonen M, Mäkelä PH. Antibody response to 14-valent pneumococcal capsular polysaccharide vaccine in pre-school age children. Pediatr Infect Dis. 1986;5:39–44.
71. O'Brien KL, Hochman M, Goldblatt D. Combined schedules of pneumococcal conjugate and polysaccharide vaccines: is hyporesponsiveness an issue? Lancet Infect Dis. 2007;7:597–606.
72. Fong SW, Qaqundah BY, Taylor WF. Developmental patterns of ABO isoagglutinins in normal children correlated with the effects of age, sex, and maternal isoagglutinins. Transfusion (Paris). 1974;14:551–9.
73. Sorensen RU, Leiva LE, Giangrosso PA, Butler B, Javier FC, Sacerdote DM, Bradford N, Moore C. Response to a heptavalent conjugate Streptococcus pneumoniae vaccine in children with recurrent infections who are unresponsive to the polysaccharide vaccine. Pediatr Infect Dis J. 1998;17:685–91.
74. Granoff DM, Gupta RK, Belshe RB, Anderson EL. Induction of immunologic refractoriness in adults by meningococcal C polysaccharide vaccination. J Infect Dis. 1998;178:870–4.

75. de Roux A, Schmöle-Thoma B, Schmöele-Thoma B, et al. Comparison of pneumococcal conjugate polysaccharide and free polysaccharide vaccines in elderly adults: conjugate vaccine elicits improved antibacterial immune responses and immunological memory. Clin Infect Dis. 2008;46:1015–23.
76. Hare ND, Smith BJ, Ballas ZK. Antibody response to pneumococcal vaccination as a function of preimmunization titer. J Allergy Clin Immunol. 2009;123:195–200.
77. Sorensen RU, Leiva LE, Javier FC, Sacerdote DM, Bradford N, Butler B, Giangrosso PA, Moore C. Influence of age on the response to Streptococcus pneumoniae vaccine in patients with recurrent infections and normal immunoglobulin concentrations. J Allergy Clin Immunol. 1998;102:215–21.
78. Fine P, Eames K, Heymann DL. "Herd Immunity": A Rough Guide. Clin Infect Dis. 2011;52:911–6.

Malignancy in Predominantly Antibody Deficiencies (PAD)

23

Claudia Wehr

23.1 Introduction

Paul Ehrlich in 1909 proposed a role of the immune system in cancer surveillance [1], a hypothesis that later was elaborated by Burnet [2]. The predisposition of primary immunodeficiency (PID) patients to malignancies has long been recognized [3]. Also patients with secondary immunodeficiency, e.g., acquired immunodeficiency syndrome, recipients of hematopoietic stem cell transplantation, and kidney transplant recipients are at increased risk for malignancies [4–6]. The importance of the immune system in controlling malignancies is currently further emphasized by the success of checkpoint inhibitor treatment, e.g., anti-PD1 antibodies in treatment of cancers. Herein, the evidence for cancer predisposition in primary *humoral* immunodeficiency is reviewed. Other primary immunodeficiencies accounting for a substantial part of cancer predisposition in PID, e.g., ataxia-telangiectasia, Nijmegen breakage syndrome, X-linked lymphoproliferative syndrome, are not in the scope of the article and have recently been reviewed elsewhere [7].

According to the current classification of the International Union of Immunological Societies Expert Committee for Primary Immunodeficiency [8],

C. Wehr
Center for Chronic Immunodeficiency (CCI), Medical Center—University of Freiburg, Faculty of Medicine, University of Freiburg, Freiburg, Germany

Department of Medicine I/Hematology, Oncology and Stem Cell Transplantation, Medical Center—University of Freiburg, Faculty of Medicine, University of Freiburg, Freiburg, Germany
e-mail: claudia.wehr@uniklinik-freiburg.de

M. M. D'Elios, M. Rizzi (eds.), *Humoral Primary Immunodeficiencies*,
Rare Diseases of the Immune System, https://doi.org/10.1007/978-3-319-91785-6_23

PAD comprises more than 30 entities (Table 23.1). Most of the entities are molecularly defined, e.g., BTK (Bruton's tyrosine kinase) mutations in X-linked agammaglobulinemia providing the means to exactly define the patient cohort. However, some entities are molecularly defined with only a few patients published, rendering epidemiological studies on cancer incidence impossible, e.g., UNG (uracil-N-glycosylase) deficiency. Common variable immunodeficiency (CVID) represents the most prevalent entity within PAD. CVID is defined according to clinical criteria with predominant hypogammaglobulinemia (https://esid.org/Working-Parties/Registry/Diagnosis-criteria) and a varying degree of T-cell deficiency in some patients [9]. This caused CVID to be used as an umbrella diagnosis for undefined PID in some of the older cohorts. About 2–10% of CVID patients—in preselected cohorts up to 30%—carry monogenetic defects [10, 11]. At the same time, it has become clear that the pathophysiology of CVID is complex and multi-facetted in the majority of patients, and some of the "monogenetic" defects turned out later to be genetic modifiers, e.g., TNFRSF13B (TACI) mutations [12]. As the field of genetics and genomics has rapidly evolved over the last years and as not all CVID patients undergo targeted or non-targeted sequencing, some molecularly defined PID might be included into CVID cohorts: NFKB1 and NFKB2 mutations and CTLA-4 and LRBA deficiency, the latter being nowadays grouped within regulator T-cell deficiencies or combined immunodeficiencies, respectively. Activating mutations in PI3K-delta lead to an immundysregulatory syndrome with a high prevalence of lymphoma [13, 14] with some of these patients formerly being subsumed under the diagnosis of CVID These aspects have to be kept in mind when interpreting registry data on CVID patients. Despite the limitations due to retrospective and/or uncontrolled studies and small patient numbers in many of the PAD subgroups, Table 23.1 summarizes the evidence for predisposition to malignancies in PAD classified according to the IUS classification [8]. CVID and BTK deficiency will be discussed separately in the text below.

Table 23.1 PAD according to IUIS classification and association with malignancy

PAD with severe reduction in all serum immunoglobulin isotypes with profoundly decreased or absent B cells	
BTK deficiency (X-linked agammaglobulinemia)	See text
μ heavy chain deficiency	Autosomal recessive agammaglobulinemia, no clear association with malignancies, case reports for gastric adenocarcinoma exist [46]
Lambda 5 deficiency	
CD79A deficiency	
CD79B deficiency	
BLNK deficiency	
PI3KR1 deficiency	
E47 transcription factor deficiency	Only few patients published, no association with malignancy reported [47, 48]
Thymoma with immunodeficiency	Good's syndrome: patients display invasive infections and autoimmunity, no malignancies besides thymoma reported [49, 50]
Severe reduction in at least two serum immunoglobulin isotypes with normal or low number of B cells	

Table 23.1 (continued)

CVID	See text
CD19 deficiency	Subsumed in CVID cohorts
CD81 deficiency	
CD20 deficiency	
CD21 deficiency	
TACI deficiency	
BAFF receptor deficiency	
TWEAK deficiency	Few patients reported, patients have recurrent warts [51] which might predispose to HPV-associated cancers
NFKB2 deficiency	No association with malignancies reported [52–54]
MOGS deficiency	Few patients reported [55, 56], early deaths
TRNT1 deficiency	Sideroblastic anemia with B-cell immunodeficiency, periodic fevers, and developmental delay, often death in first decade due to cardiomyopathy, no association with malignancy reported [57, 58]
TTC37 deficiency	Trichohepatoenteric syndrome: no association with malignancy reported [59], one case report of a patient with hepatoblastoma [60]
Severe reduction in serum IgG and IgA with normal/elevated IgM and normal numbers of B cells	
AID (activation-induced cytidine deaminase) deficiency	Autosomal recessive immunodeficiency with hyper-IgM syndrome, follicular hyperplasia in lymph nodes frequent, but no association with lymphoma or other malignancy reported [61, 62]
UNG (uracil-N-glycosylase) deficiency	Only three patients reported, follicular hyperplasia in lymph nodes is common, UNG-deficient mice are predisposed to B-cell lymphomas [62]
INO80 deficiency	Only two patients reported, leads to mild DNA repair defect, predisposition to malignancies possible [63]
MSH6 deficiency	DNA mismatch repair defect, predisposes to solid tumors (esp. HNPCC, endometrial cancer) and lymphomas [64] and Online Mendelian Inheritance in Man, OMIM®. Johns Hopkins University, Baltimore, MD. MIM number: {600,678}: {12/72015}: World Wide Web URL: https://omim.org/)
Isotype or light chain deficiencies with generally normal numbers of B cells	
Activated PI3K-delta	Increased incidence of lymphoma in 13–28% of patients [13, 14]
PI3KR1 loss of function	No malignancies reported
Ig heavy chain mutations and deletions (other than μ chain)	Can be asymptomatic, association with malignancy unknown
IGKC (kappa light chain) deficiency	Only few patients reported, all B cells express lambda light chain without clonality [65]
IgA with IgG subclass deficiency	No increased risk for neoplasms in IgA deficiency [23] reported
Specific antibody deficiency with normal Ig concentrations and normal numbers of B cells	No data available
Isolated IgG subclass deficiency	
Transient hypogammaglobulinemia of infancy with normal numbers of B cells	Prospective studies with follow-up into adulthood of this patient cohort are lacking, no association with malignancy reported
CARD11 gain of function mutations	"B cell expansion with NF-κB and T cell anergy" (BENTA) disease; one case of CLL reported, constitutive NF-κB activation might predispose to B cell lymphoma [66]

23.2 Predisposition to Malignancy in PAD

Multiple case series and registry surveys addressing the incidence of malignancies in PID were published over the last decades. Due to the rarity of PID, the results of many of the studies rely on relatively few patient numbers, and the results have to be interpreted with caution. The largest and most recent cohort on cancer epidemiology in patients with primary immunodeficiency reports data from 3658 US PID patients (USIDNET) and a control group including approximately 26% of the US population from "Surveillance, Epidemiology and End Results Program Estimated Cancer Incidence" of the National Cancer Institute [15]. Mayor et al. point out that—in contrast to many other previous registry reports—the incidence of the most common cancers in the general population (breast, colorectal, lung, prostate cancer) was not increased in PID patients, whereas the incidence of lymphoma, skin, and thyroid cancer was significantly increased compared to the general population. Data published from the Dutch national registry of PID patients [16] on 745 children and adults showed an increased incidence of lymphoma, leukemia, skin cancer, and rare solid tumors (thymus, endocrine gland) in PID patients compared to the Dutch general population. Similar findings were reported from Australian patients ($n = 1135$) from the Australasian Society of Clinical Immunology and Allergy PID Registry [17]. Of note, the relative risk increase of leukemia was in both studies based on extremely low case numbers. The increased incidence of thymoma in these cohorts most likely reflects the inclusion of patients with immunodeficiency due to thymoma and does not reflect an elevated risk of PID patients for thymoma. Consistent throughout all studies [15–18] is the increased risk of lymphoma for PID patients. Other neoplasms are most likely only increased in subgroups of PID, e.g., stomach cancer in CVID, and results from different registries vary depending on the percentages of different PIDs within the cohorts.

23.3 CVID

Malignancies are among the main causes of death in CVID patients [19–21] with gastric adenocarcinoma and lymphoma being the most common malignancies.

23.3.1 Lymphoma

The incidence of lymphoma in CVID is 7× increased for women and 8.42× increased for men [15]; other studies have found lower [17] or higher fold increases [22–24]. Lymphoma subtypes in CVID are mostly B-cell-derived high-grade non-Hodgkin lymphomas (NHL). As in the general population B-NHLs can be EBV associated in some cases, but—albeit exact statistic data are lacking—there does not seem to exist an overrepresentation of EBV-associated lymphomas in CVID [25]. This is in contrast to other combined PIDs with disturbances of T- and NK-cell surveillance (e.g., XLP1, XIAP, CD27 deficiency) where EBV-associated lymphoproliferation/malignancies are a hallmark of the disease. T-cell NHLs are rarely seen in CVID and should prompt a review of the CVID diagnostic criteria and exclusion of a DNA repair deficiency [25]. Follicular lymphoma, a low-grade lymphoma accounting for 20–25% of NHL in the normal population, has also rarely been described in CVID. If marginal zone lymphoma, another low-grade NHL, is more prevalent in CVID compared to the general population is questioned [25] albeit the hypothesis of chronic antigenic stimulation in mucosa-associated lymphoid tissues (MALT) in the context of humoral immunodeficiency leading to increased lymphoma incidence offers an attractive pathophysiological concept [26]. Treatment of NHLs in CVID can be conducted according to entity and standard hematologic protocols if there is no suspicion of a DNA repair deficiency and if the general condition and comorbidities of the patient allow for it. In contrast to treatment of non-PID lymphoma patients, it is suggested to evaluate hematopoietic stem cell transplantation in first remission [27, 28].

Establishing the diagnosis of lymphoma in CVID patients can be hampered by the fact that about ¼ of patients display benign lymphadenopathy [29] resulting from reactive lymphoid hyperplasia or granulomatous inflammation and ill-defined, irregular germinal centers [30]. Also borderline malignant lymphoproliferation can be present in CVID patients [25, 31]. For these reasons, lymph node extraction is preferred over lymph node biopsy in CVID patients with suspicion of lymphoma. Further pitfalls are expansions of oligoclonal CD8 T cells infiltrating the liver or bone marrow sometimes resembling large granular lymphocyte leukemia [25]. In summary setting both the optimal time point for lymph node excision and histologic evaluation of lymphatic proliferation in CVID is challenging and should be done by experts in the field and on an interdisciplinary basis.

23.3.2 Gastric Adenocarcinoma

In the most recent and largest analysis on cancer predisposition in PID, the incidence of stomach cancer was 5× increased in men and 4.29× in women with CVID compared to the general population [15]. Vajdic et al. reported a 7.23× increase, [17] while older studies suggested an even higher increase (10–47× fold) [23, 24]. If there is a true decline in incidence of stomach cancer in CVID due to increased treatment of *Helicobacter pylori* or if this finding results from methodological differences remains an open question. A reason for the predisposition to gastric adenocarcinoma is the high prevalence of known risk factors for gastric cancer in CVID patients compared to the general population: atrophic gastritis, *Helicobacter pylori* infections, and intestinal metaplasia [32, 33]. CVID patients develop gastric cancer earlier in life compared to non-PID patients with gastric cancer, and the most common histologic subtype is tubular adenocarcinoma [34]. Prognosis is poor and treatment is conducted according to oncological algorithms. Endoscopic screening for gastric cancer in selected CVID patients has been suggested [33] but was not formally investigated. Given the high prevalence of gastric pathology including malignancies in CVID patients, dyspepsia should prompt esophagogastroscopy without further delay.

23.4 X-Linked Agammaglobulinemia (XLA)

Mutations in Bruton's tyrosine kinase (BTK) lead to early-onset infectious susceptibility due to absence of B cells and agammaglobulinemia; a substantial part of patients suffer from autoimmune arthritis or inflammatory bowel disease [35, 36]. Cutaneous T-cell lymphomas have been reported in a few cases [37–39]. Other case reports suggest an increased incidence of gastric adenocarcinoma and colorectal cancer in XLA [40–42] and screening endoscopy revealed adenomatous polyps in two of four screened XLA patients [43]. However, these (case) studies might underlie a publication bias. While the registry study by Vajdic et al. found the relative risk of stomach cancer increased in XLA on the basis of one single case [17], others could not confirm an increased incidence of malignomas in XLA patients [44], and the largest registry study on malignancies in PID does not comment on this question due to limited number of patients in this subgroup [15]. In summary, there remains uncertainty if XLA patients are predisposed to malignancies or not.

The increased frequency of malignancy in PAD emphasizes the role of the immune system in controlling the development of malignancies but more specifically supports the hypothesis that in certain conditions B lymphocytes may be involved in this function [45]. Indeed, malignancies can constitute a late complication in PID, but they can also constitute the first manifestation of it, leading to an unusual course of the malignancy. Hence, the physician who cares for primary immune deficiency patients has to keep in mind that beyond infection and immune dysregulation, the occurrence of malignancy has to be actively searched and cared for.

References

1. Ehrlich P (1909) Ueber den jetzigen Stand der Karzinomforschung. Vortrag gehalten vor den Studenten der Amsterdamer Universitaet, Vereinigung fuer wissenschaftliche Arbeit 1 June 1908. Printed in: P. Ehrlich. Beitraege zur experimentellen Pathologie und Chemotherapie Akademische Verlagsgesellschaft, Leipzig 118–164
2. Burnet M. Cancer; a biological approach. I. The processes of control. Br Med J. 1957;1:779–86.
3. Kersey JH, Spector BD, Good RA. Primary immunodeficiency diseases and cancer: the immunodeficiency-cancer registry. Int J Cancer. 1973;12:333–47.
4. Engels EA, Pfeiffer RM, Fraumeni JF Jr, et al. Spectrum of cancer risk among US solid organ transplant recipients. JAMA. 2011;306:1891–901.
5. Shiels MS, Pfeiffer RM, Gail MH, et al. Cancer burden in the HIV-infected population in the United States. J Natl Cancer Inst. 2011;103:753–62.
6. Majhail NS. Secondary cancers following allogeneic haematopoietic cell transplantation in adults. Br J Haematol. 2011;154:301–10.
7. Hauck F, Voss R, Urban C, Seidel MG. Intrinsic and extrinsic causes of malignancies in patients with primary immunodeficiency disorders. J Allergy Clin Immunol. 2018;141:59–68.e4.
8. Picard C, Al-Herz W, Bousfiha A, et al. Primary immunodeficiency diseases: an update on the classification from the International Union of Immunological Societies Expert Committee for primary immunodeficiency 2015. J Clin Immunol. 2015;35:696–726.
9. Malphettes M, Gérard L, Carmagnat M, et al. Late-onset combined immune deficiency: a subset of common variable immunodeficiency with severe T cell defect. Clin Infect Dis. 2009;49:1329–38.

10. Bogaert DJA, Dullaers M, Lambrecht BN, et al. Genes associated with common variable immunodeficiency: one diagnosis to rule them all? J Med Genet. 2016; https://doi.org/10.1136/jmedgenet-2015-103690.
11. Maffucci P, Filion CA, Boisson B, et al. Genetic diagnosis using whole exome sequencing in common variable immunodeficiency. Front Immunol. 2016;7:220.
12. Pulvirenti F, Zuntini R, Milito C, et al. Clinical associations of Biallelic and Monoallelic TNFRSF13B variants in Italian primary antibody deficiency syndromes. J Immunol Res. 2016;2016:8390356.
13. Elkaim E, Neven B, Bruneau J, et al. Clinical and immunologic phenotype associated with activated phosphoinositide 3-kinase δ syndrome 2: a cohort study. J Allergy Clin Immunol. 2016;138:210–218e9.
14. Coulter TI, Chandra A, Bacon CM, et al. Clinical spectrum and features of activated phosphoinositide 3-kinase δ syndrome: a large patient cohort study. J Allergy Clin Immunol. 2017;139:597–606e4.
15. Mayor PC, Eng KH, Singel KL, et al. Cancer in primary immunodeficiency diseases: cancer incidence in the United States immune deficiency network registry. J Allergy Clin Immunol. 2017; https://doi.org/10.1016/j.jaci.2017.05.024.
16. Jonkman-Berk BM, van den Berg JM, Ten Berge IJM, et al. Primary immunodeficiencies in the Netherlands: national patient data demonstrate the increased risk of malignancy. Clin Immunol. 2015;156:154–62.
17. Vajdic CM, Mao L, van Leeuwen MT, et al. Are antibody deficiency disorders associated with a narrower range of cancers than other forms of immunodeficiency? Blood. 2010;116:1228–34.
18. Kersey JH, Shapiro RS, Filipovich AH. Relationship of immunodeficiency to lymphoid malignancy. Pediatr Infect Dis J. 1988;7:S10–2.
19. Quinti I, Agostini C, Tabolli S, et al. Malignancies are the major cause of death in patients with adult onset common variable immunodeficiency. Blood. 2012;120:1953–4.
20. Resnick ES, Moshier EL, Godbold JH, Cunningham-Rundles C. Morbidity and mortality in common variable immune deficiency over 4 decades. Blood. 2012;119:1650–7.
21. Gathmann B, Mahlaoui N, Gérard L, et al. European Society for Immunodeficiencies Registry Working Party. Clinical picture and treatment of 2212 patients with common variable immunodeficiency. J Allergy Clin Immunol. 2014;134:116–26.
22. Quinti I, Soresina A, Spadaro G, et al. Long-term follow-up and outcome of a large cohort of patients with common variable immunodeficiency. J Clin Immunol. 2007;27:308–16.
23. Mellemkjaer L, Hammarstrom L, Andersen V, et al. Cancer risk among patients with IgA deficiency or common variable immunodeficiency and their relatives: a combined Danish and Swedish study. Clin Exp Immunol. 2002;130:495–500.
24. Kinlen LJ, Webster AD, Bird AG, et al. Prospective study of cancer in patients with hypogammaglobulinaemia. Lancet. 1985;1:263–6.
25. Gratzinger D, Jaffe ES, Chadburn A, et al. Primary/congenital immunodeficiency: 2015 SH/EAHP workshop report-part 5. Am J Clin Pathol. 2017;147:204–16.
26. Suarez F, Lortholary O, Hermine O, Lecuit M. Infection-associated lymphomas derived from marginal zone B cells: a model of antigen-driven lymphoproliferation. Blood. 2006;107:3034–44.
27. Wehr C, Gennery AR, Lindemans C, et al. Multicenter experience in hematopoietic stem cell transplantation for serious complications of common variable immunodeficiency. J Allergy Clin Immunol. 2015;135:988–997e6.
28. Fox TA, Chakraverty R, Burns S, et al. Successful outcome following allogeneic hematopoietic stem cell transplantation in adults with primary immunodeficiency. Blood. 2018;131:917–31.
29. Wehr C, Kivioja T, Schmitt C, et al. The EUROclass trial: defining subgroups in common variable immunodeficiency. Blood. 2008;111:77–85.
30. Unger S, Seidl M, Schmitt-Graeff A, et al. Ill-defined germinal centers and severely reduced plasma cells are histological hallmarks of lymphadenopathy in patients with common variable immunodeficiency. J Clin Immunol. 2014;34:615–26.

31. da Silva SP, Resnick E, Lucas M, et al. Lymphoid proliferations of indeterminate malignant potential arising in adults with common variable immunodeficiency disorders: unusual case studies and immunohistological review in the light of possible causative events. J Clin Immunol. 2011;31:784–91.
32. Zullo A, Romiti A, Rinaldi V, et al. Gastric pathology in patients with common variable immunodeficiency. Gut. 1999;45:77–81.
33. Dhalla F, da Silva SP, Lucas M, et al. Review of gastric cancer risk factors in patients with common variable immunodeficiency disorders, resulting in a proposal for a surveillance programme. Clin Exp Immunol. 2011;165:1–7.
34. De Petris G, Dhungel BM, Chen L, Chang Y-HH. Gastric adenocarcinoma in common variable immunodeficiency: features of cancer and associated gastritis may be characteristic of the condition. Int J Surg Pathol. 2014;22:600–6.
35. Hernandez-Trujillo VP, Scalchunes C, Cunningham-Rundles C, et al. Autoimmunity and inflammation in X-linked Agammaglobulinemia. J Clin Immunol. 2014; https://doi.org/10.1007/s10875-014-0056-x.
36. Winkelstein JA, Marino MC, Lederman HM, et al. X-linked agammaglobulinemia: report on a United States registry of 201 patients. Medicine. 2006;85:193–202.
37. Gammon B, Robson A, Deonizio J, et al. CD8(+) granulomatous cutaneous T-cell lymphoma: a potential association with immunodeficiency. J Am Acad Dermatol. 2014;71:555–60.
38. Park JY, Kim YS, Shin DH, et al. Primary cutaneous peripheral T-cell lymphoma in a patient with X-linked agammaglobulinaemia. Br J Dermatol. 2011;164:677–9.
39. Kanavaros P, Rontogianni D, Hrissovergi D, et al. Extranodal cytotoxic T-cell lymphoma in a patient with X-linked agammaglobulinaemia. Leuk Lymphoma. 2001;42:235–8.
40. van der Meer JW, Weening RS, Schellekens PT, et al. Colorectal cancer in patients with X-linked agammaglobulinaemia. Lancet. 1993;341:1439–40.
41. Staines Boone AT, Torres Martínez MG, López Herrera G, et al. Gastric adenocarcinoma in the context of X-linked agammaglobulinemia: case report and review of the literature. J Clin Immunol. 2014;34:134–7.
42. Bachmeyer C, Monge M, Cazier A, et al. Gastric adenocarcinoma in a patient with X-linked agammaglobulinaemia. Eur J Gastroenterol Hepatol. 2000;12:1033–5.
43. Maarschalk-Ellerbroek LJ, Oldenburg B, Mombers IMH, et al. Outcome of screening endoscopy in common variable immunodeficiency disorder and X-linked agammaglobulinemia. Endoscopy. 2013;45:320–3.
44. Hermaszewski RA, Webster AD. Primary hypogammaglobulinaemia: a survey of clinical manifestations and complications. Q J Med. 1993;86:31–42.
45. Yuen GJ, Demissie E, Pillai S. B lymphocytes and cancer: a love-hate relationship. Trends Cancer Res. 2016;2:747–57.
46. Slotta JE, Heine S, Kauffels A, et al. Gastrectomy with isoperistaltic jejunal parallel pouch in a 15-year-old adolescent boy with gastric adenocarcinoma and autosomal recessive agammaglobulinemia. J Pediatr Surg. 2011;46:e21–4.
47. Boisson B, Wang Y-D, Bosompem A, et al. A recurrent dominant negative E47 mutation causes agammaglobulinemia and BCR– B cells. J Clin Invest. 2013;123:4781–5.
48. Dobbs AK, Bosompem A, Coustan-Smith E, et al. Agammaglobulinemia associated with BCR^- B cells and enhanced expression of CD19. Blood. 2011;118:1828–37.
49. Malphettes M, Gérard L, Galicier L, et al. Good syndrome: an adult-onset immunodeficiency remarkable for its high incidence of invasive infections and autoimmune complications. Clin Infect Dis. 2015;61:e13–9.
50. Kelleher P, Misbah SA. What is Good's syndrome? Immunological abnormalities in patients with thymoma. J Clin Pathol. 2003;56:12–6.
51. Wang H-Y, Ma CA, Zhao Y, et al. Antibody deficiency associated with an inherited autosomal dominant mutation in TWEAK. Proc Natl Acad Sci U S A. 2013;110:5127–32.
52. Brue T, Quentien M-H, Khetchoumian K, et al. Mutations in NFKB2 and potential genetic heterogeneity in patients with DAVID syndrome, having variable endocrine and immune deficiencies. BMC Med Genet. 2014;15:139.

53. Chen K, Coonrod EM, Kumánovics A, et al. Germline mutations in NFKB2 implicate the noncanonical NF-κB pathway in the pathogenesis of common variable immunodeficiency. Am J Hum Genet. 2013;93:812–24.
54. Quentien M-H, Delemer B, Papadimitriou DT, et al. Deficit in anterior pituitary function and variable immune deficiency (DAVID) in children presenting with adrenocorticotropin deficiency and severe infections. J Clin Endocrinol Metab. 2012;97:E121–8.
55. Sadat MA, Moir S, Chun T-W, et al. Glycosylation, hypogammaglobulinemia, and resistance to viral infections. N Engl J Med. 2014;370:1615–25.
56. De Praeter CM, Gerwig GJ, Bause E, et al. A novel disorder caused by defective biosynthesis of N-linked oligosaccharides due to glucosidase I deficiency. Am J Hum Genet. 2000;66:1744–56.
57. Wiseman DH, May A, Jolles S, et al. A novel syndrome of congenital sideroblastic anemia, B-cell immunodeficiency, periodic fevers, and developmental delay (SIFD). Blood. 2013;122:112–23.
58. Chakraborty PK, Schmitz-Abe K, Kennedy EK, et al. Mutations in TRNT1 cause congenital sideroblastic anemia with immunodeficiency, fevers, and developmental delay (SIFD). Blood. 2014;124:2867–71.
59. Fabre A, Martinez-Vinson C, Goulet O, Badens C. Syndromic diarrhea/Tricho-hepato-enteric syndrome. Orphanet J Rare Dis. 2013;8:5.
60. Bozzetti V, Bovo G, Vanzati A, et al. A new genetic mutation in a patient with Syndromic diarrhea and Hepatoblastoma. J Pediatr Gastroenterol Nutr. 2013;57 https://doi.org/10.1097/MPG.0b013e31825600c4.
61. Quartier P, Bustamante J, Sanal O, et al. Clinical, immunologic and genetic analysis of 29 patients with autosomal recessive hyper-IgM syndrome due to activation-induced Cytidine Deaminase deficiency. Clin Immunol. 2004;110:22–9.
62. Durandy A, Kracker S. Immunoglobulin class-switch recombination deficiencies. Arthritis Res Ther. 2012;14:218.
63. Kracker S, Di Virgilio M, Schwartzentruber J, et al. An inherited immunoglobulin class-switch recombination deficiency associated with a defect in the INO80 chromatin remodeling complex. J Allergy Clin Immunol. 2015;135:998–1007.e6.
64. Gardès P, Forveille M, Alyanakian M-A, et al. Human MSH6 deficiency is associated with impaired antibody maturation. J Immunol. 2012;188:2023–9.
65. Stavnezer-Nordgren J, Kekish O, Zegers BJ. Molecular defects in a human immunoglobulin kappa chain deficiency. Science. 1985;230:458–61.
66. Snow AL, Xiao W, Stinson JR, et al. Congenital B cell lymphocytosis explained by novel germline CARD11 mutations. J Exp Med. 2012;209:2247–61.

Humoral Primary Immunodeficiency and Autoimmune and Inflammatory Manifestations

24

Aleš Janda and Marta Rizzi

24.1 Autoimmunity and Inflammatory Manifestations in Primary Immunodeficiencies [1–4]

Primary immunodeficiencies (PIDs) are inherited disorders that are caused by impaired immune responses. They belong to the group of rare diseases. The estimated prevalence of PIDs is 4–5/100.000 live births. The conditions are inherited in polygenic as well as monogenic trait. More than 300 genes involved in the pathogenesis of PIDs have been described. Originally, the PIDs were defined by increased susceptibility to recurrent, chronic, atypical, or severe infections. However, the underlying functional impairment of the innate and/or adaptive arms of the immune system may also lead to cancers and immune diseases as allergy, inflammation, and autoimmune diseases. Indeed, the defining features of many PIDs are the autoimmune and inflammatory (A/I) conditions with or without increased susceptibility to infections. While in other PIDs, A/I occur only in a subset of patients.

The apparent paradox of under- and over-function of the immune system leading to PID and autoimmunity can be overcome by the concept of immune dysregulation. It has been clearly established that the genetic defects that affect, for example, T- and B-cell development compromise not only the ability to generate a diversified repertoire of lymphocytes capable of recognizing multiple pathogens but also impinge on mechanisms of central and peripheral tolerance, hence favoring A/I

A. Janda (✉)
Faculty of Medicine, Centre for Paediatrics, Medical Center - University of Freiburg, Freiburg im Breisgau, Germany
e-mail: ales.janda@uniklinik-freiburg.de

M. Rizzi
Faculty of Medicine, Department of Rheumatology and Clinical Immunology and Center for Chronic Immunodeficiency, Medical Center-University of Freiburg, Freiburg im Breisgau, Germany
e-mail: marta.rizzi@uniklinik-freiburg.de

M. M. D'Elios, M. Rizzi (eds.), *Humoral Primary Immunodeficiencies*,
Rare Diseases of the Immune System, https://doi.org/10.1007/978-3-319-91785-6_24

manifestations. A number of immune-related genes have been shown to be involved both in development and tolerance. The accent on the dysregulation aspect is also highly relevant for the complex therapeutic approaches combining substitutional with immunosuppressive means.

24.2 Frequency of Autoimmune and Inflammatory Manifestations in Patients with Primary Immunodeficiencies [1]

A recent extensive analysis encompassing data on more than 2000 patients with PID in French national register [1] revealed that about a quarter of those patients suffer from at least one A/I condition. The manifestations spanned through all known A/I symptoms with autoimmune cytopenia being the most frequent one, followed in frequency by gastrointestinal disorders, skin ailments, and rheumatic conditions. About a third of the affected patients did experience more than one A/I manifestation. The relative risk of developing A/I manifestation was 3- to 14-fold higher in patients with PIDs compared to the normal population. The A/I manifestations occurred throughout the life; by the age of 50 years, 40% of the patients were affected. The A/I conditions affected patients suffering from all types of PIDs (CVID, other B-cell PID, T-cell PID, innate). However, the risk of their occurrence as well as the type of A/I differed. Patients with CVID and CID carried the highest risk of developing A/I. On the other hand, the T-cell defects predisposed the patients to the earlier manifestation of A/I. T-cell PIDs were more frequently associated with immune cytopenia and rheumatologic manifestations. Interestingly, allergy was the only independent A/I risk factor other than the type of PID. In contrast to the general population, the gender bias was not observed in PID patients: males and females were equally affected with A/I symptoms. Of note, there was a similar risk of developing A/I in patients with PIDs with inherent increased susceptibility to infections as in patients with PIDs that are characterized by autoimmunity and lymphoproliferation. This fact supports the hypotheses that A/I symptoms are integral part of PIDs. Early onset of infections as well as the PID treatment (e.g., IVIg substitution) did not affect frequency of A/I. It means that in PIDs, the repeated stimulation of immune system through infections does not lead to initiation of A/I conditions. Not surprisingly, the presence of A/I conditions negatively influenced the quality of life of the patients as well as their survival. A manifestation of A/I prior HSCT was associated with worse survival after hematopoietic stem cell transplantation.

24.3 Pathophysiological Mechanisms Leading to Autoimmunity and Chronic Inflammation in Patients with Primary Antibody Deficiency [1, 5, 6]

Based on the general pathogenic mechanisms leading to autoimmunity, the molecular defects leading to primary antibody deficiency (PAD) as well as to autoimmunity and/or chronic inflammation (A/I) may be sorted according to the impact on lymphocyte development: (1) defects of early lymphocyte maturation and central tolerance and (2) defects of peripheral lymphocytes activation or development. The first group includes defects that manifests in the bone marrow or the thymus; the second one encompasses defects affecting mature lymphocytes. A few critical steps in the development of mature B cells can be identified: B-cell activation, affinity maturation and class-switch of immunoglobulin receptors, and lymphocyte trafficking. Flawless interactions between lymphocytes (especially T and B cells) are essential prerequisite of successful maturation. A number of those steps take place within germinal center response.

The molecular defects leading to PAD and/or A/I manifestation can be sorted based on the disrupted steps within the B-cell development. Defects that are primarily characterized by defective antibody production are depicted in the Table 24.1 and Fig. 24.1. Immune dysregulation conditions in which antibody deficiency is observed only in subsets of patients are listed in Table 24.2 and Fig. 24.2.

Within the defects *in early lymphocytes maturation and central tolerance*, we can distinguish defect of *lymphocyte development in the bone marrow* and in the *thymus*. When the block in B-lymphocyte development is not complete but leaky, such as in XLA or in PI3KRI deficiency or in Omenn syndrome, caused by hypomorphic defects in the enzymes involved in immunoglobulin genes recombination (e.g., *RAG1* and *RAG2*) or in DNA repair processes (e.g., Artemis), the B and or T cells that are generated are oligoclonal. Due to their low frequency and an impaired natural selection process, the cells with autoreactive T or B receptors (TCR, BCR) may survive and clonally expand. The patients will have *lymphopenia* with impaired negative selection and central tolerance and plentifully available survival factors (e.g., BAFF). Hence, the autoreactive cells benefit from the lack of competition and can expand in the periphery. The defect in the thymic function leads to defective negative selection of self-reactive T cells. This disturbance might be caused by gross structural changes of thymus as in DiGeorge syndrome (impaired development of the third and fourth branchial pouches). As the T cells are important in B-cell peripheral maturation, the patients with DiGeorge syndrome have frequently hypogammaglobulinemia.

The second group of conditions in which hypogammaglobulinemia is associated with immune dysregulation is characterized by *defect in peripheral lymphocytes maturation and activation.* The mature (follicular) B cells that leave bone marrow are "antigen inexperienced." These cells must first undergo *activation* via the B-cell receptor (BCR). The activated cells move to the germinal center where they interact with T (follicular helper) cells. The *T-B cooperation* promotes the *affinity maturation* for the antigen and *class switch* (of the immunoglobulin gene) and further development into memory and immunoglobulin-producing cells (plasma cells). This occurs in the *germinal center* (GC) response. The B cells shuttle via chemokine signals between the dark and the light zone of the germinal center to complete their maturation. The chemokine signals control also relocation of the B cells once they are selected into memory compartment. Therefore, *cell trafficking* is an essential component of a functional germinal center response. Genetic defects disturbing any of these mechanisms may impinge on the production of high-affinity

Table 24.1 Primary antibody deficiency associated with autoimmunity and immune dysregulation

Disease	Affected gene and its function	Inheritance	Autoimmune/inflammatory manifestations	Other symptoms	Phenotype OMIM no.	Ref.
1. Early lymphocyte development and central tolerance						
XLA	*BTK*; a cytoplasmic tyrosine kinase activated by cross-linking of the BCR	XL	IBD, arthritis, cytopenia		300755	[10–12]
PI3KR1 deficiency	*PI3KR;* a kinase involved in signal transduction in multiple cell types. Complete loss of PI3K p85-alpha resulting in complete loss of B-cell development	AR	IBD, EN, JIA	Neutropenia	615214	[13, 14]
Thymoma with immunodeficiency (Good syndrome)	Unknown	Unknown	Myasthenia gravis, aplastic anemia, ITP, IBD, celiac disease, adrenal insufficiency, Addison's disease, alopecia, leukopenia, pemphigoid, vitiligo, RA, Sjögren's syndrome, chronic urticaria, PSC, AIHA, myelo-radiculitis	Pure red cell aplasia, lichen planus, limbic encephalitis	Not assigned	[15]
2. B-cell activation						
Activated PI3K-δ (APDS1)	*PIK3CD*; p100 subunit of PI3K	AD, GOF	AIHA, other autoimmune cytopenia, glomerulonephritis, exocrine pancreatic insufficiency, thyroiditis, arthritis, recurrent pericarditis, gastrointestinal nodular mucosal lymphoid hyperplasia, splenomegaly, lymphadenopathy	EBV-positive lymphoma	615513	[16]

PI3KR1 deficiency (APDS2)	*PIK3R1*, LOF; p85alpha subunit	AD, LOF (leading to activation to PI3K-δ)	AIHA, ITP, Evans syndrome, insulin-dependent diabetes, arthritis, autoimmune hepatitis, chronic eczema		616005	[17]
B-cell expansion with NFKB and T-cell anergy (BENTA)	*CARD11*, GOF; scaffold for NF-κB activity in the adaptive immune response	AD	Congenital B-cell lymphocytosis; splenomegaly, hepatomegaly, lymphadenopathy, autoimmunity, ITP, AIHA	B-cell lymphoma	616452	[18–20]
3. Affinity maturation and immunoglobulin class-switch recombination						
AID deficiency	*AICDA*	AR	Diabetes mellitus, arthritis, autoimmune hepatitis, hemolytic anemia, ITP, IBD, chronic uveitis, lymphadenopathy, and germinal centers		605258	[21–23]
UNG deficiency	*UNG*	AR	Lymphoproliferation		608106	[24]
MSH6	*MSH6*; part of mismatch repair machinery, DNA repair defect	AR	SLE, vitiligo	Early onset colorectal carcinoma	Not yet assigned	[25, 26]
4. Germinal center response						
CVID	Unknown	Variable	Polyclonal lymphoproliferation, autoimmune cytopenia, and/or granulomatous disease, IBD		Not assigned	[6, 27]
CD19 deficiency	*CD19*; transmembrane protein that amplifies signal through BCR	AR	Glomerulonephritis		613493	[28]

(continued)

Table 24.1 (continued)

CD81 deficiency	*CD81*; transmembrane protein that amplifies signal through BCR	AR	Glomerulonephritis		613496	[29]
TACI deficiency	*TNFRSF13B*; a TNF receptor family member found on B cells, it is receptor for BAFF and APRIL	AD/AR/complex	Lymphoproliferation; ITP, AIHA, diabetes mellitus, vitiligo, celiac disease, arthritis, autoimmune urticaria, autoimmune hepatitis, recurrent parotitis		240500	[30]
TWEAK deficiency	*TNFSF12*; TNF-related weak inducer of apoptosis	AD	ITP		Not yet assigned	[31]
NFKB2 deficiency	*NFKB2*; an essential component of the noncanonical NF-κB pathway	AD	Alopecia	Adrenal insufficiency	615577	[32]

Adapted from Picard et al. [2]

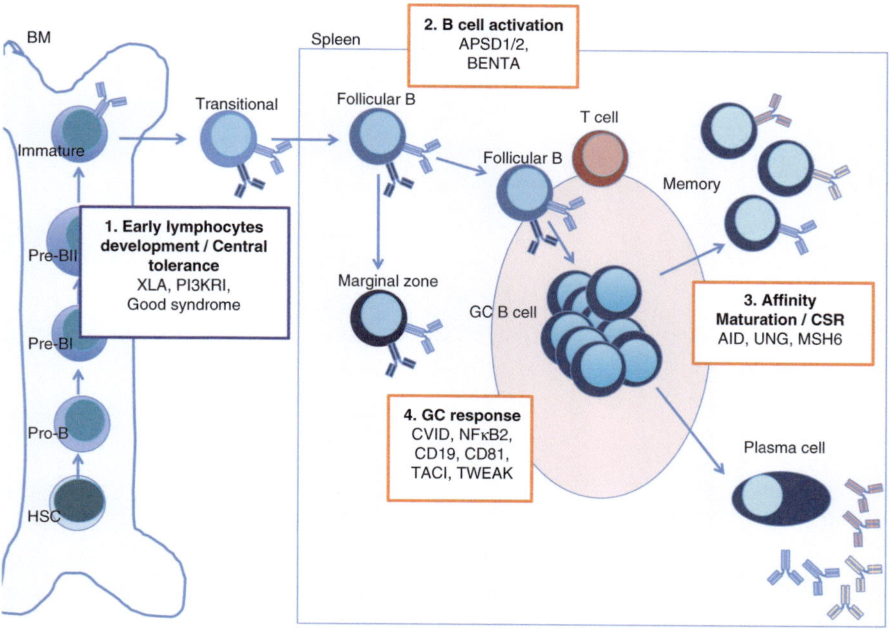

Fig. 24.1 Primary antibody deficiency associated with defect in B cell development and autoimmunity and immune dysregulation

class-switched antibodies, as well as their quality and their selection contributing to the risk of self-reactivity. Indeed, dysregulated *B-cell activation*, with hyperactivation of the BCR, has been discovered in CVID cohorts, as well as in patients suffering from other immune dysregulation syndromes (Figs. 24.1 and 24.2). In both groups hypogammaglobulinemia and A/I manifestations were present. B-cell activation is, for instance, affected by gain-of-function (GOF) mutations of B- or T-cell activation/effector molecules such as in APDS (activated PI3K-delta syndrome), in BENTA (B-cell expansion with NF-κB and T-cell anergy) or in PRKC-δ deficiency. When the signalling threshold of BCR is affected, the first phase of the immune response is disturbed, resulting in either disturbed selection of antibodies or their impaired production. Mutations in genes coding for component of the NF-κB pathway that is downstream of BCR signalling may also manifest with combination of humoral immunodeficiency and immune dysregulation, for example, mutations in genes coding for *MAP3K14*, *NEMO*, *IKBA*, or *BCL10*. Impairment of genes coding for proteins that are involved in cytoskeleton metabolism plays an important role in B-cell activation as well, as the cytoskeleton controls recruitment of signalling molecules into the lipid rafts and formation of immunological synapse. This is a case in defects in *WASP*, *DOCK2*, *DOCK8*, or *LRBA*. The cross talk between T and B cells is essential to maintain both antibody production and self-tolerance, and indeed, the defects in proteins involved in *T-B cooperation* can be associated with immune dysregulation and humoral immunity, as it is the case for deficiencies in CD40L, CD40, ICOS, CD27, and CTLA-4. One of the crucial roles of the T-cell signalling

Table 24.2 Primary immunodeficiency with autoimmunity and/or inflammatory manifestations as leading symptoms that may be associated with antibody deficiency

Disease	Affected gene and its function	Inheritance	Immunoglobulins	Autoimmune/inflammatory manifestation	Other clinical symptoms	Phenotype OMIM no.	Ref.
1. Early lymphocyte development and central tolerance							
Omenn syndrome	Hypomorphic mutations in: *RAG1*, *RAG2*, *Artemis*, *IL7RA*, *RMRP*, *ADA*, *DNA Ligase IV*, *IL2RG*, *AK2*, or genes associated with DiGeorge syndrome; some cases have no defined gene mutation	Variable	All isotypes ↓; IgE ↑	Multiple	Recurrent (severe) infections, erythroderma, eosinophilia	603554	[33, 34]
DiGeorge syndrome	Contiguous gene deletion in chromosome 22q11.2 or mutation of a gene within this deletion region, *TBX1*, encoding a transcription factor critical for development of thymus and adjacent embryonic structures	De novo haploinsufficiency or AD	All isotypes ↓/n	Cytopenia, arthritis, thyreoiditis, JIA, IBD	Hypoparathyroidism, conotruncal cardiac malformation, velopalatal insufficiency, abnormal facies, intellectual disability, and other abnormalities		[35, 36]

2. B-cell activation							
Wiskott-Aldrich syndrome	*WAS*; cytoskeletal protein important also for immune synapse	XL	IgM ↓; response to polysaccharides ↓; IgA, IgE ↑	IgA nephropathy, Henoch-Schönlein purpura, splenomegaly, IBD, dermatomyositis, AIHA, vasculitis, arthritis, eczema	Recurrent infections (bacterial, viral); thrombocytopenia with small platelets, lymphoma	300392	[37–39]
DOCK2 deficiency	*DOCK2*; required for RAC1 activation, actin polymerization, T-cell proliferation, chemokine-induced lymphocyte migration and NK-cell degranulation	AR	All isotypes ↓ /n; ↓ specific antibody response	IBD, thrombocytopenia	Infections (viral, bacterial, mycobacterial, opportunistic; vaccine strains)	616433	[39, 40]
DOCK8 deficiency	*DOCK8*; regulates actin cytoskeleton organization and STAT3 nuclear translocation	AR	IgM ↓; IgE ↑	AIHA, uveitis, SLE, arthritis, glomerulonephritis	Recurrent infections (extensive cutaneous viral and staphylococcal infections), severe atopy, eosinophilic esophagitis, malignancy	243700	[41]

(continued)

Table 24.2 (continued)

CARD11 deficiency	*CARD11*; a scaffold for NF-κB activity in the adaptive immune response	AR	All isotypes ↓	Splenomegaly, severe atopy, granulomatous inflammation, IBD, psoriasis, asthma	Recurrent infections (bacterial, *Pneumocystis jirovecii*, meningitis)	615206	[42, 43]
BCL10 deficiency	*BCL10*; encodes the B cell CLL/lymphoma 10 protein that forms a heterotrimer with Malt1and CARD family adaptors and plays a role in NF-κB signalling	AR	All isotypes ↓	IBD	Recurrent infections (bacterial, viral, fungal), epilepsy, leukoencephalopathy	616098	[44]
Anhidrotic ectodermal dysplasia with immunodeficiency, (NEMO/IKBKG deficiency)	*NEMO (IKBKG)*; modulator of NF-κB activation	XL	All isotypes ↓/n; IgM ↑/n; specific antibody response ↓; antibody response to polysaccharides ↓	IBD, AIHA	Recurrent infections (bacterial, mycobacterial, fungal), anhidrotic ectodermal dysplasia, conical teeth, variable defects of skin pigmentation	300291, 300584, 300301, 300640	[45]
Anhidrotic ectodermal dysplasia with immunodeficiency, (IKBA GOF)	*IKBA (NFKIAB)*; component of NF-κB pathway	AD	All isotypes ↓/n; IgM ↑/n; specific antibody response ↓	IBD, thyreoiditis, SLE, autoinflammation	Recurrent infections (bacterial, mycobacterial, fungal), anhidrotic ectodermal dysplasia, conical teeth, variable defects of skin pigmentation	612132	[46, 47]

NIK deficiency	*MAP3K14*; encoding NF-κB-inducing kinase	AR	All isotypes ↓	Granulomatous hepatitis, chronic diarrhea	Recurrent infections (bacterial, viral, BCG, *Cryptosporidium* spp.)	Not yet assigned	[48]
PRKC-δ/PKC-δ deficiency	*PRKCD*; member of the protein kinase C family, critical for regulation of cell survival, proliferation and apoptosis	AR	All isotypes ↓/n	SLE-like autoimmunity (nephrotic and antiphospholipid syndromes), hepatosplenomegaly, cytopenia, lymphoproliferation	Recurrent infections, EBV chronic infections	615559	[49]
3. Intercellular signalling (cooperation between T and B cells)							
CD40L deficiency	*TNFSF5*; needed for isotype switching and dendritic cell signalling; CD154, ligand for CD40	XL	IgM n/↑; other isotypes ↓	Cytopenia, hepatitis	Opportunistic infections, biliary tract, and liver disease	308230	[50]
CD40 deficiency	*TNFRSF5*; needed for isotype switching and dendritic cell signalling	AR	IgM n/↑; other isotypes ↓	Cytopenia, hepatitis	Opportunistic infections, biliary tract, and liver disease	606843	[50]
ICOS deficiency	*ICOS*; co-stimulatory molecule expressed on T cells	AR	All isotypes ↓	IBD, splenomegaly, psoriasis, arthritis, cytopenia, granulomas, eczema	Recurrent infections (mainly respiratory, gastrointestinal; rarely opportunistic), malignancy	607594	[51]

(continued)

Table 24.2 (continued)

XLP1	*SH2D1A*; adaptor protein regulating intracellular signalling	XL	All isotypes ↓/n	Vasculitis, lymphoid granulomatosis, lymphoproliferation, aplastic anemia	HLH, lymphoma, EBV susceptibility	308240	[52]
XLP2	*XIAP/BIRC4*; inhibitor of apoptosis	XL	All isotypes ↓/n	IBD, splenomegaly, lymphoproliferation, hepatitis	EBV infections, HLH	300635	[53]
CTLA4 deficiency	*CTLA4*; surface protein negatively regulating T cell activation	AD	All isotypes ↓/n	Cytopenia, IBD, type I diabetes, thyreoiditis, arthritis, psoriasis, uveitis, myasthenia gravis, lymphadenopathy, ILD, pulmonary fibrosis, splenomegaly	Malignancy	616100	[54]
LRBA deficiency	*LRBA*; may be involved in coupling signal transduction and vesicle trafficking to enable polarized secretion and/or membrane deposition of immune effector molecules	AR	IgA, IgG ↓	IBD, cytopenia, hepatosplenomegaly, thyroiditis, type I diabetes, atopy, ILD, uveitis, hepatitis, chronic urticaria	Recurrent bacterial and EBV infections	614700	[55]

CD27 deficiency	*TNFRSF7*; encoding TNF-R member superfamily required for generation and long-term maintenance of T cell immunity	AR	All isotypes ↓ (following EBV infection)	Lymphadenopathy, hepatosplenomegaly, uveitis, aplastic anemia, oral ulcers, eczema, chronic hepatitis	Clinical and immunologic features triggered by EBV infection; HLH, skin abscesses, lymphoma	615122	[56]
4. Germinal center response							
IL-21 deficiency	*IL21*; a type I cytokine produced by T cells and natural killer T cells that has pleiotropic actions on a wide range of immune and nonimmune cell types	AR	IgG ↓; IgE ↑	Severe early onset IBD, oral ulcers	Respiratory infections	615767	[57, 58]
IL-21R deficiency	*IL21R*; together with common-γ chain binds IL-21	AR	IgA, IgG ↓; IgE ↑	Hepatosplenomegaly, lymphadenopathy, discoid lupus	Recurrent infections (*Cryptosporidium* spp., *Pneumocystis* spp., mycobacterial, mainly respiratory), cholangitis	615207	[58, 59]

(continued)

Table 24.2 (continued)

STAT3 GOF	*STAT3*; transcription factor; the JAK-STAT signalling pathway transmits information from extracellular chemical signals to the nucleus resulting in DNA transcription and expression of genes involved in immunity, proliferation, differentiation, apoptosis, and oncogenesis	AD	IgG ↓	Type I diabetes, IBD, cytopenia, hypoparathyreoidismus, ILD, arthritis, lymphoproliferation	Recurrent infections	615952	[60, 61]
ALPS	*FAS (TNFRSF6)*, *FASLG (TNFSF6)*, *CASP10*, *CASP8*, *FADD;* components of FAS-signalling pathway regulating cell apoptosis and survival	AD/AR, somatic mutations	All isotypes ↓/n/↑	Cytopenia, arthritis, hepatosplenomegaly	Lymphoma	601859, 601859, 603909, 607271, 613759	[62]

Adapted from Picard et al. [2]

Abbreviations: *AD* autosomal dominant, *A/I* autoimmune and inflammatory (manifestations), *AID* activation-induced deaminase, *AIHA* autoimmune hemolytic anemia, *APECED* autoimmune polyendocrinopathy-candidiasis-ectodermal dysplasia syndrome, *APDS* activated PI3K-delta syndrome, *AR* autosomal recessive, *ALPS* autoimmune lymphoproliferative syndrome, *BAFF* B-cell activating factor, *BCR* B-cell receptor, *BENTA* B-cell expansion with NFKB and T-cell anergy, *BCG* Bacillus Calmette-Guérin, *BCR* B-cell receptor, *BCL10* B cell CLL/lymphoma 10, *BIRC4* baculoviral IAP repeat-containing protein 4, *BTK* Bruton's tyrosine kinase, *CASP 8/10* caspase 8/10, *CARD 11* caspase recruitment domain family member 11, *CMV* cytomegalovirus, *CSR* class-switch recombination, *CTLA4* cytotoxic T-lymphocyte antigen 4, *DOCK 2/8* dedicator of cytogenesis 2/8, *CVID* common variable immunodeficiency, *DMARD* disease-modifying antirheumatic drug, *EBV* Epstein-Barr virus, *EN* erythema nodosum, *FADD* FAS-associated death domain protein, *GC* germinal center, *GOF* gain-of-function, *ICOS* inducible co-stimulator, *IBD* inflammatory bowel disease, *IKBA* inhibitor of NF-κB-alpha, *IKBKG* inhibitor of nuclear factor kappa B kinase subunit gamma, *ILD* interstitial lung disease, *IPEX* immune dysregulation-polyendocrinopathy-enteropathy X-linked syndrome, *ITP* immune thrombocytopenia, *IVIg* intravenous immunoglobulin, *JIA* juvenile idiopathic arthritis, *HSCT* hematopoietic stem cell transplantation, *LRBA* lipopolysaccharide responsive beige-like anchor protein, *MAP3K13* mitogen-activated protein kinase 13, *LOF* loss-of-function, *n* normal, *MSH6* MutS, *E. coli*, homolog of, 6, *NEMO* nuclear factor-kappa B essential modulator, *NIK* NF-κB-inducing kinase, *OMIM* Online Mendelian Inheritance in Man (Database), *PAD* primary antibody deficiency, *PID* primary immunodeficiency, *PRKC/PKC* protein kinase C d, *PSC* primary sclerosing cholangitis, *RA* rheumatoid arthritis, *RAG (1,2)* recombination-activating gene (1,2), *RMRP* RNA component of mitochondrial RNA processing endoribonuclease, *SCIg* subcutaneous immunoglobulin, *SH2D1A* SH2 domain-containing protein 1A, *SHM* somatic hypermutation, *SLE* systemic lupus erythematosus, *STAT* signal transducer and activator, *TACI* transmembrane activator and CAML interactor, *TBX1* T-box transcription factor, *TCR* T-cell receptor, *NF-R* receptor for tumor necrosis factor, *TNFSF5* tumor necrosis factor superfamily 5, *TWEAK* TNF-related weak inducer of apoptosis, *UNG* uracil-DNA glycosylase, *XIAP* X-linked inhibitor of apoptosis protein, *XL* X-linked, *XLA* X-linked agammaglobulinemia, *XLP 1/2* X-linked lymphoproliferative syndrome 1/2

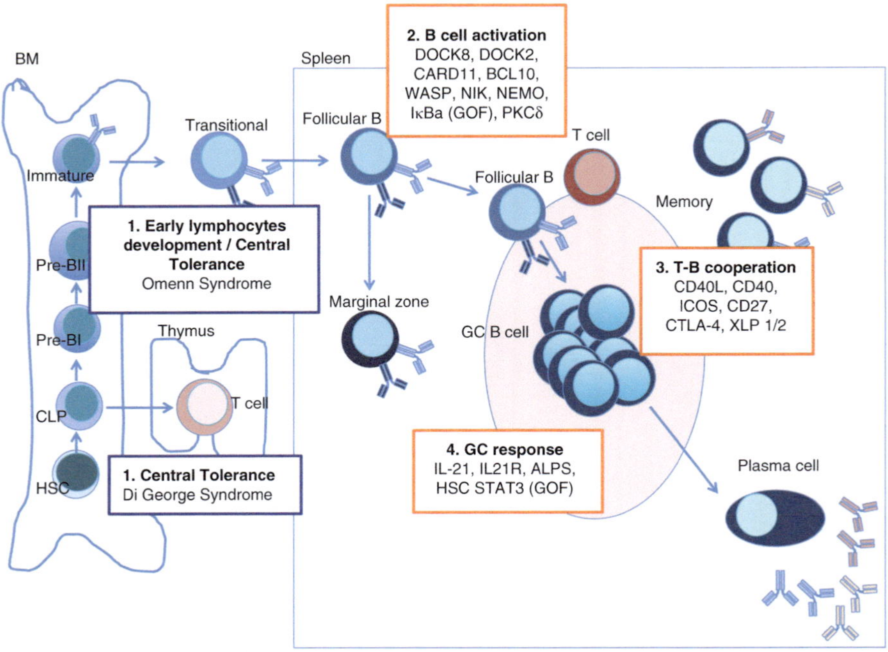

Fig. 24.2 Primary immunodeficiency with autoimmunity and/or inflammatory manifestations as leading symptoms that may be associated with defect in B-cell development and antibody deficiency

to B cells is inducing somatic hypermutation (SHM) and class-switch recombination (CSR), hence also the *defects in affinity maturation and CSR* such as genetic mutations in *AID*, or other genes involved in DNA repair such as *UNG* and *MSH6* are associated with both risk of autoimmunity and humoral immunodeficiency. The function of *GC response* is complex and requires a subtle modulation of signals mediated mainly by cytokines. Indeed, defect in cytokines (*IL21*), cytokine receptors (*IL21R*), or signalling (*STAT3* GOF) is correlated both with humoral immunodeficiency and autoimmune manifestations. The GC reaction requires also the elimination of self-reactive specificity and the positive selection of specific antibodies into the memory compartment. In this mechanism apoptosis and Fas-signalling play an important role. Mutations in *FAS* or in its downstream signalling are associated with autoimmune phenomena and in a proportion of patients with humoral immune deficiency.

There are other mechanisms leading to immune dysregulation that are not associated with primary defect in antibody-secreting function, and therefore in those cases, the immune dysregulation is not associated with hypogammaglobulinemia. Oppositely, in many of those conditions, a hypergammaglobulinemia has been described.

Within the defects of *central tolerance*, the APECED syndrome (autoimmune polyendocrinopathy-candidiasis-ectodermal dysplasia) is the most prominent representative. It is caused by defects in *AIRE*, gene expressed in medullary thymic epithelial cells encoding a transcription factor that enables expression of multiple tissue-specific antigens. This process is decisive for clonal deletion of the autoreactive T lymphocytes. Defects in this gene result in a clinically broad range of autoimmune manifestations. Defective *peripheral tolerance* is seen in IPEX (immune dysregulation, polyendocrinopathy, enteropathy, X-linked) syndrome. It is linked to the dysfunction of the transcription factor FOXP3, widely considered to be the master regulator of the regulatory T-cell lineage. It leads to the dysfunction of regulatory T cells and the subsequent autoimmunity. Further examples are defects associated with *increased type I interferon signature* that are caused by constituently increased interferon production or impairment of its degradation. The patients present most often with SLE-phenotype. Other examples are *defects of early complement components* (C1q, C1r/s, C2, C4, C3, C5-9) and *defective removal of cell debris* that are also associated with SLE-like clinical symptoms. The *congenital defects of phagocytes*, *defects in intrinsic*, *and innate immunity* and *autoinflammatory disorders* have no or only mild B-cell phenotype and tend to hypergammaglobulinemia.

Of note, there are a few defects in the B-cell development that are associated with hypogammaglobulinemia, in which no autoimmune or inflammatory phenomena have been described. This could be caused by complete block in B-cell development with no leaky phenotype. On the other side, the missing observation of A/I manifestation in these patients may be due to the low number of cases or the short observation period in case of the new defects.

24.4 Management of Patients with Primary Antibody Deficiency and Autoimmune or Inflammatory Symptoms [7–9]

The treatment of patients presenting with immunodeficiency as well as autoimmunity or chronic inflammation is challenging as it needs to preserve a balance between infection susceptibility and needs for immunosuppression.

The main pillar of the treatment of patients with antibody deficiency is the intravenous (IVIg) or subcutaneous (SCIg) *immunoglobulin substitution*. Apart from its obvious function of substituting the missing antibodies, the immunosuppressive feature of high dosing can be beneficial. Antibiotics, antiviral, and antifungal agents are frequently used in infection prophylaxis. Interestingly, there is no evidence that reduction of infection episodes contributes to the prevention of A/I manifestation in PIDs.

Steroids are a backbone of immune modulation in autoimmune diseases. Their application is, however, limited due to significant side effects. High-dose steroid therapy is lymphotoxic and may cause secondary hypogammaglobulinemia. Their application within PIDs is often restricted because of their broad immunosuppressive effect. Autoimmune cytopenia is the most frequent indication for their administration. In chronic granulomatous disease, steroids are successfully used to reduce granuloma formation due to hyperinflammation. Disease-modifying drugs (DMARDs), e.g., *methotrexate*, *hydroxychloroquine*, *ciclosporin A*, or *mycophenolate mofetil*, used ordinarily in rheumatology, are applied frequently to control the autoimmune or inflammatory symptoms within PID field, too. Those drugs reduce primarily the proliferation capacity as well as the activation of lymphocytes. They impair negatively the antibody response to antigen as well; however, they rarely cause hypogammaglobulinemia or significant increase in susceptibility to infections.

The most known representative of modern targeted therapy is *rituximab*. The depletion of B cells expressing CD20 has been first used in patients with B cell lymphomas; currently this approach inherited part of treatment of many autoimmune manifestations, especially autoimmune cytopenia. The therapeutic mechanism is based on the fact that B cells are crucial for elicitation of autoimmunity. Through elimination of all B cells, also the autoreactive cells are removed. During the repopulation it is expected that the B cells restore their tolerance to self and express non-autoreactive B-cell receptor (BCR). Nevertheless, rituximab has to be applied with caution, as a secondary antibody deficiency may be induced in predisposed individuals. The B-cell repopulation may be delayed or completely fail. This regeneration failure may damask underlying (beforehand undetected) B-cell development defect or worsen the existing one. Another surface molecule that can be specifically targeted is CTLA-4. This molecule plays an important role in interplay between T and B cells. It is a negative regulator of T-cell activation. Synthetic CTLA-4-Ig (*abatacept*) may dampen T-cell activation and reduce autoimmune and inflammatory symptoms. It is approved for usage in a number of rheumatic diseases. Its administration in the field of PID (e.g., CTLA-4 or LRBA deficiency) is, similarly as for the other targeted drugs, experimental. Inhibition of intracellular pathways can be executed via blockade of mTOR (e.g., *rapamycin* or *sirolimus*) or JAK-kinase (e.g., *baricitinib*). The immunomodulatory therapy emerge as a possible frontline therapy for PIDs with as well as without A/I manifestations.

Causative therapy in many PIDs as well as in autoimmune and inflammatory conditions is immune reconstitution via *hematopoietic stem cell transplantation* (HSCT) or *gene therapy*. Due to its still remarkable toxicity and risk of secondary hypogammaglobulinemia are those approaches reserved for the most severe cases.

24.5 Conclusion

Immunodeficiency, autoimmunity, and chronic inflammation are all caused by dysregulation of the immune system. The particular symptoms may overlap and in some cases require the same treatment, e.g., administration of immunomodulators. The clinical diagnosis of autoimmune symptoms in the context of primary antibody deficiency as well as the detection of underlying immunodeficiency in autoimmune diseases or chronic inflammatory conditions is troublesome. The presented overview of the overlapping phenotypes may serve to improved diagnostics and ease the application of targeted therapy in the indicated cases.

References

1. Fischer A, Provot J, Jais JP, et al. Autoimmune and inflammatory manifestations occur frequently in patients with primary immunodeficiencies. J Allergy Clin Immunol. 2016;140:1388–93. https://doi.org/10.1016/j.jaci.2016.12.978.
2. Picard C, Al-Herz W, Bousfiha A, et al. Primary immunodeficiency diseases: an update on the classification from the International Union of Immunological Societies Expert Committee for primary immunodeficiency 2015. J Clin Immunol. 2015;35:696–726. https://doi.org/10.1007/s10875-015-0201-1.
3. Allenspach E, Torgerson TR. Autoimmunity and primary immunodeficiency disorders. J Clin Immunol. 2016;36:57–67. https://doi.org/10.1007/s10875-016-0294-1.
4. Fodil N, Langlais D, Gros P. Primary immunodeficiencies and inflammatory disease: a growing genetic intersection. Trends Immunol. 2016;37:126–40. https://doi.org/10.1016/j.it.2015.12.006.
5. Grimbacher B, Warnatz K, Yong PFK, et al. The crossroads of autoimmunity and immunodeficiency: lessons from polygenic traits and monogenic defects. J Allergy Clin Immunol. 2016;137:3–17. https://doi.org/10.1016/j.jaci.2015.11.004.
6. Warnatz K, Voll RE. Pathogenesis of autoimmunity in common variable immunodeficiency. Front Immunol. 2012;3:1–6. https://doi.org/10.3389/fimmu.2012.00210.
7. Marciano BE, Holland SM. Primary immunodeficiency diseases: current and emerging therapeutics. Front Immunol. 2017;8:937. https://doi.org/10.3389/fimmu.2017.00937.
8. Azizi G, Ziaee V, Tavakol M, et al. Approach to the management of autoimmunity in primary immunodeficiency. Scand J Immunol. 2017;85:13–29. https://doi.org/10.1016/j.aller.2017.04.004.
9. Vignesh P, Rawat A, Singh S. An update on the use of immunomodulators in primary immunodeficiencies. Clin Rev Allergy Immunol. 2017;52:287–303. https://doi.org/10.1007/s12016-016-8591-2.
10. Pac MM, Bernatowska EA, Kierkuś J, et al. Gastrointestinal disorders next to respiratory infections as leading symptoms of X-linked agammaglobulinemia in children – 34-year experience of a single center. Arch Med Sci. 2017;2:412–7. https://doi.org/10.5114/aoms.2016.60338.
11. Barmettler S, Otani IM, Minhas J, et al. Gastrointestinal manifestations in X-linked Agammaglobulinemia. J Clin Immunol. 2017;37:287–94. https://doi.org/10.1007/s10875-017-0374-x.
12. Hernandez-Trujillo VP, Scalchunes C, Cunningham-Rundles C, et al. Autoimmunity and inflammation in X-linked agammaglobulinemia. J Clin Immunol. 2014;34:627–32. https://doi.org/10.1007/s10875-014-0056-x.
13. De La Morena M, Haire RN, Ohta Y, et al. Predominance of sterile immunoglobulin transcripts in a female phenotypically resembling Bruton's agammaglobulinemia. Eur J Immunol. 1995;25:809–15. https://doi.org/10.1002/eji.1830250327.
14. Conley ME, Dobbs AK, Quintana AM, et al. Agammaglobulinemia and absent B lineage cells in a patient lacking the p85α subunit of PI3K. J Exp Med. 2012;209:463–70. https://doi.org/10.1084/jem.20112533.
15. Jansen A, van Deuren M, Miller J, et al. Prognosis of Good syndrome: mortality and morbidity of thymoma associated immunodeficiency in perspective. Clin Immunol. 2016;171:12–7. https://doi.org/10.1016/j.clim.2016.07.025.

16. Coulter TI, Chandra A, Bacon CM, et al. Clinical spectrum and features of activated phosphoinositide 3-kinase δ syndrome: a large patient cohort study. J Allergy Clin Immunol. 2017;139:597–606.e4. https://doi.org/10.1016/j.jaci.2016.06.021.
17. Elkaim E, Neven B, Bruneau J, et al. Clinical and immunologic phenotype associated with activated phosphoinositide 3-kinase δ syndrome 2: a cohort study. J Allergy Clin Immunol. 2016;138:210–218.e9. https://doi.org/10.1016/j.jaci.2016.03.022.
18. Buchbinder D, Stinson JR, Nugent DJ, et al. Mild B-cell lymphocytosis in patients with a CARD11 C49Y mutation. J Allergy Clin Immunol. 2015;136:819–821.e1. https://doi.org/10.1016/j.jaci.2015.03.008.
19. Brohl AS, Stinson JR, Su HC, et al. Germline CARD11 mutation in a patient with severe congenital B cell lymphocytosis. J Clin Immunol. 2015;35:32–46. https://doi.org/10.1007/s10875-014-0106-4.
20. Snow AL, Xiao W, Stinson JR, et al. Congenital B cell lymphocytosis explained by novel germline CARD11 mutations. J Exp Med. 2012;209:2247–61. https://doi.org/10.1084/jem.20120831.
21. Revy P, Muto T, Levy Y, et al. Activation-Induced Cytidine Deaminase (AID) Deficiency Causes the Autosomal Recessive Form of the Hyper-IgM Syndrome (HIGM2). Cell. 2000;102:565–75. https://doi.org/10.1016/S0092-8674(00)00079-9.
22. Quartier P, Bustamante J, Sanal O, et al. Clinical, immunologic and genetic analysis of 29 patients with autosomal recessive hyper-IgM syndrome due to activation-induced cytidine deaminase deficiency. Clin Immunol. 2004;110:22–9. https://doi.org/10.1016/j.clim.2003.10.007.
23. Durandy A, Cantaert T, Kracker S, Meffre E. Potential roles of activation-induced cytidine deaminase in promotion or prevention of autoimmunity in humans. Autoimmunity. 2013;46:148–56. https://doi.org/10.3109/08916934.2012.750299.
24. Imai K, Slupphaug G, Lee W-I, et al. Human uracil–DNA glycosylase deficiency associated with profoundly impaired immunoglobulin class-switch recombination. Nat Immunol. 2003;4:1023–8. https://doi.org/10.1038/ni974.
25. Gardes P, Forveille M, Alyanakian M-A, et al. Human MSH6 deficiency is associated with impaired antibody maturation. J Immunol. 2012;188:2023–9. https://doi.org/10.4049/jimmunol.1102984.
26. Rahner N, Höefler G, Högenauer C, et al. Compound heterozygosity for two MSH6 mutations in a patient with early onset colorectal cancer, vitiligo and systemic lupus erythematosus. Am J Med Genet A. 2008;146A:1314–9. https://doi.org/10.1002/ajmg.a.32210.
27. Feuille EJ, Anooshiravani N, Sullivan KE, et al. Autoimmune cytopenias and associated conditions in CVID: a report from the USIDNET registry. J Clin Immunol. 2018;38:28–34. https://doi.org/10.1007/s10875-017-0456-9.
28. Vince N, Boutboul D, Mouillot G, et al. Defects in the CD19 complex predispose to glomerulonephritis, as well as IgG1 subclass deficiency. J Allergy Clin Immunol. 2011;127:538–541.e5. https://doi.org/10.1016/j.jaci.2010.10.019.
29. van Zelm MC, Smet J, Adams B, et al. CD81 gene defect in humans disrupts CD19 complex formation and leads to antibody deficiency. J Clin Invest. 2010;120:1265–74. https://doi.org/10.1172/JCI39748.
30. Salzer U, Bacchelli C, Buckridge S, et al. Relevance of biallelic versus monoallelic TNFRSF13B mutations in distinguishing disease-causing from risk-increasing TNFRSF13B variants in antibody deficiency syndromes. Blood. 2009;113:1967–76. https://doi.org/10.1182/blood-2008-02-141937.
31. Wang H-Y, Ma CA, Zhao Y, et al. Antibody deficiency associated with an inherited autosomal dominant mutation in TWEAK. Proc Natl Acad Sci. 2013;110:5127–32. https://doi.org/10.1073/pnas.1221211110.
32. Chen K, Coonrod EM, Kumánovics A, et al. Germline mutations in NFKB2 implicate the noncanonical NF-κB pathway in the pathogenesis of common variable immunodeficiency. Am J Hum Genet. 2013;93:812–24. https://doi.org/10.1016/j.ajhg.2013.09.009.

33. Villa A, Notarangelo LD, Roifman CM. Omenn syndrome: inflammation in leaky severe combined immunodeficiency. J Allergy Clin Immunol. 2008;122:1082–6. https://doi.org/10.1016/j.jaci.2008.09.037.
34. Niehues T, Perez-Becker R, Schuetz C. More than just SCID—the phenotypic range of combined immunodeficiencies associated with mutations in the recombinase activating genes (RAG) 1 and 2. Clin Immunol. 2010;135:183–92. https://doi.org/10.1016/j.clim.2010.01.013.
35. Patel K, Akhter J, Kobrynski L, et al. Immunoglobulin deficiencies: the B-lymphocyte side of DiGeorge syndrome. J Pediatr. 2012;161:950–3. https://doi.org/10.1016/j.jpeds.2012.06.018.
36. McLean-Tooke A, Spickett GP, Gennery AR. Immunodeficiency and autoimmunity in 22q11.2 deletion syndrome. Scand J Immunol. 2007;66:1–7. https://doi.org/10.1111/j.1365-3083.2007.01949.x.
37. Candotti F. Clinical manifestations and pathophysiological mechanisms of the Wiskott-Aldrich syndrome. J Clin Immunol. 2018;38:13–27. https://doi.org/10.1007/s10875-017-0453-z.
38. Massaad MJ, Ramesh N, Geha RS. Wiskott-Aldrich syndrome: a comprehensive review. Ann N Y Acad Sci. 2013;1285:26–43. https://doi.org/10.1111/nyas.12049.
39. Burns SO, Zarafov A, Thrasher AJ. Primary immunodeficiencies due to abnormalities of the actin cytoskeleton. Curr Opin Hematol. 2017;24:16–22. https://doi.org/10.1097/MOH.0000000000000296.
40. Dobbs K, Domínguez Conde C, Zhang S-Y, et al. Inherited DOCK2 deficiency in patients with early-onset invasive infections. N Engl J Med. 2015;372:2409–22. https://doi.org/10.1056/NEJMoa1413462.
41. Biggs CM, Keles S, Chatila TA. DOCK8 deficiency: insights into pathophysiology, clinical features and management. Clin Immunol. 2017;181:75–82. https://doi.org/10.1016/j.clim.2017.06.003.
42. Stepensky P, Keller B, Buchta M, et al. Deficiency of caspase recruitment domain family, member 11 (CARD11), causes profound combined immunodeficiency in human subjects. J Allergy Clin Immunol. 2013;131:477–485.e1. https://doi.org/10.1016/j.jaci.2012.11.050.
43. Dadi H, Jones TA, Merico D, et al. Combined immunodeficiency and atopy caused by a dominant negative mutation in caspase activation and recruitment domain family member 11 (CARD11). J Allergy Clin Immunol. 2017;141:1818. https://doi.org/10.1016/j.jaci.2017.06.047.
44. Feyder M, Goff L. Inherited BCL10 deficiency impairs hematopoietic and nonhematopoietic immunity. J Clin Invest. 2014;124:5239–48. https://doi.org/10.1172/JCI77493.
45. Fusco F, Pescatore A, Conte MI, et al. EDA-ID and IP, two faces of the same coin: how the same IKBKG/NEMO mutation affecting the NF-κB pathway can cause immunodeficiency and/or inflammation. Int Rev Immunol. 2015;34:445–59. https://doi.org/10.3109/08830185.2015.1055331.
46. Petersheim D, Massaad MJ, Lee S, et al. Mechanisms of genotype-phenotype correlation in autosomal dominant anhidrotic ectodermal dysplasia with immune deficiency canonical NF-κB pathway non-canonical NF-κB pathway. J Allergy Clin Immunol. 2017;141:1060. https://doi.org/10.1016/j.jaci.2017.05.030.
47. Boisson B, Puel A, Picard C, Casanova JL. Human IκBα gain of function: a severe and syndromic immunodeficiency. J Clin Immunol. 2017;37:397–412. https://doi.org/10.1007/s10875-017-0400-z.
48. Willmann KL, Klaver S, Do UF, et al. Biallelic loss-of-function mutation in NIK causes a primary immunodeficiency with multifaceted aberrant lymphoid immunity. Nat Commun. 2014;5:5360. https://doi.org/10.1038/ncomms6360.
49. Salzer E, Santos-Valente E, Keller B, et al. Protein kinase C δ: a gatekeeper of immune homeostasis. J Clin Immunol. 2016;36:631–40. https://doi.org/10.1007/s10875-016-0323-0.
50. Jesus AA, Duarte AJS, Oliveira JB. Autoimmunity in hyper-IgM syndrome. J Clin Immunol. 2008;28:62–6. https://doi.org/10.1007/s10875-008-9171-x.
51. Schepp J, Chou J, Skrabl-Baumgartner A, et al. 14 years after discovery: clinical follow-up on 15 patients with inducible co-stimulator deficiency. Front Immunol. 2017;8:964. https://doi.org/10.3389/fimmu.2017.00964.

52. Tangye SG. XLP: clinical features and molecular etiology due to mutations in SH2D1A encoding SAP. J Clin Immunol. 2014;34:772–9. https://doi.org/10.1007/s10875-014-0083-7.
53. Aguilar C, Latour S. X-linked inhibitor of apoptosis protein deficiency: more than an X-linked lymphoproliferative syndrome. J Clin Immunol. 2015;35:331–8. https://doi.org/10.1007/s10875-015-0141-9.
54. Verma N, Burns SO, Walker LSK, Sansom DM. Immune deficiency and autoimmunity in patients with CTLA-4 (CD152) mutations. Clin Exp Immunol. 2017;190:1–7. https://doi.org/10.1111/cei.12997.
55. Gámez-Díaz L, August D, Stepensky P, et al. The extended phenotype of LPS-responsive beige-like anchor protein (LRBA) deficiency. J Allergy Clin Immunol. 2016;137:223–30. https://doi.org/10.1016/j.jaci.2015.09.025.
56. Alkhairy OK, Perez-Becker R, Driessen GJ, et al. Novel mutations in TNFRSF7/CD27: clinical, immunologic, and genetic characterization of human CD27 deficiency. J Allergy Clin Immunol. 2015;136:703–712.e10. https://doi.org/10.1016/j.jaci.2015.02.022.
57. Salzer E, Kansu A, Sic H, et al. Early-onset inflammatory bowel disease and common variable immunodeficiency–like disease caused by IL-21 deficiency. J Allergy Clin Immunol. 2014;133:1651–1659.e12. https://doi.org/10.1016/j.jaci.2014.02.034.
58. Kotlarz D, Ziętara N, Milner JD, Klein C. Human IL-21 and IL-21R deficiencies. Curr Opin Pediatr. 2014;26:704–12. https://doi.org/10.1097/MOP.0000000000000160.
59. Kotlarz D, Ziętara N, Uzel G, et al. Loss-of-function mutations in the IL-21 receptor gene cause a primary immunodeficiency syndrome. J Exp Med. 2013;210:433–43. https://doi.org/10.1084/jem.20111229.
60. De Bruin AM, Voermans C, Nolte MA. Impact of interferon-g on hematopoiesis. Blood. 2014;124:2479–86. https://doi.org/10.1182/blood-2014-04.
61. Lorenzini T, Dotta L, Giacomelli M, et al. STAT mutations as program switchers: turning primary immunodeficiencies into autoimmune diseases. J Leukoc Biol. 2017;101:29–38. https://doi.org/10.1189/jlb.5RI0516-237RR.
62. Bride K, Teachey D. Autoimmune lymphoproliferative syndrome: more than a FAScinating disease. F1000Research. 2017;6:1928. https://doi.org/10.12688/f1000research.11545.1.

Chest Complications in Patients with Primary Antibody Deficiency Syndromes (PADS)

25

Helen M. Chapel, Consuelo Anzilotti, and Smita Y. Patel

25.1 Which Primary Antibody Deficiencies (PADS) Are Complicated by Chest Involvement?

Primary antibody deficiency syndromes (PADS) are a heterogeneous group of primary immune disorders involving only failure of antibody production (B cell failure) and not cell-mediated (T cell failure) failure, though a few innate defects are linked to antibody failure [1–3]. rAntibody failure results in recurrent or severe bacterial infections due to the inability to mount specific antibody responses and consequentially subnormal serum immunoglobulin levels [4]. The most commonly occurring of these symptomatic conditions are the common variable immunodeficiency disorders (CVID) with a prevalence of approximately 1:25,000–1:50,000 in a general population and the less common agammaglobulinemia due to mutations in the Bruton tyrosine kinase gene (*BTK*)—known as X-linked agammaglobulinemia (XLA) (Chap. 3)—or other rare genes causing B cell failure [5]. Mutations in genes involved in class switch recombination also result in B cell failure and poor IgG and IgA production but are accompanied with T cell abnormalities (Chap. 15) and so are not strictly PADS but combined immune deficiencies (CIDs). Other syndromes, some undefined and of varying severity, including partial antibody deficiencies due to missing or low levels of IgG subclasses, make up the rest of these symptomatic diseases (Chap. 17). Selective IgA deficiency (SIgAD) alone is usually asymptomatic (Chap. 16). With the exception of SIgAD, primary antibody failure syndromes result in recurrent bacterial infections of the respiratory tract and, if these are severe or prolonged infections, risk bronchiectasis. Non-infective complications, such as

H. M. Chapel, MA. MD. FRCP. FRCPath (✉) · C. Anzilotti, MD. PhD · S. Y. Patel, MBBS. BSc. MRCP. FRCPath. PhD
Primary Immunodeficiency Unit, Experimental Medicine, Nuffield Department of Medicine, John Radcliffe Hospital, University of Oxford, Oxford, UK
e-mail: helen.chapel@ndm.ox.ac.uk

M. M. D'Elios, M. Rizzi (eds.), *Humoral Primary Immunodeficiencies*,
Rare Diseases of the Immune System, https://doi.org/10.1007/978-3-319-91785-6_25

interstitial lung diseases, do not seem to be features of undefined PADs or IgA with IgG subclass deficiencies, other partial IgG deficiencies, or specific antibody deficiencies (SPAD) unless these progress to more severe defined CIDs [6].

25.2 Why Consider Chest Diseases?

The morbidity of recurrent bacterial chest infections is considerable in any population but is a cause of significant problems and mortality in those with primary antibody failure, particularly those in the more severe end of the spectrum, namely, CVIDs and XLA [7–10]. Airway infections are predominantly caused by encapsulated bacteria and can lead to persistent structural lung disease such as bronchiectasis, significantly after pneumonia in CVID patients [8]. The presence of bronchiectasis is strongly associated with mortality in both CVIDs and XLA [11, 12]. Deaths from bacterial infection are much reduced since the advent of appropriate immunoglobulin replacement therapy [11, 13].

In addition, around 15% of CVID patients suffer interstitial lung diseases that are not associated with bacterial infections, CMV, EBV, or HHV8, though the exact nature of these complications remains unknown [14]. These are usually persistent and a cause of death due to respiratory failure or infection in about half the patients. Although bacterial infections, including those in the chest, can be largely prevented with adequate immunoglobulin (Ig) replacement [11, 15, 16], interstitial lung diseases are of unknown etiology and variable histology, and treatment remains controversial.

This chapter reviews the frequency and types of chest infections, the organisms involved and appropriate therapies, the resulting bronchiectasis in some but not all PAD patients, and how to detect this. In addition we examine the interstitial lung diseases associated with CVID patients, how to investigate and classify these, and then how to consider treatment.

25.3 Chest Infections

The frequency of upper and lower tract infections in the two most common forms of symptomatic antibody failure, namely, XLA and CVID, is >98% in untreated patients. In those with less severe antibody deficiency, the frequency is unknown since there are no screening programs for IgG subclass deficiencies or specific antibody deficiencies, though anecdotal data suggests a small, selected proportion of such patients not only have recurrent chest and/or sinus infections but do respond to immunoglobulin replacement. In our experience these patients do not progress to interstitial lung diseases (ILD), though there is some data on ILD of unknown cause in a few patients with IgG subclass deficiencies [17]; whether or not this is related to recurrent infections and is therefore preventable remains unknown. Our data suggests that specific antibody deficiency (SAD) seems to presage more complex PID eventually [6].

Respiratory infections may result in bronchitis or pneumonia in the lower tract. The pathogens found most commonly are the encapsulated pyogenic bacteria, such as *Haemophilus influenzae*, *Streptococcus pneumoniae*, or *Staphylococcus,* though other organisms frequently cause infections at other sites. Rhinoviral infections are often prolonged prior to Ig therapy and may result in secondary bacterial infections in the chest. Fungi and respiratory viruses do not usually cause primary infections in patients with pure antibody failure.

Prompt antibiotics for these particular organisms, including longer courses and higher doses, are the mainstay of treatment for chest infections, in addition to prophylaxis with Ig. Microbial cultures for persistent infections, with antibiotic sensitivities, are required since organisms may often be resistant. Antibiotics with good mucosal penetration, such as azithromycin, are particularly useful for both therapy and prophylaxis (though actual evidence in unspecified PAD patients is sparse). It is helpful for patients to recognize incipient infection and to have antibiotics at home so that prompt treatment can begin at once.

Prophylactic replacement Ig reduces the frequency of all infections, including those in the chest. The Oxford data showed a reduction of all bacterial infections in 90 patients following individualized Ig replacement, to a rate of 0.02 pneumonias/patient year. Persistent infections were due to 9 patients of whom 5 were also receiving immunosuppressive drugs [11]. This data was supported by the meta-analysis of Orange et al. [15] and the information from Quinti and colleagues [18]. The Italian group showed that risk factors for pneumonia post Ig therapy include a persistently low serum IgG level (<4 g/L), low levels of IgA at diagnosis (<0.07 g/L), and bronchiectasis in CVID patients and bronchiectasis alone in XLA.

Ig therapy also reduces inflammation when used in immunomodulatory doses, though whether or not this occurs with lower replacement doses remains speculative. Prophylactic antibiotics are used in patients with severe structural damage whether due to bronchiectasis or ILD, but these patients do run the risk of resistant bacteria, so limiting the usage to patients with frequent significant infections in high-risk periods (such as winter) or rotating antibiotics are helpful strategies, though evidence is limited.

25.4 Bronchiectasis

The causes of bronchiectasis in the general population include severe infections such as pneumonia, childhood illnesses such as whooping cough and measles (now rare since widespread immunization), complications of allergy such as allergic bronchopulmonary aspergillosis, cystic fibrosis, or rare ciliary abnormalities. Smoking predisposes to bronchiectasis as well as COPD [19]. However in PAD patients, bronchiectasis is strongly associated with repeated or severe chest infections [11], though the possible contribution of smoking to bronchiectasis is not always noted in PID databases.

Not all PAD patients suffer from bronchiectasis [20]. The prevalence of bronchiectasis in PAD patients varies with the type of disease, age of the patient, geographical location, time of disease progression, and dose of Ig replacement; even in the CVID group, different centers report different percentages of patients with bronchiectasis [8]. In CVID patients this ranges from 27 to 60%, whereas in boys with

XLA, the figure is higher, between 60 and 90% [9, 21]. The precise figures for IgG subclass deficiencies or SIgAD are unknown, but bronchiectasis is unusual.

Structural damage is an infection-related complication. In CVID patients, there is a significant association of bronchiectasis with previous pneumonia but no association between bronchiectasis and the disease-related complications of CVID, i.e., cytopenias or lymphoproliferation. Lucas et al. [11] found no association in their study between bronchiectasis and low IgG or IgA levels at diagnosis, but with the Italian data [18], that of Litzman et al. [22], and in Brazil [23], there were significant associations between low IgA and bronchiectasis; these study populations had a higher prevalence of bronchiectasis than in the northern European patients, and more patients in those cohorts were smokers.

Early detection of the presence of structural lung disease is essential to ensure the correct dose of replacement Ig in order to prevent breakthrough infections, as well as setting up monitoring for progression. Persistent cough and sputum production are standard clinical signs but are not always reliable [21]. Chest X-ray (CXR) is a relatively insensitive method of detection for bronchiectasis as are pulmonary function tests (PFT) [24]. A normal lung function ($FEV_1 > 80\%$ predicted) does not preclude the presence of bronchiectasis; 59% of the patients with a normal lung function had bronchiectasis in a recent European study [21].

Imaging techniques, in particular high resolution computed tomography (HRCT), are considered the gold standard for diagnosing structural lung diseases [25]. Bronchial wall thickening, mucus plugging, and atelectasis are features of bronchiectasis. The difficulties of providing a standardized evaluation of chest CT scans in antibody deficiencies, in order to determine the exact prevalence, severity, and progression of this important infection-related complication, have been emphasized in a recent multicenter study in Europe [21]. Recently standards have been described and these should be universal [26]. Two groups have investigated magnetic resonance imaging (MRI) as an alternative that causes less radiation damage [27, 28], but there are no long-term studies for this type of monitoring as yet.

Management of bronchiectasis in PAD patients is based on protocols for bronchiectasis of other etiologies, as there is insufficient evidence relating solely to PAD patients. It is sensible to use protocols for cystic fibrosis for severe bronchiectasis and to manage the patients in conjunction with a respiratory specialist with an interest in bronchiectasis, to ensure access to physiotherapy and nebulized treatments. It is also important to consider the role of standby and/or appropriate prophylactic antibiotics, particularly in the winter months, if breakthrough infections occur. Physiotherapy is essential, and breathing exercises/brisk activities (including learning a wind instrument for reluctant teenagers) help to keep the lungs dry. Monitoring infections depends on patients keeping careful note of all infections (in upper and lower respiratory tracts), for which patient diaries are often helpful. Liaison between primary care physicians and specialist immunologists, to reconsider the dose of Ig replacement if infections recur, is crucial [29].

Longitudinal data over 22 years shows that in order to prevent breakthrough bacterial infections, a higher starting dose of Ig at 0.6 g/kg/month is needed for bronchiectatic patients [11], compared with 0.4 g/kg/month for those without bronchiectasis. As in all patients, this can be modified later depending on the frequency of infections while on Ig therapy. There is speculation as to why bronchiectatic patients need more Ig. The hypothesis that lower levels of recycling of Ig via FcRn result in the need for higher replacement is based on the finding that levels of mRNA for FcRn were reduced in 28 bronchiectatic CVID patients [30]. Furthermore FcRn mRNA levels correlated with extent of bronchiectasis and with a rapid rate of IgG decline when measured on days 7 and14 after IVIg infusion.

25.4.1 Interstitial Lung Diseases

Interstitial lung diseases (ILD) are mainly late complications in patients with the lymphoproliferative phenotype of CVID [8]. Some rare patients with partial immunoglobulin deficiencies have been described with ILD [17], but this is uncommon and not described at all in XLA.

Not all patients present with symptoms [31, 32], which makes ILD difficult to detect making a baseline HRCT obligatory in CVID patients [33].

Whereas HRCT is useful for the diagnosis of bronchiectasis, CT features indicating ILD are variable, as shown in Fig. 25.1.

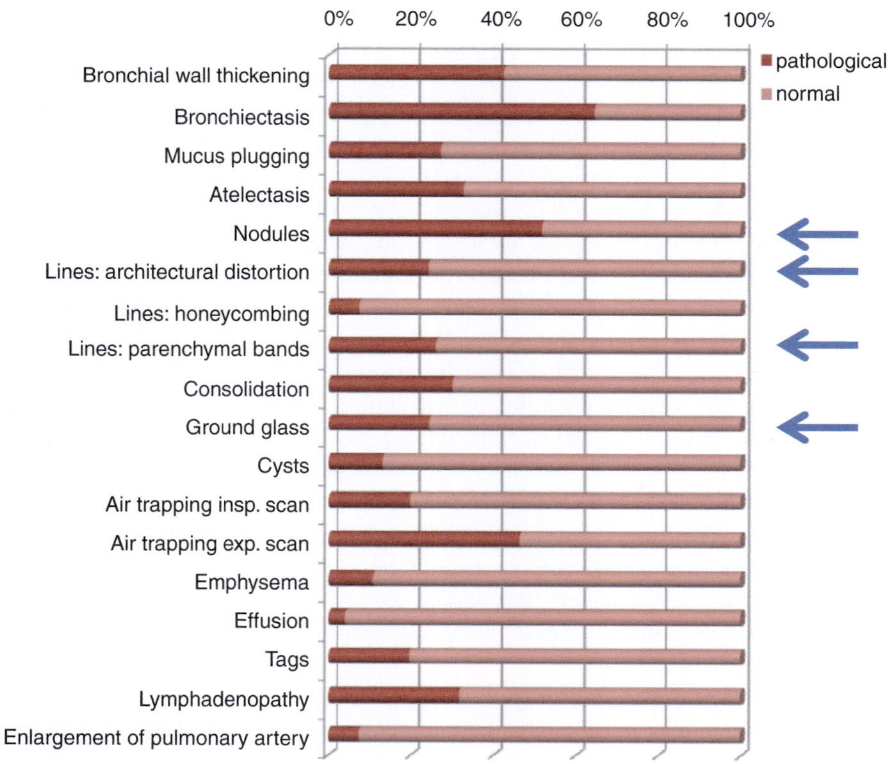

Fig. 25.1 HRCT findings in CVID patients in large study by European Chest Group [21]

The features chosen by the European Chest CT Group [21] *are those typically found in PAD patients* [23]. *The distribution of these features in CT images from 282 patients, from 15 immunodeficiency centers in 9 countries, was classified as in Fig. 25.1. The findings present in >20% of patients of 232 CVID patients are shown. Arrows indicate those that suggest ILD*

In relation to lymphoid interstitial pneumonitis, there may be architectural distortion due to lymphocytic infiltration, parenchymal bands, ground glass, or nodules.

Excessive lymphadenopathy in the chest suggests infection, lymphoid malignancy, or lymphoid dysregulation. It is important for the reporting radiologist to discuss the clinical history and to recommend biopsy if there are any positive findings.

Our findings (m/s in revision) show that there were no well-formed granulomata in our series of 29 patients biopsied between 1986 and 2016, while 11 had nodules on CT; hence we could rule out any correlation between CT nodules and the presence of granulomata. Since some patients have done well on follow-up, having recovered on corticosteroids alone and then weaned off such treatment, however, others (50%) have died within a few years of respiratory failure. There was no correlation between outcome and CT findings or histology in our CVID patients, suggesting that there is probably more than one pathology. CT must lead to biopsy—CT alone is not enough [14].

Attempts to define histological types of ILD by biopsy findings have been fraught. There is no international consensus on the reporting of chest biopsy results, and classifications are changing fairly rapidly as outcomes are slowly being related to findings. The American Thoracic Society/European Respiratory Society Classification of 2002 was updated in 2013 and has not yet been used in relation to CVID ILD, though a manuscript is in preparation (REF RICE et al.). Kokosi et al. [34] provide a useful descriptive account of the various histological patterns. However the other series of CVID patients have used different classifications. The Mount Sinai group [35] used that of Guinee [36], whereas the histological findings analyzed by Rao et al. [37] were based on the varying patterns found in their patients.

The initial term used [38] to describe ILD in CVID patients—granulomatous and lymphocytic interstitial lung disease (GLILD)—is a broad term in which GLILD is described as noninfectious, diffuse lung disease in CVID patients. The authors' initial view was that biopsies exhibited both granulomatous and lymphoproliferative histologies; however, in the Mount Sinai series [35] and in ours, well-formed granulomata are not found, and this term is now acknowledged to lack any prognostic or etiologic significance [37]. We also believe, with previous authors, that this "rather heterogeneous collection of pathologic findings and … insufficient prospective data on the natural history of this complication of CVID" is not useful, since the different histological patterns described and variations between the different admittedly small series reported so far suggest there is not a single common etiology of ILD in CVID patients.

We chose to divide the histological features in our study according to the Rao paper [37], that is, into unexplained inflammation, either bronchiolar or interstitial; lymphocytic infiltration, due predominantly to B cells or T cells; organized infiltration or diffuse sheets; granulomata; organizing pneumonia or interstitial fibrosis.

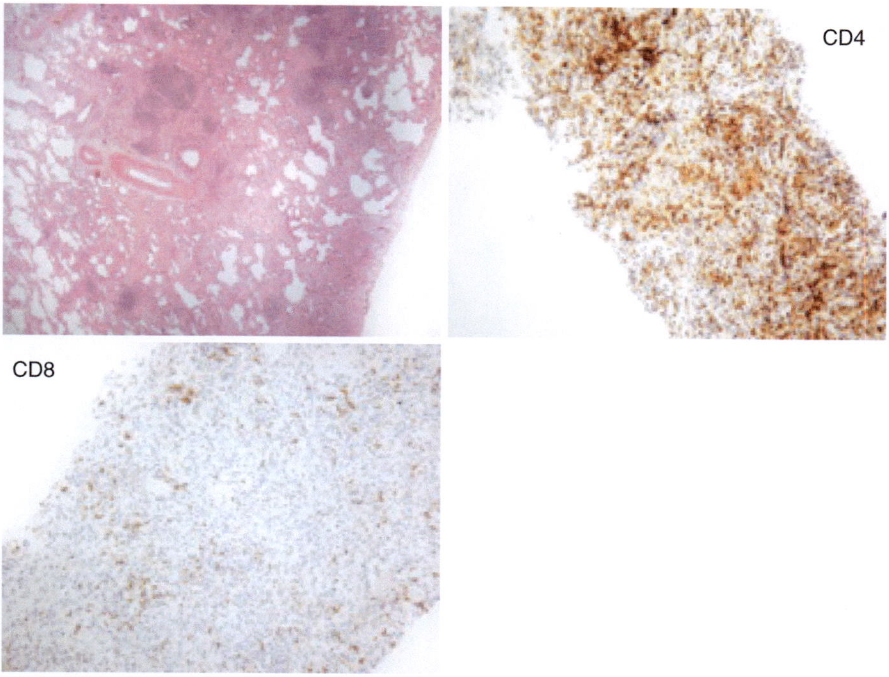

Fig. 25.2 Typical histology of lung biopsy in CVID-ILD showing infiltration of T cells and reduced lung spaces

The most common pattern in our patients and those of Maglione [35] and Rao et al. [37] is non-organized lymphocytic infiltration—see Fig. 25.2. In most cases these were T cells, with only 1/6 in the former paper and 2/16 showing B cell predominance in the latter.

In some of our patients, the infiltrating T cells were shown to be CD4 (as above), but other Oxford patients had an excess of CD8 cells on immunochemistry, suggesting a different etiology. Furthermore, although B cells are often present, only one in our series showed B cells in follicles with germinal centers (Fig. 25.3), as did 1/6 from Mount Sinai and 1/16 in Wisconsin.

However Rao also found granulomata in association with diffuse interstitial inflammation. We found no well-formed granuloma in 15 biopsies and only 1 poorly formed granuloma in 1 biopsy. This is in contrast with those found in the Wisconsin patients where the frequency of granulomata ranged from mild (1+) in 8 (50%) of 16 cases, moderate (2+) in 5 (31.25%) of 16 cases, and severe (3+) in 2 (12.5%) of 16 cases. Acid-fast bacilli and Gomori methenamine-silver stains were negative for microorganisms in all cases [37]. This suggests either different susceptibilities in our populations or different etiologies of ILD. Furthermore it is essential to review findings with clinicians, histopathologists, and radiologist together.

Only one series so far has included the patient outcomes, so we have considered this in our study. We looked at outcomes in relation to the histological findings (m/s

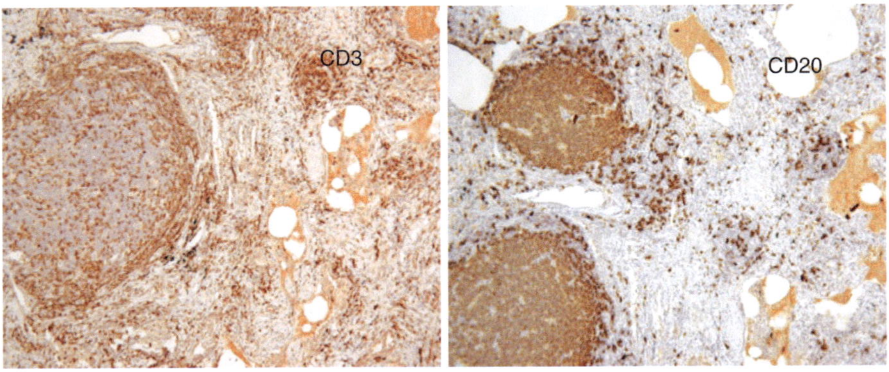

Fig. 25.3 Sparse CD3 T cells and an excess of B lymphocytes forming lymphoid follicles—courtesy of Natalja Kurjane

in revision). We had three patients who appear to have recovered ILD in that they have not received corticosteroid treatment for >6 years. We concluded that there are several different types of pathology, since not only were there different histological patterns but varying outcomes. At present it is difficult to provide a particular prognosis for an individual patient with ILD.

The question of predictive markers for ILD is important. Serum beta2 microglobulin levels are useful but not proven; raised levels indicate lymphocytic activity, and markedly increased levels suggest lymphoid hyperplasia [35, 39] in the absence of poor renal function. Reduced gas transfer also indicates ILD non-specifically and should be done regularly on all patients suspected of ILD, alongside HRCT. Not surprisingly, in a recent study [40], the presence of splenomegaly was found to be associated with ILD in CVID patients, confirming that this is part of the lymphoproliferative CVID phenotype. These authors also suggested that a history of ITP or AIHA, low serum IgA level, or percentage expansion of CD21low B cells might be useful to identify those at high risk. A case report in an atypical antibody-deficient child with ILD suggested that positron emission tomography (PET) and monitoring by CMV-specific immune response, beta2-microglobulin level, and IgM paraproteinemia were useful, but this child may have had a combined immune deficiency [41].

As with other inflammatory interstitial lung conditions, most CVID patients with ILD respond to corticosteroids in the first instance, with improvement in symptoms (if present) and less fatigue. Objectively, gas transfer levels also improve. How to treat with corticosteroids is important in patients whose immune systems are already compromised. High doses (up to 60 mg od) tapered rapidly (within 6–8 weeks) resulted, in our experience, in relapse of pre-existing HSV and candida infections. Changing to low doses (10 mg od), tapered slowly over 6–8 months, reduced these complications, and this protocol was just as effective at reducing fatigue and improving both HRCT findings and gas transfer. All patients should remain on replacement immunoglobulin therapy at 0.6 g/kg/month; there is no evidence at present that increasing the dose of therapeutic immunoglobulin is beneficial; however, those with an infective cause of ILD may respond on starting immunoglobulin [42].

A few patients have recovered from ILD, suggesting that an environmental cause such as covert infection may have accounted for rare cases of ILD in CVID patients [42]. However in most patients, ILD does relapse (suggesting immune dysregulation) and a steroid-sparing agent is required. Immunosuppressive agents used include azathioprine, particularly in patients with infiltrating T cells, rituximab for those with B cell follicles, or a combination of the two [38]. MMF has proved to be effective in some patients, both in our series and in a recent report [43]. Other agents have failed to improve ILD in CVID patients, including methotrexate (beware lung fibrosis anyway). What is the most satisfactory therapy in the long term—after steroids in the short term? Until we know the aetiologies, we have no idea, though MMF is widely used, currently it is yet unproven.

25.4.2 Other Lung Conditions

It is rare to diagnose lung cancer in antibody-deficient patients; given the infection load and repeated chest infections, patients are motivated not to smoke [44]. However, in early [17, 44] and in the more recent series [40, 44], there were predominance of smokers, many with COPD. In our series there were no smokers.

MALTOMA or NHL in the chest can be mistaken for ILD in CVID patients, in whom there is a high incidence of such malignancy anyway [25, 35]. These conditions are distinguishable on biopsy in experienced hands. MALTOMA may precede NHL by years or even decades (in two of our patients), and both are more likely to occur in CVID patients, particularly those with the cytopenic or lymphoproliferative clinical phenotypes.

Chronic infection with mycobacteria is rare in patients with pure antibody deficiency, though common in HIV and primary T cell deficiencies too. If nontuberculous mycobacteria are found, a possible T cell defect should be investigated.

25.5 Conclusions

In regard to chest complications in patients with antibody deficiency, it is really important to check the original diagnosis to ensure that the patient does not have a CID, since the chest problems are quite different in CIDs [45]. Adequate prophylactic replacement Ig has been shown to reduce the frequency of recurrent or severe chest infections, including those in the chest, and is essential for all proven antibody-deficient patients. Dosage depends on the severity of bronchiectasis and other complications and should be adjusted according to any breakthrough infections during lifelong monitoring. Prompt appropriate antibiotic treatment of breakthrough infections is essential.

Bronchiectasis as a complication of severe or recurrent pneumonia must be monitored with follow-up CT at appropriate intervals until newer imaging procedures with less radiation risk are proved to be helpful. Prophylactic antibiotics may be needed at times, and close liaison with a local chest physician is always recommended, as with ILD. Self-administered bronchial clearance will prevent many bacterial infections and help recovery of infection.

Detection of ILD in individual CVID patients is not dependent on symptoms, though new symptoms should lead to suspicion of ILD and therefore a repeat chest HRCT. Since symptoms are of little help in diagnosis of ILD, it is important to do a baseline HRCT at diagnosis, since patients with CT changes need a biopsy to confirm ILD and may require treatment to prevent progression. In particular, nodules on HRCT make biopsy obligatory—preferably by HRCT guidance—to determine the nature of these nodules which may represent actual or incipient lymphoid malignancy [33, 35] or ILD but are unlikely to be due to granuloma.

Pathologists should be asked to search for findings of ILD in particular when reporting of biopsy results in CVID patients, as well as searching for any evidence of bacterial or viral infections. Immunochemistry is essential as this may give a clue as to relevant etiology and therefore treatment; malignancy must be excluded though this requires expert interpretation [46, 47].

Lack of consistency on histological examination, other than lymphocytic infiltration, suggests different pathologies. It is essential to review findings with clinicians, radiologists, and pathologists together, for each individual patient. We also need international agreement on the histological reporting of these biopsies for comparison across databases [14]. Pathology may depend on when the biopsy is taken, so a standard protocol is needed, and patients have to be persuaded that this will enable early therapy that may provide a better outcome. Biopsies late in the disease course in five patients in our series showed interstitial fibrosis with or without organizing pneumonia; all patients died within 2 years, suggesting that these features may indicate poor prognosis.

As suggested by Harville [14], combining data sets internationally, with agreed protocols, is essential until prospective studies are set up. In the future it is hoped that genetic studies might indicate specific risk polymorphisms, but even with improved and earlier diagnosis, we still need to determine which patients require which therapeutic interventions for effective control of this often fatal complication.

With 4 images or tables

Drs *Natalja Kurjane and Uli Baumann have given permission.*

References

1. Bleesing J, Souto-Carneiro MM, Savage WJ, Brown MR, Martinez C, Yavuz S, Brenner S, Siegel RM, Horwitz ME, Lipsky PE, Malech HL, Fleisher TA. Patients with chronic granulomatous disease have a reduced peripheral blood memory B cell compartment. J Immunol. 2006;176:7096–8103.
2. Bacchelli C, Matharu K, Zarember KA, Marciano BE, Kuhns DB, Spalding C, Garofalo M, Dimaggio T, Estwick T, Huang CY, Fink D, Priel DL, Fleisher TA, Holland SM, Malech HL, Gallin JI. Cell activating factor (BAFF) is elevated in chronic granulomatous disease. Clin Immunol. 2013;148:258–64.
3. Kienzler A, van Schouwenburg PA, Taylor J, Marwah I, SharmA RU, Noakes C, Thomson K, Sadler R, Segal S, Ferry B, Taylor JC, Blair E, Chapel H, Patel SY. Hypomorphic function and somatic reversion of DOCK8 cause combined immunodeficiency without hyper-IgE. Clin Immunol. 2016;163:17–21.

4. Al-Herz W, Bousfiha A, Casanova JL, Chapel H, Conley ME, Cunningham-Rundles C, Etzioni A, Fischer A, Franco JL, Geha RS, Hammarström L, Nonoyama S, Notarangelo LG, Ochs HD, Puck JM, Roifman CM, Seger R, Tang MLK. Primary immunodeficiency diseases: an update on the classification from the International Union of Immunological Societies Expert Committee for Primary Immunodeficiency. Front Immunol. 2011;2:1–26.
5. Driessen G, van der Burg M. Primary antibody deficiencies. Eur J Pediatr. 2011;170:693–702.
6. Lopez-Granados E, Stacey M, Kienzler AK, Sierro S, Willberg CB, Fox CP, Rigaud S, Long HM, Hislop AD, Rickinson AB, Patel S, Latour S, Klenerman P, Chapel H. A mutation in X-linked inhibitor of apoptosis (G466X) leads to memory inflation of Epstein-Barr virus-specific T cells. Clin Exp Immunol. 2014;178:470–82.
7. Resnick ES, Moshier EL, Godbold JH, Cunningham-Rundles C. Morbidity and mortality in common variable immune deficiency over 4 decades. Blood. 2012;119(7):1650–7.
8. Chapel H, Lucas M, Lee M, Bjorkander J, Webster D, Grimbacher B, Fieschi C, Thon V, Abedi MR, Hammarstrom L. Common variable immunodeficiency disorders: division into distinct clinical phenotypes. Blood. 2008;112:277–86.
9. Plebani A, Soresina A, Rondelli R, Amato G, Azzari C, Cardinale F, Cazzola G, Consolini R, De Mattia D, Dell'Erba G, Duse M, Fiorini M, Martino S, Martire B, Masi M, Monafo V, Moschese V, Notarangelo LD, Orlandi P, Panei P, Pession A, Pietrogrande MC, Pignata C, Quinti I, Ragno V, Rossi P, Sciotto A, Stabile A, Italian Pediatric Group for XLA-AIEOP. Clinical, Immunological and molecular analysis in a large cohort of patients with X-linked agammaglobulinaemia: an Italian multicenter study. Clin Immunol. 2002;104:221–30.
10. Quinti I, Soresina A, Sparado G, Martino S, Donnanno S, Agostini C, Pignata P, Dammacco D, Pesce AM, Borgese F, Guerra A, Rondelli R, Plebani A. Long-term follow-up and outcome of a large cohort of patients with common variable immunodeficiency. J Clin Immunol. 2007;27:308–16.
11. Lucas M, Lee M, Lortan J, Lopez-Granados E, Misbah S, Chapel H. Infection outcomes in patients with common variable immunodeficiency disorders: relationship to immunoglobulin therapy over 22 years. J Allergy Clin Immunol. 2010;125:1354–60.
12. Winkelstein J, Marino MC, Lederman HM, Jones SM, Sullivan K, Burks AW, et al. X-linked agammaglobulinemia: report on a United States registry of 201 patients. Medicine (Baltimore). 2006;85:193–202.
13. Orange J, Belohradsky BH, Berger M, Borte M, Hagan J, Jolles S, Wasserman RL, Baggish JS, Saunders R, Grimbacher B. Evaluation of correlation between dose and clinical outcomes in subcutaneous immunoglobulin replacement therapy. Clin Exp Immunol. 2012;169:172–81.
14. Harville T. Can we effectively use radiographic imaging and clinical parameters for making an earlier diagnosis of granulomatous interstitial lung disease in patients with common variable immunodeficiency? Ann Allergy Asthma Immunol. 2017;118:529–30.
15. Orange J, Grossman WJ, Navickis RJ, Wilkes MM. Impact of trough IgG on pneumonia incidence in primary immunodeficiency: a meta-analysis of clinical studies. Clin Immunol. 2010;137:21–30.
16. Milito C, Pulvirenti F, Pesce AM, Digiulio MA, Pandolfi F, Visentini M, Quinti I. Adequate patient's outcome achieved with short immunoglobulin replacement intervals in severe antibody deficiencies. J Clin Immunol. 2014;34:813–9.
17. Popa V, Colby TV, Reich SV. Pulmonary interstitial disease in Ig deficiency. Chest. 2002;122:1594–603.
18. Quinti I, Soresina A, Guerra A, Rondelli R, Spadaro G, Agostini C, Milito C, Trombetta AC, Visentini V, Martini H, Plebani A, Fiorilli M, IPINet Investigators. Effectiveness of immunoglobulin replacement therapy on clinical outcome in patients with primary antibody deficiencies: results from a multicenter prospective cohort study. J Clin Immunol. 2011;31:315–22.
19. Ni Y, Shi G, Yu Y, Hao J, Chen T, Song H. Clinical characteristics of patients with chronic obstructive pulmonary disease with comorbid bronchiectasis: a systemic review and meta-analysis. Int J COPD. 2015;10:1465–75.
20. Stead A, Douglas JG, Broadfoot CJ, Kaminski ER, Herriot R. Humoral immunity and bronchiectasis. Clin Exp Immunol. 2002;130:325–30.

21. Schütz K, Alecsandru D, Babar J, Banerjee AK, Bondioni P, Bruining A, Chapel H, Condliffe AM, Dettmer S, Driessen G, Exley A, Farber CM, Fraioli F, Galal N, Gathmann B, Grimbacher B, Gonzalez-Granado LI, Hackett S, Haddock J, van Hagen PM, Hartmann Hurst JL, Lougaris V, Lucas M, Meyts I, Milito C, Mitrevski M, Patel S, Plebani A, Postranecka V, Quinti I, Screaton N, Serra G, Sirignano C, Soresina A, Spadaro G, Stirling R, Thon V, de Vries E, Warnatz K, Baumann U. Imaging of bronchial pathology in primary antibody deficiencies: data from the European Chest CT Group. in submission.
22. Litzman JFT, Grimbacher B, Gathmann B, Salzer U, Pavlík T, Vlcek J, Postránecká V, Trávnícková Z, Thon V. Mannose-binding lectin gene polymorphic variants predispose to the development of bronchopulmonary complications but have no influence on other clinical and laboratory symptoms or signs of common variable immunodeficiency. Clin Exp Immunol. 2008;153:324–30.
23. Costa-Carvalho B, Wandalsen GF, Pulici G, Sanchez Aranda C, Solé D. Pulmonary complications in patients with antibody deficiency. Allergol Immunopathol (Madr). 2011;39:128–32.
24. Touw CM, van de Ven AA, de Jong PA, Terheggen-Lagro S, Beek E, Sanders EA, van Montfrans JM. Detection of pulmonary complications in common variable immunodeficiency. Pediatr Allergy Immunol. 2010;21:793–805.
25. Hampson F, Chandra A, Screaton NJ, Condliffe A, Kumararatne DS, Exley AR, et al. Respiratory disease in common variable immunodeficiency and other primary immunodeficiency disorders. Clin Radiol. 2012;67:587–95.
26. Cereser L, Girometti R, d'Angelo P, De Carli M, De Pellegrin A, Zuiani C. Humoral primary immunodeficiency diseases: clinical overview and chest high-resolution computed tomography (HRCT) features in the adult population. Clinical Radiology. 2017;72:534–42.
27. Arslan S, Poyraz N, Ucar R, Yesildag M, Yesildag A, Caliskaner AZ. Magnetic resonance imaging may be a valuable radiation-free technique for lung pathologies in patients with primary immunodeficiency. J Clin Immunol. 2016;36:66–72.
28. Milito C, Pulvirenti F, Serra G, Valente M, Pesce AM, Granata G, Catalano C, Fraioli F, Quinti I. Magnetic resonance imaging may be a valuable radiation-free technique for lung pathologies in patients with primary immunodeficiency. J Clin Immunol. 2015;35:491–500.
29. Chapel H, Prevot J, Gaspar HB, Español T, Bonilla FS, Solis L, Drabwell J, Editorial Board for Working Party on Principles of Care at IPOPI. Primary immunodeficiencies – principles of care. Front Immunol. 2014.; ISSN: 1664-3224;5:627. https://doi.org/10.3389/fimmu.2014.00627.
30. Freiberger T, Grodecká L, Ravcuková B, Kurecová B, Postránecká V, Vlcek J, Jarkovský J, Thon V, Litzman J. Association of FcRn expression with lung abnormalities and IVIG catabolism in patients with common variable immunodeficiency. Clin Immunol. 2010;136:419–25.
31. Patel S, Anzilotti C, Lucas M, Jain R, Moore N, Chapel H. Outcome of interstitial lung disease in patients with common variable immunodeficiency disorders – common pathology or more than one disease? in press.
32. Kokosi M, Nicholson AG, Hansell DM, Wells AU. Rare idiopathic interstitial pneumonias: LIP and PPFE and rare histologic patterns of interstitial pneumonias: AFOP and BPIP. Respirology. 2016;21:600–14.
33. Hurst J, Verma N, Lowe D, Baxendale HE, Jolles J, Kelleher P, Longhurst HJ, Y Patel S, Renzoni EA, Sander CR, Avery GA, Babar JL, Buckland MS, Burns S, Egner W, Gompels MM, Gordins P, Haddock JA, Hart Hayman GR, Herriot R, Hoyles RK, Huissoon AP, Jacob J, Nicholson AG, Rassl DM, Sargur RB, Savic S, Seneviratne SL, Sheaff M, Vaitla PM, Walters GI, Whitehouse GL, Wright PA, Condliffe AM, BLF/UKPIN Consensus Statement on the Definition. Diagnosis and Management of Granulomatous-Lymphocytic Interstitial Lung Disease (GLILD) in Common Variable Immunodeficiency Disorders (CVID). J Allergy Clin Immunol Pract. 2017;5:938–45.
34. Kokosi M, Nicholson AG, Hansell DM, Wells AU. Respiratory. Respirology. 2016;21:600–14.
35. Maglione P, Ko HM, Beasley MB, Strauchen JA, Cunningham-Rundles C. Tertiary lymphoid neogenesis is a component of pulmonary lymphoid hyperplasia in patients with common variable immunodeficiency. J Allergy Clin Immunol. 2014;133:535–42.

36. Guinee DJ. Update on nonneoplastic pulmonary lymphoproliferative disorders and related entities. Arch Pathol Lab Med. 2010;134:691–701.
37. Rao N, Mackinnon AC, Routes JM. Granulomatous and lymphocytic interstitial lung disease: a spectrum of pulmonary histopathologic lesions in common variable immunodeficiency—histologic and immunohistochemical analyses of 16 cases. Hum Pathol. 2015;46:1306–14.
38. Chase N, Verbsky JW, Hintermeyer MK, Waukau JK, Tomita-Mitchell A, Casper JT, Singh S, Shahir KS, Tisol WB, Nugent ML, Rao RN, Mackinnon AC, Goodman LR, Simpson PM, Routes JM. Use of combination chemotherapy for treatment of granulomatous and lymphocytic interstitial lung disease (GLILD) in patients with common variable immunodeficiency (CVID). J Clin Immunol. 2013;33:30–9.
39. Chapel H, Lucas M, Patel S, Lee M, Cunningham-Rundles C, Resnick E, Gerard L, Oksenhendler E. Confirmation and improvement of criteria for clinical phenotyping in common variable immunodeficiency disorders in replicate cohorts. JACI. 2012;130:1197–8.
40. Hartono S, Motosue MS, Khan S, Rodriguez V, Iyer VN, Divekar R, Joshi AJ. Predictors of granulomatous lymphocytic interstitial lung disease in common variable immunodeficiency. Ann Allergy Asthma Immunol. 2017;118:614–20.
41. Zdziarski P, Gamian A, Dworacki G. A case report of lymphoid interstitial pneumonia in common variable immunodeficiency. Oligoclonal expansion of effector lymphocytes with preferential cytomegalovirus-specific immune response and lymphoproliferative disease promotion. Medicine (Baltimore). 2017;96:23.
42. Hasegawa M, Sakai F, Okabayashi A, Sato A, Yokohori N, Katsura H, Asano C, Kamata T, Koh E, Sekine Y, Hiroshima K, Ogura T, Takemura T. Intravenous immunoglobulin monotherapy for granulomatous lymphocytic interstitial lung disease in common variable immunodeficiency. Intern Med. 2017;56(21):2899–902. https://doi.org/10.2169/internalmedicine.7757-16.
43. Bucciol G, Petrone A, Putti MC. Efficacy of mycophenolate on lung disease and autoimmunity in children with immunodeficiency. Pediatr Pulmonol. 2017;52:E73–E6.
44. Mannina A, Chung, JH., Swigris, JJ., Solomon, JJ., Huie, TJ., Yunt, ZX., Truong, TQ., Brown, K., Achcar, RD., Olson, AL., Cox, CW., Kligerman, SJ>, Curran-Everett, D., Fernandez-Perez, ER. Clinical predictors of a diagnosis of common variable immunodeficiency-related granulomatous-lymphocytic interstitial lung disease. Ann Am Thorac Soc 2016;13:1042–1049.
45. Schussler E, Beasley MB, Maglione PJ. Lung disease in primary antibody deficiencies. J Allergy Clin Immunol Pract. 2016;4:1039–52.
46. Gompels MM, Hodges E, Lock RJ, Angus B, White H, Larkin A, Chapel HM, Spickett GP, Misbah SA, Smith JL, Associated Study Group. Lymphoproliferative disease in antibody deficiency: a multi-centre study. Clin Exp Immunol. 2003;134:314–20.
47. Dhalla F, da Silva SP, Lucas M, Travis S, Chapel H. Review of gastric cancer risk factors in patients with common variable immunodeficiency disorders, resulting in a proposal for a surveillance programme. Clin Exp Immunol. 2011;165(1):1–7.

Gastrointestinal Complications in Primary Immunoglobulin Deficiencies 26

Jiri Litzman

The gastrointestinal tract (GIT) lymphoid tissue (GALT) is the largest immune organ in the body. Because of continuous exposure to foreign antigens of both microbial and non-microbial origin, it not only forms a barrier protecting the body from pathogens but also initiates and regulates the immune response to various antigens (Chap. 2). Local inflammatory stimuli from the GIT are important for adequate immune response however may lead to various pathological states, even in patients with an otherwise "normal" immune system. In the case of immunodysregulatory disorders, including immunodeficiencies, the danger of insufficient or inadequate reactions is markedly increased, leading to various immunopathological states in many patients, some of which can frequently be observed also in immunocompetent patients. The others are relatively unusual, with a marked increase in patients with immunodeficiencies.

In patients with immunoglobulin deficiencies, the gastrointestinal tract is the second most frequently affected system, after the respiratory system. All GIT organs can be affected; however, it is mainly the stomach, small and the large intestines, and also the liver that are predominantly affected.

26.1 Prevalence of Gastrointestinal Complications in Primary Antibody Deficiencies

The frequency of gastrointestinal (GI) complications shows a large variation among studies. This is influenced by whether only clinical gastrointestinal manifestations are reported or diagnoses are based on endoscopic and histopathologic findings. The results markedly depend on the fact whether and how frequently

J. Litzman
Department of Clinical Immunology and Allergology, St Anne's University Hospital in Brno and Faculty of Medicine, Masaryk University, Brno, Czech Republic
e-mail: jiri.litzman@fnusa.cz

M. M. D'Elios, M. Rizzi (eds.), *Humoral Primary Immunodeficiencies*, Rare Diseases of the Immune System, https://doi.org/10.1007/978-3-319-91785-6_26

endoscopic investigations are performed, whether they are indicated strictly on actual clinical demand or performed routinely, as a part of clinical follow-up. Quite frequently, histologic abnormalities can be present even in patients without clinical symptoms. In a Dutch group of patients with common variable immunodeficiency disorders (CVID), endoscopy was performed in 30 patients, only 6 of whom had a previously established gastrointestinal disease. In the group of CVID patients with no previous gastrointestinal disease, only 3/24 (13%) had unremarkable endoscopic or histologic findings, while 21/24 (88%) had a pathologic histologic or endoscopic finding, the most frequent being nodular lymphoid hyperplasia (NLH - 15/24 patients, 63%) [1].

Many gastrointestinal symptoms are not present at the time of diagnosis but develop during the course of the diseases: for instance, in an Italian study, 14% of 224 CVID patients suffered from chronic diarrhea at diagnosis but 22.4% in a mean 11-year follow-up. Only in 3% of CVID patient GIT diseases were the only clinical manifestation at the time of diagnosis [2]. Also Mannon et al. showed that CVID patients with gastrointestinal symptoms differed from asymptomatic CVID patients by having a significantly longer disease duration [3]. Similarly, only 2/73 patients with X-linked agammaglobulinemia (XLA) had chronic diarrhea at diagnosis; however, it was documented in 14 of them during the mean 10-year follow-up [4].

GI complications can be observed most frequently in patients with CVID: The most extensive European survey of CVID reports enteropathy in 9% of 2212 patients [5]. An Iranian study showed GIT complaints in 19/39 (48%) patients, 11 of them (28%) suffered from chronic diarrhea [6]. Hermans reported various gastrointestinal problems (chronic diarrhea, achlorhydria) in 60% of CVID patients; 42% had malabsorption [7]. Kainulainen reported GI problems in 30 (32%) of 95 Finnish patients with CVID [8]. Hermaszewski and Webster reported diarrhea complaints in 96/240 patients with CVID [9]. In an American study, GI symptoms were present in 73/473 (15.4%) patients, and malabsorption developed in 28/473 (5.9%) patients [10]. In a Norwegian study, 48/103 (47%) CVID patients suffered from at least one predefined GI symptom (blunting [34%], pain [30%], diarrhea [26%], satiety [14%], and constipation [13%]) [11]. Compared to patients with "classical CVID," GI complications are even more frequent with patients with late-onset combined immunodeficiency (LOCID) (75 vs. 42%, $p = 0.01$) in a large French study [12].

GI complications in patients with XLA are less frequent; although a study from Poland reported various GIT symptoms in 28/44 (64%) patients, 21 (48%) suffered from recurrent diarrhea episodes [13]. Two studies are available from the USA: using the data from the US Immunodeficiency Network (USIDNet), 71/200 (35%) XLA patients had a concurrent GI manifestation, the most frequent was intermittent (38%) or chronic (26%) diarrhea, and 9.5% were reported to be suffering from enteritis and/or IBD [14]. In a previous US study, recurrent gastroenteritis was reported in 46/201 (23%) patients; in 14% recurrent gastroenteritis was present at the time of diagnosis [15]. Recurrent gastroenteritis was reported in 14/73 (19%) XLA patients in an Italian survey in [4]. Hermaszewski and Webster reported diarrhea complaints in 19/44 (43%) patients with XLA [9].

Protracted or recurrent diarrhea was observed in 24/79 (34%) patients with X-linked hyper-IgM syndrome (CD40L deficiency). If an infectious agent was determined, *Cryptosporidium* was the most frequent (21% patients) [16]. A slightly higher number of patients with diarrhea were reported by Levy et al., 31/56 patients (55.3%), leading to failure to thrive in 20 (64.5%). Again, *Cryptosporidium* was the most frequently documented etiological agent [17].

Recurrent diarrhea was present in 5/29 patients with hyper-IgM syndrome due to activation-induced cytidine deaminase (AID) deficiency [18].

A large study performed in Sweden showed increased (6.0%) inpatient and hospital-based outpatient visits because of GI infections in patients with IgA deficiency (IgAD) compared to matched controls (1.8%) [19].

26.2 Causes of GI Pathology

26.2.1 Infections

Acute, recurrent, or chronic diarrhea of infectious origin is a common manifestation in humoral immunodeficiencies. They may be caused by bacteria, viruses, or protozoa.

Gastrointestinal infections in CVID patients were more frequent in patients with undetectable IgA levels (47 [36%] out of 131 patients) than in patients with residual IgA production (19 [16%] out of 120 patients) showing the impotence of IgA, even in residual levels, in protecting against GI infections [20]. This may also explain the fact why immunoglobulin derivatives used for replacement treatment, which almost exclusively include IgG, are ineffective in preventing GI infections in hypogammaglobulinemic patients [21].

26.2.1.1 Bacterial Infections

The spectrum of bacterial infectious agents leading to diarrhea is similar to immunocompetent persons, including infections with *Campylobacter jejuni* and *Salmonella* species [20, 22, 23]. Surprisingly, despite frequent antibiotic treatment, the patients with CVID do not suffer from increased *Clostridium difficile* infection frequency. Protection by anti-*Clostridium difficile* antibodies administered in immunoglobulin derivatives used for the replacement treatment may be an explanation [24].

Infection by *Helicobacter pylori* (Hp) is also frequently observed in CVID patients, leading to atrophic gastritis resembling the autoimmune one and leading to pernicious anemia [25]. Hp infection was detectable in 14/34 (41%) CVID patients with dyspeptic symptoms [25]. Malamut et al. observed Hp infection in 8 (26.7%) of 30 patients in whom gastric biopsy was available [23]. Other combined data show an 18% prevalence, not different from the general population [26]. Hp may in CVID patients promote chronic gastritis or gastric cancer [27]. Even if adequately treated, eradicating Hp requires several courses of therapy and has a tendency to recur [2]. However Hp eradication does not lead to the retreat of gastric pathology [23].

Also the frequency of Hp-infected persons in IgAD patients did not differ from the control group (24.2 vs. 23.6%, respectively). However, comparing Hp-positive persons, IgAD patients frequently had more severe gastritis compared to the control persons (61.9 vs. 21.6%, $P < 0.001$), such as duodenal ulcers (33.3 vs. 10.8% $p = 0.01$) and also NLH (9.9% vs. none, $p = 0.011$) [28].

Bacterial overgrowth in the small intestine can commonly be observed in CVID [29, 30]. For diagnosis the hydrogen breast test can be used.

26.2.1.2 Protozoal Infections

Infection by *Giardia lamblia* is frequent in CVID but also in IgAD patients. The infection may cause watery diarrhea, abdominal cramps, and bloating. ELISA, PCR of stool samples, duodenal fluid, or duodenal biopsies increase the diagnostic sensitivity when compared to a stool's microscopic examination. Despite treatment, in CVID patients, the disease frequently has a prolonged course, showing the immunodeficient organism's disturbed ability to eradicate the protozoa [31–33]. In one study, *Giardia lamblia* infection was detected in 14/50 CVID patients, one course of nitroimidazole led to *Giardia* eradication only in 5 of them, while the remaining ones required repeated courses [23]. Chronic giardiasis leads to villous flattening similar to that that seen in celiac disease and severe malnutrition [34].

Giardia was also repeatedly described in patients with XLA [14], with X-linked hyper-IgM syndrome [16, 17], and with hyper-IgM syndrome due to AID deficiency [18].

A significant GI pathogen in patients with X-linked hyper-IgM syndrome is *Cryptosporidium*, leading not only to diarrhea but also to sclerosing cholangitis [16, 17]. *Cryptosporidium* was observed in CVID patients as well [22].

26.2.1.3 Viral Infections

The prevalence of GI viruses was shown to be increased in patients with CVID. In ome study GI viruses were identified in 12/28 (25%) CVID patients, compared to 6/66 (9%) in healthy controls. Adenovirus was the most prevalent [35]. This positivity was more common in patients with diminished serum IgA levels, and patients with GI viruses had significantly lower secretory IgA levels in their stools compared to patients without GI viruses or healthy controls [35].

Another virus associated with chronic diarrhea in CVID patients is norovirus, which was observed in stool and small bowel biopsies in eight patients with CVID enteropathy, five of them required long-term intravenous nutrition due to intestinal failure. The virus was not detectable in ten CVID patient's stools without diarrhea. In three of the affected persons, the symptoms resolved after spontaneous viral clearance (one patient) or oral ribavirin treatment (two patients) [36]. This observation lacks published confirmation from other centers. No norovirus RNA positivity was observed in GI biopsies from 52 Norwegian CVID patients with various GI symptoms [11].

Cytomegalovirus can also be a cause of chronic colitis in CVID patients [22, 37].

26.2.2 Inflammatory Complications

The second large group of complications are inflammatory disorders where autoimmunity may play various degrees of importance, sometimes more suspected than really confirmed. These include mainly atrophic gastritis, autoimmune hepatitis, CVID-associated autoimmune enteropathy, and inflammatory bowel disease (IBD).

Approximately 8–22% patients with CVID suffer from granulomatous disease [38]. Noncaseating granulomas may be present in many organs including the GIT [22]. In a large French study including 436 patients, 59 (13.5%) had granulomas in one or more organs. Of them, in nine patients where the GIT was involved, the presence of granulomas was associated with clinical symptoms such as diarrhea and weight loss [39].

The majority of these diseases will be discussed in more details in the next part of the review.

26.2.3 Malignancy

Malignancy frequency is increased, mainly in patients with CVID occurring in approximately 6–9% of the patients [40], lymphoma and gastric carcinoma being the most significantly increased [41]. This increase was not documented in IgAD or XLA.

In a study published in 1985, which included 220 patients with CVID being followed for 11 years, a 47-fold increase of gastric cancer and 30-fold increase of lymphoma compared to the general population were documented [42]. A multicenter Scandinavian study reported standardized incidence ratio (SIR) for gastric cancer 10.3 (95% confidence interval [CI], 2.1–30.2). The SIR for lymphoma was 12.1 (95% CI: 3.3–31.0). There was no cancer increase in of CVID patients' relatives suggesting that the cancer is related to the patients' immunodeficiency, but not to the genetic traits shared with their relatives. This study did not show an increased malignancy frequency in IgAD [41]. The study of Vajdic et al. from Australia showed SIR for all malignant neoplasms 1.95 (95% CI, 1.37–2.57), for non-Hodgkin lymphoma 12.1 (95% CI, 6.03–21.6), and for gastric cancer 7.23 (95% CI, 0.88–26.1) in 416 CVID patients [43]. A p53 pathway alteration in gastric mucosa was observed in 18% (6/34) of CVID patients [25]. A possible decreased risk for gastric cancer seen in CVID patients in recent years may be explained by a possible positive role for Hp infection elimination in CVID patients [10].

De Petris et al. analyzed the features of gastric adenocarcinoma in six CVID patients. These cancers were generally observed in younger patients than in the overall population with gastric cancer. These cancers were moderately to poorly differentiated of intestinal type, frequently with intratumoral lymphocytes. In no patient, Hp infection or enterochromaffin cell-like hyperplasia was observed in the fundus [44].

Although recognized as a risk factor for gastric cancer, it is probable that Hp infection does not explain the increased carcinoma risk in CVID patients, as the Hp infection does not seem to be more frequent than in the general population [27]. High pH or the presence of ethanol facilitating the penetration of N-nitroso compounds into the mucosa may contribute to cancer development in patients with chronic gastritis [27].

A population-based matched cohort study of 125 IgAD patients in Sweden showed an increased hazard ratio (HR) for any GI cancer (1.64, 95% CI = 1.07–2.50), but not HR for lymphoma [45].

26.3 Typical Gastrointestinal Complication in Concrete Primary Antibody Production Deficiencies

Regarding concrete diseases with primary disturbed antibody production (see Table 26.1), the most frequent GI complications can be seen in patients with CVID, where all types of complications may be present and frequently lead to a significant patient morbidity and sometimes also mortality. GI problems lead to decreased body mass index, iron saturation, serum albumin levels, and D-xylose absorption in affected patients [3].

In patients with XLA, predominant complications of GIT are infections, while autoimmune/inflammatory diseases are much less frequent than in CVID; the frequency of tumors is also probably not markedly increased. In patients with IgAD, markedly increased celiac disease frequency was documented [46], and also NLH, pernicious anemia, Crohn's disease, and ulcerative colitis were repeatedly reported [47–51]; however these complications are much less common than in CVID. Some patients may suffer from infectious complication.

Patients with X-linked hyper-IgM syndrome suffer from diarrhea mainly caused by *Giardia lamblia* or *Cryptosporidium parvum*. Oral ulcers, periodontitis, or anal ulcers frequently accompany neutropenia. *Cryptosporidium* may also infect a biliary tree and lead to the development of sclerosing cholangitis with progression to cirrhosis and cholangiocarcinoma [16, 17, 52]. In approximately one half of patients with protracted or recurrent diarrhea, no etiologic agent was identified [16].

Table 26.1 The most significant clinical manifestation of the most frequent primary antibody deficiencies

Immunodeficiency	Defect and pathogenesis	Major laboratory characteristics	GI complications
Common variable immunodeficiency disorders (CVID)	Various genes involved at least in a proportion of patients Pathogenesis is usually unknown and may be different in dependence of genetic defect	Decreased serum levels of IgGg and decreased IgA, and/or IgM, disturbed specific antibody response	GIT infections, NLH, villous atrophy, atrophic gastritis, IBD-like colitis, nodular regenerative hyperplasia, malignancy
X-linked agammaglobulinemia	BTK mutation, defect in B-cell development	All serum isotypes markedly decreased No B cell in the blood	GIT infections, other GE complications rare Chronic diarrhea in some patients
Selective IgA deficiency	Pathogenesis unknown	Serum IgA < 0.07 g/L; IgG and IgM not decreased	Increased frequency of celiac disease, other GE complications comparable to normal population
X-linker hyper-IgM syndrome	Deficiency of CD40L (CD154) leading to disturbed isotype switching and other T- and B-cell disturbances	Low IgG and IgA levels, normal or increased IgM levels	Cryptosporidium enteritis, sclerosing cholangitis

BTK Bruton tyrosine kinase, *GI* gastrointestinal, *GIT* gastrointestinal tract, *NLH* nodular lymphoid hyperplasia

26.3.1 Mouth Cavity and Esophagus

Oral manifestation of immunoglobulin immunodeficiencies is not frequent. Sarcoid-like granulomas [53] or necrotizing periodontitis [54] was observed in patient with CVID. In IgAD, children were documented as more frequently having caries in primary but not in permanent dentitions [55].

The esophagus is also not frequently affected in patients with humoral immunodeficiencies. However in the study of Daniels et al., in 5/10 patients prominent intraepithelial lymphocytosis and in 4/10 intraepithelial leukocytes accompanied by candida were observed in an esophageal biopsy [22].

26.3.2 Stomach

Approximately one half of CVID patients suffer from achlorhydria due to atrophic gastritis with a predominantly antral involvement. It is accompanied by an abnormal Schilling's test and decreased serum gastrin levels, resulting also in pernicious anemia syndrome [56]. No anti-gastric parietal cell antibodies or antibodies against intrinsic factors were detected in CVID [57, 58].

In an Italian study, signs of chronic gastritis were observed in routine esophagogastroduodenoscopy in 10.2% of CVID patients at diagnosis and in 21.8% in a follow-up when endoscopy was performed every 2 years in every CVID patient [2].

The histology of intestinal biopsies does not show a uniform pattern. Biopsy showed a wide spectrum of abnormalities starting from non-specific changes to pathology resembling an acute gastric GVHD pattern [59].

In 34 patients with dyspeptic problems in whom upper gastrointestinal endoscopy was performed, chronic gastritis was observed in 20, most frequently diffuse gastritis (15 patients), 9 of them had multifocal chronic gastritis, metaplasia in the antrum or the body was observed in 4 patients. In total, 14 (34%) patients were observed with a Hp infection; all had histological signs of chronic gastritis. Chronic active gastritis was more frequently observed in Hp-positive (79%) than in Hp-negative (20%) patients. Normal mucosa was observed in Hp-negative patients only [25].

A cross-sectional study of nine stomach biopsies showed morphology similar to gastric acute graft-versus-host disease (GVHD) in four cases: single cell necrosis in the glands and variable dense mononuclear cell infiltrates with obliteration of occasional glands and crypts; three of these patients had similar changes in small bowel and colon biopsies. Although less than one apoptotic body was seen in the stomach of healthy persons, in CVID patients it ranked 0 to 5 per 10 glands, similar to GVHD and human immunodeficiency virus (HIV) infection. One other biopsy showed active superficial gastritis, while two other biopsies were unremarkable. Plasma cells were notably absent in all but one biopsies [59].

In a Norwegian study, gastroscopy of 50 CVID patients showed gastric metaplasia of the duodenal bulb in 13 patients; 19 had abnormalities in the stomach—intestinal metaplasia (6), atrophic gastritis (9), and fibrosis (13) [11].

In Daniels et al.'s study, 36 gastric samples from 18 patients were available. In 12 patients lamina propria lacked plasma cells. The stomachs of 11 patients (61%) showed lymphoid aggregates; an increased apoptosis was detected in 6 patients. Four patients (22%) had lymphocytic gastritis pattern; intraepithelial neutrophils were observed in eight patients (44%) [22].

In a French study upper endoscopy showed macroscopic abnormalities in 77% of 50 patients with GI symptoms which included erythematous (27%), follicular (13%), atrophic (27%), and ulcerative (10%) gastritis [23]. Hp infection was present in eight (26.7%) patients, six of them showed intestinal metaplasia. Control endoscopy 3 years after Hp eradication still showed persistent gastric atrophy despite Hp absence [23].

As mentioned above, gastric cancer frequency is increased in CVID patients.

Gastric abnormalities seen in CVID are not observed in increased frequency in other types of primary hypogammaglobulinemia, showing that they are not related simply to immunoglobulin deficiency but probably to other mechanisms.

26.3.3 Small Intestine

Mainly in CVID patients, two typical complications can be met in the small intestine—villous flattening and nodular lymphoid hyperplasia. These complications frequently accompany each other.

26.3.3.1 Nodular Lymphoid Hyperplasia

Nodular lymphoid hyperplasia (NLH) is characterized by the presence of multiple nodules, 2–11 mm in diameter, distributed in the lamina propria or in the superficial submucosa of the small intestine but also the stomach, colon, or rectum. Histologically they are characterized by markedly hyperplastic mitotically active germinal centers and well-defined lymphocyte mantles. B cells are present but no or few plasma cells. Lamina propria and villi apart of the nodules may appear normal. NLH usually does not cause significant clinical problems but can be accompanied by abdominal pain, chronic diarrhea, bleeding, intussusception, or obstruction. The nodules cause only partial or minor disturbance of the villous pattern [60, 61].

The NLH frequency in the general population is not known but is probably low. In CVID patients, general estimation is 20% of CVID patients [61]; however, the published frequency varies between 8% (Italian study, where all CVID underwent repeated endoscopy) [2] and 53% of CVID patients in whom endoscopy was performed for various reasons [1]. Although reported, NLH is much less common in patients with IgAD [47–50] or in IgG subclass deficiency [62].

The cause of NLH is not known. Previously, *Giardia lamblia* infection was supposed to be a cause; however, Hermans et al. [7] did not observe disappearance after *Giardia lamblia* was treated with metronidazole. However, reports of endoscopic improvement after successful treatment of chronic giardiasis were published as well [33].

26.3.3.2 Villous Flattening

Chronic small bowel inflammation, sometimes referred to as CVID-associated autoimmune enteropathy, is frequently associated with unexplained chronic diarrhea, weight loss, steatorrhea, and malabsorption of minerals and fat-soluble vitamins [40]. However, the inflammation is frequently not limited to the small intestine; signs of "microscopic colitis" can be observed in these patients as well [63]. On the biopsy, villous blunting with crypt distortion is most frequently observed; however, the picture may be variable (see below). In some patients the enteropathy may have a severe course with extensive superficial and deep ulcers that may cause the perforation of the small bowel [64].

Overall prevalence in the general CVID population is not known; it depends on the cohort of patients in whom biopsy was performed, generally varying between 4 and 12% [40]. Biopsy-proven lymphocytic infiltration in lamina propria and intraepithelial mucous with villous atrophy was reported in 9% of 334 CVID patients in a European survey [65]. In patients of Persian origin, intestinal villous atrophy was observed in 11/79 CVID patients (13.9%) [66].

A histological feature frequently resembles acute intestinal GVHD. Enterocytes become flattened and vacuolized, and there is increased epithelial apoptosis. Chronic inflammation in the lamina propria lacks plasma cells and may include neutrophils [22, 23, 59, 67, 68].

In a French study, upper endoscopy performed in 41 patients with GI symptoms showed macroscopic abnormalities in the duodenum in 68% of patients: disappearance of folds and mosaic pattern (22%), nodular lymphoid hyperplasia (44%), and ulcerative duodenitis (2%). Histologically, NLH and GVH-like lesions (see below) were present in 49% and 12.2% of patients, respectively. Profound plasma cell depletion was present in 83%, villous atrophy in 51%, and chronic lymphocytic duodenitis in 56% of the patients [23].

In another study, small intestine villous atrophy was observed in 10/32 (31%) of CVID patients with gastrointestinal symptoms or anemia. Patients with villous atrophy more frequently had anemia than patients in whom villous atrophy was not observed; these patients also had lower body mass index. However, there was no significant difference in the frequency of diarrhea between these two groups [69].

Daniels reported 39 small bowel biopsies of CVID patients—paucity of B cells was present in 68%, prominent lymphoid aggregates in 47%, and increased apoptosis in 21% of patients, 25% had villous blunting and increases in IEL mimicking celiac disease, 32% had intraepithelial granulocytes, and one had collagenous colitis pattern [22].

The histologic finding of reduced plasma cells in an intestinal biopsy was significantly associated with typical CVID abnormalities: an increase of CD21low cells and decrease of switched memory cells and increases in serum levels of soluble CD14 (monocyte activation) and soluble CD25(T-cell activation) [11]. These associations were not observed with lymphoid hyperplasia or an increase in IEL cells [11].

CT or MRI can demonstrate a significant intestinal mucosal enhancement and intestinal wall thickening [67].

The mechanisms leading to CVID enteropathy are unknown; however, disturbed T-cell function was suggested as a possible mechanism [23], such as autoimmune mechanism [14]. Enteropathy was also reported in patients with chronic norovirus infection [36] and *Giardia lamblia* infection [34]. Although related to *Giardia lamblia* infection, effective treatment of *Giardia* does not lead to the disappearance of histological abnormalities [34].

The histologic picture and clinical symptoms of enteropathy associated with CVID may resemble celiac disease; meta-analysis from 2015 showed a 9.2% prevalence of possible celiac disease in CVID patients [70]. To distinguish these conditions on a biopsy, plasma cells are usually absent in CVID, compared to celiac disease where they are present [68]. Also, in contrast to celiac disease, the intraepithelial cells did not have an increased percentage of TCRγδ cells; they were predominantly CD3+ CD8+ [23]. A presence of lymphoid follicular hyperplasia also distinguishes CVID-associated enteropathy from classical celiac disease in immunocompetent patients, but as lymphoid hyperplasia and the absence of plasma cells are a typical CVID feature, these markers cannot exclude the coexistence of CVID and celiac disease [67].

In Malamut et al.'s study, findings reminiscent to celiac disease—an increased count of intraepithelial lymphocytes (IELs) (>30 IELs/100 enterocytes) were present in 31/41 (75.6%) patients with GI symptoms; it was associated with villous atrophy in 21 (68%) patients, although the atrophy was more often partial (Marsh IIIa $n = 13$) than severe (Marsh IIIb–IIIc $n = 8$). Unusual findings for celiac disease—strong neutrophil infiltration, severe rarefaction of plasma cells, and follicular lymphoid hyperplasia were present in 36%, 96%, and 55% of these patients, respectively [23].

Gene expression profiling in pars descendens of the duodenum of patients with increased IEL did not cluster with the profile of patients with untreated celiac diseases but were similar to CVID patients with a normal IEL count [11].

As patients with CVID produce small amounts of specific antibodies, including autoantibodies, determining celiac disease-associated autoantibodies (anti-tissue transglutaminase, tTG; anti-endomysium, EMA) or antibodies against gliadin has very limited significance. However, these antibodies were occasionally observed in CVID patients [23, 68].

HLADQ2/DQ8 haplotypes are used as a susceptibility marker for celiac disease, and positivity may determine patients with a probability of response to a gluten-free diet [23, 68, 71]. However, several CVID patients negative for these haplotypes may occasionally respond to a gluten-free diet [23].

Treatment of CVID colitis is problematic. Immunoglobulin treatment has no effect on GI symptoms [23]. Steroids (budesonide or prednisone) may lead to significant reduction of diarrhea and malabsorption [23, 72]. The results of treatment by infliximab are contradictory [23, 73].

Supportive treatment should include replacement by water-insoluble vitamins and antiresorptives to prevent osteoporosis. In severe cases, an elementary diet or total parenteral nutrition may be required. Treatment with antibiotics is ineffective [21].

26.3.3.3 IgAD and Celiac Disease

Celiac disease frequency in IgAD patients is increased. Meta-analysis of six previously published studies calculated a prevalence of 9.9% [70] compared to the currently calculated prevalence of 1:133 in the general population [74]. The prevalence of IgAD in celiac disease patients was calculated as 1:39 [75].

The pathogenic mechanism may not only be related to IgA production deficiency but also to shared genetic background. Although the results of different studies are contradictory, HLA-B8,DR3,DQ2 haplotype is a significant genetic risk factor for IgAD acting in a multiplicative model [76]. In celiac disease, haplotypes DQ2/DQ8 are the most important genetic predisposing factors [74].

Because of the absence of IgA production, serological tests for IgA anti-tTG or anti-EMA are not reliable; IgG antibodies against these antigens must be determined. The histopathology of celiac disease in IgAD patients is indistinguishable to the pathology seen in patients with conventional celiac disease [24].

26.3.4 Colon

Hermaszewski and Webster reported IBD (Crohn-like, ulcerous colitis-like) presence in 4% CVID patients [9] similar to Resnick et al. [10], although it may be higher. Colitis leads to diarrhea, rectal bleeding, and abdominal pain [21].

Colitis observed in patients with CVID had various histological pictures. Probably the most frequent was a picture resembling GVHD with apoptotic bodies in crypts and the loss of isolated glands. Lymphocytes on the surface were increased. The surface epithelial cells were flattened. The inflammatory infiltrate in lamina propria was predominantly composed of lymphocytes, but also macrophages were occasionally present [3, 59]. However, also other pictures may be present—acute colitis with a loss of occasional crypts or acute colitis with no single cell necrosis in the crypts and the presence of neutrophils in lamina propria and infiltrated crypt epithelium (a pattern suggestive of acute self-limited colitis) [59]. Occasionally the colitis can be consistent with the diagnosis of collagenous colitis with pseudomembrane formation [77].

Daniels et al. described sets of colon biopsies in 16 CVID patients. The paucity of plasma cells was observed in 63% and prominent apoptosis in 50% of samples, 38% biopsies had a lymphocytic colitis pattern, and two had a collagenous colitis pattern [22].

Malamut et al. reported colonoscopy results in CVID patients: inflammation, NLH, and ulcers were present in 26, 31, and 14% of patients respectively. Colonic biopsies of 35 patients showed microscopic colitis in 9 (26%) cases, Crohn's disease-like lesions in 4, and ulcerous colitis in 1. Lesions of unspecified acute colitis were present in 9 (26%), lymphoid follicular hyperplasia in 15 (43%), and GVH-like lesions in 5 (14%) patients [23].

The frequency of IBD in XLA patients is not as markedly increased as in CVID, although the frequency of 4/112 (3.6%) obtained from a web-based survey of patients with XLA in the USA was significantly above the general population's prevalence of 0.4% [78].

Treatment of colitis in CVID is similar to the treatment of other IBD. 5-Aminosalicylic acid or local steroids (budesonide) are recommended; if insufficient, immunomodulators like azathioprine/5 mercaptopurine can be used [21]. The use of infliximab is also possible in refractory cases [73].

26.3.5 Liver

The frequency of liver diseases is increased in patients with primary hypogammaglobulinemia. Twenty-seven (11.9%) out of 248 CVID patients had significant liver dysfunction in the study by Cunningham-Rundles and Bodian [79], similar to 43/473 (9.1%) in the subsequent study from the same center [10]. In the studies from the 1990s, the most frequent was chronic hepatitis C [79], which can be ascribed to hepatitis C virus transmission via immunoglobulin derivatives. Primary biliary cirrhosis [10, 79], granulomatous hepatitis [17, 79], and chronic active hepatitis [66] were also described in CVID patients.

Chronic hepatitis was present in 13/201 XLA patients, 8 of them suffering from hepatitis C [15]. Chronic active hepatitis was noticed in 2/33 XLA patients from Iran [80].

The most frequent liver complication in CVID is nodular regenerative hyperplasia (NRH). It was reported in 5% [81]–12% [82] of patients with CVID; however, the number may be underestimated. In the Oxford study, NRH was present in 13/16 patients in whom liver biopsy was performed. It was associated with hepatomegaly, granuloma elsewhere in the body, cytopenias, lymphoproliferation, and enteropathy [82]. NRH is characterized by diffuse regenerative hepatocyte nodules, less than 3 mm in diameter without fibrosis [82], the nodules compress surrounding hepatic parenchyma and the portal and central veins, which may lead to portal hypertension, esophageal varices, and splenomegaly [81]. It is not accompanied by piecemeal necrosis. It manifests by elevating alkaline phosphatase (ALP) accompanied by an increase in aspartate aminotransferase (AST)/alanine aminotransferase (ALT) levels. ALP increases to twofold above the upper limit of normal baseline. In some patients an increase in liver enzymes reaches a plateau, while in others it undergoes a further increase. An increase in AST/ALT occurs over the same period as ALP, but it is much milder. An increase of bilirubin and decrease of albumin are infrequent; however, leukopenia and thrombocytopenia due to hypersplenism may be present [81]. Some patients may have normal ALP serum levels; ALT or gamma-glutamyl transpeptidase (gGT) may be the only liver enzyme increased [82]. NRH may lead to portal hypertension with life-threatening bleeding from gastric or esophageal varices [83].

In some patients, the ALP levels gradually increase, may be fluctuating, or may decrease after an initial increase [82].

The association with autoimmune diseases, T-cell intrasinusoidal infiltration, and portal vein endotheliosis suggests a possible autoimmune mechanism [84].

NLH was observed also in patients with HIGM and XLA [84].

26.4 Conclusion

As seen in the previous text, diagnosing gastrointestinal complications in patients with humoral immunodeficiencies may be very complex and difficult, requiring the collaboration of clinical immunologists with gastroenterologists, histopathologists, X-ray specialists, microbiologists, and other medical specialists. In complicated cases, these non-immunologists must be well oriented in the problematics of immunodeficiency diseases requiring the formation of specialized centers dealing with immunodeficient patients.

References

1. Maarschalk-Ellerbroek LJ, Oldenburg B, Mombers IM, Hoepelman AI, Brosens LA, Offerhaus GJ, et al. Outcome of screening endoscopy in common variable immunodeficiency disorder and X-linked agammaglobulinemia. Endoscopy. 2013;45(4):320–3.
2. Quinti I, Soresina A, Spadaro G, Martino S, Donnanno S, Agostini C, et al. Long-term follow-up and outcome of a large cohort of patients with common variable immunodeficiency. J Clin Immunol. 2007;27(3):308–16.
3. Mannon PJ, Fuss IJ, Dill S, Friend J, Groden C, Hornung R, et al. Excess IL-12 but not IL-23 accompanies the inflammatory bowel disease associated with common variable immunodeficiency. Gastroenterology. 2006;131(3):748–56.
4. Plebani A, Soresina A, Rondelli R, Amato GM, Azzari C, Cardinale F, et al. Clinical, immunological, and molecular analysis in a large cohort of patients with X-linked agammaglobulinemia: an Italian multicenter study. Clin Immunol. 2002;104(3):221–30.
5. Gathmann B, Mahlaoui N, Gérard L, Oksenhendler E, Warnatz K, Schulze I, et al. Clinical picture and treatment of 2212 patients with common variable immunodeficiency. J Allergy Clin Immunol. 2014;134(1):116–26.
6. Khodadad A, Aghamohammadi A, Parvaneh N, Rezaei N, Mahjoob F, Bashashati M, et al. Gastrointestinal manifestations in patients with common variable immunodeficiency. Dig Dis Sci. 2007;52(11):2977–83.
7. Hermans PE, Diaz-Buxo JA, Stobo JD. Idiopathic late-onset immunoglobulin deficiency. Clinical observations in 50 patients. Am J Med. 1976;61(2):221–37.
8. Kainulainen L, Nikoskelainen J, Ruuskanen O. Diagnostic findings in 95 Finnish patients with common variable immunodeficiency. J Clin Immunol. 2001;21(2):145–9.
9. Hermaszewski RA, Webster AD. Primary hypogammaglobulinaemia: a survey of clinical manifestations and complications. Q J Med. 1993;86(1):31–42.
10. Resnick ES, Moshier EL, Godbold JH, Cunningham-Rundles C. Morbidity and mortality in common variable immune deficiency over 4 decades. Blood. 2012;119(7):1650–7.
11. Jørgensen SF, Reims HM, Frydenlund D, Holm K, Paulsen V, Michelsen AE, et al. A cross-sectional study of the prevalence of gastrointestinal symptoms and pathology in patients with common variable immunodeficiency. Am J Gastroenterol. 2016;111(10):1467–75.
12. Malphettes M, Gérard L, Carmagnat M, Mouillot G, Vince N, Boutboul D, et al. Late-onset combined immune deficiency: a subset of common variable immunodeficiency with severe T cell defect. Clin Infect Dis. 2009;49(9):1329–38.
13. Pac M, Bernatowska EA, Kierkuś J, Ryżko JP, Cielecka-Kuszyk J, Jackowska T, et al. Gastrointestinal disorders next to respiratory infections as leading symptoms of X-linked agammaglobulinemia in children – 34-year experience of a single center. Arch Med Sci. 2017;13(2):412–7.

14. Barmettler S, Otani IM, Minhas J, Abraham RS, Chang Y, Dorsey MJ, et al. Gastrointestinal manifestations in X-linked Agammaglobulinemia. J Clin Immunol. 2017;37(3):287–94.
15. Winkelstein JA, Marino MC, Lederman HM, Jones SM, Sullivan K, Burks AW, et al. X-linked agammaglobulinemia: report on a United States registry of 201 patients. Medicine (Baltimore). 2006;85(4):193–202.
16. Winkelstein JA, Marino MC, Ochs H, Fuleihan R, Scholl PR, Geha R, et al. The X-linked hyper-IgM syndrome: clinical and immunologic features of 79 patients. Medicine (Baltimore). 2003;82(6):373–84.
17. Levy J, Espanol-Boren T, Thomas C, Fischer A, Tovo P, Bordigoni P, et al. Clinical spectrum of X-linked hyper-IgM syndrome. J Pediatr. 1997;131(1 Pt 1):47–54.
18. Quartier P, Bustamante J, Sanal O, Plebani A, Debre M, Deville A, et al. Clinical, immunologic and genetic analysis of 29 patients with autosomal recessive hyper-IgM syndrome due to activation-induced cytidine deaminase deficiency. Clin Immunol. 2004;110(1):22–9.
19. Ludvigsson JF, Neovius M, Hammarström L. Risk of infections among 2100 individuals with IgA deficiency: a Nationwide Cohort Study. J Clin Immunol. 2016;36(2):134–40.
20. Oksenhendler E, Gérard L, Fieschi C, Malphettes M, Mouillot G, Jaussaud R, et al. Infections in 252 patients with common variable immunodeficiency. Clin Infect Dis. 2008;46(10): 1547–54.
21. Agarwal S, Mayer L. Pathogenesis and treatment of gastrointestinal disease in antibody deficiency syndromes. J Allergy Clin Immunol. 2009;124(4):658–64.
22. Daniels JA, Lederman HM, Maitra A, Montgomery EA. Gastrointestinal tract pathology in patients with common variable immunodeficiency (CVID): a clinicopathologic study and review. Am J Surg Pathol. 2007;31(12):1800–12.
23. Malamut G, Verkarre V, Suarez F, Viallard JF, Lascaux AS, Cosnes J, et al. The enteropathy associated with common variable immunodeficiency: the delineated frontiers with celiac disease. Am J Gastroenterol. 2010;105(10):2262–75.
24. Agarwal S, Mayer L. Diagnosis and treatment of gastrointestinal disorders in patients with primary immunodeficiency. Clin Gastroenterol Hepatol. 2013;11(9):1050–63.
25. Zullo A, Romiti A, Rinaldi V, Vecchione A, Tomao S, Aiuti F, et al. Gastric pathology in patients with common variable immunodeficiency. Gut. 1999;45(1):77–81.
26. Uzzan M, Ko HM, Mehandru S, Cunningham-Rundles C. Gastrointestinal Disorders Associated with Common Variable Immune Deficiency (CVID) and Chronic Granulomatous Disease (CGD). Curr Gastroenterol Rep. 2016;18(4):17.
27. Dhalla F, da Silva SP, Lucas M, Travis S, Chapel H. Review of gastric cancer risk factors in patients with common variable immunodeficiency disorders, resulting in a proposal for a surveillance programme. Clin Exp Immunol. 2011;165(1):1–7.
28. Magen E, Waitman DA, Goldstein N, Schlesinger M, Dickstein Y, Kahan NR. Helicobacter pylori infection in patients with selective immunoglobulin a deficiency. Clin Exp Immunol. 2016;184(3):332–7.
29. Pignata C, Budillon G, Monaco G, Nani E, Cuomo R, Parrilli G, et al. Jejunal bacterial overgrowth and intestinal permeability in children with immunodeficiency syndromes. Gut. 1990;31(8):879–82.
30. Ghoshal UC, Goel A, Ghoshal U, Jain M, Misra A, Choudhuri G. Chronic diarrhea and malabsorption due to hypogammaglobulinemia: a report on twelve patients. Indian J Gastroenterol. 2011;30(4):170–4.
31. Sawatzki M, Peter S, Hess C. Therapy-resistant diarrhea due to Giardia lamblia in a patient with common variable immunodeficiency disease. Digestion. 2007;75(2–3):101–2.
32. Paranjpe SM, Koticha A, Mehta PR. Chronic Giardiasis in a Case of Common Variable Immunodeficiency (CVID): A Case Report. J Clin Diagn Res. 2016;10(7):DD03–4.
33. Choi JH, Han DS, Kim J, Yi K, Oh YH, Kim Y. Diffuse nodular lymphoid hyperplasia of the intestine caused by common variable immunodeficiency and refractory giardiasis. Intern Med. 2017;56(3):283–7.

34. Onbaşi K, Günşar F, Sin AZ, Ardeniz O, Kokuludağ A, Sebik F. Common variable immunodeficiency (CVID) presenting with malabsorption due to giardiasis. Turk J Gastroenterol. 2005;16(2):111–3.
35. van de Ven AA, Janssen WJ, Schulz LS, van Loon AM, Voorkamp K, Sanders EA, et al. Increased prevalence of gastrointestinal viruses and diminished secretory immunoglobulin a levels in antibody deficiencies. J Clin Immunol. 2014;34(8):962–70.
36. Woodward JM, Gkrania-Klotsas E, Cordero-Ng AY, Aravinthan A, Bandoh BN, Liu H, et al. The role of chronic norovirus infection in the enteropathy associated with common variable immunodeficiency. Am J Gastroenterol. 2015;110(2):320–7.
37. Kralickova P, Mala E, Vokurkova D, Krcmova I, Pliskova L, Stepanova V, et al. Cytomegalovirus disease in patients with common variable immunodeficiency: three case reports. Int Arch Allergy Immunol. 2014;163(1):69–74.
38. Ardeniz O, Cunningham-Rundles C. Granulomatous disease in common variable immunodeficiency. Clin Immunol. 2009;133(2):198–207.
39. Boursiquot JN, Gérard L, Malphettes M, Fieschi C, Galicier L, Boutboul D, et al. Granulomatous disease in CVID: retrospective analysis of clinical characteristics and treatment efficacy in a cohort of 59 patients. J Clin Immunol. 2013;33(1):84–95.
40. Bonilla FA, Barlan I, Chapel H, Costa-Carvalho BT, Cunningham-Rundles C, de la Morena MT, et al. International Consensus Document (ICON): Common Variable Immunodeficiency Disorders. J Allergy Clin Immunol Pract. 2016;4(1):38–59.
41. Mellemkjaer L, Hammarstrom L, Andersen V, Yuen J, Heilmann C, Barington T, et al. Cancer risk among patients with IgA deficiency or common variable immunodeficiency and their relatives: a combined Danish and Swedish study. Clin Exp Immunol. 2002;130(3):495–500.
42. Kinlen LJ, Webster AD, Bird AG, Haile R, Peto J, Soothill JF, et al. Prospective study of cancer in patients with hypogammaglobulinaemia. Lancet. 1985;1(8423):263–6.
43. Vajdic CM, Mao L, van Leeuwen MT, Kirkpatrick P, Grulich AE, Riminton S. Are antibody deficiency disorders associated with a narrower range of cancers than other forms of immunodeficiency? Blood. 2010;116(8):1228–34.
44. De Petris G, Dhungel BM, Chen L, Chang YH. Gastric adenocarcinoma in common variable immunodeficiency: features of cancer and associated gastritis may be characteristic of the condition. Int J Surg Pathol. 2014;22(7):600–6.
45. Ludvigsson JF, Neovius M, Ye W, Hammarström L. IgA deficiency and risk of cancer: a population-based matched cohort study. J Clin Immunol. 2015;35(2):182–8.
46. Meini A, Pillan NM, Villanacci V, Monafo V, Ugazio AG, Plebani A. Prevalence and diagnosis of celiac disease in IgA-deficient children. Ann Allergy Asthma Immunol. 1996;77(4):333–6.
47. Jacobson KW, deShazo RD. Selective immunoglobulin A deficiency associated with modular lymphoid hyperplasia. J Allergy Clin Immunol. 1979;64(6 Pt 1):516–21.
48. Piaścik M, Rydzewska G, Pawlik M, Milewski J, Furmanek MI, Wrońska E, et al. Diffuse nodular lymphoid hyperplasia of the gastrointestinal tract in patient with selective immunoglobulin A deficiency and sarcoid-like syndrome--case report. Adv Med Sci. 2007;52:296–300.
49. Joo M, Shim SH, Chang SH, Kim H, Chi JG, Kim NH. Nodular lymphoid hyperplasia and histologic changes mimicking celiac disease, collagenous sprue, and lymphocytic colitis in a patient with selective IgA deficiency. Pathol Res Pract. 2009;205(12):876–80.
50. Postgate A, Despott E, Talbot I, Phillips R, Aylwin A, Fraser C. An unusual cause of diarrhea: diffuse intestinal nodular lymphoid hyperplasia in association with selective immunoglobulin A deficiency (with video). Gastrointest Endosc. 2009;70(1):168–9. discussion 9
51. Brandtzaeg P. Update on mucosal immunoglobulin A in gastrointestinal disease. Curr Opin Gastroenterol. 2010;26(6):554–63.
52. Leven EA, Maffucci P, Ochs HD, Scholl PR, Buckley RH, Fuleihan RL, et al. Hyper IgM syndrome: a report from the USIDNET registry. J Clin Immunol. 2016;36(5):490–501.
53. Abdel-Naser MB, Wollina U, El Hefnawi MA, Habib MA, El Okby M. Non-sarcoidal, non-tuberculoid granuloma in common variable immunodeficiency. J Drugs Dermatol. 2006;5(4):370–2.

54. Dalla Torre D, Burtscher D, Jank S, Kloss FR. Necrotizing periodontitis as a possible manifestation of common variable immunodeficiency. Int J Oral Maxillofac Surg. 2012;41(12):1546–9.
55. Tar I, Kiss C, Maródi L, Márton IJ. Oral and dental conditions of children with selective IgA deficiency. Pediatr Allergy Immunol. 2008;19(1):33–6.
56. Kalha I, Sellin JH. Common variable immunodeficiency and the gastrointestinal tract. Curr Gastroenterol Rep. 2004;6(5):377–83.
57. Twomey JJ, Jordan PH, Jarrold T, Trubowitz S, Ritz ND, Conn HO. The syndrome of immunoglobulin deficiency and pernicious anemia. A study of ten cases. Am J Med. 1969;47(3):340–50.
58. Twomey JJ, Jordan PH, Laughter AH, Meuwissen HJ, Good RA. The gastric disorder in immunoglobulin-deficient patients. Ann Intern Med. 1970;72(4):499–504.
59. Washington K, Stenzel TT, Buckley RH, Gottfried MR. Gastrointestinal pathology in patients with common variable immunodeficiency and X-linked agammaglobulinemia. Am J Surg Pathol. 1996;20(10):1240–52.
60. Webster AD, Kenwright S, Ballard J, Shiner M, Slavin G, Levi AJ, et al. Nodular lymphoid hyperplasia of the bowel in primary hypogammaglobulinaemia: study of in vivo and in vitro lymphocyte function. Gut. 1977;18(5):364–72.
61. Albuquerque A. Nodular lymphoid hyperplasia in the gastrointestinal tract in adult patients: a review. World J Gastrointest Endosc. 2014;6(11):534–40.
62. Garg V, Lipka S, Rizvon K, Singh J, Rashid S, Mustacchia P. Diffuse nodular lymphoid hyperplasia of intestine in selective IgG 2 subclass deficiency, autoimmune thyroiditis, and autoimmune hemolytic anemia: case report and literature review. J Gastrointestin Liver Dis. 2012;21(4):431–4.
63. Teahon K, Webster AD, Price AB, Weston J, Bjarnason I. Studies on the enteropathy associated with primary hypogammaglobulinaemia. Gut. 1994;35(9):1244–9.
64. Comunoglu N, Kara S, Kepil N. Inflammatory bowel disease-like colitis pathology in a patient with common variable immune deficiency. BMJ Case Rep. 2015;2015:bcr2014207177.
65. Chapel H, Lucas M, Lee M, Bjorkander J, Webster D, Grimbacher B, et al. Common variable immunodeficiency disorders: division into distinct clinical phenotypes. Blood. 2008;112(2):277–86.
66. Aghamohammadi A, Pouladi N, Parvaneh N, Yeganeh M, Movahedi M, Gharagolou M, et al. Mortality and morbidity in common variable immunodeficiency. J Trop Pediatr. 2007;53(1):32–8.
67. Woodward J, Gkrania-Klotsas E, Kumararatne D. Chronic norovirus infection and common variable immunodeficiency. Clin Exp Immunol. 2017;188(3):363–70.
68. Biagi F, Bianchi PI, Zilli A, Marchese A, Luinetti O, Lougaris V, et al. The significance of duodenal mucosal atrophy in patients with common variable immunodeficiency: a clinical and histopathologic study. Am J Clin Pathol. 2012;138(2):185–9.
69. Luzi G, Zullo A, Iebba F, Rinaldi V, Sanchez Mete L, Muscaritoli M, et al. Duodenal pathology and clinical-immunological implications in common variable immunodeficiency patients. Am J Gastroenterol. 2003;98(1):118–21.
70. Giorgio F, Principi M, Losurdo G, Piscitelli D, Iannone A, Barone M, et al. Seronegative celiac disease and immunoglobulin deficiency: where to look in the submerged iceberg? Nutrients. 2015;7(9):7486–504.
71. Venhoff N, Emmerich F, Neagu M, Salzer U, Koehn C, Driever S, et al. The role of HLA DQ2 and DQ8 in dissecting celiac-like disease in common variable immunodeficiency. J Clin Immunol. 2013;33(5):909–16.
72. Elnachef N, McMorris M, Chey WD. Successful treatment of common variable immunodeficiency disorder-associated diarrhea with budesonide: a case report. Am J Gastroenterol. 2007;102(6):1322–5.
73. Chua I, Standish R, Lear S, Harbord M, Eren E, Raeiszadeh M, et al. Anti-tumour necrosis factor-alpha therapy for severe enteropathy in patients with common variable immunodeficiency (CVID). Clin Exp Immunol. 2007;150(2):306–11.

74. Fasano A, Berti I, Gerarduzzi T, Not T, Colletti RB, Drago S, et al. Prevalence of celiac disease in at-risk and not-at-risk groups in the United States: a large multicenter study. Arch Intern Med. 2003;163(3):286–92.
75. Wang N, Shen N, Vyse TJ, Anand V, Gunnarson I, Sturfelt G, et al. Selective IgA deficiency in autoimmune diseases. Mol Med. 2011;17(11–12):1383–96.
76. Mohammadi J, Ramanujam R, Jarefors S, Rezaei N, Aghamohammadi A, Gregersen PK, et al. IgA deficiency and the MHC: assessment of relative risk and microheterogeneity within the HLA A1 B8, DR3 (8.1) haplotype. J Clin Immunol. 2010;30(1):138–43.
77. Byrne MF, Royston D, Patchett SE. Association of common variable immunodeficiency with atypical collagenous colitis. Eur J Gastroenterol Hepatol. 2003;15(9):1051–3.
78. Hernandez-Trujillo VP, Scalchunes C, Cunningham-Rundles C, Ochs HD, Bonilla FA, Paris K, et al. Autoimmunity and inflammation in X-linked agammaglobulinemia. J Clin Immunol. 2014;34(6):627–32.
79. Cunningham-Rundles C, Bodian C. Common variable immunodeficiency: clinical and immunological features of 248 patients. Clin Immunol. 1999;92(1):34–48.
80. Moin M, Aghamohammadi A, Farhoudi A, Pourpak Z, Rezaei N, Movahedi M, et al. X-linked agammaglobulinemia: a survey of 33 Iranian patients. Immunol Investig. 2004;33(1):81–93.
81. Fuss IJ, Friend J, Yang Z, He JP, Hooda L, Boyer J, et al. Nodular regenerative hyperplasia in common variable immunodeficiency. J Clin Immunol. 2013;33(4):748–58.
82. Ward C, Lucas M, Piris J, Collier J, Chapel H. Abnormal liver function in common variable immunodeficiency disorders due to nodular regenerative hyperplasia. Clin Exp Immunol. 2008;153(3):331–7.
83. Lal BK, Stanley A. Nodular regenerative hyperplasia related portal hypertension in a patient with hypogammaglobulinaemia. World J Gastroenterol. 2013;19(22):3502–4.
84. Malamut G, Ziol M, Suarez F, Beaugrand M, Viallard JF, Lascaux AS, et al. Nodular regenerative hyperplasia: the main liver disease in patients with primary hypogammaglobulinemia and hepatic abnormalities. J Hepatol. 2008;48(1):74–82.

Index

M. M. D'Elios, M. Rizzi (eds.), *Humoral Primary Immunodeficiencies*, Rare Diseases of the Immune System, https://doi.org/10.1007/978-3-319-91785-6

I

J

L

MIX
Papier aus verantwortungsvollen Quellen
Paper from responsible sources
FSC® C105338

If you have any concerns about our products,
you can contact us on
ProductSafety@springernature.com

In case Publisher is established outside the EU,
the EU authorized representative is:
Springer Nature Customer Service Center GmbH
Europaplatz 3, 69115 Heidelberg, Germany

Printed by Libri Plureos GmbH
in Hamburg, Germany